Behavior and mood disorders in focal brain lesions

This is the first clinical reference work to address specifically the relationship of focal brain dysfunction to behavioral and emotional disorders. Focal lesions produce distinctive behavioral changes, which are instructive in terms of understanding brain function as well as interpreting the symptoms of individual patients. This book offers a comprehensive account of these manifestations of brain lesions, including stroke, trauma, epilepsy, multiple sclerosis, and even neurosurgery.

A worldwide team of neuroscientists and clinicians examines the links between regional brain dysfunction and disorders of mood, thought and affect processing, and behavior. Chapters are devoted to methodological issues, to lesions of specific sites, such as the frontal lobes, basal ganglia, and thalamus, and to symptoms such as mood disorder, violent behavior, and anosognosia.

Unique in approach and authority and illustrated with informative case histories, *Behavior and Mood Disorders in Focal Brain Lesions* makes a major contribution to understanding the behavioral consequences of focal brain lesions, summarizing the current state of research, and providing the basis for improved patient care.

Julien Bogousslavsky is Professor and Chairman of Neurology at the Centre Hospitalier Universitaire Vaudois in Lausanne, Switzerland.

Jeffrey L. Cummings is Augustus S. Rose Professor of Neurology and Professor of Psychiatry and Biobehavioral Sciences at the University of California, Los Angeles.

Both editors have written extensively in neurology, neuropsychiatry, and the areas where these disciplines converge.

Behavior and mood disorders in focal brain lesions

Edited by

Julien Bogousslavsky

and

Jeffrey L. Cummings

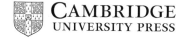

CAMBRIDGE
UNIVERSITY PRESS

PUBLISHED BY THE PRESS SYNDICATE OF THE UNIVERSITY OF CAMBRIDGE
The Pitt Building, Trumpington Street, Cambridge, United Kingdom

CAMBRIDGE UNIVERSITY PRESS
The Edinburgh Building, Cambridge CB2 2RU, UK   http://www.cup.cam.ac.uk
40 West 20th Street, New York, NY 10011-4211, USA   http://www.cup.org
10 Stamford Road, Oakleigh, Melbourne 3166, Australia
Ruiz de Alarcón 13, 28014 Madrid, Spain

First published 2000

Printed in the United Kingdom at the University Press, Cambridge

Typeface Adobe Minion 10.5/14pt.   *System* QuarkXPress® [SE]

A catalogue record for this book is available from the British Library

Library of Congress Cataloguing in Publication data

Behavior and mood disorders in focal brain lesions / edited by Julien Bogousslavsky and
Jeffrey L. Cummings.
    p. ; cm.
Includes index.
1. Clinical neuropsychology.   2. Neuropsychiatry.   3. Neurobehavioral disorders.   I.
Bogousslavsky, Julien.   II. Cummings, Jeffrey L., 1948–
[DNLM: 1. Mental Disorders – etiology.   2. Brain Diseases – complications.   3. Brain
Diseases – physiopathology.   WM 100 B419 2000]
RC386.2.B445 2000
616.89′071–dc21   99-046508

ISBN 0 521 77482 9 paperback

In the memory of my friend
Pierre-Henri Ganem
    Julien

To Inese and Juliana
    Jeffrey

Contents

Contributors

Serge Bakchine
Hôpital Maison Blanche, SHU de Reims, France

Julien Bogousslavsky
Service de Neurologie, Centre Hospitalier
Universitaire Vaudois, Lausanne, Switzerland

Caterina Breitenstein
University of Trier, Trier, Germany

Louis R. Caplan
Department of Neurology, Beth Israel Deaconess
Medical Center, Harvard University, Boston,
Massachussetts, USA

Jeffrey L. Cummings
Department of Neurology, UCLA School of
Medicine, Los Angeles, California, USA

David W. Desmond
Departments of Neurology and Pathology, SUNY
Downstate Medical Center, Brooklyn, New York,
USA

Frédéric Dubas
Service at Neurologie A, Centre Hospitalo
Universitaire, Angers, France

Terri Edwards-Lee
UCLA Medical Center and West Los Angeles
Veterans Affairs Medical Center, Los Angeles,
California, USA

Paul J. Eslinger
Section of Neurology, Department of Medicine,
Hershey Medical Center, Hershey, Pennsylvania,
USA

Frédérique Etcharry-Bouyx
Departement de Neuropsychologie, Centre
Hospitalo Universitaire, Angers, France

Laszlo Geder
Department of Behavioral Science, College of
Medicine, Pennsylvania State University, Hershey,
Pennsylvania, USA

Joseph Ghika
Department of Neurology, Centre Hospitalier
Universitaire Vaudois, Lausanne, Switzerland

Florence Ghika-Schmid
Neurologist, Lausanne, Switzerland

Jordan Grafman
Cognitive Neuroscience Section, National Institute
of Neurological Disorders and Stroke, National
Institutes of Health, Bethesda, Maryland, USA

Michael Habib
Neurological Unit and Laboratory of Cognitive
Neurology, University Hospital La Timone,
Marseille, France

Facundo Manes
Department of Psychiatry, University of Iowa
School of Medicine, Iowa City, Iowa, USA

John M. Ringman
Department of Neurology, UCLA School of
Medicine, Los Angeles, California, USA

Robert G. Robinson
Department of Psychiatry, UIHC, Iowa City, Iowa,
USA

Sergio E. Starkstein
Department of Neuropsychiatry, Raul Carrea
Institute of Neurological Research, Buenos Aires,
Argentina

Daniel Tranel
Department of Neurology, Division of Behavioral
Neurology and Cognitive Neuroscience, University
of Iowa College of Medicine, Iowa City, Iowa, USA

Diana Van Lancker
New York University, New York, USA

Patrik Vuilleumier
Institute of Cognitive Neuroscience, University
College London, London, England

Deborah L. Warden
Defense and Veterans Head Injury Program,
Walter Reed Army Medical Center, Washington
DC, USA

Atsushi Yamadori
Section of Neuropsychology, Division of Disability
Science, Tohoku University Graduate School of
Medicine, Sendai, Japan

Preface

As implied in the name, the central nervous system is a system of highly interconnected structures organized as parallel circuits of connected series of modules underlying complex human behavior and emotion. Despite the interconnected nature of the central nervous system, focal lesions produce distinctive behavioral changes and are highly instructive in terms of understanding both brain function and neurobehavioral syndromes manifested by individual patients. Studies with functional brain imaging have largely confirmed conclusions derived from observations based on the study of patients with focal lesions and investigation of brain injuries using structural and functional imaging.

The neuropsychological consequences of focal brain lesions have been relatively thoroughly studied. Memory disorders, aphasia, agnosia, apraxia, alexia, agraphia, and disorders of executive function have been intensely studied with neuropsychological and cognitive psychological approaches in the recent past. On the other hand, the emotional and behavioral consequences of focal brain lesions are more obscure and have been studied relatively little. This volume provides a comprehensive update of behavioral and emotional changes associated with focal central nervous system lesions. Abnormalities of mood, thought and affect processing, motivation, and sexual behavior are described. This volume summarizes the current state of research with regard to the behavioral and emotional consequences of localized brain lesions and provides the basis for further research and patient care.

Julien Bogousslavsky and Jeffrey L. Cummings

Acknowledgments

Dr Bogousslavsky's work in behavioral neurology has been supported by grants from the Swiss National Science Foundation (32-41950.94, 32-50728.97). He also acknowledges the continuous help and support of the medical, nursing, and administrative staff of the university Department of Neurology in Lausanne.

Dr Cummings' work has been supported by a National Institute on Aging Alzheimer's Disease Research Center grant and an Alzheimer's Disease Research Center of California grant. In addition, he gratefully acknowledges the tremendous support received from Mrs Katherine Kagan and the Sidell–Kagan Foundation. Without Mrs Kagan's enthusiasm and support of the UCLA Alzheimer's Disease Center, many fewer Alzheimer's disease and related projects would have been completed.

Dr Bogousslavsky and Dr Cummings also acknowledge their fellows and their many friends and colleagues internationally who have contributed importantly to the development of behavioral neurology and neuropsychiatry as reflected in this volume.

Emotional consequences of focal brain lesions: an overview

Jeffrey L. Cummings and Julien Bogousslavsky

Introduction

The brain mediates all cognitive activities and emotional experiences. Cognitive dysfunction following brain injury or associated with brain disease, while still incompletely understood, has been extensively studied. The aphasias, acalculias, and apraxias associated with left hemisphere injury (Levin, Goldstein and Spiers, 1993; Heilman and Gonzalez-Rothi, 1993; Benson and Ardila, 1996), the several types of agnosias associated with unilateral and bilateral brain injury (Bauer, 1993), and the amnestic syndromes associated with hippocampal dysfunction (Bauer, Tobias and Valenstein, 1993) have been the subject of numerous investigations. The emotional consequences of focal brain injury have been much less well researched. The relationships between brain dysfunction and psychosis, depression, mania, anxiety, and paraphelia are in the early phases of pathogenetic study, and more subtle changes in emotional function (such as apathy, irritability, disinhibition, and lability) are also in the initial phases of definition and descriptive linkage to regional brain dysfunction.

Investigation of the emotional correlates of regional brain dysfunction is encumbered by methodological challenges beyond those encountered in studying the relationship between cognitive impairment and brain dysfunction. Emotional disturbances are more influenced by the premorbid personality of the individual, more variable over time, and more difficult to define consistently in research investigations. On the other hand, the emotional consequences of brain dysfunction are a source of enormous distress to the patient and to the patient's family members. They may be more easily impacted through pharmacologic interventions and their importance to patient management cannot be underestimated. The recognition and treatment of these conditions constitute an important dimension of patient care. In addition, a comprehensive understanding of brain–behavior relationships depends on progress in defining the correlations between regional brain dysfunction and human emotion to complement our growing understanding of the relationship of regional brain dysfunction and intellectual disorders. The interaction of emotional and cognitive disorders also warrants study.

Regional brain dysfunction is the focus of interest in this chapter and in this volume. The pitfalls of assessing regional roles in cognition and emotion must be acknowledged. As for cognitive disorders, the occurrence of a deficit or the appearance of new, neuropsychiatric symptoms (e.g., psychosis, depression) in concert with the occurrence of focal brain lesions does not necessarily imply that a particular brain region is uniquely or even primarily involved with that specific cognitive or emotional activity. Nevertheless, there has been an encouraging concordance between models of regional brain function derived from observing patients with focal lesions and the models derived from functional brain imaging (Frith and Dolan, 1997). Extension of the lesion model to understanding human emotional function is an important first step toward establishing a neuroanatomy of emotion that can be challenged, confirmed, and remodelled based on neuroimaging, neurophysiological, neurochemical, neuropharmacological, and neuropathological research.

Focal lesions may produce local effects or may cause symptoms by disrupting functional neuronal networks. Brain regions are linked through white matter tracts into extensive circuits that mediate information processing. Some focal lesions produce signature syndromes with unique clinical symptoms arising from specific brain lesions; other brain lesions have no unique associated syndromes, and several brain lesions may produce similar clinical abnormalities. Extensive processing networks mediate the emotional functions of the nervous system, and focal lesions within the networks tend not to produce discrete localizable syndromes. The limbic system and frontal–subcortical networks are two examples of extensive brain organizational systems that mediate emotional functions (Cummings, 1993a; Mega et al., 1997).

This chapter provides an overview of the regional relationships between emotional function and brain organization. Definitions and distinctions between fundamental and instrumental functions, the integration of executive and emotional functions, relevant anatomy of the limbic system and frontal–subcortical circuitry, regional neurochemical influences based on the distribution of receptors, and clinical–regional behavioral correlations are emphasized.

Definitions of emotion

Many definitions of emotion have been proffered and none has proven completely satisfactory or has achieved consensus endorsement. *The Concise Oxford Dictionary* (Thompson, 1995) defines emotion as strong mental or instinctive feeling, such as love or fear. Rolls (1995) adopted a behavioral psychological approach in defining emotions as 'states produced by instrumental reinforcing stimuli.' Pribram and Melges (1969) recognized that there are two conceptual frames of references for emotions: (1) the social–behavioral, which includes the subjective or intrapsychic aspects of emotion, such as psychodynamic approaches, and (2) the physical, chemical, and neurological frame of reference emphasizing a physiological and neurobiological approach to emotions. Heilman (1983) adopted an operational approach to the neuropsychological study of emotion, emphasizing subjective feelings that can be expressed and behavioral and physiological changes that can be measured. Feyereisen (1989) explicitly acknowledged that 'the category of emotion may formally be described as fuzzy.' He noted different dimensions of emotion, including behaviors such as laughing, being frightened or crying; physical and mental states, such as sexual desire, doubt, and envy; and mental states such as moods or feelings of pleasure or distress.

Heilman and colleagues (Heilman, Bowers and Valenstein, 1993) also noted that there are several ways in which neurological disorders and emotions may interact: (1) changes in emotional experience and behavior can be caused directly by diseases of the nervous system; (2) patients with neurological diseases may have an emotional response to their illness, such as becoming anxious or depressed; (3) emotional states may enhance neurological symptoms, such as when anxiety aggravates a tremor; and (4) emotional states may induce neurological symptoms, such as when stress induces headaches.

For the purposes of this chapter, emotion will be defined as the experience and expression of feeling states. This definition includes sadness, elation, changes in motivation, reduced empathy or an inability to emphathetically experience another's predicted feeling state, irritability, lability, fear, anxiety, sexual desire (lust), and feelings of persecution or threat of personal harm. There are many dimensions of emotion that influence the final feeling state of the individual. These include the developmental experiences of the individual, the physiological aspects of arousal associated with many emotions, the visceral changes present with many escalated feeling states, the interaction with cognition and memory, as well as the anatomical and biochemical aspects of emotion emphasized here. Many emotions occur on a continuum from mild to extreme (such as from happiness to elation to grandiosity and mania). In the normal condition, the experience and expression of emotion are conjoined in the laughter of happiness or the crying of sadness; in neurological illnesses, experience and expression of emotion may be disassociated, such as occurs in pseudobulbar palsy, the flattened affect of parkinsonism, or the loss of inflection in aprosodia.

Another definition that bears on the terminology of this chapter is *mood*, defined as a pervasive and sustained emotion that colors the perception of the world. *Affect* refers to a pattern of observable behaviors that is typically the expression of a subjectively experienced feeling state. *Anxiety* is the apprehensive anticipation of future danger or misfortune accompanied by a feeling of dysphoria or somatic symptoms of tension. *Grandiosity* is an inflated appraisal of one's worth, power, knowledge, importance or identity. *Psychosis* may be defined restrictively as delusions or prominent hallucinations, with the hallucinations occurring in the absence of insight into their pathological nature (American Psychiatric Association, 1994).

Instrumental and fundamental functions

Albert (1978) described the neuropsychological dichotomy of instrumental functions versus fundamental functions. In this approach, instrumental functions refer to activities of communication, perception, and praxis, and deficits in these functions produce the clinical syndromes of asphasias, agnosias, and apraxias. Fundamental functions include memory, the ability to learn new information, set shifting, and rate of information processing. Fundamental functions were posited to facilitate instrumental functions.

Cummings (1990) expanded the fundamental/instrumental dichotomy to include anatomic, phylogenetic, ontogenetic, and biochemical dimensions. Instrumental functions were expanded to include language, perceptual recognition, praxis, and calculation, whereas fundamental functions included timing, arousal, attention, motor programming, motivation, mood, and emotion. The corresponding neuropsychological deficits associated with instrumental functions include aphasia, agnosia, apraxia, and acalculia. Disorders of fundamental function include slowing, forgetfulness, executive dysfunction, depression, apathy, and emotional disorders. Thus, this dichotomy of instrumental and fundamental functions created an approach to emotion with anatomic and physiologic implications.

Abnormalities of instrumental functions are prominent in cortical dementias, whereas fundamental functions are associated with subcortical, limbic, and frontal disorders. Instrumental functions are mediated by the neocortex, particularly temporal and parietal neocortex, whereas fundamental functions are mediated by prefrontal cortex, frontal–subcortical circuits, and the limbic system. White matter tracts subserving instrumental functions are discrete, well-myelinated, long, intrahemispheric and interhemispheric fibers, whereas those mediating fundamental functions are shorter, less well-myelinated projections that are more diffuse. Organizationally, instrumental functions are serial connections of functional units with well-lateralized and highly specialized functional modules. The organization of fundamental functions depends on parallel structures with overlapping functions that are less modularized. Interruption of the serial organization of instrumental functions produces signature syndromes, such as discrete aphasias, agnosias or apraxias, whereas disruption of the organization of fundamental functions produces circuit-related disorders, such as depression, apathy, and irritability and impaired executive function, that lack unique local significance.

Phylogenetically, instrumental functions are a recent evolutionary acquisition that are most well developed in humans. Fundamental functions are more primitive and present in the triune organization of the reptile brain. The ontogenetic development of instrumental functions is incomplete at birth and continues throughout childhood with maturation of the central nervous system (CNS). The anatomical structures underlying fundamental functions are largely functional at birth or soon thereafter.

The principal transmitters of instrumental functions include acetylcholine, glutamate, and gamma-aminobutyric acid (GABA). Fundamental functions are influenced more heavily by modulatory transfers, such as dopamine, norepinephrine, serotonin, and acetylcholine.

Disorders of instrumental function are largely deficit syndromes with an impairment of premorbid skills, whereas abnormalities of fundamental function may be 'productive,' with the appearance of new symptoms in concert with the CNS dysfunction, including depression, mania, psychosis, and anxiety. The existence of long, white-matter tracts associated with instrumental functions is the basis for the occurrence of disconnection syndromes that underlie some instrumental disturbances (apraxia; alexia without agraphia; conduction aphasia), whereas disconnection syndromes are unusual as the etiology of fundamental disorders.

Mesulam (1985) introduced an alternative complementary terminology suggesting that instrumental functions are 'channel dependent' whereas fundamental functions are 'state dependent.' The anatomy of channel functions is point-to-point connectivity. In state-dependent functions, there are more diffusely organized projections from the intralaminar thalamic nuclei, cholinergic neurons of the basal forebrain, neurons of the lateral and medial hypothalamus, serotonergic neurons, reticular cholinergic neurons, noradrenergic neurons, and dopaminergic neurons. These systems are characterized by a relatively small group of neurons positioned to modulate the information processing of wide regions of the cortex and thalamus. Mesulam (1985) emphasized that these modulatory projections could influence many neural operations and are poised to mediate aspects of mood, motivation, memory, arousal, and vigilance. He noted that pathways mediating state-dependent functions could influence channel-dependent functions without altering the content of the transmitted information.

Instrumental, fundamental, and executive functions

The division of neuropsychological functions into instrumental and fundamental types was a conceptual advance that has had substantial heuristic value. Current advances in understanding the behaviorally relevant organization of the nervous system allow a reformulation and extension of this framework. Progress in research concerning frontal lobe functions and frontal–subcortical circuits facilitates the reformulation of the neurological basis of emotions (Stuss and Benson, 1986; Cummings, 1993a). The original conception of fundamental functions encompassed activities of both the limbic–reticular system and the frontal–subcortical system. Sufficient information is now available to allow the recognition of three distinct domains of mental function: instrumental, fundamental, and executive/integrative. In this framework, instrumental activities include language, perceptual recognition, and praxis. Fundamental functions include speed of processing, mood, motivation, and emotion. Executive functions include abstraction, sequencing, attentional focusing, and responses to changing contingencies. When the instrumental domain is dysfunctional, the corresponding clinical syndromes associated with instrumental dysfunction are aphasia, agnosia, and aphraxia. Those disorders accompanying fundamental function disturbances include bradyphrenia, amotivational states, reduced arousal, and a variety of emotional disorders. Abnormalities of executive function include concrete thinking, distractibility, and environmental dependency. Lesions can produce signature syndromes indicative of the interruption of specific instrumental functions, whereas lesions of both fundamental and executive systems produce circuit-related symptoms.

Neuropsychiatric disorders associated with instrumental function include anosognosia; those associated with fundamental dysfunction include apathy, irritability, depression, mania, anxiety, and psychosis; and those associated with executive dysfunction may include loss of empathy. Disruption of emotional function associated with abnormal instrumental activities encompasses disorders of emotional comprehension (such as receptive aprosodia and the inability to interpret emotional facial expressions); disturbances of fundamental function produce disorders of emotional experience such as mood abnormalities and the abnormal experience of threat; disorders of emotional function associated with frontal–subcortical disorders include executive aprosodias, flattened affect, and pseudobulbar palsy.

Three dementia syndromes have also been recognized: cortical dementias (especially Alzheimer's disease) associated with disturbances of instrumental function; limbic dementias associated with temporal lobe syndromes and amygdala involvement; and frontal and subcortical syndromes associated with frontotemporal degenerations and basal ganglia diseases. Motor syndromes representative of instrumental dysfunction are the apraxias, whereas extrapyramidal syndromes are characteristic of disorders with fundamental dysfunction, and pyramidal syndromes occur with lesions of the final common pathways associated with the processing of executive function. Disconnection syndromes are typical of the instrumental level of organization and include apraxia and alexia without agraphia. Disconnection syndromes are not typical of fundamental or executive functions. Table 1.1 summarizes the clinical aspects of this tripartite approach to mental functions.

Table 1.1. Clinical features of syndromes associated with instrumental, fundamental, and executive dysfunction

Characteristics	Instrumental	Fundamental	Executive/integration
Neuropsychological functions	Language Perceptual recognition Praxis	Speed of progression Mood Motivation Emotion	Abstractions Sequencing Attentional focusing Response to changing contingencies

Neuropsychological disorders	Aphasia
	Agnosia
	Apraxia
	Signature syndromes
		Bradyphenia
		Avolition
		Reduced arousal
		Limbic system
		  syndromes
			Concrete
			Distractable
			Environmental dependency
			Frontal–subcortex circuit
			  syndromes

Neuropsychiatric conditions	Anosognosia	Deficit – apathy
		Productive:
		  irritability
		  depression
		  mania
		  anxiety
		  psychosis
		  obsessive–compulsive
		  disorder
			Deficit – loss of empathy

Emotional disorders	Disorders of emotional
	  vocal comprehension
	Receptive aprosodia
	Aprosonosia
	Difficulty understanding
	  emotional facial
	  expressions
		Disorders of emotional
		  experience – mood,
		  threat
			Disorders of emotional
			  expression (aprosodias)
			  and control
			  (pseudobulbar palsy)

Dementia associated	Cortical dementia
	  (especially
	  Alzheimer's disease)
		Limbic system dementia	Frontal and subcortical
			  dementia

Motor syndrome associated	Apraxia	Extrapyramidal disorder	Pyramidal syndromes

Disconnection syndrome	Apraxias
	Alexia without agraphia
		None	Locked-in syndrome
			  (disconnection of
			  descending pyramidal
			  pathways)

Instrumental functions are mediated predominantly by the posterior hetero-modal cortical regions. The cortical regions associated with fundamental functions include the cingulate cortex, orbitofrontal cortex, and hippocampus. Cortical regions associated with the executive function include the dorsolateral prefrontal heteromodal areas. Thalamic nuclei associated with each of the three functions include the pulvinar (instrumental function), the anterior thalamic nuclei (fundamental function), and the dorsal medial nuclei (executive function). Basal ganglia have little role in instrumental functions, but the ventral striatum, nucleus accumbens, and pallidum are intimately involved in mediating fundamental functions, and the dorsal striatum and pallidum are involved in mediating executive functions. The white matter tracts underlying instrumental function are long, well-myelinated intrahemispheric and interhemispheric fasciculi. White matter tracts related to fundamental functions include the medial forebrain bundle and other shorter, less well-myelinated tracts. White matter tracts mediating executive functions include the frontal–basal ganglionic connections and thalamofrontal projections.

The anatomical organization associated with instrumental functions is characteristically a serial linking of specialized modules. Hemispheric specialization is most marked at this level of CNS organization. In contrast, parallel circuits are characteristic of both fundamental and executive functions. There is little hemispheric specialization or lateralization of fundamental functions and a limited hemispheric specialization of executive functions.

Phylogenetically, fundamental functions are the most primitive; instrumental functions are relatively recent; and executive functions are nearly unique to humans and the most recent evolutionary acquisitions. Similarly, fundamental functions are functional at birth, whereas instrumental functions are incomplete at birth and develop throughout childhood. The anatomical pathways underlying executive functions are incompletely functional at birth, and development continues through early adulthood.

The principal neurotransmitters mediating instrumental functions are GABA and glutamate, mediating direct, fast-acting interneuronal communication. Fundamental functions depend more heavily on projection neurons of the cholinergic, dopaminergic, serotonergic, and noradrenergic systems. These are modulatory neurons that exert tonic influences. In the executive function system, both fast-acting and tonic transmitters are well represented in the circuitry.

This approach has important implications for treatment. This is limited response to pharmacologic treatment of instrumental syndromes such as aphasia, agnosia or apraxia. Emotional disorders associated with fundamental dysfunction respond well to pharmacotherapy. These disorders include psychosis, depression, mania, and anxiety. At the executive level, abnormalities of abstraction, sequencing, and environmental dependency are treatment resistant. Table 1.2 summarizes the neurobiologic aspects of the tripartite approach to mental functions.

Table 1.2. Neurobiologic characteristics of instrumental, fundamental, and executive functions

Characteristics	Instrumental	Fundamental	Executive/integration
Gray matter structures		Hippocampus cingulate	Dorsolateral prefrontal
Cortical	Posterior heteromodal cortex (six-layered)	orbitofronto cortex (three-layered and transitional)	heteromodal cortex (six-layered)
Thalamus	Pulvinar	Dorsomedial anterior	Dorsomedial
Basal ganglion	None	Ventral striatum Pallidum	Dorsal striatum Pallidum
White matter tracts	Long, intrahemispheric and interhemispheric association fibers	Medial forebrain bundle; mostly shorter tracts	Frontal–basal ganglia and thalamo-frontal connections
Organization	Serial linking of modules Hemisphere specialization (lateralization)	Little hemisphere specialization	Limited hemisphere specialization
Phylogeny	Recent evolutionary development	Primitive	Most recent evolutionary acquisition
Ontogeny	Incomplete at birth; development continues through childhood	Functional at birth	Incomplete at birth, development continues through early adulthood
Neurotransmitters			
Type	GABA Glutamate Acetylcholine	GABA Glutamate Acetylcholine Dopamine Serotonin Norepinephrine	GABA Glutamate Acetylcholine Dopamine Serotonin Norepinephrine
Primary function	Direct information transfer	Modulation	Information transfer and modulation
Speed	Fast acting	Tonic	Fast acting and tonic
Organization	Local circuit neurons	Projection neurons (brainstem and basal forebrain nuclei with widespread projections)	Local circuit cortical neurons Patch/matrix arrangement in striatum Regions receive projection neurons
Pharmacological treatment	Limited response	Responsive	Limited response

This organization of mental functions into three domains facilitates a more comprehensible approach to the discussion of the emotional disorders emphasized in this volume. The principal emotional disorders associated with instrumental dysfunction are anosognosia and associated anosognosic phenomena. There are many emotional abnormalities associated with disorders of fundamental function, including deficit syndromes such as apathy and avolition and productive syndromes such as depression, mania, psychosis, and anxiety. Emotional disorders associated with executive dysfunction have been less well studied, but empathy (the ability to imagine the emotional experience of another) is a candidate emotion for the executive system.

The anatomy described here sets up a stimulus–response channel system with thalamocortical projections mediating sensory input; long intrahemispheric projections, as well as interhemispheric projections, connecting the posterior heteromodal to frontal heteromodal cortex; and projections out via the basal ganglia and thalamus to primary motor cortex with eventual projections to bulbar and spinal motor neurons. This sensory association–motor arc is largely based on well-myelinated, long axons with excitatory and inhibitory amino acid transmitters. Information entering the nervous system, however, also spreads to the limbic cortex where emotional valence as well as memory is integrated to give the stimulus meaning and to provide a context of experience for the response. The integration of this historical–emotional information with the primary stimulus occurs in frontal heteromodal cortex and the volitional act is further modified in frontal–subcortical systems prior to exit from the nervous system via the descending pyramidal system. Thus, the frontal cortex in this schema becomes the site for the integration of emotional and cognitive information, as well as the principal region for the initiation of volitional activity.

Anatomy of emotion

The limbic system is the principal anatomical substrate of emotion. Both Thomas Willis in 1664 and Paul Broca in 1887 called attention to the anatomy of the limbic lobe comprising the cortical border that encircled the brainstem (Mega et al., 1997). Neither of these authors, however, attributed emotional function to this brain region. It was Papez (1937) who surmised that the limbic structures served the 'stream of feeling' underlying emotional expression and experience. Papez included the hippocampus, fornix, anterior thalamus, and cingulate gyrus as principal anatomical components of the limbic system.

The concept of the limbic system has been progressively expanded to include multiple brain structures in both subcortical and cortical brain regions. Table 1.3 provides a summary of structures currently included in the expanded concept of

Table 1.3. Anatomic elements of the limbic system

Hypothalamus
Hippocampus
Piriform cortex
Amygdala
Septal region in substantia innominata
Paralimbic cortex
　　Orbitofrontal cortex
　　Insula
　　Temporal pole
　　Parahippocampal gyrus
　　Cingulate cortex
Ventral striatum
Limbic thalamic nuclei
　　Medial–dorsal nuclei
　　Midline nuclei
　　Anterior nuclei
　　Lateral–dorsal nuclei

Source: From Macchi (1989); Mesulam (1985).

the limbic system as well as limbic-associated structures (Mesulam, 1985; Macchi, 1989). This extended concept of the limbic system includes the hypothalamus, hippocampus, piriform cortex, amygdala, septal nuclei and substantia innominata, paralimbic cortex (including the orbitofrontal cortex, insula, temporal pole, parahippocampal gyrus, and cingulate complex), as well as the ventral striatum, nucleus accumbens, and limbic thalamic nuclei (anterior, lateral–dorsal, midline, and dorso-medial). In addition, projections from regions in the brainstem provide critical, modulatory transmitter input into limbic system structures. These ascending projection systems include serotonergic neurons arising from the raphe, noradrenergic neurons projecting from the locus ceruleus, and dopaminergic neurons arising from the ventral tegmental area (Macchi, 1989; Cummings and Coffey, 1994).

From the perspective of understanding the emotional consequences of focal CNS lesions, the limbic structures of greatest importance are the amygdala, the cingulate cortex, the limbic components of frontal–subcortical circuits, and the limbic thalamus.

Amygdala

The principal subcortical afferents of the amygdala arise from the nucleus basalis of Meynert in the basal forebrain, the ventromedial hypothalamic nucleus, the midline thalamic nuclei, the posterior thalamic nuclei, and the substantia nigra. Cortical afferents to the amygdala arise from the anterior temporal, posterior orbitofrontal, cingulate, medial and lateral temporal, and cingulate cortex (Aggleton, 1993). The principal efferents of the amygdala include the nucleus accumbens, nucleus basalis, ventromedial hypothalamic nuclei, lateral hypothalamic region, mediodorsal nuclei of the thalamus, reticular formation, substantia nigra, and periaqueductal gray regions. The striatal efferents of the amygdala project to the nucleus accumbens and ventral portions of the putamen and ventral and caudal portions of the caudate nucleus (Russchen et al., 1985). The cortical efferent projections are most dense to the anterior temporal regions, medial posterior orbitofrontal area, and anterior cingulate. Less dense projections from the amygdala connect with wide areas of the inferior dorsolateral frontal, posterior temporal, and parieto-ocipital regions (Aggleton, 1993).

The amygdala is a complex structure with several nuclear groups within it. Each amygdaloid nucleus contains a basolateral complex, central amygdaloid group, medial amygdaloid group, and an olfactory group (Alheid and Heimer, 1988). The basolateral complex is the origin of most cortical efferents and receives most cortical afferents. It also has reciprocal projections with the mediodorsal nuclei of the thalamus (Alheid and Heimer, 1988). The central amygdaloid group is a portion of the extended amygdala which extends from the dorsal amygdala into the ventromedial part of the sublenticular area beneath the globus pallidus. The extended amygdala also contains components of the medial portion of the nucleus accumbens (Alheid and Heimer, 1988). The extended amygdala nucleus/accumbens complex is a critical area for motivational and emotional functions.

Thus, the amygdala is positioned centrally within the limbic system, receiving information from limbic and paralimbic regions and providing efferent projections to widespread limbic and paralimbic areas. The extended amygdala/nucleus accumbens complex provides the opportunity for the amygdala to influence frontal–subcortical circuits (described below) as well as regions receiving afferent from the amygdala, such as the temporal polar, inferior frontal, and anterior cingulate regions.

Cingulate

The cingulate is also an anatomically complex region with many reciprocal afferent and efferent projections (Table 1.4). An anterior infracallosal region with visceral connections, an anterior supracallosal region related to cognition, a middle skeletomotor region, and a posterior supracallosal sensory processing region have been described (Mega and Cummings, 1997). The 'visceral' region has reciprocal connections with the amygdala, orbitofrontal, and superior temporal regions and receives input from the thalamus. Its major output is to brainstem visceral nuclei.

Table 1.4. Connection of the cingulate cortex

Cingulate region	Reciprocal connections	Open afferent	Open efferent
Anterior interior (visceral) region	Basal and accessory basal amygdala Medial orbitofrontal areas 11, 12, and 13* Superior temporal pole area 38 Anterior ventral claustrum	Prefrontal areas 9 and 46 Dorsal magnocellular mediodorsal thalamus Midline and intralaminar thalamic nuclei Hippocampal CA1/ subicular sectors	Parasympathetic nucleus of solitary tract Sympathetic intermediolateral column Dorsal motor nucleus of the vagus Nucleus accumbens/ olfactory tubercle
Anterior superior (cognitive) region	Basal amygdala Prefrontal areas 8, 9, 10, and 46 Caudal orbitofrontal cortex area 12 Inferior temporal pole area 38 Anterior parahippocampal areas 35 and 36 Rostral insula Anterior medial claustrum	Dorsal parvocellular mediodorsal thalamus Midline and intralaminar thalamic nuclei Hippocampal CA1/ subicular sectors	Anterior superior temporal area 22 Parietal area 7a Dorsomedial head and body of caudate Periaqueductal gray matter Dorsomedial pontine gray matter
Middle (skeletal–motor) region	Primary motor area 4 Supplementary motor area 6 Prefrontal areas 8, 9, and 46 Parietal areas 1, 2, 3a, 5, and 7b Caudal insula	Posterior perirhinal area 35 Rostral ventroanterior thalamus Ventrolateral thalamus Basal amygdala	Lateral putamen Spinal cord Red nucleus Ventrolateral pontine gray matter
Posterior (sensory processing) region	Caudal parietal area 7 Frontal eye fields area 8 Prefrontal area 46 Posterior parahippocampal areas 35 and 36 Presubiculum Ventral caudal claustrum	Occipital area 19 Hippocampal CA1/ subicular sectors Anterior thalamus Medial pulvinar Lateral dorsal and lateral posterior thalamus	Orbitofrontal area 11 Posterior superior temporal area 22 Dorsal caudate

Note:
* Area numbers refer to Brodmann areas.
Source: Adapted by Mega and Cummings (1997).

The 'cognitive' region of the cingulate has reciprocal connections with the baso-lateral amygdala, prefrontal regions, orbitofrontal cortex, inferior temporal cortex, anterior parahippocampal regions, and rostral insula. It receives afferents from the dorsal medial thalamus, intralaminar thalamic nuclei, and hippocampus, while projecting to the anterior superior temporal regions, parietal area, dorsomedial caudate, periaqueductal gray, and pontine regions.

The 'skeletal motor' region of the cingulate has reciprocal connections with the primary motor area as well as supplementary motor area and prefrontal regions. It also has reciprocal connections with the anterior parietal and parietal association cortex, and the caudal insula. It receives afferents from the thalamus and basal lateral amygdala and has efferent projections to putamen, spinal cord, red nucleus, and pontine structures.

The 'sensory processing' region of the cingulate cortex has reciprocal connections with the caudal parietal regions, frontal eye fields, prefrontal cortex, anterior hippocampal regions, and presubiculum. It receives afferents from the occipital region, hippocampus, thalamus, and pulvinar. This region has efferents to the orbitofrontal region, posterior temporal areas, and dorsal caudate nucleus (Mega and Cummings, 1997).

The anterior cingulate (Area 24) is situated at the intersection of several distributed networks subserving internal motivation states and externally directed attentional mechanisms (Mega et al., 1997). It is critically involved in the mediation of arousal and motivational states, and as such influences widespread cognitive and emotional processing.

Frontal–subcortical circuits

Frontal–subcortical circuits provide a framework for understanding the integration of limbic and paralimbic cortical structures with limbic-associated subcortical structures. Two frontal–subcortical circuits are particularly important in this regard: the orbitofrontal–subcortical circuit and the anterior cingulate–subcortical circuit. The lateral orbital circuit originates in Brodmann's Area 10 and projects to the ventral medial sector of the caudate nucleus (ventral striatum). This caudate region projects to the dorsomedial segment of the internal globus pallidus and to the rostromedial portion of the substantia nigra reticulata. The latter two regions project in turn to the medial portions of the limbic thalamus including the ventral anterior and dorsal medial nuclei. The circuit is closed by projections from the thalamus to the lateral orbitofrontal cortex (Alexander, Mahlon and Strick, 1986; Cummings, 1993a; Mega and Cummings, 1994). This circuitry links the orbitofrontal cortex to regions with similar functions in caudate nucleus, globus pallidus, and thalamus. Interruption of this circuitry at any region has similar behavioral consequences (Cummings, 1993a).

The anterior cingulate–subcortical circuit originates in Area 24 (described above) and projects to the 'limbic striatum.' This ventral striatal area receives widespread limbic projections from the hippocampus, amygdala, and entorhinal and perirhinal cortices. In addition to its projections from the anterior cingulate region, it has input from the temporal lobe, including the temporal pole and superior and inferior temporal gyri (Alexander et al., 1986). The ventral striatum projects to ventral pallidum and to the substantia nigra, which in turn project to the mediodorsal nuclei of the thalamus. The posterior and medial portions of the mediodorsal nuclei project to the anterior cingulate area, closing the circuit (Alexander et al., 1986).

This circuitry thus links the anterior cingulate, limbic striatum, pallidum, and thalamus in a cohesive circuitry associated with limbic function. There are widespread limbic connections with both the cortex and the nucleus accumbens/ventral striatal region (Cummings, 1995).

The dorsolateral prefrontal cortex, associated with executive function, has a similar circuit structure projecting to the head of the caudate nucleus, globus pallidus, and mediodorsal nucleus. This circuit mediates executive function. Thus, lesions affecting the prefrontal cortex, caudate nucleus, globus pallidus or thalamus will produce combined cognitive and emotional disturbances because of the co-involvement of closely topographically arranged circuitry mediating cognitive and emotional functions.

Specialization within the limbic system

The functional differentiations within the limbic system exemplified by the frontal–subcortical circuits, the separation of amygdala into the basolateral nuclear group and the central amygdaloid complex/extended amygdala, and the subunits of the cingulate cortex provide a basis for understanding the differential effects of focal lesions within the limbic system. While signature syndromes indicative of injury to specific areas within the limbic system are rare, involvement of member structures within differentiated circuitry often produces behavioral markers. For example, apathy may occur with injury to any structures comprising the anterior cingulate–subcortical circuit, and disinhibition may follow injury to member structures of the orbitofrontal subcortical circuit (Cummings, 1993a; Mega and Cummings, 1994).

Regional function related to neurotransmitter projections and receptor location

Many neurotransmitter systems project to widespread cortical and subcortical regions. The nucleus basalis of Meynert sends cholinergic projections to the entire neocortex. Dopamine projections arise from the substantia nigra and ventral tegmental area. They comprise a striatal projection to putamen and caudate, a mesolimbic projection to the amygdaloid complex and related structures, and a mesocortical projection to the medial frontal lobe, anterior cingulate cortex, and medial and anterior temporal cortex. Noradrenergic projections arise from locus ceruleus and connect to a variety of brainstem regions, amygdala, septal area, hippocampal formation, and the entire neocortex. Serotonergic projections arise from the raphe nuclei and pass to the thalamus, amygdaloid complex, septal region, caudate nucleus, and neocortex (Cummings and Coffey, 1994; Nieuwenhuys, 1985).

The regional distribution of transmitter receptors superimposes a regional responsiveness on the diffuse distribution of transmitters. Thus, involvement of transmitter systems may have regional effects and treatment with neuropharmaco-logic agents related to transmitter function can provoke regional responses.

Five types of muscarinic cholinergic receptors are known. M-1 receptors are found in highest concentration in the dentate gyrus, hippocampus, and anterior olfactory nucleus. They are also detected in the upper and deeper layers of the cerebral cortex, caudate and putamen, and nucleus accumbens. The amygdala has modest M-1 receptor density. M-2 receptors are found in highest density in the parietal cortex, specific thalamic nuclei, hypothalamus, and septal nuclei. Intermediate concentrations are found in the hippocampus, dentate gyrus, caudate, putamen, frontal cortex, and nucleus accumbens. M-3 receptors are diffusely distributed at a relatively low concentration, and M-4 receptors are found primarily in the striatum. M-5 receptors have not been localized fully (Schliebs and Robner, 1995).

Two pharmacologic types of dopamine receptors are known: D-1-like receptors, comprised of D-1 and D-5 receptors; and D-2-like receptors, comprised of D-2, D-3, and D-4 receptors (Mansour and Watson, 1995). D-1-like receptors are distributed widely in the cortex, with the highest levels found in the anterior cingulate, orbitofrontal cortex, insula, and medial temporal cortex. D-2-like receptors are found primarily in the entorhinal cortex, with moderate concentrations in the anterior cingulate, orbital cortex, and insular cortex. Both D-1-like and D-2-like receptors are present within the striatum and septum.

Many types of serotonin receptors have been identified. The 5-HT_{1A} receptors are dense in the CA1 region in dentate gyri of the hippocampus. 5-HT_{1B} receptors are found in highest densities in the globus pallidus, dorsal subiculum, and substantia nigra. 5-HT_{1D} receptors are located throughout the brain and are most dense in the basal ganglia. 5-HT_2 receptors are found in the cortex and caudate nuclei (Hoyer, Palacios and Mengod, 1992; Sleight and Peroutka, 1992).

Thus, neurons may have differential responses based on these varying transmitter receptor-type densities, and regional brain responses are mediated by interventions that have differential receptor effects.

Comment

This summary of limbic structures and the differential distribution of neurotransmitters and receptors within the limbic system sets the stage for understanding the emotional consequences of focal CNS lesions. Although a few conditions, such as the Klüver–Bucy syndrome (Klüver and Bucy, 1939; Lilly et al., 1983; Ghika-Schmid et al., 1995), have high regional significance implying the involvement of bilateral anterior temporal and amygdaloid regions, most lesions of the limbic system have less specific anatomic implications. Nevertheless, circuit specificity exists in the absence of local modular specificity, and clinical syndromes have circuit-localizing significance. As noted above, apathy is observed with lesions distributed within the anterior cingulate–subcortical circuit, and disinhibition appears with lesions within the orbitofrontal–subcortical circuit (Cummings, 1993a). Depression has been implicated most frequently with lesions of the frontal cortex, anterior temporal region, or head of the caudate nucleus (Cummings, 1993b). Mania is seen most often with right-sided lesions involving the inferior medial frontal regions, perithalamic areas or basal temporal structures (Cummings and Mendez, 1984; Bogousslavsky et al., 1988). Obsessive–compulsive disorder is observed with hyperactivity of the orbitofrontal cortex in the idiopathic state and with diseases of the caudate nucleus or lesions of the globus pallidus (LaPlane et al., 1989). Hypersexuality is most often associated with lesions of the septum or anterior temporal regions (Gorman and Cummings, 1992). Functional differentiation of limbic system circuits affords an explanation for the differential emotional effects of focal limbic system lesions.

In summary, this chapter presents three types of mental functions relevant to behavior: fundamental functions, instrumental functions, and executive/integrative functions. Most emotional disorders are associated with disturbances of fundamental functions and these are mediated primarily by the limbic system and related frontal–subcortical circuits. The limbic system does not exhibit a modular organization similar to that of the cortex and, hence, unique signature syndromes are unusual. The limbic system is comprised of differentiated circuits, and focal lesions within these circuits have differing behavioral consequences.

Acknowledgments

This project was supported by a National Institute on Aging Alzheimer's Disease Center grant (AG 10123), and the Sidell–Kagan Foundation (JC), and the Swiss National Science Foundation (32-41950.94, 32-50728.97) (JB).

REFERENCES

Aggleton, J.P. (1993). The contribution of the amygdala to normal and abnormal emotional states. *Trends Neurosci* 16: 328–33.

Albert, M.L. (1978). Subcortical dementia. In *Alzheimer's Disease: Senile Dementia and Related Disorders*, Vol. 7, ed. R. Katzman, R.D. Terry and K.L. Bick, pp. 173–80. New York: Raven Press.

Alexander, G.E., Mahlon, R.D. and Strick, P.L. (1986). Parallel organization of functionally segregated circuits linking basal ganglia and cortex. *Annu Rev Neurosci* 9: 357–81.

Alheid, G.F. and Heimer, L. (1988). New perspectives in basal forebrain organization of special relevance for neuropsychiatric disorders: the striatopallidal, amygdaloid, and corticopetal components of substantia innominata. *Neuroscience* 27: 1–39.

American Psychiatric Association (1994). *Diagnostic and Statistical Manual of Mental Disorders*, 4th edn. Washington, DC: American Psychiatric Association.

Bauer, R.M. (1993). Agnosia. In *Clinical Neuropsychology*, 3rd edn, ed. K.M. Heilman and E. Valenstein, pp. 215–78. New York: Oxford University Press.

Bauer, R.M., Tobias, B. and Valenstein, E. (1993). Amnesic disorders. In *Clinical Neuropsychology*, 3rd edn, ed. K.M. Heilman and E. Valenstein, pp. 523–602. New York: Oxford University Press.

Benson, D.F. and Ardila, A. (1996). *Aphasia: a Clinical Perspective*. New York: Oxford University Press.

Bogousslavsky, J., Ferrazzini, M., Regli, F. et al. (1988). Manic delirium and frontal-like syndrome with paramedian infarction of the right thalamus. *J Neurol Neurosurg Psychiatry* 51: 116–19.

Cummings, J.L. (1990). Introduction. In *Subcortical Dementia*, ed. J.L. Cummings, pp. 3–16. New York: Oxford University Press.

Cummings, J.L. (1993a). Frontal–subcortical circuits and human behavior. *Arch Neurol* 50: 873–80.

Cummings, J.L. (1993b). The neuroanatomy of depression. *J Clin Psychiatry* 54 (Suppl.): 14–20.

Cummings, J.L. (1995). Anatomic and behavioral aspects of frontal–subcortical circuits. In *Structure and Functions of the Human Prefrontal Cortex*, ed. J. Grafman, K.J. Holyoak and F. Boller, pp. 1–13. New York: The New York Academy of Sciences.

Cummings, J.L. and Coffey, C.E. (1994). Neurobiological basis of behavior. In *The American Psychiatric Press Textbook of Geriatric Neuropsychiatry*, ed. C.E. Coffey and J.L. Cummings, pp. 71–96. Washington, DC: American Psychiatric Press.

Cummings, J.L. and Mendez, M.F. (1984). Secondary mania with focal cerebrovascular lesions. *Am J Psychiatry* 141: 1084–7.

Feyereisen, P. (1989). Theories of emotions and neuropsychological research. In *Handbook of Neuropsychology*, Vol. 3, section editors L. Squire and G. Gainotti, series editors F. Boller and J. Grafman, pp. 271–81. New York: Elsevier.

Frith, C.D. and Dolan, R.J. (1997). Higher cognitive processes. In *Human Brain Function*, ed. R.S.J. Frackowiak, K.J. Friston, C.D. Frith, R.J. Dolan and J.C. Mazziotta, pp. 329–65. San Diego: Academic Press.

Ghika-Schmid, F., Assal, G., de Tribolet, N. and Regli, F. (1995). Klüver–Bucy syndrome after left anterior temporal resection. *Neuropsychologia* 33: 101–13.

Gorman, G. and Cummings, J.L. (1992). Hypersexuality following septal injury. *Arch Neurol* 49: 308–10.

Heilman, K.M. (1983). Introduction. In *Neuropsychology of Human Emotion*, ed. K.M. Heilman and P. Satz, pp. 1–5. New York: Guilford Press.

Heilman, K.M., Bowers, D. and Valenstein, E. (1993). Emotional disorders associated with neurological diseases. In *Clinical Neuropsychology*, 3rd edn, ed. K.M. Heilman and E. Valenstein, pp. 461–97. New York: Oxford University Press.

Heilman, K.M. and Gonzalez-Rothi, L.J. (1993). Apraxia. In *Clinical Neuropsychology*, 3rd edn, ed. K.M. Heilman and E. Valenstein, pp. 141–63. New York: Oxford University Press.

Hoyer, D., Palacios, J.M. and Mengod, G. (1992). 5-HT receptor distribution in the human brain: autoradiographic studies. In *Central Serotonin Receptors and Psychotropic Drugs*, ed. C.A. Marsden and D.J. Heal, pp. 100–25. Oxford: Blackwell Scientific Publications.

Klüver, H. and Bucy, P.C. (1939). Preliminary analysis of functions of the temporal lobes in monkeys. *Arch Neurol Psychiatry* 42: 979–1000.

LaPlane, D., Levasseur, M., Pillon, B. et al. (1989). Obsessive–compulsive and other behavioral changes with bilateral basal ganglia lesions. *Brain* 112: 699–725.

Levin, H.S., Goldstein, F.C. and Spiers, P.A. (1993). Acalculia. In *Clinical Neuropsychology*, 3rd edn, ed. K.M. Heilman and E. Valenstein, pp. 91–122. New York: Oxford University Press.

Lilly, R., Cummings, J.L., Benson, D.F. et al. (1983). Clinical features of the human Klüver–Bucy syndrome. *Neurology* 33: 1141–5.

Macchi, G. (1989). Anatomical substrate of emotional reactions. In *Handbook of Neuropsychology*, Vol. 3, section editors L. Squire and G. Gainotti, series editors F. Boller and J. Grafman, pp. 283–303. New York: Elsevier.

Mansour, A. and Watson, S.J. Jr (1995). Dopamine receptor expression in the central nervous system. In *Psychopharmacology: the Fourth Generation of Progress*, ed. F.E. Bloom and D.J. Kupfer, pp. 207–19. New York: Raven Press.

Mega, M.S. and Cummings, J.L. (1994). Frontal–subcortical circuits and neuropsychiatric disorders. *J Neuropsychiatry Clin Neurosci* 6: 358–70.

Mega, M.S. and Cummings, J.L. (1997). The cingulate and cingulate syndromes. In *Contemporary Behavioral Neurology*, ed. M.R. Trimble and J.L. Cummings, pp. 189–214. Boston: Butterworth-Heinemann.

Mega, M.S., Cummings, J.L., Salloway, S. and Malloy, P. (1997). The limbic system: an anatomic, phylogenetic, and clinical perspective. *J Neuropsychiatry Clin Neurosci* 9: 315–30.

Mesulam, M-M. (1985). Patterns in behavioral neuroanatomy: association areas, the limbic system, and hemispheric specialization. In *Principles of Behavioral Neurology*, ed. M-M. Mesulam, pp. 1–70. Philadelphia: F.A. Davis Company.

Nieuwenhuys, R. (1985). *Chemoarchitecture of the Brain.* New York: Springer-Verlag.

Papez, J.W. (1937). A proposed mechanism of emotion. *Arch Neurol Psychiatry* 38: 725–33.

Pribram, K.H. and Melges, F.T. (1969). Psychophysiological basis of emotion. In *Disorders of Higher Nervous Activity*, ed. P.J. Vinken and G.W. Bruyn (in collaboration with M. Critchley and J.A.M. Frederiks), pp. 316–42. Amsterdam: North-Holland Publishing Company.

Rolls, E.T. (1995). A theory of emotion and consciousness, and its application to understanding the neural basis of emotion. In *The Cognitive Neurosciences*, ed. M.S. Gazzaniga, pp. 1091–106. Cambridge, MA: MIT Press.

Russchen, F.T., Bakst, I., Amaral, D.G. and Price, J.L. (1985). The amygdalostriatal projections in the monkey: an anterograde tracing study. *Brain Res* 329: 241–57.

Schliebs, R. and Robner, S. (1995). Distribution of muscarinic acetylcholine receptors in the CNS. In *CNS Neurotransmitters and Neuromodulators*, ed. T.W. Stone, pp. 67–83. Boca Raton, FL: CRC Press.

Sleight, A.J. and Peroutka, S.J. (1992). 5-HT receptor binding sites in the central nervous system and their distribution. In *Central Serotonin Receptors and Psychotrophic Drugs*, ed. C.A. Marsden and D.J. Heal, pp. 3–15. London: Blackwell Scientific Publications.

Stuss, D.T. and Benson, D.F. (1986). *The Frontal Lobes*. New York: Raven Press.

Thompson, D. (ed.) (1995). *The Concise Oxford Dictionary of Current English*, 9th edn. (First edited by H.W. Fowler and F.G. Fowler.) Norwalk, CT: The Easton Press.

2

The evaluation of mood and behavior in patients with focal brain lesions

David W. Desmond

Introduction

Many studies have investigated focal brain lesions as a basis for cognitive impairment but less attention has been given to their role in the etiology of mood and behavior disorders. Both as a cause and as an effect of that disparity, the measures that are available for the cognitive assessment of patients far outnumber those that might be utilized for the assessment of disorders of mood and behavior. Although there is currently greater potential for the effective pharmacologic treatment of mood and certain behavior disorders than of cognitive impairment in patients with focal brain lesions, it is likely that many patients with such disorders remain undiagnosed due to the underutilization of those standardized assessments that are available and to an understandable emphasis on the physical disabilities that may result from those lesions. Thus, this chapter describes certain of the methods that are available for the evaluation of mood and behavior disorders in patients with focal brain lesions as well as some of the difficulties inherent in the evaluation of neurologic patients with those disorders.

Overview of the characteristics of assessment tools

Although the diagnosis of major depression has frequently been based on simple clinical judgment in investigational studies, particularly those in which mood disorders were not the primary focus, scales that have been utilized to assist in that diagnosis have taken many forms, varying with regard to the following characteristics:

1 Mode of administration, i.e., is the scale administered to the patient by an examiner or is it self-administered?

2 Depth of inquiry regarding specific aspects of the syndrome of major depression, such as vegetative signs.

3 Duration of symptoms, i.e., must symptoms have been present during a specified period preceding the assessment?

4 Item scoring method, e.g., true–false, severity ratings.

5 Potential for use as a formal diagnostic tool, i.e., adherence to codified diagnostic paradigms such as the criteria presented in the *Diagnostic and Statistical Manual of Mental Disorders*, fourth edition (DSM-IV; American Psychiatric Association, 1994) versus the use of a simple cut-off score or no formal diagnostic method.

6 The complexity of the scale and the cognitive demands that it places on the patient.

In contrast, rating scales that have been developed for the assessment of behavior have typically taken the form of lists of operationally defined behavioral abnormalities that are rated as 'present' or 'absent' by a clinician or a reliable informant based on observation of the patient.

Given that the selection of a rating scale should be determined in part by the reliability and validity of that scale, a review of those concepts would be worthwhile. As summarized by Anastasi (1988), measures of reliability include the following:

1 inter-rater reliability, in which consistency between the test scores of different examiners is assessed;

2 test–retest reliability, in which consistency between scores on two administrations of a test is assessed;

3 split-half reliability, in which the comparability of two halves of a test is assessed;

4 inter-item reliability, in which the consistency among responses to all items on a test is assessed.

In general, reliability tends to be maximized by the use of highly structured interviews and operationally defined terms. Although there is no consensus on the definitions of measures of validity, Anastasi (1988) suggests that they include the following:

1 content-related validity, which results from the development of test items by experts in the field;

2 criterion-related validity, including concurrent and predictive validity, in which the effectiveness of a test in measuring an attribute is compared to an independent criterion at that time or at some point in the future;

3 construct-related validity, including convergent and discriminant validity, in which a test may be shown to measure an attribute of interest and to be unrelated to irrelevant characteristics.

Face validity, in which a set of test items may appear to be superficially relevant to a disorder of interest, can be considered to be additional informal support for the validity of a scale. While not all of these forms of reliability and validity must be documented for a test to be selected for use, some evidence of the reliability and validity of a scale in the patient population of interest should be available. Finally, it is important to note that a scale that is not reliable cannot be considered to be valid.

The description of scales that follows is not intended to be exhaustive, and other texts are available that provide more comprehensive reviews (e.g., Marsella, Hirschfeld and Katz, 1987; Beckham and Leber, 1995). Instead, scales that are popular or particularly well suited to the assessment of patients with focal brain lesions will be discussed in detail and references to alternative measures will be provided. Following a general description of the design of each scale, information regarding reliability and validity will be discussed, with an emphasis on the findings of studies of patients with focal brain lesions or other neurologic disorders when they have been performed.

Methods for the assessment of mood disorders

Diagnostic criteria

DSM-IV (American Psychiatric Association, 1994) diagnostic criteria for a Mood Disorder Due to a General Medical Condition, which would be applicable to patients with focal brain lesions, are presented in Table 2.1. Although those criteria can be used in general clinical practice, the reliability of their application can be enhanced through the use of the Structured Clinical Interview for DSM-IV Axis I Disorders (SCID-I; First et al., 1997). It is worthy of note that the diagnostic criteria presented in the *International Classification of Diseases*, 10th edition (ICD-10; World Health Organization, 1993) for an Organic Depressive Disorder (diagnosis code F06.32) are comparable to those presented in DSM-IV.

Hamilton Depression Rating Scale (Hamilton, 1960, 1967)

The Hamilton Depression Rating Scale (HDRS) is probably the most widely used rating scale for depression. In addition, it has frequently served as the 'gold standard' against which other scales have been validated. Williams (1988) developed a version of the original scale that she termed the Structured Interview Guide for the HDRS (SIGH-D) in order to enhance the reliability of its administration and scoring, but most studies have used the original HDRS without an interview guide. The HDRS and the SIGH-D consist of 21 items tapping many aspects of depressive syndromes, and 20 to 30 minutes are required for administration by a trained examiner. In the SIGH-D, questions are posed to patients with regard to their characteristics during the previous week, and follow-up questions are provided to elicit information that is directly relevant to scoring. The first question is 'What has your mood been like this past week?', for example, and it is followed by additional inquiries including 'Have you been feeling down or depressed?' and 'Have you been crying at all?' Items are scored according to the frequency and intensity of depressive symptoms. Scoring options for that first question, for example, are zero points for the absence of depression, one point for depression that is indicated only on

Table 2.1. DSM-IV diagnostic criteria for a Mood Disorder Due to a General Medical Condition (293.83)

A. A prominent and persistent disturbance in mood predominates in the clinical picture and is characterized by either (or both) of the following:
    (1) depressed mood or markedly diminished interest or pleasure in all, or almost all, activities.
    (2) elevated, expansive, or irritable mood.
B. There is evidence from the history, physical examination, or laboratory findings that the disturbance is the direct physiologic consequence of a general medical condition.
C. The disturbance is not better accounted for by another mental disorder (e.g., Adjustment Disorder With Depressed Mood in response to the stress of having a general medical condition).
D. The disturbance does not occur exclusively during the course of a delirum.
E. The symptoms cause clinically significant distress or impairment in social, occupational, or other important areas of functioning.

Specify type:
    With Depressive Features: the predominant mood is depressed but the full criteria are not met for a Major Depressive Episode.
    With Major Depressive-Like Episode: the full criteria are met for a Major Depressive Episode (296.2X), except a general medical condition is permitted as a causal factor.
    With Manic Features: the predominant mood is elevated, euphoric, or irritable.
    With Mixed Features: symptoms of both mania and depression are present but neither predominates.

Note:
If the mood disorder is not judged to be the direct physiologic consequence of the general medical condition, then the primary mood disorder (e.g., Major Depressive Episode) is recorded on Axis I and the general medical condition is recorded on Axis III.
Source: Adapted from American Psychiatric Association (1994).

questioning, two points for depression that is spontaneously reported verbally, three points for depression that is communicated nonverbally (e.g., facial expression, tendency to weep), and four points for depression that is essentially the only focus of spontaneous verbal and nonverbal communication. Studies have typically reported the total score based on the first 17 items of the scale, as recommended by Hamilton (1960), but a diagnosis of major depression conforming with DSM-III-R (American Psychiatric Association, 1987) criteria can be made if the SIGH-D is slightly modified. Cut-off scores of ≥25 for severe depression, 18 to 24 for moderate depression, 7 to 17 for mild depression, and 0 to 6 for no depression have also been proposed (Endicott et al., 1981).

Reliability and validity

Given that the HDRS is probably the most widely used rating scale for depression and that numerous studies have been performed to evaluate its characteristics, only a selection of particularly relevant reliability and validity studies will be described here. Inter-rater reliability for the original HDRS 17-item total score has been found to be acceptable in a number of studies of depressed patients (Knesevich et al., 1977; Montgomery and Åsberg, 1979; Rehm and O'Hara, 1985; Maier et al., 1988b). Based on a sample of 23 psychiatric patients with a variety of diagnoses, Williams (1988) reported four-day test–retest reliability coefficients of 0.81 for the 17-item SIGH-D scale and 0.82 for the 21-item scale, with the two assessments performed by different raters. Reliability coefficients were higher for almost all individual scale items using the SIGH-D than those that were reported by Cicchetti and Prusoff (1983) using the original HDRS without a structured interview guide. Yesavage et al. (1983) reported a split-half reliability of 0.82 and an inter-item reliability of 0.90 based on coefficient alpha in a sample of elderly subjects, the majority of whom were depressed.

In a sample of a stroke patients, Malec et al. (1990) reported an inter-rater reliability of 0.77 for the HDRS based on a Pearson correlation, with the second assessment administered within 11 days of the first assessment. In an unpublished inter-rater reliability study that we performed in 1992 (Williams et al., unpublished data), three trained research assistants and one clinical psychologist administered the SIGH-D to 32 elderly ischemic stroke patients and 20 elderly stroke-free control subjects. Intraclass correlation coefficients were excellent for the 17-item total score (i.e., 0.96 for all raters and 0.97 for the three research assistants) and all but two of the 17 individual items (i.e., observer ratings of psychomotor retardation and agitation), including items related to depressed mood and anhedonia (i.e., 0.86 and 0.87, respectively). The results were comparable when data collected from the stroke and control groups were examined separately.

Factor analysis of the HDRS in samples of depressed patients has tended to yield one primary factor that has been termed 'a unidimensional index of global depression severity' (Gibbons, Clark and Kupfer, 1993) and 'core depressive symptoms' (Faravelli, Albanesi and Poli, 1986) as well as multiple additional factors relevant to vegetative signs. It has been suggested that such a primary factor may be a better measure of depression than the total HDRS score (Gibbons, et al., 1993), in part due to the influence that somatic disorders may have on secondary factors (Linden et al., 1995). In psychiatric samples, HDRS scores have been found to be significantly correlated with global clinical ratings of the severity of depression and total scores on other scales, including the Beck Depression Inventory and the Depression Scale of the Minnesota Multiphasic Personality Inventory (Knesevich et al., 1977; Yesavage et al., 1983; Rehm and O'Hara, 1985; Faravelli et al., 1986; Maier et al., 1988a).

In patients with stroke, Agrell and Dehlin (1989) found that an HDRS cut-off score of ten yielded a sensitivity of 71% and a specificity of 87% with regard to a clinical diagnosis of depression. Similarly, Malec et al. (1990) found that the use of a cut-off score of $\geq$ eight resulted in diagnoses that were consistent with clinically diagnosed depression. Pearson correlations of 0.77, 0.74, and 0.70 have been reported for the association between HDRS total score and scores on the Geriatric Depression Scale, the Center for Epidemiologic Studies Depression Scale, and the Zung Self-Rating Depression Scale, respectively, in stroke patients (Agrell and Dehlin, 1989). Other studies of patients with stroke have found that the HDRS total score increases with the severity of depression (Ng, Chan and Straughan, 1995) and decreases in association with the effective treatment of depression (Andersen, Vestergaard and Lauritzen, 1994). Similar characteristics of the HDRS have been noted in a study of patients with closed head injury (Fedoroff et al., 1992) as well as in a number of studies of depression in patients with Alzheimer's disease (Reifler, Teri and Raskind, 1989; Fitz and Teri, 1994; Vida et al., 1994).

Beck Depression Inventory-II (Beck, Steer and Brown, 1996)

The Beck Depression Inventory-II (BDI-II) is a recent revision to the BDI-IA (Beck et al., 1979; Beck and Steer, 1987), which was itself a revision of the original BDI (Beck et al., 1961). The BDI-II was developed for the assessment of symptoms corresponding to DSM-IV criteria for the diagnosis of depressive disorders in patients aged 13 and older. It can be self-administered or administered by a trained examiner and it requires five to ten minutes for completion. The BDI-II consists of 21 items tapping symptoms such as sadness, loss of pleasure, and guilty feelings, as well as a variety of vegetative signs. Each item consists of a statement regarding the presence of a symptom during the preceding two weeks and the patient must select one of four response options, which are graded by severity. Each item is given a score ranging from zero to three, resulting in a maximum possible BDI-II score of 63. Based on study of psychiatric patients, cut-off scores of 0 to 13 for minimal or no depression, 14 to 19 for mild depression, 20 to 28 for moderate depression, and 29 to 63 for severe depression have been proposed (Beck et al., 1996).

Reliability and validity

The BDI-II manual reported a one-week test–retest reliability coefficient of 0.93 in an outpatient psychiatric sample. Internal consistency coefficients were 0.92 for a separate outpatient psychiatric sample and 0.93 for a sample of college students. Item-total correlations ranged from 0.39 to 0.70 for that outpatient sample and 0.27 to 0.74 for the college sample. Based on the original BDI, test–retest reliability coefficients of 0.79 and 0.86 based on Pearson correlations and split-half reliability coefficients of 0.58 and 0.74 based on Spearman correlations have been reported in depressed and nondepressed elderly samples, respectively (Gallagher, Nies and Thompson, 1982). Internal consistency coefficients of ≥0.73 have been reported in elderly samples (Gallagher et al., 1982; Keane and Sells, 1990) and in patients with Parkinson's disease (Levin, Llabre and Weiner, 1988).

In a sample of psychiatric patients who were diagnosed with mood disorders, anxiety disorders, adjustment disorders, or other disorders according to DSM-III-R criteria, patients with mood disorders received significantly higher BDI-II total scores than patients with other diagnoses (Beck et al., 1996). In a smaller sample of psychiatric outpatients, the correlation of BDI-II total score with HDRS total score was 0.71. Factor analysis identified two factors in samples of psychiatric outpatients and college students, which were interpreted to represent 'somatic–affective' and 'cognitive' characteristics in the former sample and 'cognitive–affective' and 'somatic' characteristics in the latter sample (Beck et al., 1996).

Until the recent publication of the BDI-II, validity studies based on patients with neurological disorders had used the original BDI and the BDI-IA. Regarding the use of the BDI with stroke patients, House et al. (1989) expressed a concern regarding a high false-positive rate for the diagnosis of depression, but another stroke study found that the BDI identified fewer cases of depression than psychiatric diagnosis but a significantly greater number of true cases of depression than a multidisciplinary nonpsychiatric rehabilitation team relying on clinical judgment (Schubert et al., 1992). In a separate study of stroke patients, median BDI-IA scores increased with the severity of depression diagnosed through the use of clinical judgment, and the correlation of BDI-IA total score with HDRS total score was 0.70 (Dam, Pedersen and Ahlgren, 1989). In prospective follow-up, BDI scores have been found to decrease from one month to one year after stroke, the decline of somatic symptoms being greater than that of cognitive–affective symptoms (House et al., 1991). Relevant to that finding, Stein et al. (1996) have suggested that a reliance on the nonsomatic items of the BDI or other depression rating scales such as the HDRS may permit a more accurate diagnosis of depression in patients after stroke and that somatic items add no incremental validity. The BDI has also been used in studies of patients with other neurological disorders, such as Parkinson's disease (Levin et al., 1988; Youngjohn et al., 1992; Tröster et al., 1995) and multiple sclerosis (Beatty et al., 1989).

Center for Epidemiologic Studies Depression Scale (Radloff, 1977)

The Center for Epidemiologic Studies Depression Scale (CES-D) was developed for use in studies of the epidemiology of depressive disorders in the general population. Although it was originally designed to be a self-report instrument, it can also be administered by lay interviewers and requires approximately 15 minutes for completion. The CES-D consists of 20 statements (e.g., 'I felt depressed,' 'My sleep was restless,' 'I did not feel like eating; my appetite was poor') and patients must determine whether each of those statements is true as applied to themselves during the previous week. Certain items are phrased in reverse format (e.g., 'I was happy') to break tendencies toward a response set. Increasing numbers of points, ranging from zero to three, are awarded for increasing severity of each symptom based on the number of days in the preceding week that the characteristic was present, and the total score on the CES-D is the sum of all item scores (range = 0 to 60).

Reliability and validity

Reliability analyses performed on multiple depressed patient and general population samples in the original study (Radloff, 1977) determined that test–retest correlations were moderate and decreased as the test–retest interval increased from one month (i.e., approximately 0.60) to one year (i.e., approximately 0.40). The internal consistency of the scale was acceptable, with all coefficient alphas ≥ 0.84 and all split-half correlations ≥ 0.76. In a study of 27 stroke patients (Shinar et al., 1986), inter-rater reliability between a nurse and a research assistant on CES-D total score was 0.76 based on a Pearson correlation. Item-total Spearman correlations ranged from 0.39 to 0.75.

Factor analysis based on general population samples in the original study (Radloff, 1977) recognized four factors, which were interpreted to represent 'depressed affect,' 'positive affect,' 'somatic and retarded activity,' and 'interpersonal characteristics,' but the high internal consistency of the scale led the author to argue against an undue emphasis on separate factors and to suggest that a simple total score be used as an estimate of the severity of depressive symptomatology. Validity studies presented in that manuscript demonstrated that depressed patient and general population samples differed significantly on CES-D total score and that the total score was significantly lower at the end of four weeks of treatment of a depressed patient sample. Correlations with HDRS total score were 0.44 on admission and 0.69 after four weeks of treatment. Age, sex, race, and education did not significantly influence the CES-D's reliability, correlation with other scales, or factor structure in the original study (Radloff, 1977), and a later study confirmed that the internal consistency and factor structure of the scale were unaffected by race or ethnicity (Roberts, 1980). Although the CES-D was not originally intended to be used for the clinical diagnosis of depression, 70% of a depressed patient sample and 21% of a general population sample scored above a cut-off score of ≥ 16 that Radloff (1977) described as 'arbitrary.'

In a sample of stroke patients (Shinar et al., 1986), correlations with CES-D total score were 0.77 for a clinical diagnosis of depression, 0.57 for HDRS total score, 0.65 for Zung Self-Rating Depression Scale total score, and 0.74 for a diagnosis based on the Present State Examination, and similar findings were reported in a later study of patients with stroke (Parikh et al., 1988). Use of a cut-off of ≥ 16 yielded a sensitivity of 73% and a specificity of 100% versus a DSM-III (American Psychiatric Association, 1980) diagnosis of depression in a sample of stroke patients (Shinar et al., 1986), and similar findings were reported in a later stroke study (Parikh et al., 1988). It should be noted that concerns have been raised regarding the diagnostic utility of the CES-D, however, suggesting that it is unable to discriminate between major depression and generalized anxiety (Breslau, 1985) and may in fact measure distress or demoralization (Vernon and Roberts, 1981).

Post-Stroke Depression Rating Scale (Gainotti et al., 1997b)

The Post-Stroke Depression Rating Scale (PSDRS) is a structured interview performed by a trained clinician and requires approximately 15 minutes for completion. It is composed of ten sections, each of which was designed to evaluate a specific aspect of the 'emotional, affective, and vegetative disorders' that the authors believed to be common among stroke patients, which are as follows: (1) depressed mood, (2) feelings of guilt, (3) thoughts of death and/or suicide, (4) vegetative disorders of sleep and appetite, (5) apathy, (6) anxiety, (7) catastrophic reactions, (8) hyperemotionality, (9) anhedonia, and (10) diurnal mood variations. Each section is scored according to symptom severity but the range of scores available in each section is variable. Regarding section 1 (depressed mood), for example, a score of zero is assigned for 'well-balanced mood, at times happier, at times worried, but not more than before illness;' a score of one is assigned for 'mood a little more sad and worried than before illness;' a score of two is assigned for 'mood clearly more oriented toward sadness and pessimism than before illness;' a score of three is assigned for 'mood clearly oriented toward sadness and pessimism, with fits of crying from time to time;' a score of four is assigned for 'very sad and disheartened mood, cries rather often and for long periods;' and a score of five is assigned for 'gloomy, black mood, cries continuously, and there is no way to hearten him/her, or so depressed and dark he/she can't even cry any more.' Patients are asked to state whether their symptoms in sections 1, 2, and 3 are related to the consequences of their stroke or independent of them. A global score is not generated. Instead, the scale provides a symptomatic profile that can be compared to other stroke patients as well as to patients with endogenous depression.

Reliability and validity

In the original study (Gainotti et al., 1997b), inter-rater reliability was assessed based on the examinations of a neurologist and a psychiatrist in a sample of 124 patients with acute stroke. Spearman rank-order correlation coefficients ranged from 0.92 for depressed mood to 0.63 for diurnal mood variation. Correlations between analogous sections of the PSDRS and the HDRS were 0.81 for depressed mood, 0.88 for suicidal thoughts, 0.77 for anxiety, 0.70 for vegetative disorders, 0.51 for apathy, and 0.42 for feelings of guilt, and the correlation between the combined analogous sections of the PSDRS and the HDRS was 0.88. Profile analysis demonstrated that the syndrome exhibited by the stroke patients in that study was significantly different from that which was exhibited by 17 patients with endogenous depression, with the profile of stroke patients distinguished by feelings of depression associated with handicap or disability, anxiety, catastrophic reactions, and hyperemotionality.

Visual analog scale (Aitken, 1969; Zealley and Aitken, 1969)

In the original administration of this measure, subjects were presented with a 100 mm long horizontal line marked 'extreme depression' or 'most depressed' at one end and 'normal mood' or 'most happy' at the opposite end, and they were asked to place a mark at the point on the scale that best represented their current feelings. Subsequent studies have used varying labels for the extremes of the 100 mm line, including 'not at all depressed' and 'extremely depressed, as bad as I could possibly feel' (House et al, 1989), 'worst mood' and 'best mood' (Luria, 1975), and, in response to the question 'How are you feeling today?,' the labels 'worst ever' and 'best ever' (Feinberg et al., 1981). Stern and Bachman (1991) presented stroke patients with a vertical line to eliminate potential bias due to hemineglect, with words and cartoon faces representing 'happy' at the top and 'sad' at the bottom. It is quite possible that those differing formats have an important but poorly understood effect on the psychometric properties of the visual analog scale. Scoring of the visual analog scale is based on the measurement of the distance from the patient's mark to the 'nondepressed' end of the scale, this objectified method ensuring that inter-rater reliability is essentially perfect. Despite the report of House et al. (1989) that stroke patients who could not complete the Beck Depression Inventory could not complete the visual analog scale and that patients without obvious cognitive impairment seemed 'bewildered' by the scale, Stern and Bachman (1991) and Gainotti et al. (1997a) have suggested that the visual analog scale may be the only usable, albeit crude, resource for the assessment of mood in patients with significant language disorders or severe cognitive impairment.

In addition to the format described above, expanded versions of the visual analog scale have been proposed (Bauer et al., 1991; Ahearn and Carroll, 1996; Nyenhuis et al., 1997). Those versions present the subject with numerous visual analog scales, each designed to assess a specific aspect of a depressive disorder. Although these expanded versions of the visual analog scale have been shown to have acceptable reliability and validity in samples of psychiatric patients, the increased demands that they impose on a patient's communicative and cognitive abilities eliminate the unique attribute that the visual analog scale possesses for use with patients with focal brain lesions.

Reliability and validity

Folstein and Luria (1973) reported one-day test–retest reliability coefficients of 0.61 and 0.73 for two samples of primarily psychiatric patients. A later study (Luria, 1975) reported two-hour test–retest reliability coefficients ranging from 0.73 to 0.91 and one-day test–retest reliability coefficients ranging from 0.56 to 0.72 in different subgroups of psychiatric patients. In a study of patients with left hemisphere lesions (Robinson and Szetela, 1981), the test–retest reliability of the visual analog scale was 0.98 based on assessments performed at the beginning and end of a long clinical interview.

Regarding validity studies, the correlation of the visual analog scale was 0.79 with HDRS total score in a sample of 13 depressed patients on admission and it was sensitive to the benficial effects of antidepressant medications (Zealley and Aitken, 1969). Folstein and Luria (1973) found that correlations of the visual analog scale were −0.46 and −0.56 with the Unhappy subscale of the Clyde Mood Scale and −0.64 and −0.67 with the Zung Self-Rating Depression Scale in two samples of primarily psychiatric patients, with those negative signs supportive of good interscale agreement. In a later study (Luria, 1975), the correlation of the visual analog scale was −0.57 with the Unhappy subscale of the Clyde Mood Scale and −0.63 with the Zung Self-Rating Depression Scale among patients with affective disorders, and the visual analog scale scores of those patients were consistent with significantly greater depression than those of patients with other psychiatric disorders. Similarly, Feinberg et al. (1981) studied patients with unipolar endogenous depression and reported Pearson correlations of −0.73 and −0.65 for visual analog scale score with HDRS total score and a clinical global rating of depression, respectively. Regarding patients with focal brain lesions, Gainotti et al. (1997a) studied a sample of 149 stroke patients and reported that the correlation of the visual analog scale with the HDRS was 0.49. In a study of patients with left hemisphere lesions (Robinson and Szetela, 1981), the correlation of the visual analog scale with the Nurse's Rating Scale was 0.60.

Additional scales for the assessment of mood

The Geriatric Depression Scale (Yesavage et al., 1983) could be a useful tool for the study of neurologic samples because its properties have been well characterized in elderly depressed patients and it de-emphasizes somatic symptoms. The Zung Self-Rating Depression Scale (Zung, 1965) is similar to the BDI-II and the CES-D but without unique attributes that would support its use in patients with neurologic disorders. Diagnostic approaches such as the Present State Examination (Wing et al., 1967) and the Schedule for Affective Disorders and Schizophrenia (Endicott and Spitzer, 1978) require lengthier subject interviews, which would probably be better dedicated to the use of the SCID-I (First et al., 1997) due to its compatibility with DSM-IV diagnoses. Other methods for the assessment of depression are more problematic and probably inappropriate for use in patients with focal brain lesions. The Minnesota Multiphasic Personality Inventory – 2 (Butcher et al., 1989) provides a clinical scale as well as multiple subscale scores relevant to depression, but its 567-item true–false format is likely to be too demanding for patients with cognitive impairment and its properties are not adequately understood in patients with neurologic disorders. Certain studies (e.g., Williams, Barlow and Agras, 1972) have used quantified observations of patient behaviors, such as reading and grooming, as markers for depression, but the interpretation of the findings of such assessments could be confounded by certain physiologic sequelae, such as hemiparesis, and other primary disorders of behavior in patients with focal brain lesions.

Methods for the assessment of behavior disorders

Diagnostic criteria

DSM-IV (American Psychiatric Association, 1994) diagnostic criteria for a Personality Change Due to a General Medical Condition, which would be applicable to patients with focal brain lesions, are presented in Table 2.2. Criterion D suggests that the use of this diagnosis could be problematic for patients with focal brain lesions who otherwise meet criteria for dementia. The diagnostic criteria presented in ICD-10 (World Health Organization, 1993) for an Organic Personality Disorder (diagnosis code F07.0) are comparable to those presented in DSM-IV.

Neuropsychiatric Inventory (Cummings et al., 1994)

The Neuropsychiatric Inventory (NPI) was developed to permit the rapid assessment of a wide range of behaviors encountered in patients with dementia of varied etiologies and to provide a method for characterizing the frequency and severity of behavioral changes. It is a structured caregiver interview that requires a minimum of seven to ten minutes for administration and, in its original format, consisted of questions tapping ten different domains of behavior (i.e., delusions, hallucinations, agitation/aggression, dysphoria, anxiety, euphoria, apathy, disinhibition, irritability/lability, and aberrant motor activity). A subsequent revision of the NPI added questions tapping the domains of nighttime behavioral disturbances and changes in appetite and eating behaviors (Cummings, 1997).

Regarding the administration of the NPI, the caregiver is asked a screening question related to the occurrence of an abnormal behavior in each domain, and seven or eight follow-up questions are presented if the caregiver responds in the

Table 2.2. DSM-IV diagnostic criteria for Personality Change Due to a General Medical Condition (310.1)

A.   A persistent personality disturbance that represents a change from the individual's previous characteristic personality pattern.

B.   There is evidence from the history, physical examination, or laboratory findings that the disturbance is the direct physiologic consequence of a general medical condition.

C.   The disturbance is not better accounted for by another mental disorder, including other Mental Disorders Due to a General Medical Condition.

D.   The disturbance does not occur exclusively during the course of a delirium and does not meet criteria for a dementia.

E.   The disturbance causes clinically significant distress or impairment in social, occupational, or other important areas of functioning.

Specify type:

   Labile Type: the predominant feature is affective lability.

   Disinhibited Type: the predominant feature is poor impulse control as evidenced by sexual indiscretions, etc.

   Aggressive Type: the predominant feature is aggressive behavior.

   Apathetic Type: the predominant feature is marked apathy and indifference.

   Paranoid Type: the predominant feature is suspiciousness or paranoid ideation.

   Other Type: the predominant feature is not one of the above.

   Combined Type: more than one feature predominates in the clinical picture.

   Unspecified Type.

Source: Adapted from American Psychiatric Association (1994).

affirmative to the screening question. Representative follow-up questions include 'Does the patient seem less spontaneous and less active than usual?,' 'Does the patient pace around the house without apparent purpose?,' and 'Does the patient talk to people who are not there?' The caregiver is asked to rate the severity (mild, moderate, or severe, with scores ranging from one to three) and frequency ('occasionally, less than once per week' through 'very frequently, once or more per day or continuously,' with scores ranging from one to four) of abnormal behavior within each domain, and scores are calculated for each domain by multiplying the severity and frequency scores for a maximum possible domain-specific score of 12. Domain-specific scores can be summed to generate a total score for the NPI. Caregiver distress can also be rated with regard to abnormalities in each behavioral domain (Cummings, 1997), with scores ranging from zero (no distress) to five (very severe or extreme distress), and total caregiver distress can be measured by summing the domain-specific distress scores.

Reliability and validity

Based on a sample of caregivers of patients with dementia in the original study (Cummings et al., 1994), frequencies of between-rater agreement ranged from 93.6% to 100% for frequency ratings and from 89.4% to 100% for severity ratings. Most of the three-week test–retest reliability coefficients for both the frequency and severity ratings were greater than 0.70. Coefficient alpha, representing the internal consistency of the overall scale, was 0.88 and varied between 0.87 and 0.88 for both the severity and frequency ratings for individual domains.

In the original study (Cummings et al., 1994), significant correlations, most of which were ≥0.60, were obtained between frequency, severity, and frquency×severity products for specific NPI domains and comparable domains of the Behavioral Pathology in Alzheimer's Disease Rating Scale and the HDRS. Scores in the delusions, anxiety, disinhibition, and aberrant motor behavior domains were significantly correlated with Mini-Mental State Examination score. Spouses of nondemented elderly control subjects were also administered the NPI. Low mean scores were obtained on the dysphoria, disinhibition, and irritability scales in that control sample, while all of the remaining scores were zero. In a study by Mega et al. (1996) comparing patients with Alzheimer's disease to a sample of normal control subjects, scores of patients with Alzheimer's disease were significantly increased in each of the ten original behavioral domains, and scores in the agitation, dysphoria, apathy, and aberrant motor behavior domains were significantly correlated with the severity of cognitive impairment. Kaufer, Cummings and Christine (1996) found that the mean NPI total score was significantly reduced (i.e., behavior improved) when patients with Alzheimer's disease were at a maximal dose of tacrine in an open-label study, with the beneficial effects most evident in the domains of hallucinations, anxiety, apathy, disinhibition, and aberrant motor behavior and in patients with moderate versus mild or severe dementia. Behavioral syndromes documented with the NPI were found to be comparable in patients from the USA, Italy, and Mexico with Alzheimer's disease, with apathy and anxiety found to be common, and disinhibition, hallucinations, and euphoria found to be uncommon (Cummings et al., 1996).

Regarding the utility of the NPI in differential diagnosis, patients with fronto-temporal dementia have been reported to have greater behavioral disturbances than patients with Alzheimer's disease, as evidenced by significantly higher total NPI scores and higher scores in the apathy, disinhibition, euphoria, and aberrant motor behavior domains (Levy et al., 1996). High apathy scores and low agitation and anxiety scores accurately distinguished patients with progressive supranuclear palsy from patients with Alzheimer's disease (Litvan et al., 1996).

Neurobehavioral Rating Scale (Levin et al., 1987)

The Neurobehavioral Rating Scale (NRS) was originally developed to assess behavioral changes resulting from head injury. Based on a structured interview focusing on the patient's self-report of symptoms and injury, self-appraisal, planning, and certain aspects of cognitive function, including orientation, memory, reasoning, and attention, the examiner evaluates specific responses and integrates behavioral observations to characterize the patient's level of function on each of 27 subscales (e.g., inattention/reduced alertness, disinhibition, decreased initiative/motivation), selecting one of seven ratings ranging from 'not present' to 'extremely severe.' Both zero to six and one to seven have been used as possible ranges of scores for those ratings. The total score on the NRS is the sum of the 27 subscale scores, and summary scores for factors that have been identified, as described below, can also be calculated.

Reliability and validity

Based on a sample of patients with closed head injury, inter-rater reliability for NRS total score was ≥ 0.88 (Levin et al., 1987), while a study of inter-rater reliability based on a sample of patients with dementia of varied etiologies reported mean Spearman rank-order correlation coefficients of 0.93 for total score, ≥ 0.74 for most factor scores, and 0.75 for item scores (Sultzer, Berisford and Gunay, 1995a).

Principal components analysis identified four factors in patients with head injury (Levin et al., 1987): 'cognition/energy,' which included items relevant to cognitive processing, behavioral slowing, and emotional withdrawal; 'metacognition,' which included items relevant to inaccurate self-appraisal, unrealistic planning, and disinhibition; 'somatic concern/anxiety,' which included items relevant to physical complaints, anxiety, depression, and irritability; and 'language,' which included items relevant to expressive and receptive language functions. Scores on Factors II and IV increased in association with the severity of the closed head injury. Subscale analysis determined that conceptual disorganization, impaired self-appraisal, poor planning, expressive language deficits, and tension were also associated with the severity of the injury. Studies have reported that the NRS can be used to track improvement (Levin et al., 1987) as well as the persistence of deficits (Dombovy and Olek, 1997) after head injury and suggested that the 'cognition/energy' factor score may be a significant predictor of a patient's ability to return to work one year after injury (Vilkki et al., 1994).

Sultzer et al. (1992) studied a sample of patients with dementia, most of whom had Alzheimer's disease, and reported a factor structure that differed from that which was reported for head-injured patients. They identified six factors: 'cognition/insight,' 'agitation/disinhibition,' 'behavioral retardation,' 'anxiety/depression,' 'verbal output disturbance,' and 'psychosis.' Evidence of the validity of the

NRS for use with dementia patients was provided by an inverse correlation between the 'cognition/insight' factor and Mini-Mental State Examination score and increasing scores on the 'cognition/insight,' 'agitation/disinhibition,' and 'verbal output disturbance' factors in association with increasing severity of dementia. Later studies by the same group found higher NRS total scores and higher 'behavioral retardation,' 'anxiety/depression,' and 'verbal output disturbance' factor scores in patients with vascular dementia compared to patients with Alzheimer's disease (Sultzer et al., 1993); significant correlations between the severity of white matter lesions in patients with vascular dementia and NRS total score, the 'verbal output disturbance' factor score, and the 'anxiety/depression' factor score, with a trend noted for its association with the 'cognition/insight' factor score (Sultzer et al., 1995b); and significant correlations between the 'agitation/disinhibition' factor score and frontal and temporal lobe metabolism, the 'psychosis' factor score and frontal lobe metabolism, and the 'anxiety/depression' factor score and parietal lobe metabolism in a sample of patients with Alzheimer's disease (Sultzer et al., 1995c).

Neuropsychology Behavior and Affect Profile (Nelson, Satz and D'Elia, 1994b)

The Neuropsychology Behavior and Affect Profile (NBAP) was designed to measure behavioral and affective changes in neurologically impaired patients. It can be administered by a trained lay examiner in approximately 20 minutes. The scale consists of 106 randomly ordered statements to which a reliable informant must respond 'yes' or 'no' with regard to the patient's characteristics (e.g., 'My relative has habits which seem odd and different,' 'My relative is excessively talkative,' 'My relative often seems unhappy'). Each statement is presented twice, once with reference to premorbid functioning ('before') and then again with reference to current functioning ('after'). Scores are generated for premorbid and current level of functioning on each of five scales: inappropriateness (e.g., unusual or bizarre behavior), indifference (e.g., anosognosia), depression, pragnosia (e.g., a defect in communicative style, such as 'missing the point of a discussion'), and mania (e.g., impulsivity, irritability, and euphoria). In addition to the 91 statements relevant to those five categories, 15 'neutral' statements to which 'no' responses would be anticipated (e.g., 'My relative enjoys gardening') were included in order to break the tendency toward a response set. Efforts have also been made to develop validity scales that might be used to detect informant bias (e.g., exaggeration, malingering; Satz et al., 1996).

Reliability and validity

Based on a sample of patients referred to an outpatient dementia clinic for evaluation (Nelson et al., 1989), two-week test–retest intraclass correlation coefficients were ≥0.92 for all of the scales for both the 'before' and 'after' administrations.

Internal consistency estimates using coefficient alpha for the 'before' administration of the NBAP were >0.70 for depression, mania, and indifference; 0.59 for inappropriateness; and 0.49 for pragnosia while all coefficients were ≥0.70 for the 'after' assessment. In a study of 70 stroke patients (Nelson et al., 1993b), internal consistency estimates using coefficient alpha were ≥0.76 for all of the scales for both the 'before' and 'after' administrations. A later publication based on a subset of that sample (Cicchetti and Nelson, 1994) reported the test–retest reliability of the scales as intraclass correlation coefficients ranging from 0.63 to 0.75 for the 'before' assessment administered two weeks and then again two months after stroke.

A validity study was performed that compared change in NBAP scores in a group of patients with dementia of varied etiologies with change in the scores of a group of elderly control subjects, whose informants completed the NBAP with regard to subject characteristics before and after retirement (Nelson et al., 1989). Univariate analyses found no significant differences between the two groups with regard to the 'before' assessment and significant elevations on all scales other than mania for the group of dementia patients in the 'after' assessment. A study based on a sample of 70 stroke patients (Nelson et al., 1993b) found that those patients received significantly higher 'after' scores on the depression, indifference, and pragnosia scales than a group of elderly control subjects, but the stroke group also received significantly higher scores on the depression, indifference, and mania scales in the 'before' assessment, for unclear reasons. A separate publication based on 56 of those patients with unilateral infarcts (Nelson et al., 1993a) reported that the depression scale score showed the greatest increase between the 'before' and 'after' assessments and that it was the highest of the scale scores in the 'after' assessment for both the left and right hemisphere stroke groups. Patients with left hemisphere stroke received higher mean scores on the depression, indifference, inappropriateness, and pragnosia scales than right hemisphere stroke patients in the 'after' assessment, but those results were not adjusted for characteristics such as volume of infarction. Although further work is needed, the NBAP may be a useful method for prospectively tracking the behavioral and affective changes of patients following stroke (Nelson et al., 1994a).

Frontal Behavioral Inventory (Kertesz, Davidson and Fox, 1997)

The Frontal Behavioral Inventory (FBI) was originally developed to provide operationalized criteria for the diagnosis of behavior disorders in patients with frontal lobe dementia. Although its characteristics have not yet been studied in patients with focal brain lesions, it would seem to hold promise for use in their evaluation. The FBI is a 24-item structured inventory of behavioral and personality characteristics that is administered by a trained clinician to a reliable informant of a patient. It requires 10–15 minutes for completion. Items fall into two general categories, those that represent negative behaviors or the lack of certain normal behaviors, and those that represent disinhibited, excess, or abnormal behaviors. Questions tap characteristics such as apathy (i.e., 'Has s/he lost interest in friends or daily activities?'), perseveration (i.e., 'Does s/he repeat or perseverate actions or remarks?'), inappropriateness (i.e., 'Has s/he kept social rules or has s/he said or done things outside what is acceptable? Has s/he been rude, or childish?'), impulsivity (i.e., 'Has s/he acted or spoken without thinking about consequences, on the spur of the moment?'), and utilization behavior (i.e., 'Does s/he seem to need to touch, feel, examine, or pick up objects within reach and sight?'), as well as other features. Certain items are phrased in reverse format to break the tendency toward a response set. The informant is asked to rate change rather than lifelong personality characteristics, and each item is given a score of zero (none of the time), one (mild or occasional), two (moderate), or three (severe or most of the time). The total score on the FBI is the sum of the item scores and ranges from 0 to 72.

Reliability and validity

A pilot study was performed based on patients with clinically diagnosed frontal lobe dementia, dementia due to Alzheimer's disease, and dementia thought to be due to depression. Formal reliability data are not yet available, but the authors stated that 'no discernible difference was observed when [the FBI was readministered] by another interviewer, who was not aware of the history or the diagnosis.' Regarding the validity of the FBI, patients with frontal lobe dementia received significantly higher total scores than patients with Alzheimer's disease or dementia thought to be due to depression, despite comparable dementia severities in the first two groups. A scattergram of patients' total scores showed no overlap between the patients with frontal lobe dementia and Alzheimer's disease and suggested that a cut-off score of ≥27 would correctly identify all patients with frontal lobe dementia. The group of patients with frontal lobe dementia received higher mean scores than the other two groups on virtually every FBI item.

Additional scales for the assessment of behavior

Measures have been developed that permit the assessment of behavior as one of multiple potentially dysfunctional domains, which may also include cognition and mood. Blessed, Tomlinson and Roth described such a scale in 1969 and it continues to be used in a number of neurologic research programs, although, typically, individual components of that scale are extracted. Similarly, a scale such as the Revised Memory and Behavior Checklist of Teri et al. (1992) can be administered. Other popular scales, such as the noncognitive component of the Alzheimer's

Disease Assessment Scale (ADAS; Rosen, Mohs and Davis, 1984) and the Behavioral Pathology in Alzheimer's Disease Rating Scale (BEHAVE-AD; Reisberg et al., 1987), were designed to assess a variety of abnormalities that might be expected in patients with Alzheimer's disease, and additional scales are available to assess a narrow range of specific behaviors that are interpersonally problematic, such as agitation and disruptive behavior (Drachman et al., 1992; Ray et al., 1992). Finally, we and other groups (e.g., Ghika-Schmid et al., 1997) are working to develop new scales that are suitable for the assessment of behavioral abnormalities in patients with stroke.

Methodologic issues in the assessment of patients with focal brain lesions

A greater number of potential methodologic problems are inherent in the assessment of mood disorders than in the assessment of behavior disorders. In large part, those problems are the result of the need to understand a patient's internal mood state, while external observation by a reliable family member or a trained examiner can provide worthwhile information regarding behavior disorders. Certain of the potential methodologic problems with regard to the assessment of mood and behavior are as follows.

Cognitive impairment

Perhaps the most challenging problem in the assessment of mood disorders in patients with focal brain lesions is posed by cognitive impairment, and, in its most severe form, dementia. In our own work (Tatemichi et al., 1992a), we have found that one in four patients aged 60 or older met modified DSM-III-R criteria for dementia three months after ischemic stroke, resulting in the readily evident methodologic problem of the assessment of the internal mood state of patients with impaired memory, insight, and judgment. Similarly, patients with left hemisphere lesions frequently exhibit impairment in expressive language skills and/or auditory comprehension, with those aphasic disorders also complicating interview-based assessments of mood.

In contrast to the use of magnetic resonance imaging to document the presence of a focal brain lesion, there is no easy solution to the problem of methods for the assessment of mood disorders in patients with dementia or aphasia. While an informant can be administered a structured interview and provide reasonably accurate information regarding superficial vegetative signs such as loss of appetite and insomnia, his or her understanding of the patient's internal mood state is likely to be limited. Alternatively, the impaired patient can be administered the interview, but the examiner's sense of the reliability of the patient should be recorded (e.g., definitely reliable, probably reliable, possibly reliable, not reliable). For such patients, the visual analog scales described earlier may be used, with the understanding that the depth of information that is obtained will be limited.

Certain vegetative signs that may be found in association with major depression are also frequently recognized in patients with dementia (e.g., anergia, insomnia, poor appetite), resulting in the additional methodologic problem of determining the true etiology of those signs. In our own work (Tatemichi et al., 1992b), we administered the HDRS to 237 elderly patients three months after stroke, with 57 (24.1%) of those patients considered to have dementia based on DSM-III-R criteria. The overall HDRS score was 5.0 ± 4.6, and it was higher among demented patients than among nondemented patients (6.2 ± 5.0 versus 4.6 ± 4.5, $p=0.03$). Significant depression, defined as a HDRS 17-item total score >11, was also more frequent among patients with dementia (17.5% versus 7.8%, $p=0.03$). We did not identify a significant difference between demented and nondemented patients with regard to depressed mood, however, while HDRS items related to psychomotor retardation, reduced work/activities, and impaired insight best distinguished between the two groups. In a multiple regression analysis, stroke severity was the most important correlate of HDRS score, while dementia status was not independently related. These findings suggest that higher HDRS scores in stroke patients with dementia can be explained by the physical and cognitive deficits that are common in patients with dementia associated with stroke rather than a disorder of mood. Alternatively, some studies have suggested that depression in the elderly is manifest more through vegetative signs than depressed mood and thus may take a form different from depression among younger individuals (NIH Consensus Development Panel on Depression in Late Life, 1992), further complicating this issue and suggesting that more work on this vexing problem is needed.

Use of informants

The primary obstacle to the use of an informant for the assessment of a mood disorder is obvious: an informant, no matter how reliable, can never have a complete understanding of a patient's internal mood state. Given that we are frequently compelled to rely on informant reports, such as when patients are demented, certain additional issues must be recognized. First, informants may also be cognitively impaired, a possibility that becomes more likely when the informant is a spouse who is in the same age group as an elderly patient. Second, even when informants are cognitively intact and reliable, consistent contact with the patient is necessary for their reports to be considered to be valid. Third, members of different racial and ethnic groups may vary in their interpretation of questions, formation of judgments, and editing of responses, potentially influencing the results of studies that rely on structured questionnaires (Warnecke et al., 1997).

Premorbid history

One of the primary goals of the study of patients with focal brain lesions is the investigation of specific associations between lesion characteristics such as location and size and the occurrence of mood and behavior disorders. Thus, it is important to have an understanding of a patient's baseline characteristics, particularly with regard to a history of depression, in order to ensure that evidence of a current disorder represents a meaningful change from a premorbid level of function. Scales such as the NPI and the NBAP are useful because they require that the informant state that a specific abnormal behavior first became evident following the onset of dementia or the occurrence of stroke. Alternatively, the base rate of a specified disorder of mood or behavior could be determined through the study of a comparable control group, or the findings of separate epidemiologic investigations of the general population could be reviewed, in order to understand fully any increase in the frequency of that disorder that might be associated with the presence of focal brain lesions.

Examiner qualifications

Although it is preferable for experienced clinicians to perform the assessments of mood and behavior disorders, cost and availability frequently necessitate the use of lay examiners. Although such examiners may fail to recognize mood and behavior disorders when they are present but subtle, it is likely that their work will be optimal when they are trained in the administration of highly structured questionnaires and provided with careful supervision and detailed manuals. The use of structured questionnaires and their associated scripts ensures that the examiner will deviate minimally from the standard protocol and reliably gather data that can be used by experienced clinicians to determine the final diagnoses.

Summary and conclusions

No scale can be optimal for every use, regardless of whether the focus is on disorders of mood or behavior. The selection of a scale should be determined by each investigator based on the specific needs and resources of the study. For certain investigations, it might be optimal for more than one scale to be used in order to derive a broader impression of a patient's characteristics. Regarding the assessment of mood, for example, the HDRS would probably provide the most rigorous evaluation of depression but it might be too cognitively demanding for some patients. Thus, a measure such as the CES-D could be added to the assessment battery, or, to select a scale from the opposite end of the spectrum of complexity, a visual analog scale could be used. Regarding the assessment of behavior disorders, it might be worthwhile to combine a scale that is primarily based on observation of a patient's behavior, such as the NRS, with an informant interview, such as the NPI or the NBAP. Finally, it is important to note that cognitive and functional abilities should also be assessed in order that those characteristics might be available to the investigator as independent variables or covariates in multivariate models exploring the correlates of mood and behavior disorders in patients with focal brain lesions.

Acknowledgments

This work was supported by Grant R01–NS26179 from the National Institutes of Health. Janet B.W. Williams and Joan T. Moroney provided helpful comments on the manuscript.

REFERENCES

Agrell, B. and Dehlin, O. (1989). Comparison of six depression rating scales in geriatric stroke patients. *Stroke* 20: 1190–4.

Ahearn, E.P. and Carroll, B.J. (1996). Short-term variability of mood ratings in unipolar and bipolar depressed patients. *J Affect Disord* 36: 107–15.

Aitken, R.C.B. (1969). Measurement of feelings using visual analogue scales. *Proc R Soc Med* 62: 989–93.

American Psychiatric Association (1980). *Diagnostic and Statistical Manual of Mental Disorders*, 3rd edn. Washington, DC: American Psychiatric Association.

American Psychiatric Association (1987). *Diagnostic and Statistical Manual of Mental Disorders*, 3rd edn, revised. Washington, DC: American Psychiatric Association.

American Psychiatric Association (1994). *Diagnostic and Statistical Manual of Mental Disorders*, 4th edn. Washington, DC: American Psychiatric Association.

Anastasi, A. (1988). *Psychological Testing*, 6th edn. New York: Macmillan Publishing Company.

Andersen, G., Vestergaard, K. and Lauritzen, L. (1994). Effective treatment of poststroke depression with the selective serotonin reuptake inhibitor citalopram. *Stroke* 25: 1099–104.

Bauer, M.S., Crits-Christoph, P., Ball, W.A. et al. (1991). Independent assessment of manic and depressive symptoms by self-rating. Scale characteristics and implications for the study of mania. *Arch Gen Psychiatry* 48: 807–12.

Beatty, W.W., Goodkin, D.E., Monson, N. and Beatty, P.A. (1989). Cognitive disturbances in patients with relapsing remitting multiple sclerosis. *Arch Neurol* 46: 1113–19.

Beck, A.T., Rush, A.J., Shaw, B.F. and Emery, G. (1979). *Cognitive Therapy of Depression.* New York: Guilford Press.

Beck, A.T. and Steer, R.A. (1987). *Manual for the Beck Depression Inventory.* San Antonio, TX: The Psychological Corporation.

Beck, A.T., Steer, R.A. and Brown, G.K. (1996). *Manual for the Beck Depression Inventory*, 2nd edn. San Antonio, TX: The Psychological Corporation.

Beck, A.T., Ward, C.H., Mendelson, M., Mock, J. and Erbaugh, J. (1961). An inventory for measuring depression. *Archives of General Psychiatry* 4: 561–71.

Beckham, E.E. and Leber, W.R. (eds.) (1995). *Handbook of Depression*, 2nd edn. New York: Guilford Press.

Blessed, G., Tomlinson, B.E. and Roth, M. (1969). The association between quantitative measures of dementia and of senile change in the cerebral grey matter of elderly subjects. *Br J Psychiatry* 114: 797–811.

Breslau, N. (1985). Depressive symptoms, major depression, and generalized anxiety: a comparison of self-reports on CES-D and results from diagnostic interviews. *Psychiatry Res* 15: 219–29.

Butcher, J.N., Dahlstrom, W.G., Graham, J.R., Tellegen, A. and Kaemmer, B. (1989). *Manual for Administration and Scoring of the Minnesota Multiphasic Personality Inventory – 2*. Minneapolis, MN: University of Minnesota Press.

Cicchetti, D.V. and Nelson, L.D. (1994). Re-examining threats to the reliability and validity of putative brain–behavior relationships: new guidelines for assessing the effect of patients lost to follow-up. *J Clin Exp Neuropsychol* 16: 339–43.

Cicchetti, D.V. and Prusoff, B.A. (1983). Reliability of depression and associated clinical symptoms. *Arch Gen Psychiatry* 40: 987–90.

Cummings, J.L. (1997). The Neuropsychiatric Inventory: assessing psychopathology in dementia patients. *Neurology* 48 (Suppl. 6): S10–S16.

Cummings, J.L., Diaz, C., Levy, M., Binetti, G. and Litvan, I. (1996). Neuropsychiatric syndromes in neurodegenerative diseases: frequency and significance. *Semin Clin Neuropsychiatry* 1: 241–7.

Cummings, J.L., Mega, M., Gray, K. et al. (1994). The Neuropsychiatric Inventory: comprehensive assessment of psychopathology in dementia. *Neurology* 44: 2308–14.

Dam, H., Pedersen, H.E. and Ahlgren, P. (1989). Depression among patients with stroke. *Acta Psychiatr Scand* 80: 118–24.

Dombovy, M.L. and Olek, A.C. (1997). Recovery and rehabilitation following traumatic brain injury. *Brain Inj* 11: 305–18.

Drachman, D.A., Swearer, J.M., O'Donnell, B.F., Mitchell, A.L. and Maloon, A. (1992). The Caregiver Obstreperous-Behavior Rating Assessment (COBRA) Scale. *J Am Geriatr Soc* 40: 463–70.

Endicott, J., Cohen, J., Nee, J., Fleiss, J. and Sarantakos, S. (1981). Hamilton Depression Rating Scale. Extracted from regular and change versions of the Schedule for Affective Disorders and Schizophrenia. *Arch Gen Psychiatry* 38: 98–103.

Endicott, J. and Spitzer, R.L. (1978). A diagnostic interview. The Schedule for Affective Disorders and Schizophrenia. *Arch Gen Psychiatry* 35: 837–44.

Faravelli, C., Albanesi, G. and Poli, E. (1986). Assessment of depression: a comparison of rating scales. *J Affect Disord* 11: 245–53.

Fedoroff, J.P., Starkstein, S.E., Forrester, A.W. et al. (1992). Depression in patients with acute traumatic brain injury. *Am J Psychiatry* 149: 918–23.

Feinberg, M., Carroll, B.J., Smouse, P.E. and Rawson, S.G. (1981). The Carroll Rating Scale for Depression. III. Comparison with other rating instruments. *Br J Psychiatry* 138: 205–9.

First, M.B., Spitzer, R.L., Gibbon, M. and Williams, J.B.W. (1997). *User's Guide for the Structured Clinical Interview for DSM-IV Axis I Disorders – Clinician Version (SCID-CV).* Washington, DC: American Psychiatric Press.

Fitz, A.G. and Teri, L. (1994). Depression, cognition, and functional ability in patients with Alzheimer's disease. *J Am Geriatr Soc* 42: 186–91.

Folstein, M.F. and Luria, R. (1973). Reliability, validity, and clinical application of the visual analogue mood scale. *Psychol Med* 3: 479–86.

Gainotti, G., Azzoni, A., Gasparini, F., Marra, C. and Razzano, C. (1997a). Relation of lesion location to verbal and nonverbal mood measures in stroke patients. *Stroke* 28: 2145–9.

Gainotti, G., Azzoni, A., Razzano, C. et al. (1997b). The Post-Stroke Depression Rating Scale: a test specifically devised to investigate affective disorders of stroke patients. *J Clin Exp Neuropsychol* 19: 340–56.

Gallagher, D., Nies, G. and Thompson, L.W. (1982). Reliability of the Beck Depression Inventory with older adults. *J Consult Clin Psychol* 50: 152–3.

Ghika-Schmid, F., Castillo, V., Neau, J.P. et al. (1997). Emotional behavior in the acute phase of stroke. The Lausanne Emotion in Stroke Study. *Neurology* 48 (Suppl.): A291.

Gibbons, R.D., Clark, D.C. and Kupfer, D.J. (1993). Exactly what does the Hamilton Depression Rating Scale measure? *J Psychiatr Res* 27: 259–73.

Hamilton, M. (1960). A rating scale for depression. *J Neurol Neurosurg Psychiatry* 23: 56–62.

Hamilton, M. (1967). Development of a rating scale for primary depressive illness. *Br J Soc Clin Psychol* 6: 278–96.

House, A., Dennis, M., Hawton, K. and Warlow, C. (1989). Methods of identifying mood disorders in stroke patients: experience in the Oxfordshire Community Stroke Project. *Age Ageing* 18: 371–9.

House, A., Dennis, M., Mogridge, L. et al. (1991). Mood disorders in the year after first stroke. *Br J Psychiatry* 158: 83–92.

Kaufer, D.I., Cummings, J.L. and Christine, D. (1996). Effect of tacrine on behavioral symptoms in Alzheimer's disease: an open-label study. *J Geriatr Psychiatry Neurol* 9: 1–6.

Keane, S.M. and Sells, S. (1990). Recognizing depression in the elderly. *J Gerontol Nurs* 16: 21–5.

Kertesz, A., Davidson, W. and Fox, H. (1997). Frontal Behavioral Inventory: diagnostic criteria for frontal lobe dementia. *Can J Neurol Sci* 24: 29–36.

Knesevich, J.W., Biggs, J.T., Clayton, P.J. and Ziegler, V.E. (1977). Validity of the Hamilton Rating Scale for Depression. *Br J Psychiatry* 131: 49–52.

Levin, B.E., Llabre, M.M. and Weiner, W.J. (1988). Parkinson's disease and depression: psychometric properties of the Beck Depression Inventory. *J Neurol Neurosurg Psychiatry* 51: 1401–4.

Levin, H.S., High, W.M., Goethe, K.E. et al. (1987). The Neurobehavioural Rating Scale: assessment of the behavioural sequelae of head injury by the clinician. *J Neurol Neurosurg Psychiatry* 50: 183–93.

Levy, M.L., Miller, B.L., Cummings, J.L., Fairbanks, L.A. and Craig, A. (1996). Alzheimer disease and frontotemporal dementias. Behavioral distinctions. *Arch Neurol* 53: 687–90.

Linden, M., Borchelt, M., Barnow, S. and Geiselmann, B. (1995). The impact of somatic morbidity on the Hamilton Depression Rating Scale in the very old. *Acta Psychiatr Scand* 92: 150–4.

Litvan, I., Mega, M.S., Cummings, J.L. and Fairbanks, L. (1996). Neuropsychiatric aspects of progressive supranuclear palsy. *Neurology* 47: 1184–9.

Luria, R.E. (1975). The validity and reliability of the Visual Analogue Mood Scale. *J Psychiatr Res* 12: 51–7.

Maier, W., Heuser, I., Philipp, M., Frommberger, U. and Demuth, W. (1988a). Improving depression severity assessment – II. Content, concurrent and external validity of three observer depression scales. *J Psychiatr Res* 22: 13–19.

Maier, W., Philipp, M., Heuser, I. et al. (1988b). Improving depression severity assessment – I. Reliability, internal validity and sensitivity to change of three observer depression scales. *J Psychiatr Res* 22: 3–12.

Malec, J.F., Richardson, J.W., Sinaki, M. and O'Brien, M.W. (1990). Types of affective response to stroke, *Arch Phys Med Rehabil* 71: 279–84.

Marsella, A.J., Hirschfeld, R.M.A. and Katz, M.M. (eds.) (1987). *The Measurement of Depression*. New York: Guilford Press.

Mega, M.S., Cummings, J.L., Fiorello, T. and Gornbein, J. (1996). The spectrum of behavioral changes in Alzheimer's disease. *Neurology* 46: 130–5.

Montgomery, S.A. and Åsberg, M. (1979). A new depression scale designed to be sensitive to change. *Br J Psychiatry* 134: 382–9.

Nelson, L.D., Cicchetti, D., Satz, P. et al. (1993a). Emotional sequelae of stroke. *Neuropsychology* 7: 553–60.

Nelson, L.D., Cicchetti, D., Satz, P., Sowa, M. and Mitrushina, M. (1994a). Emotional sequelae of stroke: a longitudinal perspective. *J Clin Exp Neuropsychol* 16: 796–806.

Nelson, L.D., Mitrushina, M., Satz, P., Sowa, M. and Cohen, S. (1993b). Cross-validation of the Neuropsychology Behavior and Affect Profile in stroke patients. *Psychol Assess* 5: 374–6.

Nelson, L., Satz, P. and D'Elia, L. (1994b). *The Neuropsychology Behavior and Affect Profile*. Palo Alto, CA: Mind Garden Press.

Nelson, L.D., Satz, P., Mitrushina, M. et al. (1989). Development and validation of the Neuropsychology Behavior and Affect Profile. *Psychol Assess* 1: 266–72.

Ng, K.C., Chan, K.L. and Straughan, P.T. (1995). A study of post-stroke depression in a rehabilitative center. *Acta Psychiatr Scand* 92: 75–9.

NIH Consensus Development Panel on Depression in Late Life (1992). Diagnosis and treatment of depression in late life. *J Am Med Assoc* 268: 1018–24.

Nyenhuis, D.L., Stern, R.A., Yamamoto, C., Luchetta, T. and Arruda, J.E. (1997). Standardization and validation of the Visual Analog Mood Scales. *Clin Neuropsychol* 11: 407–15.

Parikh, R.M., Eden, D.T., Price, T.R. and Robinson, R.G. (1988). The sensitivity and specificity of the Center for Epidemiologic Studies Depression Scale in screening for post-stroke depression. *Int J Psychiatry Med* 18: 169–81.

Radloff, L.S. (1977). The CES-D Scale: a self-report depression scale for research in the general population. *Appl Psychol Measurement* 1: 385–401.

Ray, W.A., Taylor, J.A., Lichtenstein, M.J. and Meador, K.G. (1992). The Nursing Home Behavior Problem Scale. *J Gerontol* 47: M9–M16.

Rehm, L.P. and O'Hara, M.W. (1985). Item characteristics of the Hamilton Rating Scale for Depression. *J Psychiatr Res* 19: 31–41.

Reifler, B.V., Teri, L. and Raskind, M. (1989). Double-blind trial of imipramine in Alzheimer's disease patients with and without depression. *Am J Psychiatry* 146: 45–9.

Reisberg, B., Borenstein, J., Salob, S.P. et al. (1987). Behavioral symptoms in Alzheimer's disease: phenomenology and treatment. *J Clin Psychiatry* 48 (Suppl.): 9–15.

Roberts, R.E. (1980). Reliability of the CES-D Scale in different ethnic contexts. *Psychiatry Res* 2: 125–34.

Robinson, R.G. and Szetela, B. (1981). Mood change following left hemispheric brain injury. *Ann Neurol* 9: 447–53.

Rosen, W.G., Mohs, R.C. and Davis, K.L. (1984). A new rating scale for Alzheimer's disease. *Am J Psychiatry* 141: 1356–64.

Satz, P., Holston, S.G., Uchiyama, C.L. et al. (1996). Development and evaluation of validity scales for the Neuropsychology Behavior and Affect Profile: a dissembling study. *Psychol Assess* 8: 115–24.

Schubert, D.S.P., Taylor, C., Lee, S., Mentari, A. and Tamaklo, W. (1992). Detection of depression in the stroke patient. *Psychosomatics* 33: 290–4.

Shinar, D., Gross, C.R., Price, T.R. et al. (1986). Screening for depression in stroke patients: the reliability and validity of the Center for Epidemiologic Studies Depression Scale. *Stroke* 17: 241–5.

Stein, P.N., Sliwinski, M.J., Gordon, W.A. and Hibbard, M.R. (1996). Discriminative properties of somatic and nonsomatic symptoms for post stroke depression. *Clin Neuropsychol* 10: 141–8.

Stern, R.A. and Bachman, D.L. (1991). Depressive symptoms following stroke. *Am J Psychiatry* 148: 351–6.

Sultzer, D.L., Berisford, M.A. and Gunay, I. (1995a). The Neurobehavioral Rating Scale: reliability in patients with dementia. *J Psychiatr Res* 29: 185–91.

Sultzer, D.L., Levin, H.S., Mahler, M.E., High, W.M. and Cummings, J.L. (1992). Assessment of cognitive, psychiatric, and behavioral disturbances in patients with dementia: the Neurobehavioral Rating Scale. *J Am Geriatr Soc* 40: 549–55.

Sultzer, D.L., Levin, H.S., Mahler, M.E., High, W.M. and Cummings, J.L. (1993). A comparison of psychiatric symptoms in vascular dementia and Alzheimer's disease. *Am J Psychiatry* 150: 1806–12.

Sultzer, D.L., Mahler, M.E., Cummings, J.L. et al. (1995b). Cortical abnormalities associated with subcortical lesions in vascular dementia. Clinical and positron emission tomographic findings. *Arch Neurol* 52: 773–80.

Sultzer, D.L., Mahler, M.E., Mandelkern, M.E. et al. (1995c). The relationship between psychiatric symptoms and regional cortical metabolism in Alzheimer's disease. *J Neuropsychiatry Clin Neurosci* 7: 476–84.

Tatemichi, T.K., Desmond, D.W., Mayeux, R. et al. (1992a). Dementia after stroke: baseline frequency, risks, and clinical features in a hospitalized cohort. *Neurology* 42: 1185–93.

Tatemichi, T.K., Rosenstein, B., Remien, R.H. et al. (1992b). Depression and intellectual impairment after stroke: causally linked? *Ann Neurol* 32: 267.

Teri, L., Truax, P., Logsdon, R. et al. (1992). Assessment of behavioral problems in dementia: the Revised Memory and Behavior Problems Checklist. *Psychol Aging* 7: 622–31.

Tröster, A.I., Stalp, L.D., Paolo, A.M., Fields, J.A. and Koller, W.C. (1995). Neuropsychological impairment in Parkinson's disease with and without depression. *Arch Neurol* 52: 1164–9.

Vernon, S.W. and Roberts, R.E. (1981). Measuring nonspecific psychological distress and other dimensions of psychopathology. Further observations on the problem. *Arch Gen Psychiatry* 38: 1239–47.

Vida, S., Des Rosiers, P., Carrier, L. and Gauthier, S. (1994). Depression in Alzheimer's disease: receiver operating characteristic analysis of the Cornell Scale for Depression in Dementia and the Hamilton Depression Scale. *J Geriatr Psychiatry Neurol* 7: 159–62.

Vilkki, J., Ahola, K., Holst, P. et al. (1994). Prediction of psychosocial recovery after head injury with cognitive tests and neurobehavioral ratings. *J Clin Exp Neuropsychol* 16: 325–38.

Warnecke, R.B., Johnson, T.P., Chávez, N. et al. (1997). Improving question wording in surveys of culturally diverse populations. *Ann Epidemiol* 7: 334–42.

Williams, J.B.W. (1988). A structured interview guide for the Hamilton Depression Rating Scale. *Arch Gen Psychiatry* 45: 742–7.

Williams, J.G., Barlow, A.H. and Agras, W.S. (1972). Behavioral measurement of severe depression. *Arch Gen Psychiatry* 27: 330–3.

Wing, J.K., Birley, J.L.T., Cooper, J.E., Graham, P. and Isaacs, A.D. (1967). Reliability of a procedure for measuring and classifying 'Present Psychiatric State'. *Br J Psychiatry* 113: 499–515.

World Health Organization (1993). *The ICD-10 Classification of Mental and Behavioural Disorders. Diagnostic Criteria for Research.* Geneva: World Health Organization.

Yesavage, J.A., Brink, T.L., Rose, T.L. et al. (1983). Development and validation of a geriatric depression screening scale: a preliminary report. *J Psychiatr Res* 17: 37–49.

Youngjohn, J.R., Beck, J., Jogerst, G. and Caine, C. (1992). Neuropsychological impairment, depression, and Parkinson's disease. *Neuropsychology* 6: 149–58.

Zealley, A.K. and Aitken, R.C.B. (1969). Measurement of mood. *Proc R Soc Med* 62: 993–6.

Zung, W.W.K. (1965). A self-rating depression scale. *Arch Gen Psychiatry* 12: 63–70.

3

Methodological issues in studying secondary mood disorders

Jordan Grafman and Deborah L. Warden

Introduction

This volume summarizes our current knowledge regarding the brain lateralization and topography of emotion and mood states. Whereas most of the chapters in this volume address specific forms of secondary mood disorders, including depression, mania, anxiety disorders, dysprosodias, apathy (and the evidence for the cerebral localization of each mood disorder), this chapter focuses on some of the key contentious issues that the reader should be aware of when reading the other chapters in this volume.

There are numerous challenges to studying the neurologic basis of emotions and mood states. Animal models are possible for some aspects of abnormal social behavior and emotional responsivity (Jarrell et al., 1987; Davis 1992), but are lacking for mood states. Even in humans, the conceptualization of emotions and mood states requires subjective interpretation. The lack of clear definitions of emotions and mood states that go beyond a description of feelings or tone also limits the ability of researchers to easily validate or reject even the most simple of theoretical models. Granted, there are serious theories regarding fundamental social cognitive behavior, but it is usually the observed and measured behavioral expression of emotional or mood-induced actions (or lack of action) that are utilized in these theories. Nevertheless, there are a large number of neuropsychiatric studies investigating emotion and mood state changes that follow focal brain lesions or the onset of neurodegenerative diseases. In addition, sophisticated functional neuroimaging techniques now allow for the identification of patterns of brain activity induced by mood state manipulations in patients and normal volunteers. The large number of lesion and neuroimaging studies in the literature reflects an explosion of data begging for adequate theory. This chapter emphasizes which variables are critical for the methodological interpretation of those data.

Basic concepts

A basic starting point for the neuropsychiatric investigation of mood is to select generally agreed upon definitions of mood and mood disorders, both primary and secondary, and to describe the way in which mood states interact with social and cognitive behaviors.

Definitions of mood and mood disorders

Consistency in defining mood and mood state disorders is essential if investigators are to compare results across studies and sites. Whereas in a normal individual, mood may vary depending on different internal and environmental factors (e.g., being in an irritable mood when tired or feeling sad after visiting an older loved relative who is ill), the term 'mood disorder' communicates a syndrome of abnormally disordered mood which can be characterized by enduring symptoms. These abnormal mood disorders are diagnosable on the basis of their specific symptoms, predictable longitudinal course, and treatment response.

For the purpose of defining abnormal mood, the method that is used is critical. Symptoms expressed in the context of a diagnosable and durable mood disorder may differ from those associated with transient mood states. Also, symptoms experienced during a mood disorder may vary depending on when in the course of the illness they are assessed and which treatments have been introduced prior to the evaluation. Thus, both carefully defining the study population and the assessment methods used for diagnosis become critical in establishing specific conclusions about the appearance or disappearance of mood states in the context of a mood disorder.

Primary and secondary mood disorders

Researchers have tried to identify a specific pattern of brain dysfunction for individual primary and secondary mood disorders. Primary mood disorders may differ from secondary mood disorders in their underlying pathophysiology, which has implications for any observed differences in behavior.

A primary mood disorder (e.g., major depression or mania) is due to whatever biological/genetic diathesis the individual carries, combined with whatever stressors may have contributed to the development of the mood disorder. Primary disorders have also been termed 'idiopathic,' suggesting a lack of complete knowledge regarding their pathophysiology. In the USA, the principal method used to diagnose mood disorders is the *Diagnostic and Statistical Manual* (1994). Robinson (1998) concluded that DSM III – R (the preceding edition) diagnostic criteria are also valid to diagnose depression in patients with *secondary* depression due to stroke (Fedoroff et al., 1991). Post-stroke depression shows some differences from primary major depression. Lipsey et al. (1986) reported that elderly major depressed patients had a greater frequency of loss of interest and decreased concentration than post-stroke depressed patients did. Overall, however, the symptoms of these two groups are similar enough that abandoning the DSM in the diagnostic workup of secondary mood disorders (e.g., following stroke) does not appear warranted at this time. DSM defined symptoms of depression were also found to be specific for depression in Parkinson's disease (Starkstein et al., 1990).

Secondary mood disorders can also be induced by a general medical illness, e.g., depression due to hypothyroidism. Hypothyroidism is known potentially to cause depression, and the development of depression following the development of hypothyroidism would generally be diagnosed as a secondary mood disorder. Diagnosing a secondary mood disorder with confidence can be challenging, however, and the DSM IV (1994) suggests that the existence of a known medical illness and the temporally connected development of an abnormal mood state such as depression are strongly suggestive of a secondary mood disorder.

Mood and social cognition/behavior

The relationship between mood/mood states and social or cognitive behavior is complex and compelling. That primary depression or secondary post-stroke depression may affect controlled attentional and effortful memory processes is well documented (Caine, 1981; Weingartner and Silberman, 1982). However, attention and memory deficits are not seen in all patients with abnormal or unusual mood state changes. Abnormal mood can also change the way we perceive and interact with other people, potentially leading to changes in the way social decisions are made and social interactions are conducted (Clore, Schwarz and Conway, 1994). Thus, any model attempting to argue for the brain topography or circuit of a specific mood state needs also to consider secondary or parallel social and cognitive impairments that could influence or account for the altered pattern of behavior (or in the case of a neuroimaging experiment, the altered pattern of brain activation).

Genetic and environmental factors

Although generally ignored as a factor governing the appearance of secondary mood disorders following the onset of neurological disease, the role of genes in the development of mood disorders is increasingly being understood. Like many other illnesses, mood disorders may occur more often in certain families. The genetic markers that predispose a person to a mood disorder are yet to be determined and will probably involve multiple genes. However, the genetic role in psychiatric illnesses such as alcoholism and anxiety disorders is prominent (Cloninger et al., 1998; Goate and Edenberg, 1998). Increasing evidence suggests that personality *traits* may also be influenced by genetic factors (Cloninger, Adolfsson and Svrakic, 1996; Cloninger et al., 1998), suggesting that genes play a role in normal as well as disordered mood states.

Theoretical models also exist for differential vulnerability to an illness. For example, hemoglobin AS causes severe anemia when inherited from both parents, though when inherited from only one parent, it confers some *protection* against developing malaria. Thus, the genetic make-up of the individual influences the impact that exposure to an illness (and potentially a set of experiences that might include personal loss) may have. An example of an interaction between genotype and environment is that of head injury and risk of Alzheimer's disease. An individual with the genotype of *ApoE4* who suffers a head injury has an increased risk of developing Alzheimer's disease (Tang et al., 1996).

Other research emphasizes the contribution of environmental influences. Early life stressors may increase the likelihood of depressive disorder, independent of genetics (Singer et al., 1995). The association of environmental stressors and hippocampal atrophy in post-traumatic stress disorder has been reported by Bremner and colleagues (1995, 1997). The decrease in the volume of the hippocampus is hypothesized to occur as a result of exposure to extreme stress causing the release of glucocorticoids, which at certain levels may be toxic to cells in the hippocampus (Sapolsky and Pulsinelli, 1985). This work suggests an interaction between exogenous stressors and regional neuroanatomy. Since the onset of a neurological disorder can be considered a stressor, how it interacts with subject attitude and the proclivity for developing a mood disorder should be investigated. As more associations between genotypes and mood disorders (e.g., depression) and behavior (e.g., novelty-seeking behavior) are discovered, the relationship between specific genotypes and neuroanatomical changes in both primary and secondary mood disorders will be better understood.

Mood disorders are increasingly being conceptualized as multifactorial. Any theory arguing for the neuroanatomical specificity of a mood state (or mood state change) should not only describe the specific brain areas/circuits involved in the state or change, but also consider factors such as cognitive abilities, state and trait social behaviors, the kind of environmental stressors the patient is experiencing, and genetic predisposition.

Methodological issues

Animal models

The current lack of animal models for normal and abnormal mood states limits our understanding of the role of genetics in this area of neuropsychiatry. Animal models need to be developed in order to improve the predictability of which patients are most susceptible to develop a primary or secondary mood disorder and to better characterize the various stages in the natural history of a mood disorder.

Evaluation site

Where a patient is studied can affect the kind, frequency, and reliability of behaviors elicited. Patient behavior can be studied in the most relevant context (e.g., the naturalistic settings in which the patient functions) or in the necessarily artificial setting of the clinic or laboratory. The more naturalistic the setting, the less consistency there is in measurements between subjects and across studies. In the less naturalistic setting, the patient's behavior may become consistent and more easily observable, but may not reflect what is routinely observed in the home or other setting (because of uniquely provocative stimuli that can occur outside the laboratory). The context of testing is particularly relevant for patients with frontal systems dysfunction who are influenced by the structure of the environment they find themselves in (Grafman, 1995). The more structure provided to such a patient, the less likely that certain abnormal behaviors or moods may appear.

Discrete localization versus circuit disorders

Searching for a single discrete lesion responsible for a mood state abnormality has given way to searching for dysfunction occurring in a cortical–subcortical system that includes a distributed set of brain regions (Starkstein et al., 1988b). With an increasing appreciation of the relationship between distributed neural systems and complex cognitive/social functions, the challenge to identify a set of brain regions, each of which could modify a selected aspect of a specific mood state, is beginning to be met. In an influential paper, Alexander and colleagues outlined five parallel pathways involving specific frontal cortex, striatal, and thalamic brain regions (Alexander, Crutcher and DeLong, 1990), with each pathway presumed to mediate one of the following different functions: cortical control of limb movement, eye movement, motivation, social judgment, and cognition. Cummings has promoted the relevance of impairment to one or more of these prefrontal circuits for the development of selected neuropsychiatric syndromes (Masterman and Cummings, 1997). Though these pathways do not include all anatomic areas relevant for mood state regulation (temporal lobe input, for example, in influencing social decorum, or the contribution of frontal–cerebellar pathways in influencing procedural behaviors), specifying their role in primary neuropsychiatric syndromes suggests why certain forms of secondary mood disorders may appear after the onset of certain neurological disorders. A regional analysis is still necessary to identify the specific components contributing to mood state regulation, but component identification must be put in the context of the neural pathways the components belong to, since it is likely that lesions anywhere along the pathway will produce symptoms that resemble each other.

Abnormal brain development

Some subjects may be part of a family that demonstrates a genetic predisposition to developing a *primary* mood state disorder. This genetic predisposition may be associated with developmental atypical *changes* in brain anatomy. In this case, can researchers feel confident about generalizing functional mapping inferences based on patterns of brain activation or brain damage associated with this form of mood disorder? This question is just as applicable when studying *secondary* mood disorders that are found in patients with developmental idiopathic epilepsy or other developmental neurological disorders.

Bias in patient selection

Many aspects of patient selection bias can affect the interpretation of secondary mood disorder studies. Stroke populations will be biased towards the elderly. Elderly populations will have more concomitant medical conditions, including those that may affect cerebral function, including hypertension, diabetes, and cerebrovascular disease. Validating interesting or provocative findings in different populations (e.g., younger patients or patients from different socioeconomic strata or cultures) is critical for their generalizability. To some extent, this has been accomplished in the neuropsychiatric literature. For example, Robinson et al. replicated their seminal finding that left frontal lesions lead to depression in post-stroke patients (Robinson et al., 1984) in a younger traumatically brain injured (TBI) population (Fedoroff et al., 1992). The relationship of left prefrontal cortex damage to mood state abnormality was found, however, only at the initial evaluation in TBI patients, whereas the relationship held for the stroke population at each post-stroke time interval studied. An independent replication of the association between left hemisphere lesions and depression scores has also been reported (Eastwood et al., 1989).

What is a focal lesion?

Decisions about which patients to include in a focal lesion study can affect the interpretation of a study. It is not unusual for patients having restricted left frontal lobe lesions to be grouped together with patients having a lesion that was larger than, but included, the left frontal lobe. Authors must comment on whether their findings are present in both subgroups of patients.

Diffuse brain injury

Inherent in discussing whether the localization of mood state abnormalities in TBI and stroke patients is similar is the inference that diffuse and focal brain injury may have a similar effect upon mood state regulation. The pathophysiology of TBI may include focal injury with contusions and hematomas, especially when TBI is due to a direct blow such as an assault. The most common causes of TBI, motor vehicle accidents and falls, both involve acceleration and deceleration forces, which commonly lead to diffuse axonal brain injury. Thus, if a neuropsychiatric theory of a secondary mood disorder is *only* based on patients who have focal brain damage in the presence of diffuse injury, caution is advised since the diffuse injury implies brain damage well beyond the borders of the observed focal lesion.

Neuroplasticity

A potentially interesting, but currently underspecified and unanswered, question is whether brain neuroplasticity influences mood state changes. For example, the profile of neural activation during the first few trials of a repetitive action is different from the profile of neural activation seen after the action is overlearned (Shadmehr and Holcomb, 1997; Grafman and Christen, 1999). Such long-term plasticity makes possible more efficient processing of information. One implication of current neuroplasticity theories is that repetitive emotional expression or experience may induce a change in which brain areas are optimally devoted to experiencing/interpreting that emotion in addition to increasing the ease with which that emotion may be re-experienced. Cognitive therapy is based on a similar premise, i.e., that repeated positive cognitive structuring of a situation or emotion increases a patient's ability to respond with a positive emotion subsequently, thereby combating the priming effects of past repeated negative experiences. Thus, changes in the pattern and severity of mood state disorders following neurological disease may be partly dependent on neuroplastic changes associated with both the lesion and the persistence of the patient's altered behavior.

Relevance of time after event for evaluation of mood behavior

Since the symptoms of a mood disorder may evolve over time, the timing of the evaluation may influence the results. An untreated episode of primary major depression has a variable length but may last less than 6 months (Kaplan and Sadock, 1995). Patients apparently responding to a new medication in their ninth month of a major depression may not be responding to the drug but merely showing the coincidental effect of a normal recovery from a depressive episode. These issues are not insurmountable, however, as researchers of illnesses with dynamic or fluctuating courses (such as multiple sclerosis) have developed methods to effectively study medication effects on disease activity across time (Whitaker et al., 1995).

Instruments to evaluate mood state and emotional behavior

The choice of rating scales in the research into primary and secondary mood disorders will play a role in the description of the nature and severity of the disorder. Different prevalence rates of a particular disorder, e.g., post-TBI depression, are often attributed to different study populations *and* to different rating instruments (Gualtieri, 1991). Validated instruments for a particular population being studied, moreover, are often not available. This lack of validation weakens the generalizations that can be made on the basis of a specific study's conclusions. Lack of validation undoubtedly contributes to a wide variety of instruments being used by different research groups, thus making comparisons between studies difficult.

To validate an instrument, a 'gold standard' diagnosis of the particular mood, mood disorder or emotional behavior being assessed must exist. In general, that gold standard is applying DSM criteria to the psychiatric interview (Fedoroff et al., 1992). The DSM IV (1994) states that its specific diagnostic criteria are meant to serve as a guideline to be informed by clinical judgment and should not be used in a cookbook fashion. The gold standard should be viewed as a dynamic construct so that investigators are not burdened with outdated concepts of pathophysiology and nosology. Thus, every study should make an effort to use the most appropriate (and, when necessary, novel) instrument for diagnosing mood disorders, especially when that method (or diagnostic definition) is evolving. The obvious advantage of using standardized and psychometrically sound instruments among the evaluative techniques used is that it allows appropriate comparison across studies.

Many studies of secondary mood state disorders have used the same instruments as previously used for primary mood state disorders (House et al., 1990). As long as the phenomenology is quite similar, that strategy is warranted. One potential problem is that some of the symptoms assessed in patients with a primary mood disorder may be part of the medical illness involved in the secondary mood disorder. For example, the Hamilton Depression Rating Scale asks several questions regarding somatic symptoms (e.g., fatigue, gastrointestinal complaints). A TBI patient who has sustained multiple trauma (and received an exploratory laporotomy) will probably report fatigue and gastrointestinal complaints during the postacute period. On a more positive note, Robinson (1997, 1998) suggests that using existing diagnostic criteria for major depressive disorder (i.e., DSM III–R) does not produce substantial false negatives or false positives when used to diagnose secondary depression due to TBI (or stroke).

The availability of consistent diagnostic methods and the ability to follow patients across various time periods are desirable. For example, the instrument used by Robinson and others (Jorge et al., 1993a, 1993b, 1993c) to measure mood state in TBI is a structured interview – the Present State Exam (Wing, Cooper and

Sartorius, 1974) with questions on affective and anxiety symptoms. Others have used the Structured Clinical Interview for the *Diagnostic Statistical Manual* (SCID: Spitzer et al., 1992), or relied only on clinical interviews. That these studies have yielded similar rates of mood disorder in the targeted population suggests that the researchers are studying a similar cohort.

Rather than identifying a specific DSM psychiatric diagnosis in patients with secondary mood disorders, another approach to studying mood state changes in neurological patients involves identifying the most problematic and inappropriate behaviors and rating their frequency and severity over time. This symptom description approach can be done irrespective of diagnostic criteria and still permits a rich description of the patient population. The Neuropsychiatric Inventory (NPI) (Cummings et al., 1994) was developed for this purpose. The NPI includes a set of questions about mood state and social/cognitive behaviors that is directed to the patient's spouse, significant other, or caretaker. The NPI questions were developed by Cummings and his colleagues after a careful review of the most common behavioral and mood state changes reported following stroke and other neurological disorders. While initially validated on patients with Alzheimer's disease (Cummings et al., 1994), the instrument has since been used with other patient groups (Litvan et al., 1998). The development of the NPI is a useful addition to the neurobehavioral assessment battery – providing reliable ratings of severity and frequency of moods and behaviors which may be encountered in neuropsychiatric illnesses.

Patient versus observer ratings

Determining the most appropriate informant is also important. For example, patients who experience anosognosia would not be expected to be the most accurate historians. Observer-rated instruments would be preferable in patients who may be anergic and socially withdrawn but who would attempt to rationalize or dismiss their symptoms. Some patient and observer rating instruments have been cross-validated for mood and behavioral ratings in Alzheimer's disease (Cummings et al., 1994) and one hopes that more studies comparing the ratings of patients to those of family members or other observers are conducted in studies of secondary mood disorders.

Mechanisms to evaluate localization

Modern techniques for imaging or measuring brain activity have improved their temporal and topographical resolution at breathtaking rates. This section discusses a selected range of technologies available to enable the localization of brain function in humans.

Intraoperative stimulation

Intraoperative stimulation began in the early days of modern neurosurgery and has continued to be used, though in a more limited manner. Although the localization of cognitive function may be affected by longstanding neuropathology such as epilepsy, these stimulation studies have contributed limited knowledge regarding mood or emotional perception and expression (Penfield, 1950).

WADA testing

A related area of investigation is WADA testing during preoperative evaluation for cerebral dominance in epilepsy patients. By injecting the left carotid artery with barbiturates, the left hemisphere is rendered temporarily dysfunctional, and concurrent bedside testing usually confirms the absence of spoken language in a left hemisphere-dominant individual. Terzian (1964) described a 'depressive–catastrophic' reaction in right-handed patients who had just received an amytal injection of the left carotid; patients who received a right-sided injection were more likely to display a 'euphoric–maniacal' reaction (Rossi and Rosadini, 1967). Not all studies have replicated this finding (Milner, 1967).

Focal lesion analysis

Lesion analysis is primarily responsible for our current theories of cerebral localization of depression, mania, and aggressive behavior. Even before functional neuroimaging was available, early studies of stroke patients suggested a hemispheric lateralization for mood (Ross and Rush, 1981). Gainotti reported on 160 patients with unilateral brain injury and studied their emotional reactions to failure on neuropsychological testing (Gainotti, 1972). Patients with left-sided brain lesions displayed more 'anxious–depressive' reactions, whereas patients with right-sided brain lesions more commonly demonstrated anosognosia of deficit and a tendency to joke.

The association of specific focal lesions – using computed tomography (CT) and, more recently, magnetic resonance (MR) evidence of lesion topography – with patterns of mood and behavioral scale scores has resulted in a preponderance of papers suggesting that frontal (Sinyor et al., 1986; House et al., 1990) and, more often, left frontal (Robinson et al., 1984; Robinson, 1986; Eastwood et al., 1989; Fedoroff et al., 1992) and left hemispheric (Gainotti, 1972) lesions cause depression; that damage to the right frontal lobe/right basal ganglia leads to mania (Sackeim et al., 1982; Cummings and Mendez, 1984; Starkstein et al., 1987, 1988a); and that ventromedial frontal lobe damage leads to aggressive behaviors (Heinrichs, 1989; Grafman et al., 1996). However, not all lesion studies concur with the finding of some studies of penetrating head-injured veterans that indicated a significant association between right hemisphere lesions and depressive symptoms (Lishman,

1968; Grafman et al., 1986; House et al., 1990), possibly because of differences in the instruments used, subjects studied, and time of assessment.

The optimal patient group should have single focal lesions only. Stroke patients often have underlying cerebrovascular pathology, and may have multiple sites of cerebral dysfunction contributing to possible behavioral or mood effects (Bolla-Wilson et al., 1989). TBI patients may have evidence of both focal lesions and diffuse axonal injury. Although left frontal localization for modulation of depressive affect was first noted in stroke patients, this finding was replicated in an evaluation of TBI patients (Fedoroff et al., 1992). Replication of findings is critical to establish an agreed upon role for a cerebral sector in mood state modulation (Fedoroff et al., 1991).

Anterior left frontal and basal ganglia lesions are associated with the development of secondary depression. Other studies note the association of obsessive–compulsive disorder (OCD) symptomatology and neurologic disorders involving the extrapyramidal motor system, including Sydenham's chorea, Tourette's syndrome, Parkinson's disease, and even closed head injury. Multiple studies also suggest that dysfunctional orbitofrontal cortex and caudate nuclei can lead to the development of OCD. It is curious that a wider array of secondary mood state disorders has not been reported since so many brain areas are involved in various neurological disorders.

Functional imaging

Functional imaging studies offer convergent evidence about the role of various cerebral structures in mood state regulation (Mozley et al., 1996). Positron emission tomography (PET) studies in depression have shown, in general, abnormal hypometabolism in the prefrontal, cingulate, and amygdalar regions (Drevets, 1998). That these anatomic regions are involved in depression is also supported by human lesion data (Robinson, 1997). Some studies have also shown changes in limbic structures, although adequate replication of these results is lacking. PET studies have implicated dysfunction in the orbito-frontal-striatal circuit in primary OCD. Primary OCD patients exhibited abnormally increased metabolic activity in the left orbital gyrus and both caudate nuclei compared to normal controls and unipolar depressed controls (Baxter et al., 1992). In partnership with lesion studies, functional neuroimaging will facilitate our ability to associate specific patterns of brain activity with the modulation of specific mood states.

Effects of interventions to improve mood states in brain-damaged patients

Although an early study questioned the efficacy of antidepressants in post-stroke depression (Robinson, 1986), positive studies have since been reported (Lipsey et al., 1984). In an early report of the efficacy of Valproate in treating primary mania, patients with post-TBI mania were included (Pope et al., 1988). Functional imaging has been applied to patients with depression *treated* with pharmacotherapy. Recent functional neuroimaging evidence indicates that pharmacologic treatment can induce normalization of brain activation in brain regions that had shown abnormal activation before treatment (Buchsbaum et al., 1997; Kalin et al., 1997).

This same change from pretreatment abnormal brain activity was also shown in a group of OCD patients treated with a selective serotonin reuptake inhibitor (SSRI) (Baxter et al., 1992). Behavioral therapy in non-brain-injured OCD patients has also been associated with a normalization of PET activity in the head of the caudate body.

Thus, it is important for researchers to report explicitly the type and number of interventions patients in their study sample received and whether they were receiving any of the interventions at the time of the study, since there is evidence that such interventions may affect the pattern of brain activity observed in functional neuroimaging experiments as well as the interpretation of lesion study findings.

Future considerations

Readers of this volume are interested in the relationship of mood state to neuroanatomy, the clinical evaluation and treatment of mood state disorders secondary to brain lesions or impairment, and perhaps even in the search for what represents a mood state in terms of both neural mechanisms and a cognitive description. Mood states modulate cognitive processes such as memory, reasoning, social behavior, and decision making. Since mood has a role in normal cognitive processing, its impairment has a critical effect on postmorbid cognitive processing. Yet, because a clear and concise definition of what a mood state is still eludes us, we need to be especially careful in interpreting studies that attempt to understand how the brain modulates mood. We caution readers to look carefully at each study or set of studies contained in the chapters in this volume, so as to be able to abstract generally accepted findings from those that are more controversial and deserve further study. Table 3.1 lists a set of cautions that should accompany the reader's critical thinking.

Where do we go from here? Some of the answers to this question are obvious. The reductionist molecular approach follows a clearly defined path. We need to learn more about the pattern of cellular and neurotransmitter changes that are associated with normal and abnormal mood state changes and if there are genetic determinants that can forecast a person's susceptibility to secondary mood disorders. We need to clarify exactly what a mood state implies minus its cognitive and behavioral effects. That is, we need to determine if a mood state is simply a tonic modulating autonomic signal that carries great weight in a distributed network

Table 3.1. Methodological issues

Variable	How measured or described?	Comments
Diagnosis	Psychiatric interview or mood state scales	Was the DSM, ICD, or another diagnostic scheme used?
Impact	Scales or interview	Impact of diagnosis on social behavior?
Symptoms	Observed or reported	How reliable is symptom report? How is it recorded?
Neural correlates	Component location or an impaired circuit?	What is the researcher's *a priori* theoretical view?
Nature of lesion	Focal or diffuse	How are lesion location, volume, and progression estimated?
Duration of lesion	Time since onset of disorder	Patient performance may differ depending on when evaluated
Interventions	Pharmacologic or behavioral interventions	When were they initiated – before or concurrent with evaluation?
Normal volunteer selection	Medical and behavioral examination	Are normal subjects truly normal? How careful was the screening? How are they matched with the patients?
Patient selection	Characteristics	Age, education, vocation, gender, handedness, cultural background, risk for other disorders all have to be considered
Cognition	Interview or neuropsychological testing	Cognitive deficits can impact upon subject ability to express or remember mood
Theoretical agenda	Theory or model	Is it a scientifically testable model (can it be validated or rejected) or is it based on *post-hoc* analyses only?

which includes social knowledge, decision-making rules and other representational knowledge, or is something more tangible and cognitive. It would also be advantageous to understand clearly the neural distribution of the synapses that carry a particular modulator's message (i.e., mood state). That would certainly help clarify the functional breadth of the distributed network of which a particular modulator was a member (depression versus anxiety coding). Although brain lesions cause both temporary and more persistent changes in mood state, being able to distinguish quickly between these two forms of secondary mood state change would be helpful in setting treatment priorities. Finally, it is clear that we need convergent evidence from a variety of sources to make sense of neuropsychiatric data. That is, only by integrating results from molecular and genetic experiments, lesion studies, functional neuroimaging research, evaluation and treatment of patients with psychiatric disorders not due to brain lesions, studies of fluctuating moods in normal volunteers, and from the social and emotional research emerging from the discipline of psychology can we come to a complete understanding of the neuroscientific basis of mood states.

REFERENCES

Alexander, G.E., Crutcher, M.D. and DeLong, M.R. (1990). Basal ganglia–thalamocortical circuits: parallel substrates for motor, oculomotor, 'prefrontal' and 'limbic' functions. *Prog Brain Res* 85: 119–46.

Baxter L.R. Jr., Schwartz, J.M., Bergman, K.S. et al. (1992). Caudate glucose metabolic rate changes with both drug and behavioral therapy for obsessive–compulsive disorder. *Arch Gen Psychiatry* 49: 681–9.

Bolla-Wilson, K., Robinson, R.G., Starkstein, S.E. et al. (1989). Lateralization of dementia of depression in stroke patients. *Am J Psychiatry* 146: 627–34.

Bremner, J.D., Randall, P., Scott, T.M. et al. (1995). MRI-based measurement of hippocampal volume in patients with combat-related posttraumatic stress disorder. *Am J Psychiatry* 152: 973–81.

Bremner, J.D., Randall, P., Vermetten, E. et al. (1997). Magnetic resonance imaging-based measurement of hippocampal volume in posttraumatic stress disorder related to childhood physical and sexual abuse – a preliminary report. *Biol Psychiatry* 41: 23–32.

Buchsbaum, M.S., Wu, J., Siegel, B.V. et al. (1997). Effect of sertraline on regional metabolic rate in patients with affective disorder. *Biol Psychiatry* 41: 15–22.

Caine, E.D. (1981). Pseudodementia. Current concepts and future directions. *Arch Gen Psychiatry* 38: 1359–64.

Cloninger, C.R., Adolfsson, R. and Svrakic, N.M. (1996). Mapping genes for human personality (news). *Nat Genet* 12: 3–4.

Cloninger, C.R., Van Eerdewegh, P., Goate, A. et al. (1998). Anxiety proneness linked to epistatic loci in genome scan of human personality traits. *Am J Med Genet* 81: 313–17.

Clore, G.L., Schwarz, N. and Conway, M. (1994). Affective causes and consequences of social information processing. In *Handbook of Social Cognition*, ed. R.S. Wyer Jr and T.K. Srull, pp. 323–417. Hillsdale, NJ: Lawrence Erlbaum Associates.

Cummings, J.L., Mega, M., Gray, K. et al. (1994). The Neuropsychiatric Inventory: comprehensive assessment of psychopathology in dementia. *Neurology* 44: 2308–14.

Cummings, J.L. and Mendez, M.F. (1984). Secondary mania with focal cerebrovascular lesions. *Am J Psychiatry* 141: 1084–7.

Davis, M. (1992). The role of the amygdala in conditioned fear. In *The Amygdala: Neurobiological Aspects of Emotion, Memory, and Mental Dysfunction*, ed. J.P. Aggleton, pp. 255–306. New York: Wiley-Liss.

Diagnostic and Statistical Manual of Mental Disorders-IV (1994). Washington, DC: American Psychiatric Association.

Drevets, W.C. (1998). Functional neuroimaging studies of depression: the anatomy of melancholia. *Annu Rev Med* 49: 341–61.

Eastwood, M.R., Rifat, S.L., Nobbs, H. and Ruderman, J. (1989). Mood disorder following cerebrovascular accident. *Br J Psychiatry* 154: 195–200.

Fedoroff, J.P., Starkstein, S.E., Parikh, R.M. et al. (1991). Are depressive symptoms nonspecific in patients with acute stroke? *Am J Psychiatry* 148: 1172–6.

Fedoroff, J.P., Starkstein, S.E., Forrester, A.W. et al. (1992). Depression in patients with acute traumatic brain injury. *Am J Psychiatry* 149: 918–23.

Gainotti, G. (1972). Emotional behavior and hemispheric side of lesion. *Cortex* 8: 41–55.

Goate, A.M. and Edenberg, H.J. (1998). The genetics of alcoholism. *Curr Opin Genet Dev* 8: 282–6.

Grafman, J. (1995). Similarities and distinctions among current models of prefrontal cortical functions. *Ann NY Acad Sci* 769: 337–68.

Grafman, J. and Christen, Y., eds. (1999). *Neuronal Plasticity: Building a Bridge from the Laboratory to the Clinic.* Research and Perspectives in Neurosciences. Berlin: Springer-Verlag.

Grafman, J., Schwab, K., Warden, D. et al. (1996). Frontal lobe injuries, violence, and aggression: a report of the Vietnam Head Injury Study. *Neurology* 46: 1231–8.

Grafman, J., Vance, S.C., Weingartner, H., Salazar, A.M. and Amin, D. (1986). The effects of lateralized frontal lesions on mood regulation. *Brain* 109: 1127–48.

Gualtieri, C.T. (1991). *Neuropsychiatry and Behavioral Pharmacology.* New York: Springer-Verlag.

Heinrichs, R.W. (1989). Frontal cerebral lesions and violent incidents in chronic neuropsychiatric patients. *Biol Psychiatry* 25: 174–8.

House, A., Dennis, M., Warlow, C., Hawton, K. and Molyneux, A. (1990). Mood disorders after stroke and their relation to lesion location. A CT scan study. *Brain* 113: 1113–29.

Jarrell, T.W., Gentile, C.G., Romanski, L.M., McCabe, P.M. and Schneiderman, N. (1987). Involvement of cortical and thalamic auditory regions in retention of differential bradycardiac conditioning to acoustic conditioned stimuli in rabbits. *Brain Res* 412: 285–94.

Jorge, R.E., Robinson, R.G. and Arndt, S. et al. (1993a). Are there symptoms that are specific for depressed mood in patients with traumatic brain injury? *J Nerv Ment Disord* 181: 91–9.

Jorge, R.E., Robinson, R.G., Arndt, S.V. et al. (1993b). Comparison between acute- and delayed-onset depression following traumatic brain injury. *J Neuropsychiatry Clin Neurosci* 5: 43–9.

Jorge, R.E., Robinson, R.G., Starkstein, S.E. et al. (1993c). Secondary mania following traumatic brain injury. *Am J Psychiatry* 150: 916–21.

Kalin, N., Davidson, R., Irwin, W. et al. (1997). Functional magnetic resonance imaging studies of emotional processing in normal and depressed patients: effects of Venlafaxine. *J Clin Psychiatry* 58 (Suppl. 16): 32–9.

Kaplan, H.I. and Sadock, B.J. (1995). *Comprehensive Textbook of Psychiatry/VI.* Baltimore: Williams and Wilkins.

Lipsey, J.R., Robinson, R.G., Pearlson, G.D., Rao, K. and Price, T.R. (1984). Nortriptyline treatment of post-stroke depression: a double-blind study. *Lancet* 1: 297–300.

Lipsey, J.R., Spencer, W.C., Rabins, P.V. and Robinson, R.G. (1986). Phenomenological comparison of poststroke depression and functional depression. *Am J Psychiatry* 143: 527–9.

Lishman, W.A. (1968). Brain damage in relation to psychiatric disability after head injury. *Br J Psychiatry* 114: 373–410.

Litvan, I., Paulsen, J.S., Mega, M.S. and Cummings, J.L. (1998). Neuropsychiatric assessment of patients with hyperkinetic and hypokinetic movement disorders. *Arch Neurol* 55: 1313–19.

Masterman, D.L. and Cummings, J.L. (1997). Frontal–subcortical circuits: the anatomic basis of executive, social and motivated behaviors. *J Psychopharmacol* 11: 107–14.

Milner, B. (1967). Discussion of the subject: experimental analysis of cerebral dominance in man. In *Brain Mechanisms underlying Speech and Language*, ed. C.H. Millikan and F.L. Darley, pp. 122–45. New York: Grune and Stratton.

Mozley, P.D., Hornig-Rohan, M., Woda, A.M. et al. (1996). Cerebral HMPAO SPECT in patients with major depression and healthy volunteers. *Prog Neuropsychopharmacol Biol Psychiatry* 20: 443–58.

Penfield, W. (1950). *The Cerebral Cortex of Man; a Clinical Study of Localization of Function*. New York: Macmillan.

Pope, H.G. Jr., McElroy, S.L., Satlin, A. et al. (1988). Head injury, bipolar disorder, and response to valproate. *Comp Psychiatry* 29: 34–8.

Robinson, R.G. (1986). Post-stroke mood disorders. *Hosp Pract* 21: 83–9.

Robinson, R.G. (1997). Neuropsychiatric consequences of stroke. *Annu Rev Med* 48: 217–29.

Robinson, R.G. (1998). *The Clinical Neuropsychiatry of Stroke*. Cambridge, UK: Cambridge University Press.

Robinson, R.G., Kubos, K.L., Starr, L.B. et al. (1984). Mood disorders in stroke patients. Importance of location of lesion. *Brain* 107 (Part 1): 81–93.

Ross, E.D. and Rush, A.J. (1981). Diagnosis and neuroanatomical correlates of depression in brain-damaged patients. Implications for a neurology of depression. *Arch Gen Psychiatry* 38: 1344–54.

Rossi, G.F. and Rosadini, G. (1967). Experimental analysis of cerebral dominance in man. In *Brain Mechanisms underlying Speech and Language*, ed. C.H. Millikan and F.J. Darley. New York: Grune and Stratton.

Sackeim, H.A., Greenberg, M.S., Weiman, A.L. et al. (1982). Hemispheric asymmetry in the expression of positive and negative emotions. Neurologic evidence. *Arch Neurol* 39: 210–18.

Sapolsky, R.M. and Pulsinelli, W.A. (1985). Glucocorticoids potentiate ischemic injury to neurons: therapeutic implications. *Science* 229: 1397–400.

Shadmehr, R. and Holcomb, H.H. (1997). Neural correlates of motor memory consolidation. *Science* 277: 821–5.

Singer, M.I., Anglin, T.M., Song, L.Y. and Lunghofer, L. (1995). Adolescents' exposure to violence and associated symptoms of psychological trauma. *J Am Med Assoc* 273: 477–82.

Sinyor, D., Jacques, P., Kaloupek, D.G. et al. (1986). Poststroke depression and lesion location. An attempted replication. *Brain* 109 (Part 3): 537–46.

Spitzer, R.L., Williams, J.B., Gibbon, M. and First, M.B. (1992). The Structured Clinical Interview for DSM III-R (SCID). I: History, rationale, and description. *Arch Gen Psychiatry* 49: 624–9.

Starkstein, S.E., Boston, J.D. and Robinson, R.G. (1988a). Mechanisms of mania after brain injury. 12 case reports and review of the literature. *J Nerv Ment Disord* 176: 87–100.

Starkstein, S.E., Pearlson, G.D., Boston, J. and Robinson, R.G. (1987). Mania after brain injury. A controlled study of causative factors. *Arch Neurol* 44: 1069–73.

Starkstein, S.E., Preziosi, T.J., Bolduc, P.L. and Robinson, R.G. (1990). Depression in Parkinson's disease. *J Nerv Ment Disord* 178: 27–31.

Starkstein, S.E., Robinson, R.G., Berthier, M.L. et al. (1988b). Differential mood changes following basal ganglia vs thalamic lesions. *Arch Neurol* 45: 725–30.

Tang, M.X., Maestre, G., Tsai, W.G. et al. (1996). Effect of age, ethnicity, and head injury on the association between APOE genotypes and Alzheimer's disease. *Ann NY Acad Sci* 802: 6–15.

Terzian, L. (1964). Behavioral and EEG effects of intracarotid sodium amytal injection. *Acta Neurochir* 12: 230–9.

Weingartner, H., and Silberman, E. (1982). Models of cognitive impairment: cognitive changes in depression. *Psychopharmacol Bull* 18: 27–42.

Whitaker, J.N., McFarland, H.F., Rudge, P. and Rheingold, S.C. (1995). Outcomes assessment in multiple sclerosis clinical trials: a critical analysis. *Mult Scler* 1: 37–47.

Wing, J.K., Cooper, J.E. and Sartorius, S.N. (1974). *Measurement and Classification of Psychiatric Symptoms: an Instruction Manual for the PSE and CATEGO Program.* Cambridge, UK: Cambridge University Press.

4

Emotional behavior in acute brain lesions

Florence Ghika-Schmid and Julien Bogousslavsky

Introduction

Little is known about the emotional and related behavioral changes in acute focal lesions, although they may be associated with specific prognostic correlates. Although already recognized by Bleuler in 1924, depression and, more generally, mood disorders following cerebral lesions have been studied systematically only during the last 20 years. The initial studies of emotional disorders following brain injuries included patients with various lesions such as surgical incisions, traumatic closed head injuries, penetrating head injury, and stroke, making it difficult to determine the location of the lesion in each case. For this methodological reason, the most precise evaluation of mood disorders following acute brain lesion has been made in stroke studies. Although these studies suggest a critical role of the anterior left hemisphere in depression, some authors deny a causal contribution of lesion location to depression. The predominant role of the right hemisphere in secondary mania is well recognized, but a consensus is still lacking and further studies are needed to determine the clinico-topographic correlation of disorders such as apathy, anxiety, catastrophic reaction, and pathological laughing and crying sometimes encountered after stroke. These affective disorders are important to consider in stroke patients, since they may negatively influence neurological recovery and may be responsive to treatment.

Specific emotional behaviors, such as disinhibition, denial, indifference, overt sadness, and aggressiveness, often occur during the days immediately following stroke. They can be overlooked if not searched for systematically with appropriately designed scales. Some of these early behaviors, such as denial, may be related to the late development of depression and anxiety. Prospective studies of mood changes during and *immediately after stroke* have not yet been performed. Such studies on large samples of patients may permit the delineation of which of these acute emotional behavioral changes are markers for the delayed development of emotional disturbances.

Some stroke subtypes, such as cardioembolic stroke, may have a specific pattern of early emotional behavior. Stroke occurrence itself may be related to an individual vulnerability different from that of stress, as in carotid artery disease.

In stroke, early disregard of the symptoms by patients or their relatives may delay consultation and compromise acute management with new developing techniques, such as thrombolysis. Even after improvement, some patients with denial may require considerable persuasion to enrol in stroke prevention therapy or be reluctant to accept rehabilitation. However, in spite of the important impact on management, little is known about the subjective experience of acute stroke patients.

The current data of the ongoing Lausanne Emotion in Stroke Study (LEASS) show that early emotional behavior can be quantified in acute stroke. Further analyses on a larger sample of patients may allow us to delineate which are the best markers of ulterior development of depression or anxiety and to perform detailed clinico-topographical correlation.

Depression

Diagnosis

The standardized diagnostic criteria of the DSM-IV for mood disorders are appropriate for stroke, since post-stroke depression has a symptomatic profile similar to that of primary depression (Starkstein and Robinson, 1989). Adapted depression rating scales, such as the Hamilton Scale for Depression, can be useful tools, with the cut-off score for post-stroke depression being suggested as 13 (Andersen et al., 1994c). Other scales have been developed that are more directly aimed at the evaluation of post-stroke depression (Gainotti et al., 1997b). However, these different scales include features such as anxiety and catastrophic reaction, which may be specific clinical syndromes (see below). Special attention should be paid to autonomic disturbances, such as abnormal sleep patterns, decreased appetite and libido, vegetative anxious signs, and subjective anergia (Fedoroff et al., 1991). No definite relationship has been established between the severity of neurological impairment and the presence of depressive features (Herrmann et al., 1995), but the negative influence of depression on neurological recovery is well recognized (Starkstein and Robinson, 1989; Parikh et al., 1990; Morris et al., 1992).

Risk factors, early prognostic markers, prevalence, and evolution

Among the risk factors for the development of post-stroke depression, pre-existing cerebral atrophy has been suggested, but remains controversial (Starkstein et al., 1988c; Morris et al., 1990; Herrmann et al., 1995; Astrom, 1996). An increased frequency of personal or familial history of psychiatric disorders was found in patients with post-stroke depression, suggesting a personal or genetic predisposition (Starkstein and Robinson, 1989; Morris et al., 1990; Andersen et al., 1995;

Starkstein, 1998). Intellectual impairment may also explain some of the variation in mood scales (Andersen et al., 1995).

These various risk factors may be differentially implicated in the development of depression a certain period of time after stroke (Astrom, Adolfsson and Asplund, 1993). The potential role of very acute, or 'during stroke,' behavioral changes as markers for the ulterior development of mood disorder is the subject of an ongoing study (the Lausanne Emotion in Acute Stroke Study: Ghika-Schmid et al., 1996, 1997). A wide range of emotional reactions can already be present during the days immediately following acute stroke and include: overt sadness, passivity, aggressiveness, indifference, disinhibition, denial, adaptation, and abnormal sleep or feeding patterns. These reactions can be quantified using a specifically designed scale (Behavioral Index Form: Table 4.1), and may be predictors of the later development of depression. These behavioral reactions should be distinguished from the patients' subjective experience. Indeed, in a prospective study on 53 patients with strokes in the anterior (32) or posterior (21) circulation (17 right, 33 left, three bilateral), acute behavioral denial was related to less frequent subjective experience of fear, and to delayed depression, and was independent of anosognosia. Other emotion reactions, including happiness, sadness, irascibility, were dissociated from the patients' subjective experience (Ghika-Schmid et al., 1998). The prevalence of depression in the acute phase of stroke is about 40% (20% major depression, 20% minor depression) (Ebrahim, Barer and Nouri, 1987; Starkstein and Robinson, 1989; Starkstein, 1998) whereas estimates made in the chronic phases range between 18% and 54% (Sinyor et al., 1986; Eastwood et al., 1989; Astrom et al., 1993; Sharpe et al., 1994; Burvill et al., 1995a). The period of maximal prevalence and the evolution vary in the different studies: post-stroke depression may be especially frequent in the acute phase of stroke, but can also occur one to two years after stroke and, if left untreated, may last for up to one year (Starkstein and Robinson, 1989; Morris et al., 1990; House et al., 1991; Astrom et al., 1993; Burvill et al., 1995; Starkstein, 1998). The evolution may be dependent on stroke location and a better prognosis of depression was found following stroke in the posterior circulation (Starkstein et al., 1988b).

Lesion location

The left frontal anterior region, both the dorsolateral prefrontal cortex and subcortical region, was found to be important for depression in left hemisphere-damaged patients (Starkstein and Robinson, 1989; Astrom et al., 1993; Herrmann, Bartels and Wallesch, 1993; Starkstein, 1998). The severity of depression may be associated with lesion proximity to the frontal pole in the left hemisphere, in cortical or subcortical location (Starkstein and Robinson, 1989). Among patients with right hemisphere stroke who developed depression, a positive association with a

Table 4.1. Emotional behavior index

A Overt sadness	F Denial
cries	minimized
looks sad	denial of all symptoms
complains	partial denial
shouts	G Adaptation
whines	smiles
B Passivity	socializes
gives up	quiet
isolated	asks sensible demands
C Aggression	pudic
tensed	interested
agitated	looks serious
angry	sensitive to what happens
rebellious	helpful
oppositional	active collaboration
aggressive	expressive
revolted	clean, self-attentive
D Indifference	obeys
indifferent	H Abnormal sleep/feeding
neglected	
apathic	
E Dishinhibition	
jokes	
disinhibited	
laughs	
impatient	

posterior lesion was found (Starkstein and Robinson, 1989; Starkstein, 1998). However, although an association was found between major depressive disorder and left lentiform nucleus lesion, no significant difference between depression scores in left and right hemisphere lesions or a correlation between the severity of depression and the anterior location or volume of the lesion was seen in 47 patients during acute stroke (Herrmann et al., 1995). Moreover, severity of depression is not always proportional to the distance of the lesion from the frontal pole, suggesting a more complex nature of association (Sinyor et al., 1986). Thus, an association between left-sided lesions and depression and right-sided lesions and hypomania is not a constant finding (Folstein, Maiberger and McHugh, 1977; House et al., 1990). Some authors even suggest that lesion location may not be a prime etiological factor for post-stroke depression (Andersen et al., 1995; Burvill et al., 1996; Gainotti et al., 1997a). In the Lausanne Emotion in Acute Stroke Study

(Ghika-Schmid et al., 1996, 1997b), the use of previously developed precise templates of the vascular territories may shed some new light on this issue. On the other hand, electrophysiological evidence for a crucial role of left frontal activation of 'positive affects' (Davidson et al., 1987) and rapid-rate transcranial magnetic stimulation, showing a lateralized control of mood, following prefrontal cortex stimulation in normal volunteers (Pasqual-Leone et al., 1996), argue for the 'localizing' thesis.

The *hypothetical mechanisms* considered by those authors supporting the role of lesion location are based on the observation of a higher incidence of familial psychiatric disorders in patients with right posterior lesions, which might suggest differential vulnerability to depression for right and left lesions (Starkstein and Robinson, 1989). Positron emission tomography (PET) studies showed a possible compensatory up-regulation of 5-HT2 (serotonin) receptors in the right hemisphere after stroke, which is not seen after left-sided lesions (Mayberg et al., 1988). Animal studies also showed a lateralized biochemical response to ischemia, suggesting asymmetry in the human biological response to injury, which supports these views (Robinson, 1979). However, the finding of temporolimbic hypoperfusion in patients with depression and subcortical stroke suggests that alternative mechanisms should be considered (Grasso et al., 1994). Various mechanisms have been suggested to link depression and coronary heart disease, such as changes in lipid metabolism, and in catecholamine–corticoid and serotonergic modulations, and altered sympathetic arousal in patients with depression leading to arrhythmia (Wassertheil-Smoller et al., 1996). Identical physiopathological mechanisms might be present in patients with post-stroke depression. In an similar way, post-stroke depression may be related to a higher secondary occurrence of hypertension (Jonas, Franks and Ingram, 1997).

Treatment

Nortriptyline, trazodone and serotonin reuptake inhibitors (Lipsey et al., 1984; Reding et al., 1986; Andersen et al., 1994b) were shown to be effective in randomized, placebo-controlled studies of post-stroke depression (Table 4.2). Because of the high frequency of their contraindication and adverse effects (orthostatic hypotension, atrioventricular block), tricyclic antidepressants are not the first choice in cerebrovascular patients (Gustafson et al., 1995). Serotonin reuptake inhibitors may be the best choice (Reding et al., 1986; Andersen et al., 1994b); however, adverse reactions such as fluoxetine-induced mania can occur in patients with post-stroke depression (Berthier and Kulisevsky, 1993). Open trials have suggested the potential benefit of psychostimulants (methylphenidate), but further controlled studies are required to reach a conclusion (Gustafson et al., 1995). Imipramine and mianserine have been effective in trials, and imipramine probably has a combined action on the noradrenergic and especially the serotoninergic

Table 4.2. The main studied treatments of post-stroke depression

Double-blind, placebo controlled
Nortriptyline
Trazodone
Serotonin reuptake inhibitors
Citalopram
Open studies
Methylphenidate
Imipramine
Mianserine
Moclobemide

systems (Gustafson et al., 1995). The potential benefit of electroconvulsive therapy warrants confirmation (Currier, Murray and Welch, 1992; Gustafson et al., 1995). Treatment for spasticity, psychological assistance, and social support should not be neglected (Angeleri et al., 1993). The presence of negative affective signs which are responsive to treatment may also lengthen hospital stay (Galynker et al., 1997). The mortality rate is higher in stroke patients with initial depression (70%) than without (40%), even when signs of depression were no longer present at the time of death (Morris et al., 1993a). The suicidal rate remains low; when present, its risk factors are insomnia and cognitive impairment (Kishi, Kosier and Robinson, 1996).

Fear and anxiety

Generalities

The occurrence of fear or anxiety in reaction to a stressful challenge is determined in part by the social context in which it occurs and the social status of the individual, such as whether he or she is dominant or subordinate (McEwen, 1996). The effect of a potentially stress-evoking situation on the nervous system is influenced by genetic predisposition, biological development, sex, and learned experience (McEwen, 1996). An unforeseen stress source induces physiological arousal. A threat may induce a high-cost response such as aggression, or, if no response is possible, displaced aggression, helplessness, or hopelessness, with altered physiological responses (McEwen, 1996). Alcohol and substance abuse as well as risk-taking behaviors are other coping alternatives (Sher, 1987; McEwen, 1996).

The central nucleus of the amygdala is an important neural control center for fear and conditioned fear (Aggleton, 1992). It projects to cardiovascular, facial, autonomic, respiratory, and neuroendocrine control centers in the brain that affect cardiovascular, gastrointestinal, and adrenocortical activity, facial expression, and social interaction, and cause arousal (McEwen, 1996). The hippocampus also plays an important role in controlling the secretion of adrenal steroids and in processing spatial–temporal aspects of a changing environment, and possibly in the auditory processing of fear (Eichenbaum and Otto, 1992; McEwen, 1996).

Definitions

Historically, the word fear evolved from the Old English word *faer*, which meant peril or calamity. The word anxiety originated from the Latin word *anxius*, which means troubled in mind, solicitous, or uneasy.

Fear is an emotional state involving physiological arousal (e.g., increased heart rate), verbal reports of distress (e.g., apprehension, worry), overt behavior (e.g., avoidance), and cognitive disruption (e.g., hyperawareness about possible threat cues in the environment), typically triggered by specific objects or situations. It is a fundamental emotion, present across ages, cultures, ethnic groups, and species. Its function is often described as an alarm system activating the organism in response to threat (McNeil, Turk and Ries, 1994).

Anxiety involves the same emotional state but with a lesser mobilization for physical action. It is characterized by feelings of distress and worry, maladaptive shifts in attention due to off-target thinking, and the perception that aversive events are occurring in an unpredictable and uncontrollable manner. It is associated with more cognitive symptoms, and less visceral activation. Cues for its manifestation are more diffuse and changeable relative to fear (McNeil et al., 1994). Anxiety is the second most prevalent mood disorder following stroke, being found in 3.5% to 24% of patients (Starkstein et al., 1990b; Castillo et al., 1993; Burvill et al., 1995b; Astrom, 1996; Starkstein, 1998). It is frequently associated with depression (Castillo, Schultz and Robinson, 1995; Astrom, 1996). Restricted criteria from the DSM III-R have been proposed to diagnose anxiety in stroke patients, but duration of symptoms was not included as we wished to use the criteria for assessment immediately after stroke (Castillo et al., 1993). A personal history of alcohol abuse may be a significant association (Castillo et al., 1993), as well as cerebral atrophy (Astrom, 1996). According to a recent study, combination of anxiety and depression is more frequent after left cortical stroke, whereas anxiety without depression is mainly seen following right hemisphere lesion (Castillo et al., 1993). Comorbidity with depression may impair the prognosis of depression (Astrom, 1996).

Relationship to acute focal brain lesion

Stroke incidence may be related to an individual vulnerability different from that of mental stress, as shown in patients with carotid artery disease (Barnett et al.,

1997). Indeed, cardiovascular reactivity can be assessed by measuring hemo-dynamic changes during a frustrating cognitive task such as the Stroop Color Word Interference Task. In 136 untreated subjects followed for two years, a significant change in systolic blood pressure during the task was a strong predictor of the rate of progression of carotid arteriosclerosis measured with Doppler ultrasound (Barnett et al., 1997). In the clinical setting, patients with high blood pressure in a doctor's office may be at similar risk. In animals, exposure to social stress and challenges to dominance are associated with coronary atherosclerosis (Spence, 1996).

Individual and cultural variability in the appraisal of emotion certainly plays an important role in these phenomena and deserves further study. When faced with the same situation, different people often respond with different emotions. This general statement may be painfully self-evident, but appraisal theories go beyond the general statement to specify the differences (Ellsworth, 1991). For example, a person who characteristically sees his or her misfortunes as caused by bad luck may be more prone to depression, while one who attributes these to other people's malice may be more prone to aggression (Roseman, 1984). Among the Utku Eskimos, feelings of anger are strongly condemned (Briggs, 1970), but in certain Arab groups, a man's failure to respond with anger is seen as dishonorable (Abu-Lughod, 1986).

It is clear that much of atherosclerosis is genetic, the candidate gene ranging from lipoprotein lipase to angiotensin receptor gene, for example (Spence, 1996). Thus, the study of vascular reactivity could be a new tool for investigating the genetics of atherosclerosis. Moreover, a significantly increased incidence of stroke was found in men reporting a high level of stress (Harmsen et al., 1990).

Life experiences such as grief, mourning, loss of status or self-esteem, or threat of injury involve a response of overwhelming excitation or acceptance and may be associated with neurovegetative responses that may lead to lethal cardiac events, particularly in individuals with pre-existing cardiovascular disease (Engel, 1971). Similar phenomena may be important in cerebrovascular disease, as well as certain at-risk personality features, including a behavior pattern that ensures the attainment of self-set goals, difficulty in the control of anger, and object-related style characterized by the assumption of personal responsibility for the gratification of one's needs. The systematic study of the personality characteristics of 32 men who experienced ischemic stroke occurring within a period of sustained emotional disturbance showed that some features appeared with unexpected frequency (Adler, MacRitchie and Engel, 1971). These included: (a) a pressure to keep busy; (b) a self-image of an active, hard worker; (c) high standards and a pronounced sense of responsibility; (d) a sense of urgency, time pressure, and a need to fulfil goals; and (e) a sense of determination and strong will (Adler et al., 1971). Of these 32 patients, 28 reported that they were concerned with controlling the expression of their anger, which was aroused mostly by a feeling of not being able to control their environment or their own bodies, which frustrated their attempts to fulfil self-set goals (Adler et al., 1971). In that group of patients, the onset of stroke at the moment of an intense peak of emotion was unusual, occurring only twice (Adler et al., 1971). These findings of the psychological characteristics of stroke patients were very similar to what is reported for coronary patients, such as angina pectoris occurring in a 'keen and ambitious man, the indicator of whose engines is always set at *full speed ahead*' (Adler et al., 1971; Osler, 1896, 1910). The main drawback of this study is its retrospective nature, leading to possible distortion by the interviewer. In a meta-analysis of the relation between psychological factors and coronary heart disease, reliable association was found for 'type A behavior' (referring to a person who is involved in an aggressive and incessant struggle to achieve more and more in less and less time) for anger, hostility, and aggression, but also for depression and anxiety (Booth-Kewley and Friedman, 1987). This suggests that coronary proneness may not involve the expected hurried, impatient workaholic, but instead someone with one or more negative emotions. Other studies have emphasized the importance of hostility, especially an antagonistic interactional style, rather than the whole set of behaviors associated with type A behavior, as a risk factor for coronary heart disease. A new, experimental approach to applying the appraisal theories of emotions may prove useful in better characterizing the individual balance between fear, anger, and anxiety in such a setting as well as in stroke (Scherer, 1984; Ellsworth, 1991). A relationship may exist between fear and anxiety, and anger. These three emotional states are common responses to stressful situations and are often difficult to distinguish because all involve unpleasant feelings and physiological arousal. Some evidence suggests that anxiety and fear can be differentiated from anger according to feelings along the dominance–submissiveness continuum. People who are angry may feel in control of events, while people who are anxious or fearful may feel out of control or vulnerable. Physiologically, fear and anxiety have been associated with increased skin conductance and respiratory rate, while anger has been involved in increased diastolic blood pressure (McNeil et al., 1994).

The repeated and successful practice of courageous behavior leads to a decrease in verbal reports of fear and physiological responsivity, which can lead to a state of fearlessness (McNeil et al., 1994). Stress could also affect the metabolic control of diabetes by changes in compliance behavior and neurohumoral axis, but the findings supporting these hypotheses remain contradictory (Barglow et al., 1984).

Thus, the relative importance of personality features and emotional reaction, both in cardiovascular and in cerebrovascular diseases, remains debated. Precise prospective data on the emotional profile of patients with acute stroke may allow a better understanding of their characteristics and implications.

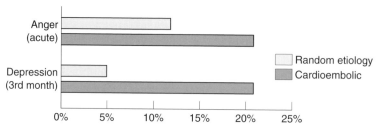

Fig. 4.1   Frequency of anger in acute stroke and post-stroke depression in patients with cardioembolic versus non-cardioembolic stroke.

Preliminary data from the Lausanne Emotion in Acute Stroke Study (Ghika-Schmid et al., 1999) suggest that patients with acute cardioembolic stroke may have a specific pattern of early emotional disturbances. Among 85 patients, 23 (13 men, 10 women, age 66 ± 17 years) had cardioembolic sources, 15 had stroke in the middle cerebral artery territory, and 8 in the posterior circulation (10 right, 13 left). They presented acute emotional reactions of disinhibition (12), denial (6), indifference (7), overt sadness (6), and aggressiveness (5). On questioning, 6 patients expressed fear, 5 anger, 14 joy, and 8 sadness. In the third month, 12 (52%) patients were: anxious (4), anxiodepressive (3), or depressed (5). Compared to 55 patients with stroke of random etiology (Ghika-Schmid et al., 1997b), they expressed more anger during the acute phase (21% versus 12%) and displayed more depression at three months (21% versus 5%) (Fig. 4.1). No other between-group difference was observed. These data suggest that, during the acute period, patients with cardioembolic stroke express anger more often than the overall stroke population. This may be related to specific personality features such as difficulty in the control of anger, and may suggest that such a behavioral pattern indicates a risk for cardioembolic events. In the third month, patients with cardioembolic stroke had a higher incidence of depressive, but not anxious, manifestations. Thus, the expression of post-stroke affective disorders may be different in relation to different stroke etiologies. This may be due to pre-existing personality features favoring a peculiar stroke mechanism, such as cardiac embolism.

Pseudodepressive manifestations

Abulia

The clinical characterization of apathy, or abulia, has been debated in the literature, and includes features such as flat affect, short and delayed answers, hypophonia, reduced motor responses, fixed gaze and blank face, perseverations, and lack of awareness of condition (Fisher, 1995). Clinical scales, which can be useful diagnostic and follow-up tools, have been developed (Starkstein, 1998). Abulia is related to the disruption, at various anatomical sites, of frontosubcortical pathways such as anterior cingulate and capsular lesions (Starkstein et al., 1993a; Fisher, 1995). Apathy was reported as more frequent following stroke in the posterior arm of the internal capsule in the left hemisphere, probably because anterior cerebral artery stroke with cingulate involvement is rare (Starkstein et al., 1993a). Major depression is significantly more frequent in patients with apathy (Starkstein et al., 1993a), but should be distinguished from it (Marin, Firinciogullari and Biedrzycki, 1993). Post-stroke apathy may be significantly associated with age and more severe impairment in activities of daily living and cognitive functions (Starkstein, 1998), and with frontal and anterior temporal reduction in cerebral blood flow measured by ^{133}Xe inhalation. The therapeutic potential of agents such as bromocriptine or methylphenidate has been suggested (Muller and Von Cramon, 1994; Watanabe et al., 1995).

Loss of psychic self-activation

Apathetic, aspontaneous, indifferent behavior, with loss of motor and affective drive, and reversible when patients are repeatedly stimulated by another person, can be seen in toxic bilateral subcortical lesions involving the pallidum or putamen and in bithalamic infarct (Laplane, 1990; Bogousslavsky et al., 1991). Occasionally, loss of psychic self-activation following bilateral thalamic infarct of venous origin may be accompanied by *obsessive–compulsive behaviors* (Bogousslavsky, 1993; personal observation), similar to the effects seen following bilateral basal ganglia involvement due to encephalitis, anoxia, disulfiram, carbon monoxide intoxication or trauma (Ali-Cherif et al., 1984; Laplane, 1994). Obsessive–compulsive behavior may be due to dysfunction of the fronto-striato-pallido frontal circuit (Laplane, 1994), and the occurrence of identical symptoms after bilateral thalamic stroke suggests an additional thalamic connection to this circuit. Patients with obsessive–compulsive behavior have a low affective resonance to their symptoms and loss of projection of themselves into the future that is different from the depressive state, but sometimes associated with it (Laplane, 1994).

Pathological laughing and crying

This is characteristically unrelated to the patient's inner emotional state. It can occur independently of depression (Robinson et al., 1993), although this point remains controversial (Andersen et al., 1995). A corresponding lesion location is not clear (Robinson et al., 1993; Derex et al., 1997), although bilateral pontine lesions have been emphasized (Andersen et al., 1994a). Unilateral lesion, especially if subcortical, might be sufficient. Pathological laughing and crying is often delayed (Berthier et al., 1996), suggesting a mechanism similar to that of delayed-on set movement disorders. Symptomatic improvement has been reported with serotonin reuptake agents and tricyclics (Robinson et al., 1993; Andersen et al., 1994b), being consistent with the hypothesis of stroke-induced partial involvement of the serotoninergic raphe nuclei in the brainstem or their ascending projection to the brain hemispheres (Andersen et al., 1994c; Derex et al., 1997). *Emotional lability* may follow stroke, mainly if the anterior regions of both cerebral hemispheres are involved (Morris et al., 1993).

Catastrophic reactions

First recognized by Babinski in 1914, catastrophic reactions were defined by Goldstein (1939) as an inability to cope when confronted with the deficit, with short-lasting sudden bursts of tears, refusal, and irritation. They were initially reported predominantly in patients with left hemispheric lesions (Gainotti, 1972). However, recent studies have failed to demonstrate significant hemispheric involvement differences, but rather suggest a preferential basal ganglia involvement (Starkstein et al., 1993a). Catastrophic reactions may be associated with a positive personal and familial history of psychiatric disorder, increased frequency of major depression, and lower scores of daily living activity (Starkstein et al., 1993b).

Mania

Mania, characterized by signs such as inflated self-esteem or grandiosity, decreased need for sleep, distractibility, flight of ideas, and excessive involvement in pleasurable activities with potential painful consequences (DSM IV), is a rare occurrence following stroke. Starkstein et al. (1987) found the prevalence of manic patients among a consecutive series of more than 300 patients with acute stroke to be 1%. In manic syndromes following cerebral injury, lesions were located mainly in the right hemisphere and involved the thalamus (Cummings and Mendez, 1984; Bogousslavsky et al., 1988a; Starkstein et al., 1988), right temporal lobe (Starkstein et al., 1988b), head of the caudate (Starkstein et al., 1990c) or, bilaterally, the frontal cortex (Starkstein et al., 1988c). As for major depression, silent cerebral infarcts may play a role in the occurrence of late-onset mania (Fujikawa, Yamawaki and Touhouda, 1995). Hypometabolism involving the right inferior temporal lobe was seen in a PET study of two patients with lesions of the right head of the caudate (Starkstein et al., 1990d), leading to the hypothesis of a direct or indirect role (diaschisis) of the right inferior temporal lobe in secondary mania. In primary mania, decreased blood flow to the right temporal lobe has also been found (Migliorelli et al., 1993). Post-stroke mania has been reported in patients previously free of psychiatric conditions but with a family history of psychiatric disease (Starkstein et al., 1987; Robinson et al., 1988). In a patient with previous recurrent episodes of mania, a dramatic change in symptoms with the appearance of persisting hyperthymia has been reported following a right thalamic infarct (Vuilleumier et al., 1998). A dual mechanism of depression and mania, the former being associated with left and anterior lesions and the second with right hemisphere lesions, may be related to a differential neuromodulation by serotoninergic agents and a differential adaptive mechanism of S2 receptors in both hemispheres (Starkstein et al., 1989). The influence of a positive family history of psychiatric disorders in right-side-damaged patients with secondary mood disorders suggests a genetic predisposition in this population (Robinson et al., 1988).

Aggressive burst

Bursts of anger may occur following stroke, accompanied by behaviors ranging from shouting to violence (Paradiso, Robinson and Arndt, 1996). These behaviors seem to occur more commonly in patients with higher Hamilton scores and greater cognitive impairment (Paradiso et al., 1996). They are more frequent following left hemisphere stroke (Paradiso et al., 1996).

Post-stroke psychosis

Hallucinations or paranoid delusions occur more often in older patients, with a positive personal and family history of psychosis in 50% of cases (Starkstein, 1998). The ventricular to brain ratio in these patients is often decreased, suggesting subcortical atrophy (Starkstein, 1998). The lesion can be parieto-temporal, occipital, frontal, or subcortical in the right hemisphere, or pontine (Kim et al., 1995; Starkstein, 1998).

Acute behavioral reactions, subjective experience, and nosognosia

In stroke, early disregard of the symptoms by patients and their relatives may delay consultation and compromise acute management and early treatment with thrombolysis (Grotta and Bratina, 1995). Even after they improve, some patients may require much persuasion to enrol in follow-up and stroke prevention therapy. Moreover, patients with denial of hemiplegia are often reluctant to accept rehabilitation, sometimes to a point of refusing to use a cane to walk (Ullman et al., 1960; Prigatano and Schacter, 1991). However, in spite of this important impact on management, little is known about the subjective experience of stroke patients. In his detailed self-observation of motor hemiplegia, dysarthria and modification of handwriting following infarction in the right internal capsule and surroundings, Brodal (1973) mentioned his 'incontinence of emotional expression' and his 'painful awareness of no longer being what he used to be.' Although a couple of historical stroke patients, such as Auguste Forel, have pointed to the potential importance of patients' self-evaluation, studies of subjective experience in stroke remained exceptional (Ullman et al., 1960; Ullman and Gruen, 1961; Alajouanine and Lhermitte, 1964). Systematic prospective studies are required to evaluate the influence of subjective experience, especially in the acute phase of stroke when this aspect may be overlooked.

Since the initial descriptions, the terms anosognosia and denial have been used interchangeably, although some authors have preferred denial, to emphasize that the notion is wider than the initially recognized anosognosia for hemiplegia or hemianopia (Anton, 1889; Babinski, 1914; Prigatano and Schacter, 1991). Denial is the product of an interaction in which the observer interprets the patient's behavior. The type of interview can influence the degree of denial (Prigatano and Schacter, 1991). Some authors have proposed scales aimed at quantifying the severity of anosognosia (Prigatano and Schacter, 1991). On the other hand, the various entities often lumped together in the terms denial or anosognosia should be separated from each other. In order to differentiate between the patient's own appreciation of his or her condition and observed behavior, the terms *anosognosia/anosodiaphoria* can be reserved for the patients' own assessment of their deficits during questioning, while *denial reactions* can be used to describe activities observed by an external examiner, such as attempts to stand in spite of hemiplegia. In addition, *subjective experience*, defined as the patients' own appreciation of their affective state (happiness, sadness, anger or fear), should be emphasized.

In a recent study assessing subjective experience in acute stroke to correlate it with stroke features, acute emotional behavior, and impact on medical care seeking, we studied all patients with acute first-ever stroke. During the first four days, we rated subjective experience (happiness, sadness, irascibility, fear), mood (Hamilton) and behavioral reactions using a specifically designed scale. Fifty-three patients (30 men, 23 women, 60 ± 19 years) completed three-month follow-up. Strokes were in the anterior (32/53) or posterior (21/53) circulation (17 right, 33 left, three bilateral). Seventeen (32%) patients failed to seek medical care spontaneously (Ghika-Schmid et al., 1998).

Anosognosia and anosodiaphoria

Anosognosia has been shown to be frequent in right-sided lesions, but may also develop after left-sided lesions. Anosodiaphoria was even reported to be more frequent following left strokes (Ghika-Schmid et al., 1998b). The lack of recognition of the deficit was manifested in various functions, such as hemianopia, dysarthria, aphasia, or sensory loss (Prigatano and Schacter, 1991). Babinski (1914) noted that patients with right hemisphere lesions may display euphoria and indifference towards their symptoms (anosodiaphoria and anosognosia). Gainotti suggested that depression in patients with right hemisphere lesions may be underdiagnosed due to a tendency to denial and failure to express affects. However, no significant difference was found in depression scores between patients with anosognosia for hemiplegia (common with right parieto-temporal or basal ganglia involvement) and patients who were nosognosic, suggesting that anosognosic patients do not deny depression (Starkstein et al., 1990b). Thus, anosognosia, neglect, and major depression may coexist. A longitudinal case study suggested that they are independent phenomena (Starkstein et al., 1990c). The coexistence of anosognosia and depression challenges the psychological theory of depression (Ramasubbu, 1994).

Behavioral reactions of denial

Acute behavioral signs of denial were independent of anosognosia. They were not related to the side of the lesion, but were significantly more frequent in patients with deep lesions on either side. This confirms a clear distinction between the behavioral manifestations of denial and nosognosia. It suggests that these two aspects may also be independent in terms of their neuroanatomic substrate, since nosognosia, but not behavioral signs of denial, related to the side of the lesion. This may apply a dissociation between behavioral display and awareness of physical impairment. Thus, the behavioral signs of denial and nosognosia should be distinguished in further studies; their confusion may have accounted for some of the discrepancies in the literature (Ullman and Gruen, 1961). Denial reactions were inversely correlated to subjective experience of fear. The possibility of a relationship between anxiety, fear, and denial has been raised, but has remained ambiguous (Ullman et al., 1960). In Ullman's widow patient, the rejection of denial (realizing that her paralyzed arm was not her dead husband's) decreased her fear. In contrast, in another patient, initial feelings of fright were relieved by the identification of the arm upon her breast (her arm) as that of her husband (Ullman et al., 1960). The presence of denial may be related to a reduction of the patient's experience of fear (Ghika-Schmid et al., 1998a). An impact of denial on the patient's outcome, as shown by a worsening record of employment, has been reported in follow-up studies of patients with head injury (Prigatano and Schacter, 1991). The presence of an acute denial reaction may be correlated with delayed occurrence of depression and anxiety (Ghika-Schmid et al., 1999).

Subjective experience

For all emotions other than fear (joy, sadness, and anger), the patients' subjective experience was not related to the behavior displayed during the acute phase of stroke (Ghika-Schmid et al., 1998, 1999). Such an independence of nosognosia from the emotional reactions supports a similar dissociation observed over time in a prospective longitudinal single case study (Starkstein et al., 1990b). The coexistence of anosognosia and depression challenges the psychological theory of depression (Ramasubbu, 1994). This seems to confirm the hypothesis that a decreased experience of fear may relate to the manifestation of denial, which is sometimes interpreted as a defense mechanism. Fear may be mediated by a different neuronal network, accounting for the dissociation we observed between subjective experience of fear (which related to behavior of denial) and the independent subjective experience of other emotions in regard to the observed behavioral response. Indeed, impaired recognition of fear in emotional faces has been noted in patients with selective bilateral damage to the amygdala (Adolphs et al., 1994; Calder et al., 1996), whereas the hippocampus and adjacent white matter may play a crucial role in the auditory perception of fear (Ghika-Schmid et al., 1997b; Fig. 4.2). This suggests that there may be multiple emotion systems for different aspects of emotion (Adolphs et al., 1994; Damasio, 1994; Adolphs et al., 1995). Abnormal fear reactions may be related to affective disorders such as anxiety and stress (Le Doux, 1996).

Recall of the acute event

A third of the patients could only partially recall or did not recall at all the acute event (Ghika-Schmid et al., 1999). These results are consistent with a study on patients showing dramatic recovery following thrombolysis (Grotta and Bratina, 1995). This impaired recall of the acute phase certainly adds to the difficulties encountered in trying to motivate patients to enrol in regular follow-up.

Medical care seeking

Patients with preserved nosognosia did spontaneously better at seeking medical attention on their own initiative than those with anosognosia, suggesting that a lack of insight may indeed be the cause of the failure to consult. The presence of a subjective experience was related to appropriate care seeking; its impairment may contribute, as for anosognosia, to increased delay in seeking consultation.

In conclusion, acute behavioral signs of denial may be regarded as markers of delayed post-stroke depression and anxiety. Patients with acute behavioral denial reactions may have a decreased frequency of subjective experience of fear. Preserved subjective experience of fear relates to appropriate care seeking and its impairment may contribute, as for anosognosia, to increased delay in seeking consultation. All other emotional reactions seem to be dissociated from the patients' subjective experience, suggesting that emotional behavior should be distinguished from the subjective emotional experience, which may be closer to affective disorders. This distinction, which was not made in earlier studies (Ullman and Gruen, 1961), should be confirmed in further studies.

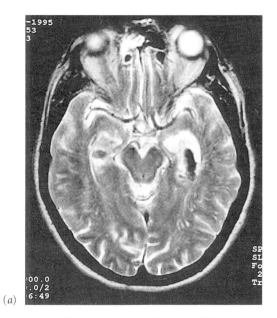

(a)

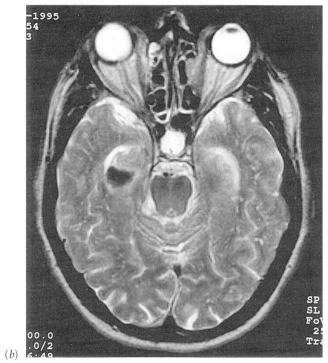

(b)

Fig. 4.2   Mediotemporal lesion in a patient with impaired auditory perception of fear.

Mood disorders and cognition in acute brain lesions

On rare occasions, the relationship between mood disorders and cognitive impairment has been studied in stroke (Bolla-Wilson et al., 1989; Herrmann et al., 1993; Downhill and Robinson, 1994; Iacoboni et al., 1995). Studies based on the Mini-Mental State Examination are not sufficient because this test mainly depends on language abilities and left hemispheric function and does not allow a proper estimation of cognitive function due to right hemisphere lesion. A study using a complete neuropsychological battery of tests has shown impaired orientation, language, and visuo-perceptive and executive functions in left hemisphere-damaged, depressed patients, whereas no significant correlation between depression and a specific cognitive defect was found in right hemisphere patients (Bolla-Wilson et al., 1989). Post-stroke depression might contribute to cognitive impairment in the late phase after stroke (Iacoboni et al., 1995). Further studies are needed to confirm these findings and to demonstrate a possible improvement of cognitive symptoms following treatment. Moreover, the possibility of a positive adrenergic effect on neurological signs and cognition following physical therapy has been suggested (Feeney, 1997). As the diagnosis of depression for patients with aphasia is difficult, these patients have been excluded from most studies of post-stroke depression. Patients with nonfluent aphasia may show a higher frequency of depression than patients with fluent aphsia, but this may be related to the sharing of a lesion location (left frontal) between nonfluent aphasia and depression (Starkstein and Robinson, 1989; Herrmann et al., 1993; Starkstein, 1998).

Cognitive functions and mood may be related to each other and share common neuronal networks and neurotransmitter systems. However, the way in which these different brain functions interact and their relationship to the possible occurrence and clinical features of post-stroke mood disorder are far from understood and require further investigation.

Mood and emotional perception and expression

Emotional aptitudes in patients with acute brain lesions and their relationship to mood disorder and cognition have rarely been studied (Starkstein et al., 1994). Emotional aprosody may not necessarily be associated with post-stroke depression (Starkstein et al., 1994). One limitation of the study by Starkstein et al. (1994) was the exclusion of patients with comprehension disorder, which may explain the finding of an association between aprosody and right hemisphere lesion; this observation therefore needs to be confirmed. A relationship between memory dysfunction and emotional perception is suggested by studies on the role of the amygdala in acquiring and storing long-term associative memory to link sensory information and affective significance (Ono, Nishijo and Uwano, 1995). The role of the lateral nucleus of the amygdala in fear is recognized in animals (Le Doux, 1996). Recognition of fear in emotional faces may be mediated by the amygdala (Adolphs et al., 1994; Calder et al., 1996). Animal studies suggest that the emotional functions of the amygdala and hippocampus may be relayed through amygdala–hippocampal interconnections (Aggleton, 1986), and recent observations suggest that the amygdala may process emotional aspects of events (Starter and Markowitsch, 1985). These studies on the role of the amygdala in fear challenge the septohippocampal theories of fear and anxiety (Gray, 1987). On detailed testing of the *recognition of facial and vocal expression of emotion* (Ekman and Friesen, 1971; Pittam and Scherer, 1993) an impairment of the vocal perception of fear, but not that of other emotions such as joy, sadness, and anger, was found in a patient with bihippocampal hemorrhage (see Fig. 4.2), probably due to Urbach–Wiethe disease. Such selective impairment of fear perception was not present in the recognition of facial expression of emotion. Thus, emotional perception varies according to the different aspects of emotions and the different modality of presentation (faces versus voices). Evidence about the origin and universality of the production of particular facial expressions (Ekman and Friesen, 1971) initially led to the claim of the existence of a 'specialized perceptual system tuned to the peculiar movements that signal them' (Etcoff and Magee, 1992). However, our findings suggest the possibility of a distinct processing of emotion according to the modality of perception. They are consistent with the idea that there may be multiple emotion systems for different aspects of emotion (Adolphs et al., 1994, 1995; Damasio, 1994). Moreover, our studies suggest that the hippocampus and adjacent white matter may play a critical role in the *recognition of fear in vocal expression*, possibly dissociated from that of other emotions.

A critical role of the right hemisphere in acquired deficit of emotional expression and comprehension (prosody, emotional faces, and lexical emotional expression) has been suggested by numerous studies (Heilman, Scholes and Watson, 1975; Ross and Mesulam, 1979; De Kosky et al., 1980; Cicone, Waper and Gardner, 1980; Ross, 1981; Weintraub, Mesulam and Kramer, 1981; Borod et al., 1988, 1992; Bowers et al., 1985; Ahern et al., 1991), but remains controversial (Stone et al., 1996). Other authors emphasized the role of basal ganglia (Cancelliere and Kertesz, 1990). A relative superiority of the visuospatial (70) versus verbal (54) IQ on the Weschler Memory Scale was observed in a patient with bihippocampal hemorrhage and impaired recognition of fear in vocal expression. This finding is not suggestive of a predominantly right-sided dysfunction. Data from tachistoscopic presentation of emotional faces in the right and left hemisphere also challenge the view that the right hemisphere is uniquely involved in all emotional behavior (Davidson et al., 1987). In Klüver–Bucy syndrome (a syndrome first described in rhesus monkeys following bilateral temporal lobectomy, with a tendency to examine all objects orally, loss of anger and fear responses, and increased sexual activity) an interesting feature has been called 'psychic blindness.' In the human, psychic blindness may be characterized by an inability to differentiate strangers from friends. It may be associated with sensory agnosia. Cummings and Duchen (1981) suggested that sensory agnosia results from disruption of the temporal neocortex or its connections, and that the other components of the syndrome (hyperorality, hypersexuality) are caused by disturbances of the amygdala functions. Loss of recognition of people has been reported following lesions in the anterior temporal region and in the limbic structures of the mesial temporal region (Corkin, 1984; Damasio, 1989). One patient was unable to learn the identity of the face he had first come into contact with after he sustained bilateral ablation of entorhinal cortex and hippocampus (Corkin, 1984). Another patient with bilateral mesial limbic system structures and bilateral higher-order neocortical damage was unable to recognize the identity of the people she met, not only in the visual modality, but also with the help of vocal or sensory clues (Damasio, 1985). These findings support the critical role of the anterior temporal lobe in the formation of binding codes, which allow the reconstruction and retrieval of unique memories (Damasio, 1989). The rare occurrence of complete Klüver–Bucy syndrome after a lesion restricted to the left temporal region (Fig. 4.3) may suggest that some aspects of facial recognition such as a sense of familiarity may require the integrity of the left temporal mesial region. This may represent a network distinct from the one involved with the recognition of facial expression, which may relate more specifically with the function of the right fusiform gyrus (Allison, 1994).

Summary

Studies in patients with focal acute brain lesion suggest that the left frontal anterior region, both dorsolateral prefrontal cortex and white matter, may be strategically important for depression (Starkstein and Robinson, 1989; Bogousslavsky, 1993; Astrom et al., 1993; Starkstein, 1998). These findings could not always be replicated (Folstein et al., 1977; House et al., 1990; Bogousslavsky, 1993), and some authors even deny any causal contribution of lesion location to depression (Burvill et al 1996; Gainotti et al., 1997a). In secondary mania, lesion location was mainly in the right hemisphere (Cummings and Mendez, 1984; Bogousslavsky et al., 1988b; Starkstein et al., 1990b), but a consensus is still lacking concerning a possible clinico-topographical correlation of disorders such as apathy, anxiety, catastrophic reaction, and pathological laughing and crying, sometimes encountered after stroke. Important methodological problems and difficulties in comparing the data certainly account for some of the discrepancies found in the literature. Psychiatric

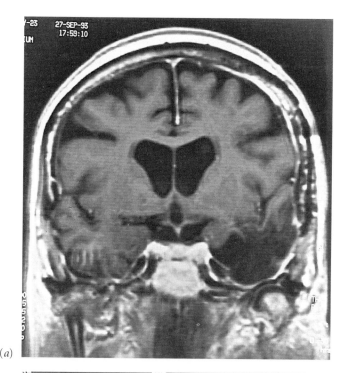

(a)

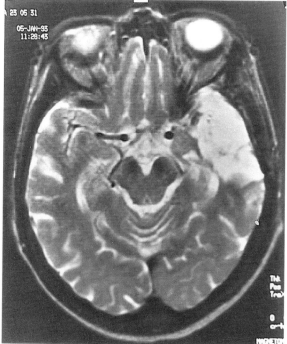

(b)

Fig. 4.3   Unilateral damage to the left temporal lobe in a patient with Klüver–Bucy syndrome.

diagnosis has not always been made using standardized criteria (DSM III-R or DSM IV). The prevalence and correlation of mood disorders may change over time, and studies considering only the acute or chronic phase might not be accurate (Starkstein, 1998). The psychiatric assessment of aphasic patients remains problematic, although these patients may be evaluated through their behavioral changes, such as sleep and food intake (Ross and Rush, 1981). The exclusion of aphasic patients from studies may induce a bias. Studies including patients with previous stroke or multiple lesions may introduce confusing variables in trying to correlate clinical and topographic information (Starkstein and Robinson, 1989; Starkstein, 1998). Also, the classification of stroke subtype and localization has been variable and often simplistic, leading to much difficulty in repeating studies. Further studies using precise templates of vascular involvement in large series of patients are still needed to clarify these points. The systematic study of mood change during and immediately after stroke, as assessed in the on-going Lausanne Emotion in Acute Stroke Study (Ghika-Schmid et al., 1996, 1997, 1999), remains poorly studied. However, early thymic alterations may be useful markers of the late functional prognosis. Appropriately designed scales, such as the Behavioral Index Form, make it possible to quantify early emotional reactions (Ghika-Schmid et al., 1996, 1997b). Systematic studies on larger samples of patients may allow the delineation of acute emotional behavioral changes, which may be markers for the delayed occurrence of emotional disturbances.

Studies in animals suggest that stress-induced biological modification of the hippocampal and hypothalamic responsiveness to glutamate may play a critical functional role (Bartanusz et al., 1995). In humans, a selective reduction in a serotonin metabolite (5HIAA) was found in the cerebrospinal fluid of depressed, but not of nondepressed, post-stroke patients, supporting the hypothesis of a serotoninergic mechanism in post-stroke depression (Bryer et al., 1992). Studies on the overall stroke population showed a higher level of glutamate and glycine in the plasma and cerebrospinal fluid of patients with large cerebral infarcts, cortical infarcts, and severe neurological deficit, supporting the concept of the excitotoxic activity of glycine and glutamate in these patients (Castillo et al., 1996). These findings suggest not only that neuroexcitatory amino acids may be a useful parameter to monitor the severity of stroke, but also that measurement of other metabolites such as serotonin metabolites might allow more selective measures of the differential biological response in patients prone to develop post-stroke mood disorders. Further systematic studies, with careful monitoring of stroke and measurement of monoamine metabolites and neuroexcitatory amino acids, may give a better understanding of the biological mechanism underlining post-stroke emotional disturbances.

In conclusion, although most lesion studies on mood disorder agree on the critical role of the anterior left hemisphere in depression and the predominant role of the right hemisphere in manic syndromes, controversy exists concerning the exact clinical characterization of post-stroke mood disorders in relation to the site of the lesion. Further studies are needed to determine the clinico-topographic correlation and to define predictors of handicap in connection with the different patterns of emotional behavior.

REFERENCES

Abu-Lughod, J. (1986). *Veiled Sentiments.* Berkeley, CA: University of California Press.

Adler, R., MacRichtie, K. and Engel, G.L. (1971). Psychologic processes and ischemic stroke (occlusive cerebrovascular disease) I. Observation on 32 men with 35 strokes. *Psychosom Med* 33: 1–29.

Adolphs, R., Tranel, D., Damasio, H. and Damasio, A. (1994). Impaired recognition of emotion in facial expressions following bilateral damage to the human amygdala. *Nature* 372: 669–72.

Adolphs, R., Tranel, D., Damasio, H. and Damasio, A.R. (1995). Fear and the human amygdala. *J Neurosci* 15(9): 5879–91.

Aggleton, J.P. (1986). A description of the amygdalo-hippocampal interconnections in the macaque monkey. *Exp Brain Res* 64: 515–26.

Aggleton, J.P. (1992). *The Amygdala.* New York: Wiley.

Ahern, G.L., Schomer, D.L., Kleefield, J. et al. (1991). RH advantage for evaluating emotional facial expressions. *Cortex* 27: 193–202.

Alajouanine, T. and Lhermitte, F. (1964). Essai d'introspection de l'aphasie (l'aphasie vue par les aphasiques). *Rev Neurol* 110(6): 609–21.

Ali-Chérif, A., Royère, M.L., Gosset, A. et al. (1984). Troubles du comportement et de l'activité mentale après intoxication oxycarbonée. Lésions pallidales bilatérales. *Rev Neurol* 1400: 32–40.

Allison (1994). N200 in fusiform and inferior temporal gyri. Face specific potential. *Clin Neurol* 15: 730–7.

Andersen, G., Ingeman-Nielsen,M., Verstergaard, K. and Riis, J.O. (1994a). Pathoanatomic correlation between poststroke pathological crying and damage to brain areas involved in serotoninergic neurotransmission. *Stroke* 25: 1050–2.

Andersen, G., Vestergaard, K., Ingemann-Nielsen, M. and Lauritzen, L. (1995). Risk factors for post-stroke depression. *Acta Psychiatri Scand* 92: 193–8.

Andersen, G., Vestergaard, K. and Lauritzen, L. (1994b). Effective treatment of post-stroke depression with the selective reuptake inhibitor citalopram. *Stroke* 25: 1099–104.

Andersen, G., Vestergaard, K., Riis, J. and Lauritzen, L. (1994c). Incidence of post-stroke depression during the first year in a large unselected stroke population determined using a valid standarized rating scale. *Acta Psychiatr Scand* 90: 190–5.

Angeleri, F., Angeleri, V.A., Foschi, N., Giaquinto, S. and Nolfe, G. (1993). The influence of depression, social activity, and family stress on functional outcome after stroke. *Stroke* 24: 1478–83.

Anton, F. (1889). Uber die selbstwahrnehemungen der Herderkrankungen des gehirns durch den Kranken bei Rindenblindheit und Rindentaubheit. *Arch Psychiatry* 32: 86–127.

Astrom, M. (1996). Generalized anxiety disorder in stroke patients. A 3-year longitudinal study. *Stroke* 27: 270–5.

Astrom, M., Adolfsson, R. and Asplund, K. (1993). Major depression in stroke patients. A 3-year longitudinal study. *Stroke* 24: 976–82.

Babinski, J. (1914). Contribution à l'étude des troubles mentaux dans l'hémiplegie organique cérébrale (anosognosie). *Rev Neurol* 27: 845–8.

Barglow, P., Hatcher, R., Edidin, D.V. and Sloan-Rossiter, D. (1984). Stress and metabolic control in diabetes: psychosomatic evidence and evaluation of methods. *Psychosom Med* 46: 127–44.

Barnett, P.A., Spence, D., Maruck, S.B. and Jennings, J.R. (1997). Psychological stress and the progression of carotid artery disease. *J Hypertension* 15: 49–55.

Bartanusz, V., Aubry, J.M., Pagliusi, S. et al. (1995). Stress-induced changes in messenger RNA levels of N-methyl-D-aspartate and AMPA receptor subunit in selected regions of the rat hippocampus and hypothalamus. *Neuroscience* 66: 247–52.

Berthier, M.L. and Kulisevsky, J. (1993). Fluoxetine-induced mania in a patient with post-stroke depression (letter). *Br J Psychiatry* 163: 698–9.

Berthier, M.L., Kulisevsky, J., Gironell, A. and Fernandez Benitez, J.A. (1996). Poststroke bipolar affective disorder: clinical subtypes, concurrent movement disorders, and anatomical correlates. *J Neuropsychiatry Clin Neurosci* 8: 160–70.

Bleuler, E. (1924). *Textbook of Psychiatry*. New York: Macmillan.

Bogousslavsky, J. (1993). Troubles thymiques et accidents vasculaires cérébraux. *Rev Neuropsychol* 3: 257–69.

Bogousslavsky, J., Ferrazzini, M., Regli, F. et al. (1988a). Manic-like delirium and frontal-like syndrome with paramedian infarction of the right thalamus. *J Neurol Neurosurg Psychiatry* 51: 116–19.

Bogousslavsky, J., Regli, F., Delaloye, B. et al. (1991). Loss of psychic self-activation with bithalamic infarction. Neurobehavioural, CT, MRI and SPECT correlates. *Acta Neurol Scand* 83: 309–16.

Bogousslavsky, J., Regli, F. and Uské, A. (1988b). Thalamic infarcts: clinical syndromes, etiology, and prognosis. *Neurology* 38: 837–48.

Bolla-Wilson, K., Robinson, R.G., Starkstein, S.E., Boston, J. and Price, T.R. (1989). Lateralization of dementia of depression in stroke patients. *Am J Psychiatry* 146: 627–34.

Booth-Kewley, S. and Friedman, H.S. (1987). Psychological predictors of heart disease: a quantitative review. *Psychol Bull* 101: 343–62.

Borod, J.C., Andelman, F., Obler, L.K., Tweedy, J.R. and Welkowitz, J. (1992). Right hemisphere specialization for the identification of emotional words and sentences: evidence from stroke patients. *Neuropsychologia* 30: 827–44.

Borod, J.C., Koff, E., Lorch, M.P., Nicholas, M. and Welkowitz, J. (1988). Emotional and non-emotional facial behaviour in patients with unilateral brain damage. *J Neurology Neurosurg Psychiatry* 51: 826–32.

Bowers, D., Bauer, R.M., Coslett, H.B. and Heilman, K.M. (1985). Processing of faces by patients with unilateral hemispheric lesions. I. Dissociation between judgments of facial affect and facial identity. *Brain Cogn* 4: 258–72.

Briggs, J.L. (1970). *Never in Anger: Portrait of an Eskimo Family*. Cambridge, MA: Harvard University Press.

Brodal, A. (1973). Self-observation and neuro-anatomical consideration after stroke. *Brain* 96: 675–94.

Bryer, J.B., Starkstein, S.E., Vtypka, V., Price, T.R. and Robinson, R.G. (1992). Reduction of CSF monoamine metabolites in poststroke depression: a preliminary report. *J Neuropsychiatry Clin Neurosci* 4: 440–2.

Burvill, P.W., Johnson, G.A., Chakera, T.M.H. et al. (1996). The place of site of lesion in the etiology of post-stroke depression. *Cerebrovasc Dis* 6: 208–15.

Burvill, P.W., Johnson, G.A., Jamrozik, K.D. et al. (1995a). Prevalence of depression after stroke: the Perth Community Stroke Study. *Br J Psychiatry* 166: 320–7.

Burvill, P.W., Johnson, G.A., Jamrozik, K.D. et al. (1995b). Anxiety disorders after stroke: results from the Perth Community Stroke Study. *Br J Psychiatry* 166: 328–32.

Calder, A.J., Young, A.W., Rowland, D. et al. (1996). Facial emotion recognition after bilateral amygdala damage: differentially severe impairment of fear. *Cogn Neuropsychol* 13(5): 699–745.

Cancelliere, A.E.B. and Kertesz, A. (1990). Lesion localization in acquired deficits of emotional expression and comprehension. *Brain Cogn* 13: 133–47.

Castillo, J., Davalos, A., Naveiro, J. and Noya, M. (1996). Neuroexcitatory amino acids and their relation to infarct size and neurological deficit in ischemic stroke. *Stroke* 27: 1060–5.

Castillo, C.S., Schultz, S.K. and Robinson, R.G. (1995). Clinical correlates of early-onset and late-onset poststroke generalized anxiety. *Am J Psychiatry* 152: 1174–9.

Castillo, C.S., Starkstein, S.E., Fedoroff, J.P., Price, T.R. and Robinson, R.G. (1993). Generalized anxiety disorder after stroke. *J Nerv Ment Dis* 181: 100–6.

Cicone, M., Waper, W. and Gardner, H. (1980). Sensitivity to emotional expressions and situation in organic patients. *Cortex* 16: 145–58.

Corkin, S. (1984). Lasting consequences of bilateral medial temporal lobectomy: clinical course and experimental findings in HM. *Semin Neurol* 4: 249–59.

Cummings, J.L. and Duchen, L.W. (1981). Klüver–Bucy syndrome in Pick's disease: clinical and pathologic correlations. *Neurology* 31: 1415–22.

Cummings, J.L. and Mendez, M.F. (1984). Secondary mania with focal cerebrovascular lesions. *Am J Psychiatry* 141: 1084–7.

Currier, M.B., Murray, G.B. and Welch, C.C. (1992). Electroconvulsive therapy for post-stroke depressed geriatric patients. *J Neuropsychiatry Clin Neurosci* 4: 140–4.

Damasio, A. (1989). Multiregional retroactivation: a systems level model for some neural substrates of cognition. *Cognition* 33: 25–62.

Damasio, A. (1985). Prosopagnosia. *Trends Neurosci* 8: 132–5.

Damasio, A.R. (1994). *Emotion, Reason and the Human Brain*. New York: GP Putman Sons.

Davidson, R.J., Mednick, D., Moss, E., Saron, C. and Schaffer, C.E. (1987). Ratings of emotion in faces are influenced by the visual field to which stimuli are presented. *Brain Cogn* 6: 403–11.

De Kosky, S., Heilman, K., Bowers, D. and Valenstein, E. (1980). Recognition and discrimination of emotional faces and pictures. *Brain Lang* 9: 206–14.

Derex, L., Ostrowsky, K., Nighoghossian, N. and Trouillas, P. (1997). Severe pathological crying after left anterior choroidal artery infarct. Reversibility with paroxetine treatment. *Stroke* 28: 1464–9.

Downhill, J.E. Jr. and Robinson, R.G. (1994). Longitudinal assessment of depression and cognitive impairment following stroke. *J Nerv Ment Dis* 182: 425–31.

Eastwood, M.R., Rifat, S.L., Nobbs, H. and Ruderman, J. (1989). Mood disorder following cerebrovascular accident. *Br J Psychiatry* 154: 195–200.

Ebrahim, S., Barer, D. and Nouri, F. (1987). Affective illness after stroke. *Br J Psychiatry* 151: 52–6.

Eichenbaum, H. and Otto, T. (1992). The hippocampus. What does it do? *Behav Neurol Biol* 57: 2–36.

Ekman, P. and Friesen, W.V. (1971). Constants across cultures in the face and emotion. *J Person Soc Psychol* 17: 124–9.

Ellsworth, P.C. (1991). Some implication of the cognitive appraisal theories of emotion. In *International Review of the Studies on Emotion*, Vol. 1, ed. K.T. Strongman, pp. 53–67. New York: John Wiley & Sons Ltd.

Engel, G.L. (1971). Sudden and rapid death during psychological stress. Folklore or folk wisdom? *Ann Intern Med* 74: 771–82.

Etcoff, N.L. and Magee, J.J. (1992). Categorical perception of facial expression. *Cognition* 44: 227–40.

Fedoroff, J.P., Starkstein, S.E., Price, T.R. and Robinson, R.G. (1991). Are depressive symptoms non-specific in patients with acute stroke? *Am J Psychiatry* 148: 1172–6.

Feeney, D.M. (1997). From laboratory to clinic: noradrenergic enhancement of physical therapy for stroke or trauma patients. *Adv Neurol* 3: 383–94.

Fisher, C.M. (1995). Abulia. In *Stroke Syndromes*, ed. J. Bogousslavsky and L. Caplan, pp. 182–7. Cambridge: Cambridge University Press.

Folstein, M.F., Maiberger, R. and McHugh, P.R. (1977). Mood disorder as specific complication of stroke. *J Neurol Neurosurg Psychiatry* 40: 1018–20.

Fujikawa, T., Yamawaki, S. and Touhouda, Y. (1995). Silent cerebral infarctions in patients with late-onset mania. *Stroke* 26: 946–9.

Galynker, I., Prikhojan, A., Phillips, E. et al. (1997). Negative symptoms in stroke patients and length of hospital stay. *J Nerv Ment Dis* 185: 616–21.

Gainotti, G. (1972). Emotional behavior and hemispheric side of the lesion. *Cortex* 8: 41–55.

Gainotti, G., Azzoni, A., Gasparini, F., Marra, C. and Razzano, C. (1997a). Relation of lesion location to verbal and nonverbal mood measures in stroke patients. *Stroke* 28: 2145–9.

Gainotti, G., Azzoni, A., Razzano, C. et al. (1997b). The Post-Stroke Depression Scale: a test specifically devised to investigate affective disorders of stroke patients. *J Clin Exp Neuropsychol* 19: 340–56.

Ghika-Schmid, F., Castillo, V., Neau, J.P. et al. (1996). Emotional behavior in acute stroke. The Lausanne Emotion in Stroke Study. *Cerebrovasc Dis* 6 (Suppl. 2): 122.

Ghika-Schmid, F., Ghika, J., Regli, F. and Bogousslavsky, J. (1997a). Abnormal movements during and after acute stroke. The Lausanne Stroke Registry. *J Neurol Sci* 146: 109–16.

Ghika-Schmid, F., Ghika, J., Vuilleumier, P. et al. (1997b). Bihippocampal damage with emotional dysfunction. Impaired perception of fear. *Eur Neurol* 38: 276–83.

Ghika-Schmid, F., van Melle, G., Guex, P. and Bogousslavsky, J. (1998). Early emotional behavior in acute cardioembolic stroke. Specific emotional features. *Eur J Neurol* S38.

Ghika-Schmid, F., van Melle, G., Guex, P. and Bogousslavsky, J. (1999). Subjective experience and behavior in acute stroke. The Lausanne Emotion in Acute Stroke Study. *Neurology* 52: 22–8.

Goldstein, K. (1939). *The Organism: a Holistic Approach to Biology Derived from Pathological Data in Man.* New York: American Books.

Grasso, M.G., Pantano, P., Ricci, M. et al. (1994). Mesial temporal cortex hypoperfusion is associated with depression in subcortical stroke. *Stroke* 25: 980–5.

Gray, J.A. (1987). *The Psychology of Fear and Stress.* New York: Oxford University Press.

Grotta, J. and Bratina, P. (1995). Subjective experiences of 24 patients dramatically recovering from stroke. *Stroke* 26: 1285–8.

Gustafson, Y., Nilsson, I., Mattsson, M., Astrom, M. and Bucht, G. (1995). Epidemiology and treatment of post-stroke depression. (Review.) *Drugs & Aging* 7: 298–309.

Harmsen, P., Rosengren, A., Tsipogianni, A. and Wilhelmsen, L. (1990). Risk factors for stroke in middle-aged men in Goteborg, Sweden. *Stroke* 21: 223–9.

Heilman, K.M., Scholes, R. and Watson, R.T. (1975). Auditory affective agnosia: disturbed comprehension of affective speech. *J Neurol Neurosurg Psychiatry* 38: 69.

Herrmann, M., Bartels, C., Schumacher, M. and Wallesch, C.W. (1995). Poststroke depression. Is there a pathoanatomic correlate for depression in the postacute stage of stroke? *Stroke* 26: 850–6.

Herrmann, M., Bartels C. and Wallesch, C.W. (1993). Depression in acute and chronic aphasia: symptoms, pathoanatomical–clinical correlations and functional implications. *J Neurol Neurosurg Psychiatry* 56: 672–8.

House, A., Dennis, M., Warlow, C., Hawton, K. and Molyneux, A. (1990). Mood disorders after stroke and their relation to lesion location. A CT scan study. *Brain* 113: 1113–29.

Iacoboni, M., Padovani, A., Di Piero, V. and Lenzi, G.L. (1995). Post-stroke depression: relationships with morphological damage and cognition over time. *Italian J Neurol Sci* 16: 209–16.

Jonas, B.S., Franks, P. and Ingram, D.D. (1997). Are symptoms of anxiety and depression risk factors for hypertension? Longitudinal evidence from the National Health and Nutrition Examination Survey I. Epidemiologic Follow-up Study. *Arch Fam Med* 6: 43–9.

Kim, S.J., Lee, J.H., Joo, H.I. and Myoung, C.L. (1995). Syndromes of pontine base infarction. *Stroke* 26: 950–5.

Kishi, Y., Kosier, J.T. and Robinson, R.G. (1996). Suicidal plans in patients with acute stroke. *J Nerv Ment Dis* 184: 274–80.

Laplane, D. (1990). La perte d'auto activation psychique. *Rev Neurol* 146: 6–7, 397–404.

Laplane, D. (1994). Obsessions et compulsion par lésions des noyaux gris centraux. *Rev Neurol* 150: 8–9, 594–8.

Le Doux, J.E. (1996). In search of an emotional system in the brain: leaping from fear to emotion and consciousness. In *The Cognitive Neurosciences*, ed. M.S. Gazzaniga, pp. 1049–61. Cambridge, MA: MIT Press.

Lipsey, J.R., Robinson, R.G., Pearlson, G.D., Rao, K. and Price, T.R. (1984). Nortriptyline treatment of post-stroke depression: a double blind treatment trial. *Lancet* S2: 297–300.

Marin, R.S., Firinciogullari, S. and Biedrzycki, R.C. (1993). The sources of convergence between measures of apathy and depression. *J Affect Disord* 28: 117–24.

Mayberg, H.S., Robinson, R.G., Wong, D.F. et al. (1988). PET imaging of cortical S2 serotonin receptors after stroke: lateralized changes and relationship to depression. *Am J Psychiatry* 145: 937–43.

McEwen, B. (1996). Stressful experience, brain and emotions: developmental genetic and hormonal influences. In *The Cognitive Neurosciences*, ed. M.S. Gazzaniga, pp. 1117–35. Cambridge, MA: MIT Press.

McNeil, D.W., Turk, C.L. and Ries, B.J. (1994). Anxiety and fear. In *Encyclopedia of Human Behavior*, ed. V.S. Ramachandran, pp. 151–63. New York: Academic Press.

Migliorelli, R., Starkstein, S.E., Teson, A. et al. (1993). SPECT findings in patients with primary mania. *J Neuropsychiatry Clin Neurosci* 5: 379–83.

Morris, P.L., Robinson, R.G., Andrzejewski, P., Samuels, J. and Price, T.R. (1993a). Association of depression with 10-year poststroke mortality (see comments). *Am J Psychiatry* 150: 124–9.

Morris, P.L.P., Robinson, R.G. and Raphael, B. (1990). Prevalence and course of depressive disorders in hospitalized stroke patients. *Int J Psychiatry Med* 20: 349–64.

Morris, P.L., Robinson, R.G. and Raphael, B. (1993b). Emotional lability after stroke. *Aust NZ J Psychiatry* 27: 601–5.

Muller, U. and Von Cramon, D.Y. (1994). The therapeutic potential of bromocriptine in neuropsychological rehabilitation of patients with acquired brain damage. *Prog Neuropsychopharmacol Biol Psychiatry* 18(7): 1103–20.

Ono, T., Nishijo, H. and Uwano, T. (1995). Amygdala role in conditioned associative learning. (Review). *Prog Neurobiol* 46: 401–22.

Osler, W. (1896). Lectures on angina pectoris and allied states. *NY J Med* 4: 224.

Osler, W. (1910). Angina pectoris. *The Lancet* 1: 297.

Paradiso, S., Robinson, R.G. and Arndt, S. (1996). Self-reported aggressive behavior in patients with stroke. *J Nerv Ment Dis* 184: 746–53.

Parikh, R.M., Robinson, R.G., Lipsey, J.R. et al. (1990). The impact of poststroke depression on recovery in activities of daily living over a 2-year follow-up. *Arch Neurol* 47: 785–9.

Pasqual-Leone, A., Catala, M.D., Pascual-Leone Pasqual, A. (1996). Lateralized effect of rapid-rate transcranial magnetic stimulation of the prefrontal cortex on mood. *Neurology* 46: 499–502.

Pittam, J. and Scherer, K.R. (1993). Vocal expression and communication of emotion. In *Handbook of Emotions*, ed. M. Lewis and J.M. Haviland, pp. 112–19. New York: Guilford Press.

Prigatano, G.P. and Schacter, D.L. (1991). *Awareness of Deficit after Brain Injury. Clinical and Theoretical Issues.* New York: Oxford University Press.

Ramasubbu, R. (1994). Denial of illness and depression in stroke (letter; comment). *Stroke* 25: 226–7.

Reding, J.J., Orto, L.A., Winter, S.W. et al. (1986). Antidepressant therapy after stroke: a double blind trial. *Arch Neurol* 43: 763–5.

Robinson, R.G., Boston, J.D., Starkstein, S.E. and Price, T.R. (1988). Comparison of mania and depression after brain injury: causal factors. *Am J Psychiatry* 145: 172–8.

Robsinson, R.G., Parikh, R.M., Lipsey, J.R., Starkstein, S.E. and Price, T.R. (1993). Pathological laughing and crying following stroke: validation of a measurement scale and a double-blind treatment study (see comments). *Am Psychiatry* 150: 286–93.

Roseman, I. (1984). Cognitive determinants of emotion: a structural theory. In Shaver, P. *Review of Personality and Social Psychology*, Vol. 5: *Emotions, Relationships and Health*, ed. P. Shaver, pp. 11–36. Beverley Hills: Sage.

Ross, E.D. (1981). The aprosodias. Functional–anatomic organization of the affective components of language in the RH. *Arch Neurol* 38: 561–9.

Ross, E.D. and Mesulam, M.M. (1979). Dominant language functions of the RH? Prosody and emotional gesturing. *Arch Neurol* 36: 144–8.

Ross, E.D. and Rush, A.J. (1981). Diagnosis and neuroanatomical correlates of depression in brain-damaged patients. Implications for a neurology of depression. *Arch Gen Psychiatry* 38: 1344–54.

Scherer, K.R. (1984). On the nature and function of emotions: a component process approach. In Approaches to Emotion, ed. K.R. Scherer and P. Ekman, pp. 293–317. Hillsdale, NJ: Erlbaum.

Sharpe, M., Hawton, K., Seagroatt, V. et al. (1994). Depressive disorders in long-term survivors of stroke. Associations with demographic and social factors, functional status, and brain lesion volume. *Br J Psychiatry* 164: 380–6.

Sher, K.J. (1987). Stress response dampering. In *Psychological Theories of Drinking and Alcoholism*, ed. H.T. Bland and K.E. Leonard, pp. 227–71. New York: Guilford Press.

Sinyor, D., Jaques, P., Kaloupek, D.G. et al. (1986). Poststroke depression and lesion location. An attempted replication. *Brain* 109: 537–46.

Spence, J.D. (1996). Cerebral consequences of hypertension. *J Hypertension* 14 (Suppl. 5): S139–45.

Starkstein, S.E. (1998). Mood disorders after stroke. In *Cerebrovascular Disease*, ed. M. Grinsberg and J. Bogousslavsky, pp. 131–8. Oxford: Blackwell Science.

Starkstein, S.E., Berthier, M.L., Fedoroff, P., Price, T.R. and Robinson, R.G. (1990a). Anosognosia and major depression in 2 patients with cerebrovascular lesions. *Neurology* 40: 1380–2.

Starkstein, S.E., Boston, J.D. and Robinson, R.G. (1988a). Mechanisms of mania after brain injury. 12 case reports and review of the literature. (Review). *J Nerv Ment Dis* 176: 87–100.

Starkstein, S.E., Cohen, B.S., Fedoroff, P. et al. (1990b). Relationship between anxiety disorders and depressive disorders in patients with cerebrovascular injury. *Arch Gen Psychiatry* 47: 246–51.

Starkstein, S.E., Fedoroff, J.P., Price, T.R., Leiguarda, R. and Robinson, R.G. (1993a). Apathy following cerebrovascular lesions. *Stroke* 24: 1625–30.

Starkstein, S.E., Fedoroff, J.P., Price, T.R., Leiguarda, R. and Robinson, R.G. (1993b). Catastrophic reaction after cerebrovascular lesions: frequency, correlates, and validation of a scale. *J Neuropsychiatry Clin Neurosci* 5: 189–94.

Starkstein, S.E., Federoff, J.P., Price, T.R., Leiguarda, R.C. and Robinson, R.G. (1994). Neuropsychological and neuroradiological correlates of emotional prosody comprehension. *Neurology* 44: 515–22.

Starkstein, S.E., Mayberg, H.S., Berthier, M.L. et al. (1990c). Mania after brain injury: neuroradiological and metabolic findings. *Ann Neurol* 27: 652–9.

Starkstein, S.E., Pearlson, G.D., Boston, J. and Robinson, R.G. (1987). Mania after brain injury. A controlled study of causative factors. *Arch Neurol* 44: 1069–73.

Starkstein, S.E. and Robinson, R.G. (1989). Affective disorders and cerebral vascular disease. (Review). *Br J Psychiatry* 154: 170–82.

Starkstein, S.E. and Robinson, R.G. (1990). Depression following cerebrovascular lesions. (Review). *Semin Neurol* 10: 247–53.

Starkstein, S.E., Robinson, R.G., Berthier, M.L. and Price, T.R. (1988b). Depressive disorders following stroke in the posterior circulation as compared with middle cerebral artery infarcts. *Brain* 111: 375–87.

Starkstein, S.E., Robinson, R.G. and Price, T.R. (1988c). Comparison of patients with and without post-stroke major depression matched for size and location of the lesion. *Arch Gen Psychiatry* 45: 247–52.

Starter, M. and Markowitsch, H.J. (1985). The amygdala's role in human mnemonic processing. *Cortex* 21: 7–24.

Stone, V.E., Nisenson, L., Eliassen, J.C. and Gazzaniga, M.S. (1996). Left hemisphere representation of emotional facial expressions. *Neuropsychologia* 34: 23–9.

Ullman, M., Ashenhurst, E.M., Hurwitz, L.J. and Gruen, A. (1960). Motivational and structural factors in the denial of hemiplegia. *Arch Neurol* 3: 306–18.

Ullman, M. and Gruen, A. (1961). Behavioral change in patients with strokes. *Am J Psychiatry* 117: 1004–9.

Vuilleumier, P., Ghika-Schmid, F., Bogousslavsky, J., Assal, G. and Regli, F. (1998). Persistent recurrence of hypomania and prosoaffective agnosia in a patient with right thalamic infarct. *Neuropsychiatry Neuropsychol Behav Neurol* 12: 120–30.

Wassertheil-Smoller, S., Applegate, W.B., Berge, K. et al. (1996). Change in depression as a precursor of cardiovascular events. SHEP Cooperative Research Group (Systolic Hypertension in the Elderly). *Arch Int Med* 156: 553–61.

Watanabe, M.D., Martin, E.M., DeLeon, O.A. et al. (1995). Successful methylphenidate treatment of apathy after subcortical infarcts. *J Neuropsychiatry Clin Neurosci* 7(4): 502–4.

Weintraub, S., Mesulam, M.M. and Kramer, L. (1981). Disturbances in prosody. A right-hemisphere contribution to language. *Arch Neurol* 38: 742–4.

5

Depression and lesion location in stroke

Robert G. Robinson

Introduction

The relationship between depressive disorder and lesion location has been, perhaps, the most controversial area of research in the field of post-stroke mood disorders. Although the association between specific clinical symptomatology and lesion location is one of the fundamental goals of clinical practice in neurology, this has rarely been the case with psychiatric disorders. Cognitive functions such as visual spatial reasoning, auditory comprehension, speech production, and extent and severity of motor or sensory impairment are all symptoms of stroke which are commonly used by clinicians to localize lesions to particular brain regions. There is, however, no known neuropathology consistently associated with primary mood disorders (i.e., mood disorders not associated with a physical illness), and, even among secondary mood disorders (i.e., mood disorders associated with a physical illness) the idea that there may be a focal neuropathology associated with the development of major depression has led to both surprise and skepticism.

Our finding of a clinical–pathological correlation between the severity of depression, as measured by depression rating scales, and the distance of the lesion from the frontal pole on a computerized tomography (CT) scan image, as measured by the distance in millimeters between the anterior border of the lesion and the frontal pole, was first reported in 1981 by Robinson and Szetela. We reported an inverse correlation between the overall severity of depressive symptoms, determined by combining three depression rating scales, and the distance of the anterior border of the lesion from the frontal pole normalized to the overall anterior to posterior length of the brain. Since then, this finding has turned out to be one of the most robust and consistently replicated clinical – pathological correlations reported in psychiatry. This phenomenon is discussed in greater detail in the section on the relationship between depression and anterior–posterior lesion location, but the ability to study the relationship between symptomatology and lesion location is

An earlier version of this chapter was published in *The Clinical Neuropsychiatry of Stroke* by Robert G. Robinson, Cambridge University Press, 1998, and is reproduced here with the agreement of the publishers.

one of the benefits of studying mood disorders in patients with stroke lesions. Because studies of patients with primary mood disorders have not been able to associate clinical symptoms with focal neuropathology, utilizing patients with known neuropathological disorders to examine potential clinical–pathological relationships in mood disorders may provide more insights than are possible with studies of primary disorders. These kinds of studies of patients with brain lesions might ultimately provide a basis for identifying the location of more subtle neuropathology in patients with primary mood disorders. In fact, reports using positron emission tomography (PET) brain imaging techniques have identified metabolic and blood flow abnormalities in the left prefrontal cortex of patients with primary major depression (Baxter et al., 1989; Martinot et al., 1990; Bench et al., 1992; Drevets et al., 1992). These studies demonstrate the potential for validating the neuroanatomical mechanism of mood disorders based on the convergence of findings from studies utilizing patients with post-stroke depression and patients with primary mood disorders.

Effects of interhemispheric and intrahemispheric lesion location

The effect of unilateral ischemic lesions on depression was examined in a series of patients with no risk factors for depression admitted to hospital after an acute stroke lesion (Robinson et al., 1984a). All patients were right-handed and had a single stroke lesion of the right or left hemisphere which was visible on a CT scan. Patients were included only if they had no previous personal or family history of psychiatric disorder. The background characteristics of these patients are shown in Table 5.1.

Major or minor depression was found in 14 of 22 patients with left hemisphere lesions and two of 14 patients with right hemisphere lesions ($p<0.01$) (Robinson et al., 1984a). In addition to the increased frequency of depression in patients with left hemisphere lesions, the intrahemispheric lesion location was also an important determinant of the frequency of depression. Among ten patients who had left *anterior* lesions (i.e., the anterior border of the lesion was *rostral* to 40% of the overall anterior–posterior length of the brain on CT scan), six had depression as compared to only one of eight patients with left posterior lesions (i.e., the anterior border of the lesion was caudal to 40% of the anterior–posterior distance, $p<0.05$). The percentage of patients with depressive disorder among those with lesions of each quadrant of the brain are shown in Fig. 5.1. Thus, patients with left anterior hemisphere injuries were found to have a significant greater frequency of major depression than patients with any other lesion location.

This issue was also looked at in another study of 45 patients with single lesions restricted to either cortical or subcortical structures in the right or left hemisphere

Table 5.1. Characteristics of single-lesion patients

Characteristic	Left hemisphere (n=22)	Right hemisphere (n=14)
Age (mean±SD in years)	57±12	61±10
Gender (% male)	53	73
Race (% white)	33	37
Socioeconomic class (Hollingshead IV or V) mean	40	45
Marital status (% married)	90	82
No. of children (mean±SD)	1.6±3.9	2.5±2.1
Origin (% rural)	33	54
No. of siblings (mean±SD)	4.5±3.9	4.8±4.0
Tobacco use (% 1 pack/day or greater)	57	46
Previous medical illness (%) (life threatening)	10	27
Time since stroke (mean no. of days±SD)	12±12	10±7

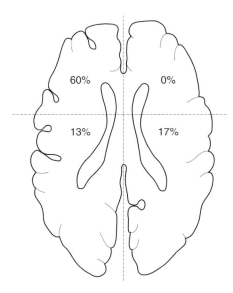

Fig. 5.1   Schematic axial slice of the brain at the level of the body of the lateral ventricles. The brain is shown divided into four quadrants, and the numbers indicate the percentage of patients who had major depression during the acute post-stroke period following a lesion whose anterior border lay within that quadrant. Patients with left anterior lesions had a significantly higher frequency of major depression than patients with any other lesion location. (From Robinson et al., 1984a.)

Table 5.2. Characteristics of patients: lesion location

Characteristic	L Cortical (n=16)	R Cortical (n=9)	L Subcortical (n=13)	R Subcortical (n=7)
Age (mean ± SD in years)	59 ± 12	54 ± 13	63 ± 12	54 ± 8
Gender (% male)	60	88	54	57
Race (% black)	50	33	80	100
Marital status (% married)	87	100	100	86
Mean no. of children	2	2	3	3
Origin (% rural)	27	11	31	14
Mean no. of siblings	3	3	4	3
Tobacco use (% > pack/day)	44	22	23	29
Previous medical illness (% life threatening)	25	22	28	29
Time since stroke (mean days ± SD)	23 ± 25	18 ± 14	19 ± 21	20 ± 19
Education (mean no. of years ± SD)	9 ± 3	11 ± 4	9 ± 3	8 ± 3
Family history of psychiatric disorder (% positive)	6	23	11	14
Personal history of psychiatric disorder (% positive)				
Alcholism	19	15	11	28
Other	6	0	11	14

(Starkstein et al., 1987). The background characteristics of these patients, who are grouped according to whether they had a cortical or subcortical lesion location, are shown in Table 5.2. Patients were included only if they had single lesions on CT scan which were exclusively limited to either the subcortical gray nuclei or the cerebral cortex and underlying white matter. Patients with subcortical lesions had infarcts limited to the basal ganglia, thalamus, or white matter of the internal capsule without any involvement of cortical gray matter or subcortical white matter. Patients with cortical lesions had ischemic damage of the cerebral cortical gray matter or underlying white matter.

We found that 44% of patients with left cortical lesions were depressed (i.e., four of 16 had major and three of 16 had minor depression) and 39% of patients with left subcortical lesions were similarly depressed (i.e., four of 13 with major and one of 13 with minor depression). In contrast, only 11% of patients with right cortical lesions (none of nine with major, one of nine with minor depression) and 14% of patients with right subcortical lesions were depressed (one of seven with major, none of seven with minor depression) (Fig. 5.2). Patients with lesions of the left

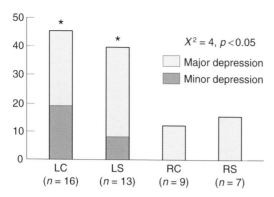

Fig. 5.2   The percentage of patients with major or minor depression grouped according to stroke lesion location. Patients with either left cortical or left subcortical lesions had a significantly higher frequency of major depression during the acute post-stroke period than patients with right hemisphere lesions. LC=left cortical, LS=left subcortical, RC= right cortical, RS=right subcortical. (From Starkstein et al., 1987.)

hemisphere had significantly higher rates of depression than patients with right hemisphere lesions, regardless of the cortical or subcortical location of the lesion ($p<0.01$).

The patients were further grouped according to whether they had anterior or posterior lesions (i.e., anterior lesions were defined as lesions in which the rostral border was less than 40% of the overall anterior–posterior length of the brain on CT scan; posterior lesions were defined as lesions in which the rostral border was located at more than 40% of the anterior–posterior dimension). All five patients with left cortical anterior lesions involving the frontal lobe had depression (three major, two minor depression) as compared to only two out of 11 patients with left cortical posterior lesions involving the temporal, parietal, and/or occipital cortex (one major, one minor depression, $p<0.01$). Moreover, four of the six patients with left subcortical anterior lesions had major depression (none had minor depression) as compared to one minor depression (none with major depression) among seven patients with left subcortical posterior lesions ($p<0.01$).

A subsequent study (Starkstein et al., 1988a), which included the 20 patients with subcortical lesions from the previous study as well as five new patients, examined the relationship between lesions of specific subcortical nuclei and depression. Patients were included if they had a single stroke lesion limited entirely to the basal ganglia/internal capsule or thalamus of the right or left hemisphere with no evidence of other brain lesions. The frequency of major or minor depression in each group is shown in Fig. 5.3. Basal ganglia (caudate and/or putamen) lesions produced major depression in seven out of eight patients with left hemisphere lesions but in only one of seven patients with right hemisphere lesions. None of the

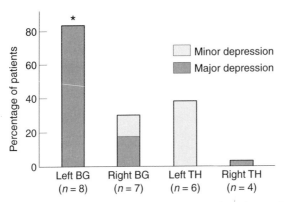

Fig. 5.3   The percentage of patients with major or minor depression based on the location of their subcortical lesions. Patients with left basal ganglia lesions had a significantly higher frequency of major depression than those with any other lesion location. BG = basal ganglia, TH = thalamus. (From Starkstein et al., 1988a.)

patients with left ($n=6$) or right ($n=4$) thalamic lesions had major depression ($p<0.001$).

Studies by other investigators have sometimes shown similar lateralized effects of stroke lesions, but sometimes have not. The variable which seemed most likely to account for differences in findings between studies was 'time since stroke.' For example, in contrast to our studies of acute stroke patients examined one to two weeks following stroke, a study of 88 Australian patients seen in a rehabilitation hospital 8.4 weeks (average) following stroke found that 43% of patients with left hemisphere lesions had a major or minor depression and 38% of patients with right hemisphere lesions had depression (Morris et al., 1990). Similarly, Eastwood et al. (1989) examined 87 patients admitted to a rehabilitation hospital 12 weeks (average) after stroke. Of 28 patients with left hemisphere lesions, 50% had either major or minor depression, while among 45 patients with right hemisphere stroke 62% had major or minor depression. Thus, both of these studies which examined patients in rehabilitation hospitals at approximately two to three months post-stroke failed to show a lateralized effect of hemispheric brain injury on the frequency of depression.

House et al. (1990) examined 95 patients at one month after their first episode of stroke (no variance in this time was reported). Another 33 patients were seen for the first time at six months following stroke. Of the 40 patients with a lesion visible on CT scan involving one cerebral hemisphere, one of 19 patients (5%) with a left hemisphere lesion, and three of 21 patients (14%) with a right hemisphere lesion, had major depression. When patients were grouped according to whether they had an anterior or posterior lesion, one out of eight (13%) patients with left anterior, and none of seven with right anterior lesions had major depression. Among patients with posterior hemisphere lesions, none of five with left posterior, and three of eight (38%) with right posterior lesions had depression. At six months (combining 33 new patients at follow-up with the original patients), three out of nine patients (33%) with left anterior, two out of seven (29%) with right anterior, none of ten with left posterior, and two of 22 (9%) with right posterior lesions had major depression. Thus, although there was a tendency for right posterior lesions to be associated with major depression (at one month this was significant; i.e., $p < 0.05$, compared to the association between major depression and lesions of the right anterior plus left posterior hemispheres), the small number of major depressions (i.e., 10%) made this difficult to evaluate. The fact that no intrahemispheric lesion location was associated with depression at six months was consistent with the idea that laterality and intrahemisphere lesion location are associated with major depression only during the acute stroke period.

Dam, Pedersen and Ahlgren (1989) examined 92 patients at between eight and 1280 days post-stroke (median 35 days). Out of 92 patients, 28 (30%) had major ($n = 17$) or minor ($n = 11$) depression. Although the relationship between the diagnosis of depression and the location of the intrahemispheric lesion was not investigated, patients with lesions involving the right frontal cortex ($n = 16$) had significantly higher Hamilton depression scores (median 8) than those with any other lesion location. Furthermore, the mean Hamilton depression score was highest (NS) in patients who were 181–360 days post-stroke. This study involved such a mix of acute-stage and chronic-stage stroke patients without giving their diagnosis at each stage that it is difficult to determine whether these findings would support the hypothesis of a lateralized effect on depression of left anterior lesions during the acute stroke period.

In contrast to these studies, which failed to show a lateralized effect of hemispheric brain injury on mood, a study by Astrom, Adolfsson and Asplund (1993), examining 44 patients during the acute hospitalization from stroke (mean ten days post-stroke), found that 67% of 21 patients with left hemisphere stroke had major depression compared with only 9% of 23 patients with right hemisphere stroke ($p < 0.001$). When the anterior–posterior location of the lesion was examined (anterior lesions were defined in the same way as in our studies), 86% of 14 patients with left anterior lesions had major depression compared with only 28% of seven patients with left posterior lesions ($p = 0.017$). When these same patients were examined three months later, however, the frequency of depression in patients with right hemisphere lesions had significantly increased from 9% to 36% and the difference in the frequency of depression between patients with right or left hemisphere injury was no longer statistically significant.

Similarly, Herrmann, Bartels and Wallesch (1993) examined 21 acute ($<$ three months post-stroke) and 21 chronic (<six months post-stroke) aphasic patients with single left hemisphere lesions. Definite major depression, using research diagnostic criteria (RDC) classification, was found in five patients with acute stroke but in no patients with chronic stroke ($p<0.05$). Major (definite or probable) depression or minor depression was found in seven out of ten nonfluent aphasia patients who had CT-verified acute left frontal stroke lesions. This rate of depression was also significantly greater than that found in patients with CT-verified left posterior lesions and fluent aphasia (none of seven patients, $p<0.01$).

Changes over time in lesion locations associated with depression

We have recently examined the relationship between location of brain injury and depression over the first two years following stroke. Using the same population of stroke patients with follow-up (i.e., 142 patients) we identified patients who had a single stroke lesion involving either the right or left middle cerebral artery distribution that was visible on CT scan and who had had a follow-up evaluation either at three or six months (short-term follow-up) or at 12 or 24 months (long-term follow-up). Of 60 possible patients who met these qualifications, 41 were seen at short-term follow-up and 46 were seen at long-term follow-up. There were no statistically significant differences between the short-term and long-term follow-up groups in terms of age, gender, race, marital status, education, socioeconomic status, frequency of family or personal psychiatric history or prevalence of major or minor depression (39% of the short-term follow-up patients and 43% of the long-term follow-up patients had in-hospital major or minor depression). The frequency of depression in patients with right and left hemisphere lesions during the initial evaluation and at the short-term and long-term follow-up is shown in Fig. 5.4. During the initial evaluation, patients with left hemisphere stroke had a significantly higher prevalence of both major and minor depression (as defined by DSM-IV criteria) than patients with right hemisphere stroke ($p=0.0006$) (Fig. 5.4). At short-term and long-term follow-up, however, there were no significant differences between right and left hemisphere lesion groups in terms of the frequency of major or minor depression (Fig. 5.4).

These studies involving patients over the first two years post-stroke support the importance of intrahemispheric lesion location in determining the frequency of major depression during the acute stroke period. The failure by other investigators to find a lateralized effect of both hemispheric and intrahemispheric lesion location was probably the result of examining patients who were beyond the first few weeks following their stroke.

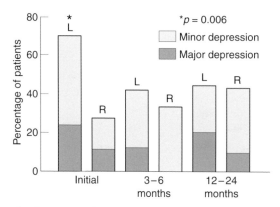

Fig. 5.4   The frequency of major and minor depression defined by DSM-IV criteria associated with single lesions of the right or left hemisphere during the acute stroke period and at follow-up. The lateralized effects of left hemisphere lesions on both major and minor depression was found only during the acute stroke period. At short-term and long-term follow-up, there were no hemispheric lesion effects on the frequency of depression.

Correlation between severity of depression and anterior–posterior location

Perhaps the most remarkable finding from the studies of lesion location in patients with post-stroke depression is the statistically significant correlation between the severity of depression and the proximity of the lesion to the frontal pole. This correlation was first reported in 1981 in a study which compared the severity of depression between patients with traumatic brain injury (TBI) ($n=11$) and stroke ($n=18$) (Fig. 5.5; Robinson and Szetela, 1981). All patients had brain lesions demonstrable on CT scan which involved the left hemisphere. Although patients with stroke had more severe depressive symptoms compared with patients with TBI, for a combined group of 16 patients with either stroke or TBI lesions which extended into the frontal lobe (i.e., the anterior border of the lesion was rostral to 60% of the overall anterior–posterior length of the brain), there was significant inverse correlation between the severity of depression and the distance between the anterior border of the lesion and the frontal pole (Pearson correlation coefficient $r=-0.76$, $p<0.001$) (Fig. 5.5). Thus, for a combined group of patients with either stroke or TBI, the closer the lesion was to the frontal pole the more severe the associated depressive symptoms.

This finding does not appear to be as sensitive to time since stroke as the laterality finding, and numberous subsequent studies have reported similar findings. One subsequent study (Robinson et al., 1984b), which has already been described, involved 36 patients with single stroke lesions of the right ($n=14$) or left ($n=22$) hemisphere demonstrable on CT scan. All patients were right-handed with no previous history of stroke or other brain lesions and had no risk factors for depression

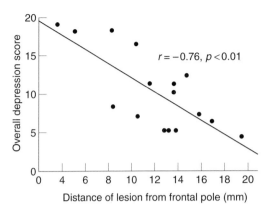

Fig. 5.5   Scattergram showing the correlation between severity of depression (overall score based on a combination of Hamilton Depression, Zung Depression, and Nurses' Rating Scale scores) and proximity of the anterior border of the lesion to the frontal pole as measured on CT scan. Patients all had left hemisphere lesions secondary to stroke or traumatic brain injury. (From Robinson and Szetela, 1981.)

such as previous personal or family history of psychiatric disorder. Patients were examined at an average of 12 days after their stroke. Among patients with left-sided lesions whose anterior border was rostral to 40% of the overall anterior–posterior brain distance, there was a significant inverse correlation between the severity of depressive symptoms–as measured by a combined score on the Zung depression scale, Hamilton depression scale, and total score on the present state examination – and the distance between the lesion and the frontal pole (Fig. 5.6). Thus, for patients with left anterior lesions (i.e., less than 40% of the anterior–posterior distance), lesions closer to the frontal pole were associated with more severe depressive symptoms compared with lesions further from the frontal pole. In the right hemisphere, however, the correlation was in the opposite direction, with more posterior lesions being associated with more severe depressive symptoms (Fig. 5.6). Although the correlation was strongest in patients with left anterior lesions, if patients with left posterior lesions (i.e., anterior border of the lesion was caudal to 40% of the overall anterior–posterior length of the brain) were included (total increased from 11 to 22), the correlation decreased to $r = -0.54$ but remained significant ($p < 0.01$). A similar correlation between severity of depression and distance of the lesion from the frontal pole was also found in the previously described study of patients with cortical lesions (i.e., lesions restricted to the cortex) of the left hemisphere ($n = 16$; $r = -0.52$, $p < 0.05$) (Fig. 5.7) or subcortical lesions (i.e., lesions only involving subcortical gray matter) of the left hemisphere ($n = 13$; $r = -0.68$, $p < 0.01$) (Fig. 5.8; Starkstein et al., 1987). We have also found a similar correlation between the proximity of the lesion to the frontal pole and the severity

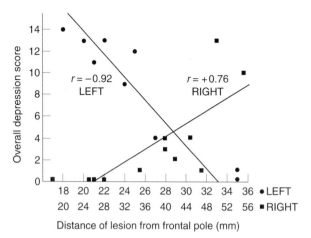

Fig. 5.6   Scattergram showing the correlation between severity of depression (overall score based on a combination of Hamilton Depression and Present State Examination scores) and proximity of the anterior border of the lesion to the frontal pole. Patients had single lesions of the right or left hemisphere and no risk factors (i.e., family or personal history of psychiatric disorder) for depression and were right-handed. Left hemisphere lesions were all anterior to 40% of the overall anterior–posterior brain measurement. The severity of depression increased with the proximity of the lesion to the frontal pole in patients with left hemisphere lesions; however, for those with right hemisphere lesions, depression increased with the proximity to the occipital pole. (From Robinson et al., 1984a).

of depression in left-handed patients with single left hemisphere lesions ($n = 13$; $r = -0.78$, $p < 0.01$) (Robinson et al., 1985).

Similar correlations have now been reported by investigators in Canada, UK, Germany, and Australia (Fig. 5.9). Some investigators found that the correlation between the severity of depression and the proximity of the lesion to the frontal pole applied to combined right and left hemisphere lesion groups (Sinyor et al., 1986; House et al., 1990), while others found this to be the case only among patients with left-sided lesions (Eastwood et al., 1989; Morris et al., 1992). The investigators who found significant correlations among patients with either right or left hemisphere lesions, studied subjects who were more than one month post-stroke. An increase in the frequency of depression among patients with right hemisphere lesions between the acute post-stroke period and at three months post-stroke (e.g., Astrom et al., 1993, found an increase from 9% during the acute stroke period to 36% at three months follow-up) may explain why some studies found a correlation for both right and left hemisphere lesions while other studies (found significant correlations only for patients with left hemisphere lesions (i.e., acute patients).

The remarkable aspect of this finding, however, is that every study which has examined the relationship between the severity of depression and the proximity of

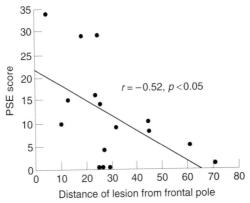

$r = -0.52, p < 0.05$

Fig. 5.7   Scattergram showing the correlation between severity of depression (overall score based on the Present State Examination, PSE) and proximity of the anterior border of the lesion to the frontal pole. Distance is expressed as percentage of the total A-P distance. Data are from patients who had lesions restricted to the cortex of the left hemisphere and/or the underlying white matter. (From Starkstein et al., 1987.)

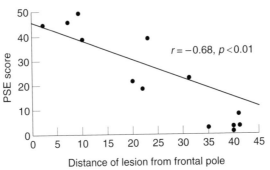

$r = -0.68, p < 0.01$

Fig. 5.8   Scattergram showing the correlation between severity of depression (overall score based on a combination of Hamilton Depression and Present State Examination scores) and proximity of the anterior border of the lesion to the frontal pole. Distance is expressed as percentage of the total A-P distance. Patients all had subcortical lesions restricted to the basal ganglia, thalamus, or internal capsule. (From Starkstein et al., 1987.)

the lesion to the frontal pole during the first six months post-stroke has found a statistically significant inverse correlation (Fig. 5.9). Although studies differ in the reported strength of the correlation and, therefore, in the amount of variance in the severity of depression which could be explained by anterior–posterior lesion location, this phenomenon has emerged as one of the most consistent and robust clinical–pathological correlations ever described in neuropsychiatry. This is certainly a phenomenon which is deserving of further research. There is likely to be an

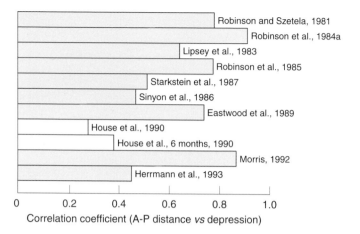

Correlation coefficient (A-P distance *vs* depression)

Fig. 5.9   Magnitude of correlation coefficients between severity of depression and proximity of the lesion to the frontal pole (left hemisphere or combined left and right hemisphere lesion data) for all studies which have examined this correlation. All correlations were statistically significant and ranged in magnitude so that between 8% and 80% of the variance in depression severity can be explained.

important physiological or anatomical factor which underlies this clinical–pathological correlation and may provide important clues concerning the neural mechanisms involved in depressive disorder. This neural mechanism may be relevant both to post-stroke depression and to primary depressive disorder.

As with other findings in post-stroke depression, the correlation between the proximity of the lesion to the frontal pole and the severity of depression changes over time (Robinson et al., 1986; Parikh et al., 1987). In the two-year longitudinal study previously described (i.e., 103 acute stroke patients with follow-up data including positive single lesion CT scan for 30 patients), we found significant inverse correlations between the severity of depression and the proximity of the lesion to the frontal pole in patients with left hemisphere lesions in hospital as well as at six months ($n=9$) and one year ($n=6$) post-stroke (Fig. 5.10). At two years post-stroke ($n=7$), however, there was no significant correlation between anterior–posterior lesion location and the severity of depression.

Because of the relatively small numbers in our previous assessment, we have examined the relationship between the severity of depressive symptoms and the proximity of the lesion to the frontal pole in our overall population of 140 patients seen for follow-up (Shimoda and Robinson, 1999). This represents the total number of patients seen in follow-up from the original 103 patients plus a second group of 112 new patients. We obtained CT scans showing single lesions and follow-up data for 60 of these patients. Correlations between the severity of depression, as measured by the total score on the present state examination, and the

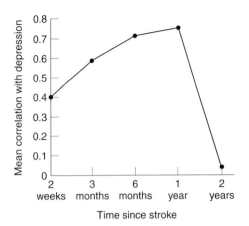

Fig. 5.10   Changes over the first two years following stroke in the correlation between the proximity of the left hemisphere lesion to the frontal pole (measured at the time of the acute stroke) and severity of depression (measured at 3, 6, 12, or 24 months post-stroke). The correlations were statistically significant during the first year post-stroke, but were no longer significant at two years post-stroke. (From Parikh et al., 1988.)

proximity of the lesion to the frontal pole are shown in Fig. 5.11. During the initial evaluation, there was a significant correlation between the severity of depression and the proximity of the lesion to the left frontal pole ($n=34$). There was also a significant correlation between the severity of depression and left hemisphere lesion volume ($r=0.4$, $p<0.05$). There were no significant correlations, however, between the severity of depression and the proximity of the lesion to the frontal pole or lesion volume among patients with right hemisphere lesions ($n=26$) (lesion volume $r=0.13$, $p=$NS).

At short-term follow-up, there continued to be a significant correlation between the severity of depression and the distance between the anterior border of the lesion and the frontal pole, as well as a significant correlation between the severity of depression and lesion volume for patients with left hemisphere lesions ($n=26$). In contrast to the acute stroke period, at short-term follow-up, among patients with right hemisphere lesions, there was a significant correlation between the severity of depression and the proximity of the lesion to the frontal pole ($n=15$) (Fig. 5.11). There was, however, no significant correlation between depression severity and lesion volume ($r=0.23$, $p=$NS). In addition, a two-way analysis of variance (ANOVA) of Hamilton depression scores examining the factors of right or left hemisphere lesion location and cortical or subcortical lesion location demonstrated a significant interaction ($p=0.04$). Left cortical lesions were associated with the most severe depression scores.

At long-term follow-up (i.e., 12–24 months), there was no significant correlation

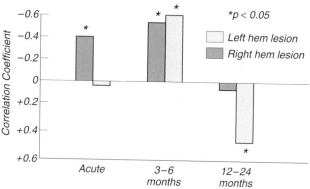

Fig. 5.11　Spearman correlation coefficients between severity of depression, as measured by PSE total score, and distance of the lesion from the frontal pole, as measured on CT scan. A negative correlation indicates that depression increased with proximity of the lesion to the frontal pole, and a positive correlation indicates that depression increased with the proximity of the lesion to the occipital pole. During the acute stroke period, depression severity correlated with the proximity of the lesion to the frontal pole, but only among patients with left hemisphere lesions. During short-term follow-up, the proximity of the lesion to the frontal pole was correlated with more severe depression for both right and left hemisphere lesions. At long-term follow-up, severity of depression was significantly correlated with the proximity of the lesion to the occipital pole (i.e., lesions further away from the frontal pole), but only for patients with right hemisphere lesions. These findings demonstrate the dynamic nature of clinical–pathological correlations in post-stroke depression.

between the severity of depression as measured by the present state examination score and the proximity of the lesion to the frontal pole or lesion volume among patients with left hemisphere stroke ($n=25$). Among patients were right hemisphere stroke ($n=21$), however, lesion volume was correlated with the severity of depression (lesion volume $r=0.53$, $p=0.04$). Moreover, in contrast to previous results, severity of depression among patents with right hemisphere stroke was now correlated with the proximity of the lesion to the occipital pole (i.e., lesions further from the frontal pole were associated with more severe depression). A two-way ANOVA or Hamilton depression scores among patients at long-term follow-up showed no significant effect of either right or left hemisphere lesion location or cortical or subcortical lesion location, or their interaction, on the severity of depression.

This study found an intriguing, temporally dependent relationship between depression and lesion volume and lesion location. The association of depression with left anterior lesions was present only during the acute post-stroke period. By three to six months post-stroke, depression was related to the proximity of the lesion to the frontal pole in both the right and left hemisphere lesion patients. At long-term follow-up (12–24 months), however, depression was associated with lesion volume but then the severity of depression correlated with the proximity of the lesion to the occipital pole, but only among patients with right hemisphere stroke.

These findings are consistent with results reported by Schwartz et al. (1993) and Sharpe et al. (1994), i.e., that mood disorders after the acute stroke period and at long-term follow-up are correlated with right hemisphere lesion volume. Schwartz et al. (1993) examined 91 men undergoing stroke rehabilitation who were between one and 103 months post-stroke. Hamilton depression scores were significantly correlated with the position of the posterior lesion border in the right hemisphere and lesion volume. Sharpe et al. examined 60 surviving patients from a community study of individuals with first stroke who had a single brain lesion identified by CT scan. Patients were interviewed between three and five years following their stroke. A logistical regression analysis was performed examining the relationship between the existence of depression and demographic characteristics, personal and family history of psychiatric disorder, social relationships and living arrangements, functional impairment, cognitive impairment, and lesion volume. Independent associations with the existence of a DSM-III-R depression (five patients with major depression, six patients with dysthymia) were found for the severity of functional impairment (activities of daily living), female gender and lesion volume. Lesion volume showed an odds ratio of 6.9 (95% confidence 1.0–50), indicating that depressed patients were more than six times as likely to have a large lesion than nondepressed patients.

These findings of the dynamic nature of the relationship between the severity of depression and lesion characteristics also help to explain discrepancies between studies reported in the literature. House et al. (1990) and Sinyor et al. (1986) reported significant correlations between the proximity of the lesion to the frontal pole and the severity of depression for both right and left hemisphere lesions. In the House study, the correlation of total present state examination score and the proximity of the lesion to the frontal pole for combined right and left hemisphere lesions was $r = -0.25$, $p < 0.05$ for 40 patients at one month and $r = -0.28$, $p = 0.01$ for 63 patients at six months. Sinyor et al. (1986) found a correlation of $r = -0.37$, $p < 0.05$ for 33 patients with right or left hemisphere lesions. Dam et al. (1989) reported higher mean Hamilton scores in patients with right compared to left frontal lesions; however, these patients were examined between <three months and >two years since their stroke. In contrast, our patients and Astrom's patients were examined within the first two weeks post-stroke. Thus, the lack of agreement in the literature as well as the reported association between both left and right hemisphere lesions with post-stroke depression appear to be a consequence of the time at which patients were examined following their stroke. The increased frequency of major and minor depressions among patients with left anterior lesions has been found to be a phenomenon of the acute stroke period (i.e., the first three weeks post-stroke). The correlation between depression severity and the proximity of the lesion to the frontal pole, however, has been found to be a phenomenon of the first six months post-stroke.

A brief explanation of the hypothesized mechanism that we have proposed for this phenomenon may help to highlight the potential importance of this finding. The biogenic-amine-containing neurons which contain the neurotransmitter nor-epinephrine or serotonin have cell bodies located in the brain stem and send axonal projections rostrally toward the frontal pole. These ascending axons project through the median forebrain bundle into the deep layers of cortex in the frontal pole. The axons then arc posteriorly around the corpus callosum and run in the deep layers of the cortex anteriorly to posteriorly, sending arborizing branches into the superficial cortical layers. Lesions which are more anterior will disrupt more downstream (posterior) terminals than the more posterior lesions. This kind of anatomy might explain why a linear correlation exists between anterior lesion location and the severity of depression. Greater depletions of downstream (i.e., parietal or temporal) concentrations of norepinephrine or serotonin might lead to the development of depressive symptoms. Other anatomically based explanations might also be proposed, such as interruption of different types of cortical–cortical projections or frontal–temporal–basal ganglia connections. The anatomical structures involved in this correlation, however, may represent an important mechanism of primary as well as post-stroke depression.

Another interesting issue is why this temporal dynamic occurs in the relationship between the severity of depression and lesion location. It suggests that if physiological changes, including depletion of biogenic amines, occur in patients with left anterior lesions and lead to depression, these changes are hemisphere specific for only a few weeks. By two to three months following stroke (i.e., short-term follow-up), similar or alternative mechanisms occur in patients with right frontal lesions which lead to correlations of depression severity with the proximity of the lesion to the frontal pole in both right and left hemisphere lesion patients. The finding that depression was related to right posterior lesion location and lesion volume at long-term follow-up may emphasize the importance of impairment of right posterior hemisphere functions in the mechanism of depression in the chronic post-stroke period. Right hemisphere functions, such as spatial orientation, nonverbal memory and reasoning, as well as facial recognition, may be impaired. These impairments might then lead to a breakdown in the patients' ability to care for themselves or their social relationships and lead to depression. Alternatively, chronic dysfunction of the right hemisphere, which may play an important long-term role in emotion regulation, may be responsible for this finding. Whatever the explanation, however, this change in the dynamic relationship between lesion location and the severity of depression emphasizes the need to carefully control for the time since stroke when clinical–pathological correlations with depression are being examined. These findings also emphasize the fact that, for at least one to two years following stroke, changes are occurring which affect the relationship between depression and lesion location.

Relationship between depression and middle cerebral artery versus posterior circulation stroke

Although brain stem and cerebellar strokes are much less common that cerebral hemisphere strokes, they, nevertheless, constitute an important group of brain infarcts. In contrast to the motor and sensory symptoms that are common in patients with hemispheric infarcts involving the middle cerebral artery, patients with infarcts of the vertebral-basilar artery have symptoms of cranial nerve dysfunction, such as dysphagia or diplopia, or cerebellar dysfunction, such as ataxias or intention tremor. We examined patients with cerebral-basilar strokes to determine whether there was a difference between depression associated with infarcts of the posterior circulation (i.e., vertebral-basilar arteries supplying the brain stem, cerebellum, thalamus, and posterior hemispheres) and infarcts of the middle cerebral artery circulation (i.e., large areas of frontal, temporal, and parietal cortex, and subcortical structures including the basal ganglia). This study compared 37 consecutive patients with clinical findings or CT scan evidence indicating a first episode stroke in the posterior circulation with a consecutive series of 42 patients with single stroke lesions involving the middle cerebral artery territory. The background characteristics of these patients are shown in Table 5.3. All patients were evaluated during the first 30 days following stroke except for two patients with posterior circulation infarcts who were assessed during the second month post-stroke.

Neurological findings from each group are also shown in Table 5.3. Based on clinical signs or CT scan imaging, 39% of the patients with posterior circulation lesions (PC group) had cerebellar involvement, 30% had midbrain lesions, 26% had lesions of the pons, 22% had paramedian infarcts of the tegmentum, and 9% had lateral medullary infarcts. Among patients with middle cerebral artery infarcts (MCA group), 55% had left hemisphere lesions and 45% had right hemisphere lesions.

Among the 37 patients in the PC group, 27% were found to be depressed immediately after the acute lesion (four had DSM-III major and six had DSM-III minor depression). Among the 42 patients with MCA lesions, 48% developed depression immediately after the acute infarct (11 had major depression, and nine had minor

Table 5.3. Characteristics of posterior circulation lesion patients

Characteristic	PC group ($n=37$)	MCA group ($n=42$)
Age (years $\pm$ SD)	60.4 $\pm$ 13.5	59.7 $\pm$ 12.1
Gender (% female)	30	42
Race (% black)	62	64
Socioeconomic status (% Hollingshead class IV or V)	65	69
Marital status (% married)	51	50
No. of children (mean)	2	3
Education (mean years $\pm$ SD)	8.8 $\pm$ 4.4	9.8 $\pm$ 3.7
Tobacco (% smoking more than one pack/day)	19	38
Alcoholism (% hospitalized because of alcholism)	8	5
Familial history of psychiatric disorders (% positive)	11	5
Personal history of psychiatric disorders (% positive)	11	12
Previous medical illness (% with life-threatening illness)	18	14
Neurological findings		
Paresis (%)	57	81
Mild	32	50
Moderate	19	21
Severe	5	10
Sensory deficits (%)	35	38
Visual field deficits (%)	38	14
Cranial nerve involvement (%)	41	0
Cerebellar signs (%)	24	0
Aphasia (%)	3	21
Broca	0	10
Wernicke	0	5
Anomia	3	7
Lesions on CT scan (%)	49	71

Notes:
PC = posterior circulation.
MCA = middle cerebral artery.

depression). This higher frequency of depression among the MCA compared with the PC group just failed to reach statistical significance ($p=0.054$).

At six months follow-up, 82% of the patients with MCA lesions who were depressed (major or minor) in hospital remained depressed (Fig. 5.12). Among patients with PC lesions who were depressed (major or minor) at the in-hospital evaluation, only 20% remained depressed at the six months follow-up ($p<0.05$). At one or two years follow-up, the percentage of patients with continued

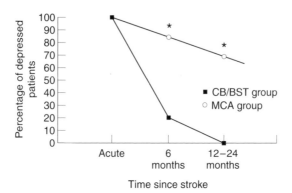

Fig. 5.12   The percentage of patients with depression after an acute stroke who remained
depressed at six months and at the one-year or two-year follow-up. Patients with
brainstem or cerebellar infarcts (CB/BST) recovered from depression (without treatment)
significantly more quickly than patients with left or right middle cerebral artery (MCA; i.e.,
hemispheric) infarcts. (From Starkstein et al., 1988a.)

depression was 68% for the MCA group and zero for the PC group ($p < 0.05$).
Although the significantly shorter course of depression in the PC as compared to
the MCA group might be hypothesized to result from the PC group having smaller
lesion volumes than the MCA group, there was no significant correlation between
lesion volume and the severity of depression for the combined group of MCA and
PC lesion patients either in hospital or at one-year or two-year follow-up.

The relationship between depression and impairment was examined by dividing
MCA and PC lesion patients into groups of those with major depression, minor
depression, or no depression. Among patients with PC lesions, neither intergroup
comparisons using ANOVA (e.g., Mini-Mental State Examination scores across the
three diagnostic groups) nor dimensional comparisons using correlational analysis (e.g. Hamilton depression score correlated with Mini-Mental State
Examination score) demonstrated a significant relationship between depression
(diagnosis or severity) and cognitive impairment (measured by the Mini-Mental
State Examination), activities of daily living (measured by the Johns Hopkins
Functioning Inventory, JHFI, or social support (measured by the Social
Functioning examination). Among the patients with MCA lesions, however, those
with major depression had significantly higher (i.e., more impaired) JHFI scores
(activities of daily living) than patients with minor depression or no mood disorder ($p < 0.05$).

The finding that patients with cerebellar-brain stem lesions had significantly
shorter durations of depression than patients with MCA distribution lesions suggests that the mechanism of depression may be different in these two groups of
patients. We suggested that one possible explanation for this shorter course of

depression following brain stem lesions was that PC lesions produce less injury to the biogenic amine pathways compared with hemispheric MCA lesions. As indicated in the previous section, the norepinephrinergic and serotonergic cell bodies located in the locus ceruleus or raphe nucleus project both to rostral and caudal brain regions (Morrison, Molliver and Grzanna, 1979). Interruption of these *ascending* norepinephrinergic or serotonergic pathways in the basal ganglia or cerebral cortex could lead to widespread dysfunction of the biogenic amine system in uninjured downstream areas of cortex. This could ultimately lead to clinical symptoms of depression. Similarly, brain stem lesions which interrupt *descending* norepinephrinergic projections into the lower brain stem, spinal cord or cerebellum might lead to biogenic amine dysfunction in noninjured brain regions and ultimately to the clinical symptoms of depression. Relatively small brain stem lesions, however, might cause less disruption than MCA infarcts to the biogenic amine neurons. This might lead to shorter duration depressions.

In summary, depressions associated with posterior circulation lesions (i.e., cerebellar/brain stem lesions) are less frequent than depressions associated with the cerebral hemisphere infarcts (e.g., 11% of PC lesion patients had major depression compared with 26% of those with MCA lesions) and are significantly shorter in duration than depressions associated with MCA lesions. Although there are no known differences in the clinical syndromes of major or minor depression associated with PC or MCA lesions, differences in the duration of depression suggest that the mechanisms leading to depression may be different following MCA hemispheric lesions compared with those following PC brain stem or cerebellar lesions.

Depression associated with right hemisphere lesions

Although the frequency of major depression in the acute post-stroke period has been found in several studies to be greater following left frontal cortical or left basal ganglia lesions than for any other lesion location, depressions do occur in many patients with right hemisphere lesions during both the acute and chronic post-stroke periods. We, therefore, examined the clinical correlates of depression associated with right hemisphere lesions to compare them with the clinical correlates of left hemisphere lesion location. This work comprised a study of a consecutive series of 93 patients who had single acute stroke lesions of the right hemisphere. Lesion location was based on CT findings and/or clinical diagnosis and patients were included only if there was no previous history or CT scan evidence of prior brain injury.

The background characteristics of the study population are shown in Table 5.4. The 93 acute stroke patients consisted of both males and females in their late 50s and early 60s, primarily from lower socioeconomic classes (i.e., Hollingshead class

Table 5.4. Characteristics of right hemisphere lesion patients

Characteristic	Right hemisphere				Left hemisphere
	No depression ($n=46$)	Undue cheerfulness ($n=19$)	Major depression ($n=17$)	Minor depression ($n=11$)	Major depression ($n=27$)
Age (mean ± SD in years)	64 ± 10	60 ± 14	60 ± 11	62 ± 8	56 ± 13
Gender (% female)	35	42	47	36	52
Race (% black)	65	74	41	55	59
Socioeconomic status: Hollingshead class IV or V		87	74	82	89
Marital status (% married)	54	37	42	36	44
Handedness (% right-handed)	87	90	100	100	89
Education (mean no. of years ± SD)	6.5 ± 3.7	8.2 ± 4.3	8.4 ± 3.4	8.8 ± 3.5	9.3 ± 2.8
Familial history of psychiatric disorders (% positive)*	6	5	29	9	4
Personal history of psychiatric disorders (% positive)	15	5	29	36	6
Time since stroke (mean no. of days ± SD)	13 ± 12	11 ± 6	16 ± 9	20 ± 18	14 ± 11

Notes:
*$p<0.05$.

IV and class V). There were 46 patients with no mood disturbance, 17 patients with major depression, 11 patients with minor depression, and 19 patients with undue cheerfulness. The classification of 'undue cheerfulness' was based on either a self-report of elevated or expansive mood or clinical observation of inappropriately cheerful affect or disinhibited behavior during the structured interview of the present state examination. These symptoms or behavior also had to occur in the absence of feelings of sadness or depression.

One of the major findings was that patients with major depression had a significantly higher frequency of psychiatric disorder among their first-degree or second-degree relatives (i.e., 29% with 55% of these being alcoholism and 45% depression) compared with other diagnostic groups (i.e., 6% for no diagnosis to 9% for minor depression, $p<0.05$, Fig. 5.13). In order to determine whether the significantly higher rate of psychiatric disorder among family members of patients with major depression was specific for patients with right hemisphere lesions, we compared the frequency of positive family psychiatric history among patients with major depression following right hemisphere stroke to the frequency among 27

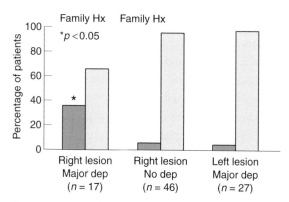

Fig. 5.13   The percentage of patients with and without a family history (Hx) of psychiatric disorder (defined by having seen a professional for treatment of an emotional disorder) following an acute right hemisphere infarction. Patients with major depression following a right hemisphere lesion were significantly more likely to have a family history of psychiatric disorder than those without major depression or patients with major depression following a left hemisphere lesion. These data suggest that some post-stroke depressions may be related to genetic vulnerability and that the factors associated with major depression following right or left hemisphere lesions may be different.

patients with major depression following left hemisphere stroke (Fig. 5.13). Patients with major depression following right hemisphere lesions showed a significantly higher frequency of family history of psychiatric disorders compared with patients with major depression following left hemisphere lesions ($p<0.05$).

The only other investigators to examine this issue were Morris et al. (1990). A study of 88 Australian patients in a rehabilitation hospital found a significantly higher frequency of family history of psychiatric disorder among patients with major depression (i.e., 11 of 16, or 69%) compared to patients with minor depression (i.e., five of 18, or 28%) or no depression (i.e., 20 of 54 or 37%, $p<0.03$). Patients with major depression following right hemisphere lesions had a positive family history in 71% of the cases (i.e., five of seven). This frequency, however, was not different from that of patients with major depression following left hemisphere lesions (i.e., 67%, or six of nine patients). These patients, however, were examined at an average of 8.4 weeks following stroke when more 'delayed-onset' cases of depression had developed compared to our acute post-stroke study.

In addition to the association of major depression with an increased family history of psychiatric disorders among patients with right hemisphere lesions, we also examined the relationship between diagnosis and lesion volume and location (Starkstein et al., 1989). There were no significant differences in lesion volume among patients with major or minor depression, undue cheerfulness, or no mood disorder. Therefore, the size of the infarct did not appear to be related to depression. Patients with undue cheerfulness, however, showed a significantly higher frequency of lesions involving the right frontal operculum compared with depressed (major and minor) and nondepressed patients. Of 12 patients with undue cheerfulness, five had right frontal opercular lesions compared with four of 25 nondepressed and one of 17 depressed patients ($p<0.05$). On the other hand, patients with depression (both major and minor) showed a significantly higher frequency of lesions involving either the right parietal cortex (i.e., six of nine with major depression and five of eight with minor depression compared to one of 12 with undue cheerfulness and nine of 25 with no depression; $p=0.02$) or the right dorsal lateral frontal cortex (i.e., two of nine with major depression and four of eight with minor depression compared to none of 12 with undue cheerfulness and one of 25 with no depression; $p<0.01$) than nondepressed or unduly cheerful patients.

Patients with right hemisphere lesions have also been investigated for depression by other researchers Finset et al. (1989) found that among 42 patients with CT-verified single right hemisphere lesions, ischemic damage involving white matter underlying the parietal cortex was associated with a higher frequency of depression (five of 13 patients) than lesions in any other location in the right hemisphere (seven of 29 patients, $p<0.02$). House et al. (1990) reported on a group of 21 patients with CT-verified right hemisphere lesions examined one month following their first stroke. Of the three patients with major depression following a right hemisphere lesion, all of them had a right posterior lesion (i.e., three major depressions of eight patients with right posterior injury) compared with none of the patients with right anterior ($n=7$) or right intermediate ($n=6$) lesion locations ($p<0.03$). Sinyor et al. (1986) examined 16 patients with single CT-verified right hemisphere lesions studied an average of 56 days post-stroke. There was a significant quadratic relationship between depression scores and the distance between the anterior border of the lesion and the frontal pole in patients with right hemisphere lesions (i.e., patients with the most anterior and most posterior lesions of the right hemisphere had the highest depression scores, $p<0.05$). Another study, by Stern and Bachman (1991), examined 19 patients with CT-verified single right hemisphere lesions an average of 16 months post-stroke. Lesions were classified as dorsal or ventral, frontal or nonfrontal. Dysphoric mood was significantly more severe in patients with right ventral nonfrontal as compared with right ventral frontal lesions. This suggests that right temporal lesions are associated with depressed mood. Finally, Astrom et al. (1993) and Eastwood et al. (1989) found no association between lesion location in the right hemisphere and the existence of post-stroke depression. Astrom et al. (1993) found only two cases of major depression among 23 patients with single acute stroke lesions of the right hemisphere. They reported no lesion localization findings for these two patients. Eastwood et al. (1989) found 18 cases of major or minor depression among 27 patients with single right hemisphere lesions but found no difference in the distance between the anterior border of the lesion and the frontal pole or in lesion volume between depressed and nondepressed patients. This finding, however, could have resulted from patients with the most anterior and most posterior lesions of the right hemisphere having more severe depression than patients with intermediate lesion locations.

Conclusion

In summary, the clinical and pathological correlates of depression among patients with right hemisphere stroke appear to be different from those found among patients with left hemisphere stroke. We found that a family history of psychiatric disorder was significantly more frequent among patients with acute-onset major depression following right compared with left hemisphere stroke. It seems likely that a positive family history of depression or anxiety disorder would increase the likelihood of depression occurring independently of lesion location (i.e., a vulnerability that could be provoked by any major stress). However, if left frontal or basal ganglia lesions provoke depression through a different mechanism (i.e., physiological or biochemical response to a strategic brain lesion), as we have previously suggested, the percentage of major depression associated with a positive family history following right hemisphere lesions would be expected to be higher than the percentage of major depressions and positive family history among patients with left hemisphere lesions. Since the overall rate of positive family history was 12% compared with Morris' overall rate of 41%, the higher rate in the Morris study may have overwhelmed the laterality effect.

Across several studies, there has been a relatively consistent finding that both major and minor depressions are associated with posterior lesions of the right hemisphere. These posterior lesions have sometimes been localized to ventral or deep portions of the right hemisphere and sometimes associated with parietal and sometimes with temporal lesions. In addition, right anterior lesions have also been associated with depression in several studies. The mechanism by which right posterior (and perhaps anterior frontal) lesions may lead to depression is an issue that deserves future investigation.

REFERENCES

Astrom, M., Adolfsson, R. and Asplund, K. (1993). Major depression in stroke patients: a 3-year longitudinal study. *Stroke* 24: 976–82.

Baxter, L.R., Schwartz, J.M., Phelps, M.E. et al. (1989). Reduction of prefrontal cortex glucose metabolism common to three types of depression. *Arch Gen Psychiatry* 46: 243–50.

Bench, C.J., Friston, K.J., Brown, R.G. et al. (1992). The anatomy of melancholia – focal abnormalities of cerebral blood flow in major depression. *Psychol Med* 22: 607–15.

Dam, H., Pedersen, H.E. and Ahlgren, P. (1989). Depression among patients with stroke. *Acta Psychiatr Scand* 80: 118–24.

Drevets, W.C., Videen, T.O., Price, J.L. et al. (1992). A functional anatomical study of unipolar depression. *J Neurosci* 12: 3628–41.

Eastwood, M.R., Rifat, S.L., Nobbs, H. and Ruderman, J. (1989). Mood disorder following cerebrovascular accident. *Br J Psychiatry* 154: 195–200.

Finset, A., Goffeng, L., Landro, N.I. and Haakonsen, M. (1989). Depressed mood and intrahemispheric location of lesion in right hemisphere stroke patients. *Scan J Rehabil Med* 21: 1–6.

Herrmann, M., Bartels, C. and Wallesch, C-W., (1993). Depression in acute and chronic aphasia: symptoms, pathoanatomical–clinical correlations and functional implications. *J Neurol Neurosurg Psychiatry* 56: 672–8.

House, A., Dennis, M., Warlow, C., Hawton, K. and Molyneux, K. (1990). Mood disorders after stroke and their relation to lesion location. A CT scan study. *Brain* 113: 1113–30.

Lipsey, J.R., Robinson, R.G., Pearlson, G.D., Rao, K. and Price, T.R. (1983). Mood change following bilateral hemisphere brain injury. *Br J Psychiatry* 143: 266–73.

Martinot, J.H., Hardy, P., Feline, A. et al. (1990). Left prefrontal glucose hypometabolism in the depressed state: a confirmation. *Am J Psychiatry* 147: 1313–17.

Morris, P.L.P., Robinson, R.G. and Raphael, B. (1990). Prevalence and course of depressive disorders in hospitalized stroke patients. *Int J Psychiatr Med* 20: 349–64.

Morris, P.L.P., Robinson, R.G. and Raphael, B. (1992). Lesion location and depression in hospitalized stroke patients: evidence supporting a specific relationship in the left hemisphere. *Neuropsychiatr Neuropsychol Behav Neurol* 3: 75–82.

Morrison, J.H., Molliver, M.E. and Grzanna, R. (1979). Noradrenergic innervation of the cerebral cortex: widespread effects of local cortical lesions. *Science* 205: 313–16.

Parikh, R.M., Lipsey, J.R., Robinson, R.G. and Price, T.R. (1987). A two-year longitudinal study of poststroke mood disorders: dynamic changes in correlates of depression at one and two years follow-up. *Stroke* 18: 579–84.

Parikh, R.M., Lipsey, J.R., Robinson, R.G. and Price, T.R. (1988). A two-year longitudinal study of poststroke mood disorders: prognostic factors related to one and two years outcome. *Int J Psychiatr Med* 18: 45–56.

Robinson, R.G., Kubos, K.L., Starr, L.B., Rao, K. and Price, T.R. (1984a). Mood disorders in stroke patients: importance of location of lesion. *Brain* 107: 81–93.

Robinson, R.G., Lipsey, J.R., Bolla-Wilson, K. et al. (1985). Mood disorders in left handed stroke patients. *Am J Psychiatry* 142: 1424–9.

Robinson, R.G., Lipsey, J.R., Rao, K. and Price, T.R. (1986). A two year longitudinal study of poststroke mood disorders: a comparison of acute onset with delayed onset depression. *Am J Psychiatry* 143: 1238–44.

Robinson, R.G., Starr, L.B., Lipsey, J.R., Rao, K. and Price, T.R. (1984b). A two year longitudinal study of poststroke mood disorders: dynamic changes in associated variables over the first six months of follow-up. *Stroke* 15: 510–17.

Robinson, R.G. and Szetela, B. (1981). Mood change following left hemispheric brain injury. *Ann Neurol* 9: 447–53.

Schwartz, J.A., Speed, N.M., Brunberg, J.A. et al. (1993). Depression in stroke rehabilitation. *Biol Psychiatry* 33: 694–9.

Sharpe, M., Hawton, K., Seagroatt, V. et al. (1994). Depressive disorders in long-term survivors of stroke: associations with demographic and social factors, functional status, and brain lesion volume. *Br J Psychiatry* 164: 380–6.

Shimoda, K. and Robinson, R.G. (1999). The relationship between post-stroke depression and lesion location in long term followup. *Biol Psychiatry* 45: 187–92.

Sinyor, D., Jacques, P., Kaloupek, D.G. et al. (1986). Poststroke depression and lesion location: an attempted replication. *Brain* 109: 539–46.

Starkstein, S.E., Robinson, R.G., Berthier, M.L., Parikh, R.M. and Price, T.R. (1988a). Differential mood changes following basal ganglia versus thalamic lesions. *Arch Neurol* 45: 723–30.

Starkstein, S.E., Robinson, R.G., Berthier, M.L. and Price, T.R. (1988b). Depressive disorders following posterior circulation compared with middle cerebral artery infarcts. *Brain* 111: 375–87.

Starkstein, S.E., Robinson, R.G., Honig, M.A. et al. (1989). Mood changes after right hemisphere lesion. *Br J Psychiatry* 155: 79–85.

Starkstein, S.E., Robinson, R.G. and Price, T.R. (1987). Comparison of cortical and subcortical lesions in the production of post-stroke mood disorders. *Brain* 110: 1045–59.

Stern, R.A. and Bachman, D.L. (1991). Depressive symptoms following stroke. *Am J Psychiatry* 148: 351–6.

6

Mood and behavior in disorders of the basal ganglia

Joseph Ghika

Introduction: general concepts, anatomy, physiology, and neurochemistry

The basal ganglia have been associated with motor control since Wilson's Croonian lecture (1925), but Kleist (1922), and later others, extended their role to behavior, cognitive functions, emotions, motivation, reward, personality and character (for a summary, see Weiner and Lang, 1995). With their strategic location within the brain, and their rich and reciprocal connection with cortical sensorimotor areas, but also with limbic, paralimbic, midbrain, and diencephalic structures, the basal ganglia have all the rationale for processing the interface between internal personal drives (basic instincts, mood, motivations, needs) and the external world's stimuli, i.e., the modulation and motor expression of emotions, moods, needs, drives or motivation and cognition through corticospinal volitional axial and distal pathways (Kuypers, 1982), but also through emotional limbic motor-visceromotor pathways (Holstege, 1992).

Fronto-subcortical circuits

The basal ganglia are included in retroactive loops on cortical activity and cannot any more be considered functional as separate anatomical entities. Therefore, a lesion at any level of this network can be followed by a common syndromic symptomatology. After a first attempt by Kleist (1922), Alexander et al. (1986) described five frontal-based ganglia-thalamocortical segregated and parallel loops (there are probably more to discover), which have been designated as motor, oculomotor, dorsolateral prefrontal (DLPF), orbitofrontal (OF), and anterior cingulate (AC) fronto-subcortical circuits, which participate in the frontal management of primitive unmodulated drives and behaviors, that are ingrained in limbic, thalamic, and paralimbic structures. Each of these circuits has two pathways, one direct, projecting from the cortex to the caudate, external pallidum, internal pallidum/substantia nigra, and one indirect pathway, from external pallidum to the subthalamic nucleus and back to the internal pallidum, from where both circuits project together to the ventrolateral thalamic nucleus and back to their respective cortical areas.

The key role of the basal ganglia is their action as a filter, or gate processor on convergent motor, mood, and cognitive behavior (for a review, see Kimura and Graybiel, 1995). The overall activity of the basal ganglia is dichotomic, binary, organized within reciprocal zones of excitation and inhibition: either a release or activation, mediated by the direct pathways, promoting activity in recurrent, positive feedback loops, helped by dopamine, which also inhibits the indirect (inhibitory) pathway, or an inhibition or deficit, generated by the indirect inhibitor pathways, leading to the suppression of unwanted movements, thoughts, behaviors, or emotions. The clinical translation of either activation or inhibition of general motility is, respectively, dyskinesia (chorea, ballism, dystonia, akathisia, tics, etc.) or hypo/akinetic motor syndromes (parkinsonism, apathy, akinetic mutism, or motor neglect); on mood, the dichotomic clinical picture is depression or mania and anxiety disorders; on cognition, the clinical presentation is either increased organization (obsessive slowness, obsessive–compulsive disorder) or loss of control (dysexecutive syndrome, attention deficit hyperactivity disorder, loss of attention or confusion, bradyphrenia); on behaviors (and personality) the clinical translation is increased control (obsessive–compulsive disorder) or decreased control (disinhibition syndromes, disorders of impulse control, self-injurious behaviors, impulsivity, echophenomena, paliphenomena, or coprophenomena, stereotypies, perseverations, environment dependency, hyperactivity or attention deficit hyperactivity disorder).

The reality of direct inhibitory and indirect net excitatory pathways has been recently questioned (Parent and Hazrati, 1995a, 1995b), as has their strict segregation in parallel circuits throughout their courses, funneling separate convergent cortico-cortical and cortico-limbic information. Two of these circuits are predominantly involved in motor functions and three in nonmotor functions (behavioral, affective, cognitive functions). All circuits converge on thalamic nuclei, before they go back to their cortical area of origin. The ventrolateral thalamic nucleus (VL) is the main relay of motor circuits. The magnocellular dorsomedial (DM) thalamus is involved in limbic functions, the parvocellular part in cognitive functions. Therefore, the frontal cortex is an integrator of information coming from the external world (processed in the parietal areas), and the internal needs or drives (hypothalamic and limbic structures), using different parallel, separate fronto-subcortical circuits travelling as closed loops, converging to thalamic nuclei. These closed-loop circuits are named after their cortical origin and projection.

The two motor circuits, which will not be concentrated on here, are:

1 The motor circuit, originating in the supplementary motor area (SMA), mainly involved in motor and psychic initiation. The indirect pathway

(SMA–caudate–internal pallidum–VL thalamocortical) is probably responsible for most of the akinetic and axial features of the parkinsonian syndrome, motor neglect, and part of akinetic mutic syndromes together with the anterior cingulate circuit (see below). The direct pathway (SMA–caudate–external pallidum–subthalamic nucleus (STN)-internal pallidum–VL thalamo–cortical pathway) is probably responsible for dyskinesias.

2 The oculomotor circuit, originating in the frontal eye field (FEF, area 8), following the same direct (FEF–caudate–pallidum) and indirect (FEF–caudate–external pallidum–STN–internal pallidum) pathways' organization, finally to converge on VL thalamic nucleus and back to FEF. It organizes saccades, antisaccades, memory-guided eye movements, stability of gaze in the presence of external stimuli, oculomotor exploration, and directional orientation of gaze, and perhaps spontaneity of saccades (supplementary eye field area) and oculogyric crises, and perhaps influences the rate of blinking.

The three nonmotor circuits, which are the main focus of our attention here are:

1 The AC pathway, originating in area 24 of the cingulum, but also in area 28 (entorhinal), 35 (perirhinal), hippocampus, area 12 (orbitofrontal), amygdala, parafascicular thalamus, raphe, and ventral tegmental area of midbrain, and projects to the ventro-medial striatum (caudoputamen) and accumbens, olfactory tubercle, rostromedial globus pallidus internus, ventral pallidum, rostrocaudal substantia nigra for the direct pathway, and from ventral striatum to the rostral pole of the globus pallidus externus, medial STN and ventral pallidum for the indirect pathway. Both pathways converge to the magnocellular DM of the thalamus and project back to the same cortical area. The AC pathway allows intentional selection of environmental stimuli based on internal relevance, integration of emotional information with motivation and spontaneity (akinetic mutism, abulia, apathy, psychic emptiness, aspontaneity, indifference), together with the DLPF circuit and inhibition of programs strategies (perseveration). A lesion at any level of this circuit (anterior cingulum, caudate, pallidum, thalamus, and interconnecting pathways) is therefore followed by similar motor and cognitive dysfunction, going from apathy, abulia and loss of psychic autoactivation to akinetic mutism, catalepsy, and catatonia.

2 The dorsolateral prefrontal circuit, originating in areas 9–14, 24, 25, 32, 45–47, with contributions from 7a (superior parietal lobule, visual stimuli, visually guided reaching, visuospatial strategies), but also from parafascicular thalamus, dopaminergic, serotoninergic norepinephrinergic brainstem nuclei and cholinergic diencephalic nuclei, and limbic structures (hippocampal complex, amygdala, parahippocampal, cingulate, subiculum cortices, thalamic ventral anterior, dorsomedial, anteromedial, intralaminar and pulvinar nuclei, and ventral striatum). It projects to the dorsolateral head of the caudate, the lateral aspect of

mediodorsal pallidus internus, and rostrolateral substantia nigra reticulata for the direct pathway, to the dorsolateral external globus pallidus and lateral subthalamic nucleus, globus pallidus internus, and pars reticulata of the substantia nigra (SNr) for the indirect pathway. From there, both pathways terminate in the parvocellular portion of the pars anterior of the ventrolateralis (VoA) and DM thalamic nuclei and project back to the same cortical areas. The function of this circuit is called executive, i.e., it is responsible for the processing of multimodal information input (throughout its wide connections with associative cortical areas, not with the primary sensorimotor cortex) in the executive control of action. Its role consists of matching goal-oriented behavior with emotional and instinctual motivation and reward, in the context of external stimuli and circumstances and mnemonic (experience) inputs. Its role is therefore major in gating and focusing attention, considering saliency of inputs, emotional, mnemonic, motivational and motor behavior with respect to a goal-oriented adequate behavior in response to internal and external stimuli. This includes the solving of complex problems, the learning of new information, the copying of complicated figures, the shifting and maintaining of behavioral sets appropriately, the usage of verbal skills to guide behaviors, the activation of remote procedural memories, the fluency of word and action, the organization of strategies and constructional behaviors, the anticipation, planning, and monitoring of actions by using feedback and memory, the focusing of the attention by keeping the independence from environmental contingencies. The clinical expression of the dysexecutive syndrome is difficulty in anticipating, executing, planning, switching, sequencing, monitoring, and using of feedback, i.e., mental flexibility and attentional deficits syndromes, together with OF areas.

3 The orbito-frontal (OF) circuit originates in OF areas 10, 11, 12, but also area 22 of superior temporal lobe, entorhinal cortex, parafascicular thalamus, amygdala, area 12 (gyrus rectus) and 25 (medial posterior frontal) and 32 (inferorostral cingulate), area 9, 33, insula, temporal pole (38), substantia nigra reticulata (SNr), and raphe nuclei of brainstem. Efferences from OF cortex are directed to the ventromedial caudate and accumbens, the ventral portion of the globus pallidus internus, and rostromedial SNr (direct pathway), the dorsal globus pallidus externus, the lateral subthalamic nucleus and pallidus internus and substantia reticulata of the nigra (indirect pathway). Both circuits end in the medial portion of the magnocellular VA and inferomedial sector of the magnocellular DM nuclei of the thalamus and go back to the OF cortex. The role of this circuit is the integration of mood, emotional tone, and instinctive behaviors, with situational and social critical restraint, environment, and goal of action. Consecutive clinical syndromes resulting from a dysfunction in this circuit are disinhibition syndromes: irritability, lability, tactlessness, fatuous euphoria, impulsivity, undue familiarity, jocularity, witzelsucht, moria, empathy, or increased behavior control

diseases, such as in obsessive–compulsive disorders with overconcern, and disorders of impulse control and antisocial behavior (pathological gambling, binge eating, kleptomania, arsonism, exhibitionism or sexual behavior disorders, hyperactivity, risk taking, etc.), and manic and hyperactivity syndromes.

There are probably (many?) other circuits to add, like the one described for motor speech (Damasio et al., 1984), probably originating near the supplementary frontal area, including fronto-opercular and Broca's area, mostly responsible for motor and emotional aspects of speech (aspontaneity, mutism, loss of fluency, short sentences, hypophonia, dysarthria, aprosody, festination, palilalia or, on the contrary, echolalia, coprolalia, logorrhea, vocal tics, klazomania). We should probably also add two further frontal striato-limbo-thalamo-mesencephalo-frontal circuits, anterior temporal-striato-limbo-temporal and insulo-claustro-hypothalamo-limbo-insular, and perhaps many others, such as the ones described by Livingston (1977) and Blumer and Benson (1975), i.e., the medial prefrontal-cingulate hippocampus circuit, important in regulating depression, and the lateral orbito-frontal-tempora-amygdala circuit regulating mood (depression, anxiety, phobias, and mania). Their connection with the ventral striatum is not yet described.

Control of behavior

The role of the basal ganglia in behavior is now well asserted, but our understanding is still preliminary (for a review, see Saint-Cyr et al., 1995). Basal ganglia are not the site of computation of behaviors, but the anatomical site of selection, modulation, and integration of behaviors, i.e., a sort of sensory analyzer for motor systems' gating of relevant sensory information. The striatum processes the contextual analysis, samples the information from almost the entire cortex through spiny neurons, chooses the expression of ritualistic behaviors, and integrates the sensory information for an appropriate behavior. Basal ganglia operate, therefore, at a high level of central nervous system (CNS) integration of sensorimotor functions, controlling some of the organism–environment interrelationships, the context-regulated balance between approach and avoidance reactions, affective reactions, preparation or setting up for performance (response set) and tasks requiring a high level of cognition (cognitive set). A high level of integration means that the basal ganglia operate upon performances not only triggered reflexly but also internally or volitionally.

The striatum integrates cortical and subcortical information with consecutive alteration of the cortical threshold for initiation of movement, emotions cognition and behavior, i.e., the pathogenesis of motor behavioral, psychic, cognitive, and mood akinesia or hyperkinesia. The basal ganglia facilitate the execution of action (dorsolateral prefrontal circuit), determine parameters and prepare movements, promote automaticity, organize sequences of behaviors, participate in learning and planning, motivate (anterior cingulate circuit), allow the integration of limbic-emotional processing and sensorimotor input into behavior (OF circuit), scale the magnitude of muscle activity and specifications of movement parameters, organize anticipatory reflexes, and select strategies, habits or innate behavioral routines or patterns that do not rely on conscious recall for skilled execution. Basal ganglia build up sequences of behavior into meaningful, goal-directed repertoires, and promote adaptation to novel circumstances and reward-based learning (for reviews, see Brooks, 1995; Kimura and Graybiel, 1995; Saint-Cyr et al., 1995).

Sensory processing of the basal ganglia is known from their contribution in noci-ception and pain, controlling pain behavior, sensory–discriminative, affective and cognitive dimensions of pain, and modulating nociceptive information for higher cortical areas (for a review, see Chudler and Dong, 1995). In movement disorders, there are a number of conditions in which the patient is aware of an unpleasant sen-sation, mostly described as a compulsion or an urge to move in response to this urging 'sensation.' Tics (premonitory urges, sensory tics) (Leckman et al., 1993), mental counting, painful legs, and moving toes, akathisia, impulsions, and com-pulsions are examples. There are also well-documented sensory syndromes in par-kinsonism or dystonia. The effect of L-dopa on the modulation of pain is well known. Orienting behaviors to external sensory stimuli are also controlled by the basal ganglia, with consecutive translation in frontal environment dependency syn-dromes (Lhermitte, 1986), but also exploratory movements, especially locomotion, supposed to be processed in accumbens and subpallidal regions. The caudate nucleus modulates polysensory activity via the thalamic connections with predom-inance of inhibition and therefore mediates high forms of attention. Thus, it is not surprising that lack of striatal inhibition has been found to have some contribution to the attention deficit hyperactivity disorders.

Another implication of sensory processing in the basal ganglia is their analysis of the context of action, via multisensory associative areas input. The striatum is responsible for a coherent, goal-oriented and context-adequate (socially and situ-ationally correct) motor behavior and emotional output, as processed in the frontal cortices, with suppression of unwanted or inappropriate obsessions, compulsions, impulsions, basic instincts or needs, as seen in obsessive–compulsive disorders, dis-eases of impulse control, and disinhibition syndromes (Alexander et al., 1986). Compensatory cortical areas are the OF cortex and cingulum.

The limbic input conveys information related to reinforcement and incentive directly to the striatum or indirectly via nigrostriatal dopamine pathways. Generation, maintenance, shifting, and selection blending of motor behavior, mental, and emotional sets explain why the basal ganglia can play a role not only in executive functions, abulic-athymormic and akinetic syndromes, but also in mood disorders. Preparation and initiation of action, in a behavioral context-dependent manner (external sensory, reward, task-related, reinforcement or incentive) (Kimura and Graybiel, 1995), explain their role in apathy and slowing of information processing (bradyphrenia, subcortical dementia). The recognition of limbic-hypothalamic motor integration, or needs or drive-induced behaviors, is best seen in the locomotion component of 'fight and flight' reactions, 'food procurement,' sexual and greed behaviors, (Hess, 1954), and also in the motor expression of emotions of face and limbs (mimic, gestures, prosody) and their overall autonomic and endocrine responses. This results from a highly integrated neuronal pathway including the limbic and paralimbic structures, hypothalamus, ventral striatum-accumbens, septum, DM thalamus, ganglia, brainstem (especially pedunculopontine nucleus of locomotion, reticular system and motor nuclei) and motor insular cortices (Morgenson, 1987).

Control of emotions

The role of the basal ganglia in emotions is starting to be understood. Mood disorders (depression, bipolar mood disorders, mania, anxiety) are well known in almost all diseases involving the basal ganglia, such as parkinsonism, Huntington's disease, idiopathic basal ganglia calcifications, etc. Emotions are complex, multicomponental, processes. The exact definitions of mood, affect, and emotion are still missing, but emotions have an at least five-dimensional recognized expression (Izard, 1977; LeDoux, 1993; Ross et al., 1994; Heilman, 1994):

1 a mental experience, or feeling, with primary emotions (euphoria, sadness, fear, anger), social emotions (doubt, rage, surprise, disgust) and, when lasting, mood states constitute frank disorders such as mania or elation, depression, anxiety, aggressivity, indifference;

2 an arousal reaction (interest, motivation, or indifference);

3 a motor expression or emotional displays (emotional mimic, gesture, vocalization, prosody, verbal–semantic emotional expression of sentences, flight, withdrawal, freezing, approach, aggression, interest, suspicion, indifference, sham);

4 an autonomic visceral and somatic emotional expression, or emotional indicators (heart rate, capillary circulation, sweating, lacrimation, pupillary size, xerostomia or salivation, striction of throat, tightness of breathing, sphincters, tremor);

5 an emotional cognition system: emotional memory and mental imaging, motor expression (prosodia, kinesics, syntactic, mimic), and recognition system (emotional gnosias).

Primary, formal, or basic alterations of emotion can be seen in patients with lesions of the basal forebrain, temporomedial limbic, diencephalic and brainstem (respiratory nuclei, periaqueductal gray matter, locus ceruleus, raphe nuclei, reticular formation etc.) lesions (Brown, 1967) and in schizophrenia. 'Sham' emotions with motor and autonomic behavioral expression without internal or emotional experience can be induced by hypothalamic stimulation (White, 1940). Motor emotional expression of sadness without internal feeling has been reported in a patient with right opercular lesion (Ross and Mesulam, 1979). Experiental feelings of emotion without motor or vegetative indicators can be observed in patients with epileptic seizures starting in the limbic (amygdala), OF, and anterior temporal region. The hippocampus is responsible for processing of the information coming from the extrapersonal surrounding, whereas the amygdala processes affective and experimental internal tone (LeDoux, 1993). Direct connection with these deep temporal structures with neocortex, posterior (experiential) and anterior (expressive) insula and neocortical areas of expression of emotion (prosodia, kinesics, mimic) are responsible for primary (right hemisphere dominance) or social (left hemisphere dominance) emotions (for a review, see Ross et al., 1994) and emotional cognition (expression, comprehension, memory, and mental imagery of emotional semantics). The basal ganglia, as a part of these modular systems or pathways (fronto-subcortical pathways, temporolimbic etc.), can reproduce parts of these deficits, but their major role in emotion is modulation, execution, spontaneity, shifting, flexibility, adaptation to the context, motivation (as a part of emotional intelligence), basic motor processing of emotions (mimic, prosody, gestures, postures), emotional motor expression (Ross et al., 1994) and gnosias (Buck and Duffy, 1980) and perhaps memory and mental imaging (LeDoux, 1993), with a probable similar left–right dominance as in hemispheric functions, rather than their intimate computing.

Mood and motor behaviors are two synchronous, parallel aspects of a common neurological process, and, therefore, cannot be artificially separated, as they have been in the past. There are many examples that illustrate this statement. Psychiatric diseases, such as schizophrenia, depression, obsessive–compulsive disorders or anxiety, for example, have well-recognized patterns of abnormal motor expression (Rogers, 1985). Similarly, in movement disorders such as Parkinson's disease, Huntington's disease, Wilson's disease, dystonia, Gilles de la Tourette's syndrome and many others, mood and 'psychiatric features' are an inherent part of the clinical picture (for a review, see Cummings, 1995). In the same way, the influence of emotion and stress on the expression of many movement disorders such as tics, tremor or other dyskinesias is well documented (Larmande et al., 1993). Parkinsonian patients experience motor fluctuations and mood swings as well as behavioral autonomic, visceral, and painful fluctuations (Nissenbaum et al., 1987). Similarly, the adverse events of psychiatric medication are often movement disorders, and the treatment of parkinsonism or dyskinesias can lead to drug-induced psychiatric syndromes (Steck, 1927). Movements are performed in response to internal cues or drives (mood, emotions, will) as well as in response to external stimuli drives, but sometimes 'involuntarily' or 'automatically.' They are highly influenced by mood states (see Bipolar mood disorders), and the motor expressions of mood states can induce emotions in another person, such as in dialogue, conferences, or concerts, for example. It is therefore suspected that both movement disorders and many psychiatric disorders may be shared by common, intimately connected, mechanisms, and the common present concept of movement disorders as diseases of the motor pathways and psychiatric diseases as functional pathology is challenged by present knowledge acquired in both fields. This suggests that a disorder of psychomotility has to be assessed in both dimensions carefully, rather than by introducing artificial, unrealistic barriers between the symptoms of a common entity. Moreover, motor and behavior aspects of emotions are intimately integrated with cognition, with a major input of basal ganglia in this connection.

Control of cognition

The basal ganglia also comprise a highly dynamic control system in cognition, involved in modulation of attention, and the building up, storage, retrieval, execution, motivation, shifting, and motor expression of behavioral activities (Barat et al., 1978; Damasio et al., 1984; Rafal et al., 1984; Saint-Cyr et al., 1988; Kimura and Graybiel, 1995; Graybiel, 1995; Brooks, 1995). They encompass concepts such as focused attention, goal-directed execution, skilled action, habit formation, selection or planification of behaviors in relation to internal, memory-related or rewarding system function, stimuli relevant response, organization of sequences, selection and inhibitions of motor programs, imaged movements and mental rehearsal of behavior, as well as new tasks' preparation, planning, decision, but not learning, adaptative motor control, sensorimotor association learning, locomotion, representation of both innate and learned movement sequences, and organization of behavioral context-dependent manners. Memory and learning are also processed in the basal ganglia, especially procedural learning and memory (Phillips and Carr, 1987; Saint-Cyr et al., 1988; Taylor et al., 1990) and habits. The frontal cortex acts when new rules need to be learned and older ones rejected, whereas the basal ganglia potentiate previously learned rules based on environmental context and reinforcement history. They also have a role in the motor and emotional processing of written and oral language (Barat et al., 1978; Damasio et al., 1984; Mehler, 1987; Martinez-Vila et al., 1988).

Some involvement of basal ganglia in delirium, psychosis, and schizophrenia is also suspected (Figiel et al., 1990). The mechanisms are still obscure.

Neurotransmission

Neurotransmission in the basal ganglia is highly complex within these circuits, but the major characteristics of the present understanding can be summarized as follows (for a review, see Graybiel, 1990). The cortex sends excitatory glutama-tergic fibers to the caudate, putamen, and ventral striatum. Cells in the striatum are divided into two distinct organizational systems: the striosomes and the matrix. The striosomes receive medial prefrontal cortical inputs, whereas the matrix receives mostly glutamatergic afferences from the sensorimotor cortex, lateral frontal, parietal, and temporal lobes, and dopaminergic projections from the dorsal part of the substantia nigra pars compacta. The matrix is rich in acetylcholine inhibitory interneurons, serotonin, and receives high inputs from the sensori-motor cortex and dopaminergic modulation from the dorsal part of the nigra pars compacta. GABA-ergic and substance P output from the matrix is to the external and internal globus pallidus, and pars reticulata of the nigra (direct pathway) is reg-ulated by dopamine D1 receptors by dorsal substantia nigra compacta. GABA-ergic-enkephaline output to the external globus pallidus (indirect pathway) and the subthalamic nucleus is regulated though dopamine D2 receptors, also from dorsal substantia nigra compacta. The latter nucleus projects to globus pallidus internus and substantia nigra reticulata through excitatory glutamatergic projections. The final common ouput globus pallidus-internus/substantia nigra reticulata then pro-jects inhibitory GABA fibers to a specific VL thalamus area, which in turn sends a final excitatory glutamatergic response to the cortex. Striosomes, poor in acetyl-choline, dopamine, and serotonin, receive dense glutamatergic input from the OF and insular cortex, and receive their dopaminergic input from the ventral tier of the substantia nigra compacta. GABA-ergic output from the striosomes goes to the medial portion of the pars compacta of the nigra and back to OF cortex.

Dopaminergic projections from substantia nigra compacta inhibit the indirect pathways of the fronto-subcortical circuits via D2 receptors (mostly in striatal matrix), and activate the direct pathways through D1 receptors (mostly in strio-somes). As the substantia nigra receives inputs from the limbic areas, there is an anatomical substrate in order to explain the limbic emotional influence on motor executive activity, cognition, and motivation.

Cholinergic projections from the pedunculopontine nucleus and cholinergic reticular nuclei of the brainstem to the thalamic nuclei activate cortical areas, but the cholinergic interneurons of fronto-subcortical circuits (DM thalamus, VA thal-amus, reticular nuclei responsible for cognitive functions) are under the influence of the basal forebrain nuclei, including the septal nuclei, the nuclei of diagonal band of Broca, and the basal nucleus of Meynert. Acetylcholine facilitates thalamic activation of the cortex.

Serotoninergic nuclei of the brainstem diffusely influence basal ganglia differently through their multiple subtypes of receptors. 5HT1 and 5HT1d are abundant all over the basal ganglia and substantia nigra, 5Ht2 is moderately abun-dant in caudate, putamen, and accumbens, whereas 5HT1a is in low levels; 5Ht1c is dense in pallidum, but less in caudate, putamen, and accumbens nucleus, and 5HT3 is especially found in the matrix and anterior cingulate, hippocampus, septum, and amygdala.

Mood, behavioral, and cognitive syndromes of the basal ganglia

Abulic and akinetic syndromes: the anterior cingulate pathway syndrome

The AC syndrome is a behavioral, thymic, and cognitive syndrome. Apathy (Marin, 1991), abulia (Fisher, 1995), loss of psychic autoactivation or pure psychic akinesia (Hauptmann, 1922; for a review, see Laplane, 1990), loss of action initiation and maintaining (Ali-Chérif et al., 1984), athymormic syndromes (Dide and Guiraud, 1922; Habib and Poncet, 1988), and in their extreme expression, at the other end of the spectrum, akinetic mutism (Ross and Stewart, 1981), and catatonia (Kahlbaum, 1973) represent a continuum of wakeful states of mood, behavior and cognitive aspontaneity, apathy, with indifference to basic instincts, needs (such as hunger, thirst) and pain accompanied by the absence of spontaneous motor and psychic initiative (mental or ideation emptiness), more or less profound loss of projection into the future, motivation and initiative, the absence of spontaneous verbalization or response to questions, laconic responses to questions, general loss of spontaneous motor activity, with apragmatism, loss of initiative, a trouble of affects with indifference to emotional stimuli and loss of expression of emotion. Dissociation between dramatic decrease in spontaneous mental, emotional, or motor activity (gestural, linguistic, mimic akinesia) and almost normal productions given in response to external stimuli or orders or social stimuli is striking. Patients are aware of these changes, are not depressed or anxious, and do not make any plans or projects. A striking feature is mental emptiness (absence of spontaneous thought). In some patients, compulsive activity or stereotyped movements were observed on incitation. This loss of motivation is not attributable to emotional stress, intellectual impairment, or diminished level of consciousness. Catatoniform syndromes (Kahlbaum, 1973) associate abnormal tonic persistence of awkward voluntary or passively imposed postures (catalepsy) with immobility and mutism, resistance to forced movements, insensitivity to pain, and sometimes stereotypia.

Akinesia is another aspect of the same basic process. Loss of spontaneous activity, facial, gestural, and speech motor and emotional expression, increased reaction time, and loss of adventitious synkinetic movements are well known features of parkinsonism, but also of motor neglect with decrease in spontaneous, explorative, or responsive activity, reluctance to move, delay in initiating activity and reaching maximal strength (Valenstein and Heilman, 1981).

Any of the above-mentioned syndromes, from apathy to akinetic mutism or catatonia, can result from focal lesions at any level of the AC circuit, from anterior cingulate (generally transient), medial frontal cortex (including SMA), caudate, putamen, pallidum, and thalamic and diencephalic relays, including white matter pathways, especially when bilateral (see Cummings, 1995, for a review), except for caudate (for a review, see Bhatia and Marsden, 1994). There are several reports of bilateral striatal (caudate and putamen) lesions associated with athymormic syndromes, including striatal or pallidal necrosis, anoxic or toxic lesions, infarcts, hematomas, trauma, abcesses, tumors, or idiopathic calcifications (Laplane et al., 1982, 1984, 1988a, 1989, 1992; Levin et al., 1983; Ali-Chérif et al., 1984; Williams et al., 1988; Asakura et al., 1989; Desi et al., 1990; Laplane, 1990; Trillet et al., 1990; Macucci et al., 1991; Wang, 1991; Lehembe and Graux, 1992; Hayashi et al., 1993; Mrabet et al., 1994; Smadja et al., 1995). Some of them were accompanied by compulsory symptoms such as compulsive counting (Laplane et al., 1984; Lehembe and Graux, 1992), typing (Williams et al. 1988), or compulsive stereotypic pedalling, pacing, thumb sucking, scratching, arythmomania, mastication, bruxism (Trillet et al., 1990), obsessive–compulsive disorder (Smadja et al., 1995), and some degree of parkinsonism (akinesia, loss of arm swing, rigidity, micrographia, slow steps, amimia). These were mostly bilateral caudate and putamen (plus anterior internal capsule), or bilateral pallidal or lenticular lesions. Alexander (1995) described an infarct involving the substantia nigra with obsessive–compulsive disorder.

Drugs such as dopamine agonists (bromocriptine, pergolide, amantadine, lergotrile, ropinrole), selegiline, amphetamine, methylphenidate, buprorion have sometimes been useful in treating these states of apathy, but not L-dopa.

Disinhibition syndromes

The determination of adequacy of time, place, and strategy of environmentally elicited behaviors are processed in the OF cortex. Disconnection from this cortical area of the limbic structures results in a disinhibition syndrome, such as the OF disinhibition syndrome, hyperactivity, agitation, akathisia, attention deficit hyperactivity disorder, mania (right hemisphere), disorders of impulse control, or, in the case of hyperfunctioning of OF cortex, increased inhibition such as in obsessive–compulsive disorders.

The OF disinhibition syndrome

The OF disinhibition syndrome is characterized by 'witzelsucht,' jocularity, moria, socially inappropriate sexual and aggressive behaviors, improper sexual remarks and gestures, risk-taking behaviors, antisocial acts, emotional lability, impulsivity, inattention, and distractibility. Sometimes, patients are irritable to trivial stimuli and respond with outbursts of anger. Increased motor activity, hypomania, or mania may be seen. Changes in personality with outspoken, tactless, elevated mood, loss of conscientiousness, interest, initiative, and irresponsibility have all been reported (for a review, see Cummings, 1995), but also perseverative behavior, inappropriate response to environment, inappropriate emotional display, difficulty in executing new or unpredicted situations. Patients are placed in a state 'in which experience and thought processes have lost their power to raise echoes from the interoceptive depths, and thus lost their power to guide' (Nauta, 1986, pp. 130–1). Cognitively, patients show disruption of delayed response to task, with sometimes irrelevant tactics, and are slow in planification. They lack an internal cue and depend on external cues (Taylor et al., 1990).

Examples of disinhibition syndromes have been reported with focal lesions at all levels of the OF circuit, including OF cortex, ventral striatum and pallidum, nucleus accumbens, DM thalamus and interconnecting pathways. Bilateral (Richfield et al., 1987; Starkstein et al., 1988d) or large unilateral caudate lesions (Mendez et al., 1989) and other diseases involving basal ganglia, such as Huntington's disease, Tourette's disease, parkinsonism, Wilson's disease, and Sydenham's chorea, can present with an OF disinhibition syndrome (see below).

Treatment of the disinhibition syndrome includes propranolol, carbamazepine, sodium valproate, lithium, benzodiazepines, or neuroleptics. Impulsive aggression can be treated wth 5HT2 downregulation. Serotonergic agonists (clomipramine, fluoxetine) may be effective in impulsive or aggressive behaviors, or sexual disinhibition. Propranolol and pindolol may also be useful, possibly through their 5HT1a agonist properties.

Obsessive–compulsive disorder

Obsessive–compulsive disorder, first described by Taylor et al. (1990) as 'scrupules,' has been called 'religious melancholy,' 'reasoning monomanias or partial deliria,' 'folie circulaire,', 'obsessive representation,' 'ruminative sickness or Grübelsucht,' 'delire du toucher – touching madness,' 'abortive insanity,' 'neurasthenic madness,' 'imperative ideas,' compulsive neurosis and obsessional neurosis, and obsessivoid state (for a historical review, see Hunter and MacAlpine, 1963).

Obsessions are recurrent, persistent, intrusive, reiterating, stereotyped, mental experiences (ideas, thoughts, images, premonitory urges or feelings, desires, doubts, images, or impulses) with a compelling quality, which constantly intrude into consciousness and activity and interfere with life functioning, with persistence of insight. Patients do not experience them as voluntarily produced, and should recognize them as irrational, senseless, alien, absurd, repugnant, abnormal, and not the result of mind control or some form of thought insertion, and try to resist them up to some point; they are unable to prevent them occurring. Patients are disrupted by these recurrent internal thoughts, a subjective sense of compulsion overriding an internal resistance.

When the obsession leads to an act, it is called compulsion, which is a repetitive, purposeful, and intentional action, performed in a response to an obsession, in order to prevent discomfort or some dreaded event or situation. The repetitive, ritualistic, excessive, unnecessary, and seemingly purposeless motor behaviors, performed in a stereotyped fashion according to certain rules, resulting from strong subjective urges, are still under the individual's control. The activity is not connected realistically with what it is designed to prevent, and the person recognizes the behavior as excessive or unreasonable. Obsessions and compulsions cluster around a few themes in general, mostly centered on the person or the person's home. They include contamination, aggressive thoughts, exactness, symmetry, exact scheduling of time, security (door, gas, or water taps, windows, lights, plugs, cigarettes), filth (speck on clothes, dirtiness), somatic worries about a severe illness, harm, responsibility for death or injury, danger, or doubt, sexual, religious worries or violence, and cognitive rituals in which a discrete number of steps has to be performed and must be redone when any deviation occurs in the process. Compulsions commonly include cleaning, washing, grooming, checking, ordering, counting, hoarding, repeating, collecting, but also pure obsessions, obsessional slowness, and inability to make decisions. The majority of patients have more than one obsessional expression, for example 76% of checkers complained of doubting, 58% of slowness, 55% of cleaning; 61% of cleaners also reported doubting, 54% slowness, 60% checking rituals; 65% of slow patients also reported doubting, 60% checking, and 50% cleaning.

When obsessions and compulsions cause distress, are time consuming ($>$one hour/day), or significantly interfere with the person's life and/or relationships, they meet the criteria for obsessive–compulsive disorder.

Obsessive–compulsive disorder is an idiopathic, genetic disease, which can be recognized in 2% of the general population. It usually occurs in early adulthood, rarely in late life. One-third of the cases identified in adults started during childhood or adolescence, and two-thirds of the children with this disorder will keep some degree of symptomatology in adulthood. In adults, the remission rate is 30%; 20% reported a duration of more than ten years; 30% less than one year. In 29–61% of patients, the condition continued with no improvement. Obsessive–compulsive disorder has an episodic, chronic, or remitting course, and can be associated with major depression (30%), simple phobias (27%), panic disorders (14%), agoraphobia (9%), and Gilles de la Tourette's syndrome, but many investigators consider that the disorder could be one end of the spectrum of clinical expression of Tourette's disease.

In a third of children with obsessive–compulsive disorder, soft neurological signs are described, all of them being compatible with a fronto-subcortical motor dysfunction. The signs include alterations of postural control, tone, gait, equilibrium, spontaneous movement, speech, eye movements, facial motility, arm and hand posture, mirror movements, fine motor incoordination, difficulty with rhythms, sensory deficits (graphesthesia), choreiform movements or tics (Rasmussen and Eisen, 1992).

Sometimes, some degree of magical logic is found, concerning the prevention of danger or harm, forestalling an unpleasant event, the restoration of safety, avoiding punishment, criticism, guilt, or fear. Attempts to suppress the compulsive behavior lead to anxiety, and patients eventually give up resisting. Patients do not derive pleasure from carrying out the activity, although it often provides a release of tension. In 33% of obsessive–compulsive disorders, schizotypic personality is found.

Cognitive dysfunction, especially frontal lobe dysexecutive syndrome, is found in a majority of patients with obsessive–compulsive disorder, suggestive of predominant left fronto-subcortical dysfunction, especially of caudate (Flor-Henry, 1990), with reduced verbal fluency, impaired shifting or sequencing of cognitive set, indecision, difficulty in initiating goal-directed actions, performing two tasks simultaneously, suppressing intrusive and perseverative behaviors, but also deficient memory for details, attention and learning difficulties, poor visuospatial processing, recall and cube drawing, speech abnormalities (receptive speech, better than normal verbal performance), and confabulations (see Alarcon et al., 1994, for review). Obsessional slowness (Rachman, 1974) is found in 30% of cases, in addition to the dysexecutive syndrome, and 72% had reduced work capacity due to the disorder. A peculiar personality profile is also described, with a celibacy rate of 72% (Coryell, 1981).

The earliest association between a neurologic disease and obsessive–compulsive disorder was made in von Economo's encephalitis. Obsessive–compulsive disorder, or symptomatic obsessive–compulsive disorder, has been associated with focal lesions at any level of the OF fronto-subcortical circuit: left, right, or bilateral frontal, basal ganglia (bilateral striatum or pallidum), thalamus and interconnected pathways, or anterior cingulum. Lesions of the striatum (caudo-putamen) are often reported, bilaterally (Brickner et al., 1940; Mena et al., 1967; Laplane et al., 1981, 1984, 1988a, 1992; Pulst et al., 1983; Ali-Chérif et al., 1984; Behar et al., 1984; Weilberg et al., 1986; Stahl, 1988; Williams et al., 1988; Croisile et al., 1989; Modell et al., 1989; Trillet et al., 1990; Laplane, 1994; Ghika et al., 1999a) more often than unilaterally (Tonkonogy and Barreira, 1989; Flor-Henry, 1990; Rapoport, 1990) or of the bilateral (Laplane et al. 1989, 1992) more often than of unilateral lentiform nucleus (Turecki et al., 1993; Laplane, 1994), or bilateral putamen (Ali-Chérif et al., 1984; Laplane et al., 1992).

When no lesion was obvious, as in obsessive–compulsive disorder, quantitative radiological studies of basal ganglia with computerized tomography (CT) (Behar et al., 1984; Luxenberg et al., 1988; Stein et al., 1993) or magnetic resonance imaging (MRI) scan (Garber et al., 1989; Scarone et al., 1992; Calabrese et al., 1993; Zitterl et al., 1994; Robinson et al., 1995) showed bilateral smaller caudate nuclei (Luxenberg et al., 1988; Robinson et al., 1995), no change (Garber et al., 1989; Kellner et al., 1991; Stein et al., 1993), or increased volume of the head of caudate nucleus (Scarone et al., 1992), unilateral atrophy of the head of left caudate and putamen (Luxenberg et al., 1988; Robinson et al., 1995), or abnormal T1 signal in frontal white matter, basal ganglia, or thalamus (Garber et al., 1989; Calabrese et al., 1993; Vincent et al., 1994; Zitterl et al., 1994).

Metabolic or blood flow studies showed interesting, but sometimes contradictory, results, even by the same groups. Findings and methods across studies are heterogeneous, but a convergent pattern (see Berthier et al., 1996b, for review) tending to describe increased metabolism or blood flow was shown in OF areas (left, right, or bilaterally), DLPF cortex (right, left, or bilaterally), anterior and posterior cingulate, and other areas (right sensorimotor, dorsal parietal, and superior temporal cortex), but also in the basal ganglia, in bilateral caudate nuclei (Modell et al., 1989; Benkelfat et al., 1990; Machlin et al., 1991; Rubin et al., 1992; McGuire et al., 1994; Molina et al., 1995), sometimes predominantly on the right. Increased metabolism has been also described in putamen (Benkelfat et al., 1990), and increased metabolism in pallidum (Laplane et al., 1989) and thalamus. A few studies are at variance with these results, describing decreased metabolism in mediofrontal cortex, sensorimotor, parietal, and temporal cortical areas, normal or even decreased blood flow or metabolism in caudate and putamen (Nordahl et al., 1989; Martinot et al., 1990; Harris et al., 1994; Perani et al., 1995).

Symptom provocation may increase right caudate metabolism, whereas effective treatment decreases the metabolic rate, especially on the right caudate, left caudate, and bilateral caudate (Baxter et al., 1985). Others report no change in the basal ganglia after treatment but a reduction from baseline in bilateral or right OF regions and cingulate (Zohar et al., 1989; Benkelfat et al., 1990; Hoehn-Saric et al., 1991; McGuire et al., 1994).

Functional MRI (f-MRI) (Breiter et al., 1996), allowing repeated studies in the same patients without harm, showed results consistent with previous positron emission tomography (PET) and single-positron emission computerized tomography (SPECT) studies. Bilateral anterior and posterior medial orbital gyri, bilateral superior, middle, and inferior frontal gyri, bilateral anterior cingulate cortex, bilateral temporal cortex, right caudate, left lenticulate nucleus, left insula and bilateral amygdaloid nucleus were hyperactive in more than 70% of the patients when compared to controls. Paralimbic and limbic activations were more prominent with f-MRI than with PET or SPECT studies. This shows that isocortical (lateral frontal), paralimbic (medial OF gyrus, anterior cingulate, temporal cortex, insula), limbic (amygdaloid nucleus), and striatal regions (caudate and lenticular nucleus) are activated, involving systems associated with cognition, emotion, and motor behavior.

Patients with diseases of the basal ganglia often shown obsessive–compulsive disorder. Associations between this disorder and previous encephalitis lethargica and other meningoencephalitis of the basal ganglia, head trauma (3.4%), striatal necrosis, strokes, carbon monoxide or manganese intoxication, perinatal anoxia, tumors, head trauma, basal ganglia calcification, Tourette's (50–75%), Huntington's, Wilson's, Parkinson's diseases, Sydenham's chorea, progressive supranuclear palsy, neuroacanthocytosis, focal dystonia, and with drugs acting on monoamines such as cocaine, amphetamine, levodopa, and dopamine agonists, are described below in more detail.

Based on all this information, it is hypothesized that obsessive–compulsive disorder results from some degree of neurofunctional abnormality in the OF-basal ganglia-limbic-cortical circuits (Modell et al., 1989; Flor-Henry, 1990; Alarcon et al., 1994; Baxter, 1994; Cummings, 1995). In obsessive–compulsive disorder, an aberrant positive feedback loop develops in the fronto-thalamic loop, due to a loss of inhibition (negative gating, filtering) by the ventral striatum-accumbens complex, and perhaps also anterior cingulum on the thalamic DM-OF cortex drive, allowing incoherent goal-oriented and context-oriented behavioral and emotional output, or, clinically, inappropriate obsessive–compulsive, emotional–behavioral drive. Automatic execution of learned sensorimotor programs, thought, and emotions are spontaneously repetitively generated by the ventral striatum and accumbens nucleus and the increased metabolism of the OF cortex would be the compensating mechanism. The cingulate gyrus seems also to play a major role in the regulation of automatic behaviors through its association with the septohippocampal and thalamo-cortical systems (Martuza et al., 1990).

Serotonergic neurotransmission seems to play a major role in obsessive–compulsive disorder (Winslow and Insel, 1990), but also dopamine and possibly norepinephrine. Complex repetitive behaviors and obsessive–compulsive disorder have been described after intoxication with amphetamine, cocaine, L-dopa, and mCPP (serotonin agonist). Treatment of the disorder shows that selective serotonin reuptake inhibitors (SSRIs) are effective in more than 50% of the patients, with a reduction by 30–50% of the severity of symptoms. Drugs that are reported to be effective include clomipramine, imipramine, doxepin, amitriptyline, chlorimipramine, guanfacine, nardil, desipramine, fluoxetine, sertraline, fluvoxamine, fenfluramine, citalopram, trazodone, zimelidine, buspirone, monoamine oxidase inhibitors, nardil, amphetamines, naloxone, clonidine, yohimbine, clonazepam, selegiline, L-tryptophan, and antiandrogenic treatment (Jenike, 1992). The addition of lithium, buspirone, or diazepam, but also of neuroleptics may be necessary in refractory cases (40–60% of the patients reacted with SSRI). There have been open-label studies showing the effectiveness of monotherapy with neuroleptic patients with obsessive–compulsive disorder. In Tourette's syndrome, obsessive–compulsive disorder is typically resistant to neuroleptics alone.

Psychosurgery has been used in refractory cases (for a review, see Martuza et al., 1990; Hay et al., 1993). Cingulatomy, limbic leukotomy, orbitomedial lesions, subcaudate tractotomy, bimedial leukotomy, anterior capsulotomy, and medical thalamotomy have been used with reported success. Considerable ethical and scientific problems are raised in the interpretation of results. Small series, incomplete assessments, short-duration follow-up, and poor use of control groups impair the validity of reported results. Benefits range from 25% to 100%, with a mean of 60%.

Disorders of impulse control or conduct disorders, impulsions and impulsivity

Another class of disinihibition syndrome, or perhaps another end of the spectrum of obsessive–compulsive disorder, comprises disorders of impulse control, or conduct or impulse disorders (Frosch and Wortis, 1954). These disorders consist of a failure to resist an impulse, drive or temptation to perform some act that is harmful to the person or to others, with or without conscious resistance to the impulse and with or without premeditation. An increasing sense of tension, or arousal, is present before committing the act.

Impulsions are repetitive intentional actions performed according to certain rules, in a stereotyped fashion. The behavior is performed automatically, without purpose or as the consequence of the failure to resist an impulse or a temptation to perform some act that is harmful to the individual or to others. Pleasure, gratification, or relief is felt during the act; feelings of guilt and regret arise later (Hoogduin, 1986), but the person recognizes the behavior as unrealistic or excessive. Impulsions are more sudden and less predictable than compulsions. When impulsions cause distress, are time consuming (>one hour/day) or significantly interfere with the person's life and/or relationships, they meet the criteria for disorder of impulse control.

A subjective urge to perform tics is well known in tic disorders such as Tourette's syndrome, akathisia, restless legs, painful legs, and moving toes. Impulsiveness can be part of the obsessive–compulsive disorder (Hoehn-Saric and Barksdale, 1983), compulsive shopping, substance abuse, and dependence disorders (Scott, 1983; Lesieur et al., 1986; Modell et al., 1990), kleptomania (Bradford and Balmaceda, 1983; Goldman, 1991), pyromania (Scott, 1978), intermittent explosive disorder, sudden mood swings, catathymic crises, or episodic dyscontrol syndrome (Bach-y-Rita et al., 1971), isolated explosive disorder, sociopathy, self-harm

(Winchel and Stanley, 1991) risk taking (Spittle et al., 1976; Schalling et al., 1984), sexual obsessions and compulsions (intrusive, repetitive, and vivid sexual images, compulsive masturbation or other sexual behavior, including paraphilias, voyeurism, and exhibitionism) (Coleman, 1990), and other personality disorders, but they can also be associated as in multi-impulsive patients.

Body dysmorphic disorder (dysmorphobia) (Andreasen and Bardach, 1977) may also be included here, consisting of preoccupation with an imagined defect in one's appearance, often leading to surgical procedures or compulsive rituals in order to conceal the perceived defect. Obsessive–compulsive disorder, mirror checking, make-up rituals, excessive physician visits, avoidance behavior, anxiety, narcissism, social phobia, hypochondriacal traits, and depression are often associated. No metabolic study has been reported so far.

Craving and loss of control in alcohol abuse (Modell et al., 1990) have also been considered as an impulse disorder with basal ganglia/limbic striatal and thalamo-cortical dysfunction, especially the ventral striatal dopaminergic circuit. Craving has been hypothesized as arising from overactivity within the fronto-thalamic circuit resulting from a decrease in dopamine in the ventrotegmental-accumbens pathway (hypodopaminergic state), which can be reversed by the rewarding dopaminergic stimulation resulting from the ingestion of alcohol. Striatal serotonin seems also to be increased during abstinence, and SSRI decreases the consumption of ethanol in humans (Modell et al., 1990). PET studies showed lower metabolic rates in the basal ganglia, thalamus, and numerous cortical areas in chronic drinkers, but studies during withdrawal show conflicting results.

Pathological gambling (Moran, 1970; Lesieur et al., 1986) is also considered as an impulse disorder. Metabolites of norepinephrine (3-methoxy-4-hydroxy-phenylglycol) and norepiphrine were increased in the cerebrospiral fluid of pathological gamblers, but there was no decrease in 5HT metabolites (5HIAA) as in obsessive–compulsive disorder; however, no blood flow or metabolic study has been reported so far.

Eating disorders (anorexia, bulimia, binge eating) and purging, and stercoral compulsion (George et al., 1990) are associated with obsessive–compulsive disorder in 54% of cases, with kleptomania in 54% and substance abuse. Andreason et al. (1992) showed increased metabolism in basal ganglia of anorexic patients with bulimic symptoms of bingeing and purging. Lehembe and Graux (1992) described lacunar striatal infarcts in association with stercoral compulsion.

Moral or religious scrupulosity (Hoffnung et al., 1989) is an excessive observance of moral and religious teaching to a degree that far exceeds the expected practice of an individual's moral or religious reference group, and which is very difficult to accomplish, becoming a source of great anxiety to the person and his or her social network. Obsessive–compulsive disorder is often associated. The intense fear of violating a moral or religious code, the need to avoid potential danger, and compulsive checking are time consuming for the patients. There are no quantitative MRI, blood flow, or metabolic studies so far available.

Trichotillomania (Hallopeau, 1889) is an under-recognized disorder affecting 3% of the population, characterized by repetitive urges to pull one's own hair and often associated with paresthesia. Pulling hair is frequently associated with pleasure and the relief of these urges (Minichiello et al., 1994), with resulting hair loss or definitive baldness. Ninety percent of those affected are females, who usually have no other compulsions, impulsions, or obsessions. In severe cases, people spend many hours of the day and night pulling out their hairs, one at a time, the feel of regrowing stubble inducing an irresistible impulse to pull. When severe, it can lead to denuded eyebrows and eyelashes, and large bald patches. First considered as a habit disorder, a manifestation of intrapsychic conflict, a personality disorder, or a secondary manifestation of psychosis, it is now classified as an impulse control disorder and is not associated with obsessions (Demaret, 1973; George et al., 1990). O'Sullivan et al. (1997), in a morphometric MRI study, found a 13% smaller left putamen volume and lenticulate (10%), and Swedo et al. (1991) found results similar to obsessive–compulsive disorder on PET study.

Nailbiting (onychophagia) can be present in up to 25% of people (Leonard et al., 1991), 19% have motor tics or bodily manipulations such as thumb sucking or nose picking, finger and hand biting with excoriations, scars, and keloids. Considered as trivial or a sign of anxiety, it is often associated with motor restlessness. No blood flow or metabolic study has been reported so far.

Self-injurious behavior (automutilation) is a peculiar form of disinhibition syndrome or compulsion. Dopamine, serotonin and tachykinins and endorphins seem to be major players in the neurotransmission of automutilation (Sivam, 1996). Impulsive suicide, head banging, perioral, finger, or lip biting, burning, punching, pummelling, slapping, scratching, tongue and cheek biting, tooth extraction, eye poking or pressing, putting the head or hand through windows, walking into obstacles, reckless driving etc., are well known in diseases involving basal ganglia such as choreoacanthocytosis, Tourette's syndrome, Lesh–Nyhan, and Cornelia de Lange syndromes, onychophagia, trichotillomania, and other disorders of impulse control (see above and below), and mood disorders such as depression and mania. Dopamine agonists, SSRIs, clonidine, naloxone, and beta-blockers may be useful.

Hetero-injurious behaviors such as hitting, pinching, burning etc., are also seen in these diseases (Tourette's syndrome, Huntington's chorea, Wilson's disease).

Coprohenomena are impulsive motor (copropraxia, manipulation of excrements), vocal (swearing), or psychic (mental obscenities) behaviors that are frequently seen in Tourette's syndrome (see below), as well as in dementia. Focal lesions have not been reported.

Serotonin seems to have a major role in the pathophysiology of impulsive disorders, together with norepinephrine and dopamine. Clomipramine, fluoxetine, fluvoxamine or other SSRIs, pimozide, buspirone, and lithium are helpful in all of the above-mentioned disorders, as they are in obsessive–compulsive disorder, but sometimes propranolol, carbamazepine, fluprazine or pimozide or other serenics can be helpful.

Repetitive and compulsive behavior, motor and mental stereotypies, and perseverations

Other classes of disinhibition syndromes are repetitive behaviors (for a review, see Sandson and Albert, 1987; Ford, 1991), which have been reported in 78% of 46 proven pathological cases of frontal lobe degeneration, which are often accompanied by minimal lesions of the basal ganglia (including Pick's disease, non-Alzheimer fronto-temporal dementia, progressive subcortical gliosis, amyotrophic lateral sclerosis–dementia syndrome) (Akelaitis, 1994). The behaviors range from motor stereotypies (Guirand, 1936) to complex obsessive–compulsive disorder and akathisia. They include purposeless repetitive behaviors, restlessness, wandering, pacing, repetitively tearing stuffing from mattress, picking at clothing, rubbing a hand, continuous masturbation, repetitively turning a light switch on and off, stereotyped gestures, ritualistic activities, repetitive autoenemas, hoarding of paper scraps or matches, echolalia, echopraxia, palilalia, stereotyped utterances of sounds, syllables, words or sentence(s), prayers, stories, questions, greetings, counting, continuous singing, mannerisms, stereotyped behavior, perseverations, rigid programming of household tasks and social functions, incessant cigarette smoking, and compulsions. Unlike patients with idiopathic obsessive–compulsive disorder, these patients showed substantial cognitive impairment and no insight into the irrational nature of their repetitive behaviors or thoughts. Combined damage of the frontal lobe, caudate nucleus, and globus pallidus is reported in the majority of the cases on pathology, and, when performed, SPECT or PET scan showed reduced metabolism or blood flow in the fronto-temporal cortex and caudate nuclei (Ames et al., 1994).

Perseverations are stereotyped movements that are not accompanied by mental content suggestive of obsession, with the individual being unable to direct his or her activities in response to external stimuli, and usually having insight into his or her behavior (Sandson and Albert, 1987). Repetition is an important aspect of motor behavior, from walking to repetitive hand movements. Fixed action pattern can be triggered by environmental stimuli. Flexible, self-initiated and voluntary behavior is a more recent acquisition in phylogenesis. Pathological repetition can result from overexcitation of motor programs or from loss of inhibitory mechanism from internal or voluntary command. No obvious external incentive is at the origin of sterotypy. Perseveration and stereotypy are the clinical expression of repetitious behaviors such as tics and motor rituals, but also of rumination, fixation, and inflexibility. Perseverations result from a restriction of choices of action such that behavior is repetitive but not excessive. Slow mental changes are perseverative. According to Goldberg (1986), there are several levels of perseveration. The lowest level is productive stereotypy, 'motor perseveration,' in which the patient continues to make the same movement when asked to do only one (e.g., continues to make many circles when asked to do only one). The second level, 'task-specific perseveration,' results from the inability to change or sequence different patterns when asked (perseverating in making circles when asked to draw a circle then a square). In the higher level, 'set perseveration,' the patient stays in the same category of motor program when asked to change it semantically (perseverating in drawing a circle then a square when asked to draw a circle then write the word square).

Ideatory perseverations, as well as perseverations in drawing and speech, have been reported with caudate lesions (Cambier et al., 1979), frontal lobe lesions, metabolic encephalopathies, and temporo-parietal lobe lesions (Allison, 1966; Cambier et al., 1988). Difficulty in maintaining semantic set, or mental focus, and ideatory perseveration show that the caudate nucleus has a role to play in the preliminary selection before organizing the speech process, including realization and sequencing of phonemes, choice of words, and syntactic organization of the sentence. Graphomania (compulsive writing) or arithmomania (compulsive counting) has also been described in caudate lesions (Cambier et al., 1979). Arithmetic, language, and visuospatial tasks perseverations have been found with basal ganglia encephalitis (Peatfield, 1987).

Stereotypy (which refers to motor acts) is at a higher level of severity than perseveration (which refers to mental states). Stereotypy is an excessive repetition of motor acts, a 'higher rates of activity but in a decreasing number of response categories.' Simple motor stereotypy (Ali-Cherif et al., 1984; Trillet et al., 1990), complex (Luria, 1978) or purely mental stereotypies such as arithmomania and stercoral compulsion, have been found in multiple lacunes of the striatum (Lehembe and Graux, 1992) and accompany athymormic states (Laplane et al., 1988a, 1988b, 1989; Laplane, 1994). If stereotypy is considered as a consequence of failure to use sensory input into the direct behavior, environmentally induced stereotypy, such as confinement stereotypy with to-and-fro pacing, or deprivation stereotypy, such as congenitally blind or mentally deficient children, are well known. Stereotypies may be accompanied by a variable level of volition and insight and can be found in schizophrenics, autism, obsessive–compulsive disorder, addiction, frontal lobe lesions, Parkinson's disease, Tourette's syndrome, postencephalitic states, amphetamine abuse, or with L-dopa. Stereotyped rocking and twirling, unusual hand and arm movements, and arm flipping are seen in normal children, especially before sleep, and sometimes in adults. Severe stereotypies including self-injury such as head banging, self-biting, or eye poking can be seen in autistic patients, schizophrenics, mentally retarded individuals, acanthocytosis, Lesch–Nyhan syndrome, Tourette's syndrome, and amphetamine and cocaine psychosis (see below).

Pali-phenomena are motor (palipraxia), vocal (palilalia), or psychic (mental palilalia), repetitive of initial movements, words or thoughts, which are frequently reported in Tourette's syndrome (see below). Focal lesions have not yet been reported.

Stimulus-bound or environment-dependency behavior, echophenomena

Another disinhibition syndrome is the environment-dependency syndrome. Denny Brown (1962) described animals with bilateral lesions of the head of the caudate 'visually determined cortical automatisms, with forced delicate, labile, but stereotyped' obligatory fixed responses to a visual stimulus. Lhermitte (1986) later called this behavior 'environment-dependency syndrome,' which he found in patients with frontal lesions, but this behavior has been now recognized in association with lesions at all levels of the fronto-subcortical circuits, i.e., caudate, lenticular, thalamic, and their interconnecting pathways. The environment-dependency syndrome is thought to result from a disconnection between prefrontal cortex and parietal regions (Lhermitte, 1986). This may reflect a difficulty or a disconnection between internally driven behaviors and external (environmental)-driven stimuli, leading to stereotyped behaviors. Environment-dependency syndrome has been reported in progressive supranuclear palsy and in vascular diseases involving the basal ganglia (see below).

Echo-phenomena are impulsive behaviors that consist in motor (echopraxia), vocal (echolalia), or mental (mental echopraxia or echolalia) copy of the examiner's gestures or speech, or a semantic echoing such as in echoing approval (Ghika et al., 1996). Frequently seen in patients with Tourette's syndrome (see below), it can also be seen in vascular or fronto-temporal dementias and parkinsonism (see below).

Hypermetamorphosis, or mandatory exploration of high-stimulus items in the environment, observed in Klüver–Bucy syndrome or bilateral temporal lobe injury (for a review, see Lilly et al., 1983), lacks the ritualistic stereotypy of repetitive behaviors and obsessive–compulsive disorder and is more spontaneous than the compulsive behaviors or environmental dependency or imitation and utilization behaviors that can also be seen in frontal lobe degenerations. Compulsive eating (hyperphagia) and hyperorality or oral exploration are also part of this syndrome.

Agitation and hyperactivity

Agitation and hyperactivity are somewhat nonspecific symptoms, perhaps due to dopamine and norepinephrine dysfunction, mostly seen with frontal lesions. Agitation and hyperactivity have, however, been described with caudate (Cambier et al., 1979; Caplan et al., 1990), subthalamic (Trillet et al., 1995), and thalamic lesions (Bogousslavsky et al., 1988). Agitation and hyperactivity are seen in akathisia – feeling an urge to move, restlessness, and various expressions of hyperactivity including pacing, walking, sitting up and down, talking, smoking etc. sometimes accompanied by disorders of impulse control, generally due to neuroleptic or L-dopa treatment, cocaine, amphetamines, head trauma, subthalamic lesions, and withdrawal (Haskovec, 1901) – as well as in attention deficit hyperactivity disorder (see below).

Hyperkinetic mutism (Inbody and Jankovic, 1986) is a peculiar form of agitation and mutism. This syndrome was described in a case of idiopathic basal ganglia calcification. Logorrhea has been described with striatal lesions (Trillet et al., 1990).

Hyperactivity is also part of mania (see below), graphomania (compulsive writing, seen in caudate lesions, see below), trichotillomania (see above), arithmomania, and mental play (repetitive, useless thoughts or images, intended as a pastime, see Tourette's syndrome).

Mood and affective disorders

Emotions are the result of an external or internal input. The integrative circuitry of emotion is thought to depend on a set of structures of the limbic system, including the amygdala, the septum, the hippocampus, the cingulate and related cortices. The performance of emotional motor expression (mimic, gesture, prosody) is considered to be processed in the paralimbic cortex and basal ganglia, whereas autonomic and endocrine features arise from the hypothalamic region. Transfer of information from the limbic system to the basal ganglia is probably processed at the level of the accumbens nucleus (Nauta, 1986), with some regulation by the mesencephalic dopaminergic pathways.

Motor manifestations of mood disorders are often discounted clinically. Patients with mania are physically hyperactive, with pacing and running, becoming involved in all kinds of activities, including buying, calling, and talking, but also their speech and overall activities are faster and their affective expression and gestures are exaggerated. Depressives, on the other hand, show a loss of emotion or a sad face, bowed posture, slow gestures, and sparse verbal output with hypophonia, shuffling gait, and psychomotor retardation. Anxiety is well recognized, with a peculiar pattern of mimickry including widening of the palpebral fissures and widening of the eyebrows, furrowing of the forehead, and tachypnea, as well as autonomic features such as perspiration, dry mouth, tachycardia and tachypnea, tremor, and pacing.

The correlation of some patterns of emotional states and behaviors with the laterality of the lesions has been well known since its description by Goldstein (1939), and left hemispheric lesions are associated with depressive–catastrophic reactions (Flor-Henry, 1979; Robinson et al., 1984, 1988), while indifference or mania prevails in right hemispheric lesions (Gainotti, 1972). Livingston (1977) and Blumer and Benson (1975) described two separate parallel fronto-limbo-hypo-thalamic-mesencephalic circuits for emotional control, the medial prefrontal-cingulate-hippocampal circuit regulating what is understood clinically to be depression, and the lateral orbito-frontal-temporal amygdala circuit regulating anxiety and mania.

Disorders involving the basal ganglia are known to affect both emotional states and emotional expression, and perhaps emotional comprehension. Mood disorders (depression, mania, or bipolar disorders) are well known in diseases involving basal ganglia.

Depression

Major primary unipolar depression afflicts 2–7% of the general population at any time, and includes low mood, insomnia, reduced appetite, weight loss, a decreased feeling of energy (anergia), psychomotor retardation, difficulty concentrating. forgetfulness, anhedonia, loss of interest in sex, feelings of worthlessness, pathological guilt, and thoughts about suicide. Patients with late-onset depression have more frequent hypochondriacal ideation, early insomnia, agitation, preoccupation with guilt and feces than do patients with early-onset depression.

In unipolar depression, CT and MRI imaging are mostly unremarkable. Morphometric studies showed reduction of the volume of the basal ganglia (caudate and putamen) on MRI bilaterally in patients with major depression (Mendez et al., 1989; Husain et al., 1991; Krishnan et al., 1992; Coffey et al., 1993; Videbech, 1997), or subcortical atrophy (Starkstein et al., 1988c), increased rate of white matter and periventricular hyperintensities (50–60% of the patients versus 5% of controls), some of them involving the basal ganglia, especially the caudate (for reviews, see Figiel et al., 1990; Dupont et al., 1995, Videbech, 1997), or enlarged ventricles (Kellner et al., 1991). Patients with basal ganglia lesions, particularly of the caudate, experienced more adverse events (especially delirium after ECT: Figiel et al., 1990). Other morphometric abnormalities were found, within or outside fronto-subcortical circuits, including a smaller mean total frontal lobe volume (7% smaller on CT), smaller cerebellum, especially vermis, and larger sulci.

Metabolic and blood blow PET and SPECT studies in unipolar depression also showed decreased metabolism in left fronto-subcortical and paralimbic circuits, left anterior cingulate and left anterolateral and dorsolateral; prefrontal cortex, but also inferior frontal and superior temporal and parietal cortex, and caudate (Buchsbaum et al., 1986), which normalized after therapy. In activation studies, left anterolateral prefrontal cortex or left anterior cingulate, left medial frontal and anterior limbic system (George, 1994) were activated when subjects were asked to think sad thoughts.

Frontal lobe dysfunction, especially dysexecutive dysfunction, is well documented in depression (for a review, see Mayberg, 1994; Mayberg et al., 1994), generally supporting the association of depression with a dysfunction in fronto-striatal and basal-limbic pathways, with left-side predominance.

Secondary or symptomatic depression is well studied in stroke. Focal lesions in fronto-subcortical and paralimbic subcortical circuits are described in left frontal, striatal strokes, especially when involving the head of the caudate, thalamus, and bilateral subcortical white matter hyperintensities on T2 MR imaging, with frontal and parietal predominance and basal ganglia. In subcortical strokes, when basal ganglia are involved, the best predictor for depression is the left frontal lobe, especially when anterior subcortical structures are involved, i.e., caudate, lenticular, anterior arm of internal capsule (Starkstein et al., 1988d; Robinson and Starkstein, 1990; Krishnan et al., 1992; Bogousslavsky, 1993; Berthier et al., 1996a). In the elderly, depression is often associated with white matter lesions in subcortical frontal areas and basal ganglia, and with a decrease in the volume of putamen (Husain et al., 1991). Vascular diseases with important frontal and striatal involvement, such as Binswanger's disease and multilacunar states, often cause depression and emotional lability. Depression was minor or major, but a gradient of severity of depression was found for more anteriorly located lesions. Depression is also a well-known feature in diseases involving basal ganglia, such as Huntington's chorea and Parkinson's disease, in HIV patients with basal ganglia lesions, Sydenham's chorea, Tourette's syndrome, basal ganglia calcification, tumors, and head injury (see below). Dopamine, norepinephrine, and serotonin are major neurotransmitters in the pathology and treatment of depression.

Anxiety disorders

Anxiety (worry, fear, uneasiness about what may happen, with feelings of intense malaise accompanied by autonomic features such as palpitations, perspiration, tremor, shortness of breath, and feelings of constriction in the throat, thorax or abdomen), panic attacks (paroxysmal extreme anxiety of limited duration), and phobias (persistent irrational fear of objects, persons, situations) are frequent findings in basal ganglia diseases such as parkinsonism, Huntington's disease, Wilson's disease, Sydenham's chorea, basal ganglia calcifications etc. (see below).

In anxiety, there is decreased glucose metabolism in frontal lobe, inferior temporal lobe, or left middle temporal lobe (Buchsbaum et al., 1986), but increased activity in the right posterior cingulate and basal ganglia.

Mania

Primary mania includes symptoms such as euphoria, irritability, flight of ideas, hyperactivity, logorrhea, decreased need for sleep, distractibility, impaired judgment, hypersexuality, spending and travelling sprees, hypergraphia, excessive phone calling, an increase in time spent working, excessive rate of speech, racing thoughts, increased motivation, and grandiosity. Mania can exist as unipolar disease. In general, no lesion is found on CT or MRI. SPECT and PET metabolic and blood flow studies in mania showed lower perfusion or decreased metabolism of the right hemisphere, especially in temporobasal portions, but no change in the basal ganglia, even though the lesions involved the head of the right caudate. In unipolar secondary mania, focal lesions, such as strokes, trauma or tumors, were reported in the right hemisphere, involving OF cortex, head of caudate, or striatum, limbic or limbic-associated areas, lateral basotemporal, amygdala, thalamus, diencephalon, and substantia nigra, and interconnecting white matter, i.e. also in fronto-subcortical-limbic paralimbic circuits (see Starkstein et al., 1990a).

Secondary or symptomatic mania has been reported after head trauma or with tumors, but occurs more frequently in patients with a positive family history. Other disease of the basal ganglia may present with mania, including Huntington's disease, Wilson's disease, calcification of basal ganglia, stroke, hemorrhage, abscess of the thalamus or subthalamic nucleus (see below).

Bipolar mood disorders

In familial or idiopathic bipolar mood disorders, cycles of depression alternate with mania. If most CT or MRI studies are unremarkable in bipolar depression, CT morphometric studies showed increased density of right and left caudate, and ventricular enlargement (Beats et al., 1991). Similar MRI studies showed conflicting results: smaller volumes of caudate or putamen bilaterally were described by some authors (Husain et al., 1991; Swayze et al., 1992), larger caudate volume by others (Aylward et al., 1994), or no difference in the volume of basal ganglia between bipolar patients and controls (Strakowski et al., 1993; Dupont et al., 1995). Conflicting results are also given about increases in ventricular size or cortical atrophy (reported in up to a third of patients), smaller cerebellum, temporal lobe, and hippocampus, and increased rates (69–72%) of white matter and periventricular hyperintensities on T2, some of them involving basal ganglia (for a review, see Figiel et al. 1990; contested by Altschuler et al., 1995). Metabolic PET studies showed decreased metabolism in the left DLPF cortex and head of caudate, with an anterior–posterior ratio in favor of anterior structures (Baxter et al., 1985).

When focal lesions were found in secondary or symptomatic bipolar mood disorders, they were mostly localized in thalamus and caudate (Starkstein et al., 1990a, 1991), periventricular white matter (44% versus 6% of controls), internal capsule, and brainstem. In post-stroke bipolar secondary mania, a high incidence of movement disorders has been reported, and a variable incidence of family history of affective disorder (0–44%). Bipolar mood disorders have been reported in diseases of basal ganglia such as Tourette's syndrome, Huntington's disease, and basal ganglia calcification (see below).

Emotional lability

Emotional lability is a feature of the corticobulbar syndrome, but is frequently found in basal ganglia diseases and vascular dementia, even in the absence of a frank corticobulbar or bilateral corticospinal syndrome. The physiopathology is not well understood, but fronto-subcortical limbic circuits have not been comprehensively investigated with regard to this symptomatology.

Emotional blunting, indifference, apathy, anhedonia

Emotional blunting is a feature of the anterior cingulate syndrome (see above). Anhedonia (loss of pleasure in life) is a frequent finding in parkinsonism. The rewarding network, including nucleus accumbens and substantia nigra, but also motivational areas of the cingulate are the main relays of the involved circuitry that is suspected to account for this symptomatology.

Intermittent explosive disorder

Disorders of impulse control may be associated with violent expression of emotions, especially rage, but also with rapid mood swings as in intermittent explosive disorders (see above).

Disorders of emotional communication (cognition)

Amimia (loss of spontaneous emotional face expression) is a classical feature in parkinsonism (Rinn, 1984). Deficit in emotional facial communication, for both expression and comprehension, has been found in diseases of the basal ganglia such as Parkinson's disease and Huntington's disease (Blonder et al., 1989; Buck and Duffy, 1980; Borod et al., 1986; Katsikis and Pilowsky, 1991; Jacobs et al., 1995a, 1995b; Smith et al., 1988). Similar deficits in emotional communication of speech (motor and sensory aprosodia, syntactic aprosodia) have also been reported in Parkinson's disease (Canter, 1963; Scott et al., 1984; Blonder et al., 1989) and Huntington's disease (Speedie et al., 1990). Abnormal kinesia for emotional gestures and postures is also found, but has not been studied in detail, as well as alexithymia (the inability to describe emotions orally). Abnormalities in emotional memory or mental imaging have not been studied in much detail so far (Jacobs et al., 1995a). The underlying deficits in motor expression of the limbs are the same as those for mimicry and limb motions, i.e., akinesia (aspontaneity), bradykinesia, hypokinesia, hypometria, impersistence, perseveration, stereotypia, echoing phenomena, and hyperkinesia.

Cognitive syndromes of basal ganglia

Subcortical dementia was first defined by Albert et al. (1974) in order to describe a cognitive dysfunction including impairment of memory and learning, slowness of intellectual processing (bradyphrenia), difficulty in manipulating knowledge (dysexecutive syndrome, procedural memory problems), inertia, apathy, loss of motivation (anterior cingulate syndrome), mood disorders (including depression, bipolar moods, or emotional lability), and deficits in attention and arousal. As will be seen in the following paragraphs, these are mixed clinical pictures associating syndromes of the AC, OF, DLPF, speech, and limbic fronto-subcortical circuits. Language, praxias, gnosias, and perception are characteristically not involved, except in their motor and emotional expression.

The dorsolateral prefrontal syndrome: dysexecutive syndrome

Executive functions include anticipation, goal selection, planning, monitoring, and use of feedback (Stuss and Benson, 1986). Patients with a dysexecutive syndrome have an inability to execute goal-oriented strategies and to cope with complex activities in daily living. The syndrome involves loss of mental flexibility, difficulty with novel manipulation, sequential processing, major problems in performing two or several activities at the same time, problems when learning and copying tasks, a loss of adequate interaction with the environment, difficulty focusing, sustaining, shifting attention and inhibiting distractive responses to changing tasks, reduced fluency for speech and action, psychomotor akinesia, slowness or aspontaneity, psychomotor impersistence or perseverations, loss of abstract thinking and appreciation of abstract sets, difficulty with decisions, anticipation and foresight, problems generating hypotheses, searching strategies, organizing programming, decreased executive capacity to put the present sensory stimuli in the context of prior experience rather than respond to the stimuli themselves (environment dependency and social constraints), decreased self-awareness and judgment, decreased appreciation of abstract sets, and poor control of basic knowledge and cognitive processes. Behavioral deficits from a dysfunction at any level of the DLPF fronto-subcortical motor circuit result in a dysexecutive motor syndrome, but also in changes in personality, social behavior, emotional blunting, irritability, and difficulty in regulating behavior to the context rather than to the stimulus.

Focal lesions at any level from DLPF cortex, caudate, putamen, pallidum, thalamus and interconnecting pathways, generally bilateral (see Cummings, 1995, for a review), have been followed by dysexecutive syndromes, such as bilateral globus pallidus hemorrhages (Strub, 1989), left or bilateral paramedian–dorsomedian thalamic hemorrhages, but are also well known in diseases of the basal ganglia such as parkinsonism, Huntington's chorea, idiopathic calcification of the basal ganglia, Wilson's disease, lacunar states etc. (see below).

Norepinephrinergic fibers originating from the locus ceruleus seem to play a significant role in arousal and excitability. Dopaminergic mesocortical (frontal, pyriform, entorhinal) and mesolimbic systems (DM thalamus, DLPF cortex) also contribute in large measure to initiation, planning, temporal organization, and integration of motor behaviors. Serotonin has a more diffuse pattern, with a contribution to the processing of sensory information; acetylcholine from the nucleus basalis of Meynert plays its role in attention and memory; and GABA, mostly in cortical interneurons is involved in the modulation of excitatory neurotransmission. Drugs that are recognized to improve executive functions are monoamine oxidase inhibitors, clonidine, guanfacine, idazoxan, methylphenidate, and dextroamphetamine, showing that the norepinephrinergic system is an important modulator of the frontal lobe. Serotoninergic selective serotoninergic reuptake inhibitors (SSRIs) have tangential benefit only.

Attention-deficit hyperactivity disorder

This is a disinhibition and cognitive disorder associating developmentally inappropriate attention, impulsivity, and motor restlessness, and, often, delinquency. A form without hyperactivity is also described (Hynd et al., 1993). Attention-deficit hyperactivity disorder is the most common neuropsychiatric disorder of school-age children (2–5%). It is two to three times more common in males than in females. It is a major partner in developmental learning disorders. Forty to sixty percent of affected children will continue to have symptoms in adulthood. Patients have great difficulty regulating their behavior and are more active than their peers, as especially manifested at school, on car trips, in church etc. They are impulsive, demanding, inattentive, hyperactive, emotionally labile, and have learning disabilities. Patients are unable to use knowledge 'on line' to adjust their behavior, despite their intelligence and knowledge. They have difficulty in processing environmental stimuli, or are easily distracted by surrounding events. They are extremely sensitive to light, noise, and physical discomfort, and seek a quiet environment to be able to concentrate. They have response inhibition deficits, misestimate time intervals, and have impaired self-regulation of arousal, anger, and environmental factors. They also often seek highly stimulating environments, are prone to tantrums and anger, and are impulsive.

Associated dysexecutive dysfunction is well documented in patients with attention deficit hyperactivity disorder. They lack insight, have perseverative response tendencies, disinhibition or failure to inhibit impulsive responding, increased sensibility to external stimuli, poor attention and decreased capacity to plan and organize a course of action and follow it through.

Dysfunction of fronto-striatal pathways is supposed, based on clinical, MRI, and blood flow and metabolic studies (for a review, see Benson, 1991). A global decrease in brain metabolism of about 30% was found by one group (Zametkin et al., 1993), and decreased metabolism in the left anterior frontal lobe, superior prefrontal cortex, sensorimotor, and premotor cortex was described by others (Lou et al., 1989). The latter was reversed by dextroamphetamine, and perhaps by frontal maturation (after 12–15 years of age), but not by methylphenidate (Zametkin et al., 1993). Basal ganglia abnormalities have been described on morphometric studies, showing smaller right than left caudate and pallidum on MRI (about 5% in volume), i.e., reversed normal asymmetry (Filipek et al., 1987; Hynd et al., 1993; Castellanos et al., 1996; Aylward et al., 1994; Mataro et al., 1997), correlating with PET studies (Lou et al., 1989; Castellanos et al., 1994).

Secondary or symptomatic attention deficit hyperactivity disorder is found in diseases involving the basal ganglia, such as Tourette's syndrome, obsessive–compulsive disorder, anxiety disorders, antisocial behavior, drug addiction, after birth hypoxic injury or meningoencephalitis, lead poisoning, and head injury (see below).

Loss of inhibition of the right prefrontal cortex and caudate control of inhibition tasks (response selection and inhibition tasks), suppressing attentional and behavioral responses, is suspected in attention deficit hyperactivity disorder. Similar findings have been found in Tourette's syndrome (Singer et al., 1993; see below). A dysfunction in the arousal and rewarding system, probably distributed between OF limbic accumbens and DLPF fronto-striatal circuits, especially on the right hemisphere (Lou et al., 1989; Hynd et al., 1993; Zametkin et al., 1993), i.e., arousal and rewarding systems, driven by dopaminergic activity, modulated by norepinephrinergic and serotoninergic neurotransmission, is the present understanding of this disorder.

Dopamine and norepinephrine are important neurotransmitters, which are probably decreased in attention deficit hyperactivity disorder. Amphetamines and methylphenidate are recognized treatments (Zametkin et al., 1993).

Motor and emotional modulation of speech, writing, and other higher 'cortical' functions

A peculiar type of aphasia is encountered in lesions of the left basal ganglia, especially when the head of caudate and anterior part of the internal capsule are involved, but also the putamen. It combines features of Wernicke's aphasia (deficient auditory comprehension), dysarthria, hypophonia, with generally fluent speech, intact or impaired repetition (Damasio et al., 1984). When the thalamus and subthalamic nuclei are involved, logorrhea may be found (Barat et al., 1978; Brunner et al., 1982; Damasio et al., 1984; Fromm et al., 1985), or hypophonia. Diseases of the basal ganglia such as parkinsonism and Huntington's chorea have been associated with disorders of the motor aspects of speech, including loss of spontaneity, festination, pallilalia, decreased fluency, perseverations, intrusions, shorter sentences, hypophonia, silent hesitation at the beginning of sentences, and also other frontal or mnesic dysfunction of speech (see below). Similarly, abnormalities of written language such as isolated micrographia have been described in association with basal ganglia lesions (Martinez-Vila et al., 1988).

Slowing of mental process (bradyphrenia) is probably a mixture of DLPF and AC syndromes, and is often encountered in parkinsonism and vascular dementia (see below).

Delirium

Delirium is a state of decreased ability to maintain or shift attention in response to stimuli, associated with a disorganization of thinking and at least two of: decreased arousal, alteration of perception or interpretation, delusion, hallucinations, increased or decreased psychomotor activity, and disorientation.

The possible significance of basal ganglia lesions in the physiopathology of delirium has been raised by a few studies. Figiel et al. (1990) reported that all patients over 45 years who were taking antidepressant medication or had electroconvulsive therapy (ECT) had basal ganglia lesions on MRI. Mori and Yamadori (1987) noted that in 24 of 25 patients who developed delirium after right middle cerebral artery infarct, the latter involved the basal ganglia. Caplan et al. (1990) reported delirium in four of eight patients with right caudate infarct, and Stein et al. (1984), Weisberg (1984), and Pedrazzi et al. (1990) reported it in association with caudate hemorrhage. Trzepacz et al. (1989) suggested that delirium associated with endstage liver disease might be due to subcortical dysfunction. Delirium is a frequent finding in Binswanger's disease and lacunar states, and an abnormal T2 signal on MRI is often seen, involving the basal ganglia (see below).

Mental slowing, bradyphrenia, mental emptiness, obsessional slowness, apathetic dementia

'Akinesia or bradykinesia of thinking or mental processing' is a major feature of the anterior cingulate syndrome, in which patients describe mental emptiness and, in bradyphrenia of parkinsonism and 'subcortical dementia' (Albert, 1974) or the obsessional slowness of obsessive-compulsive disorder (see above). An apathetic form of dementia is described in the terminal phases of Huntington's disease (see below).

Flight of ideas, mental automatism, hallucinations, delusions, and psychosis

'Hyperkinesia of thinking process' is reflected in mania with flight of ideas, difficulty in focusing attention, and elation, but also in mental automatisms seen in Tourette's syndrome such as coprophenomena, paliphenomena, or echophenomena, mental play, and frank psychosis with hallucinations and delusions, as it can be seen in most diseases of the basal ganglia (see below).

In summary, the basal ganglia, with their anatomic location between the neocortex and limbic and paralimbic areas, play a major role in matching external and internal drives with cognitive and behavioral motor and emotional processing. With their basic overall bipolar effect of either activation or inhibition, they play a role in the servo-assistance in motor, cognitive, and affective functions, especially on frontal processing such as executive functions, decision making, self-awareness, spontaneity, social behavior, attention and motivation, but also on regulation of limbic, hypothalamic temporal, and brainstem emotional expression of mood and behavior.

Mood and behavior according to basal ganglia nuclei: topographical anatomo-clinical correlations

Caudate nucleus

Isolated lesions of the caudate nucleus are associated with behavioral or mood disturbances in about three-quarters of the cases. Unilateral lesions (Croisile et al., 1989; Mendez et al., 1989; Caplan et al., 1990; Pedrazzi et al., 1990) presented with confusion, abulia or apathy (left caudate) (Croisile et al., 1989), transient mutism (Pedrazzi et al., 1990), alternating abulia and hyperkinesia, disinhibited behavior (left more than right caudate) (Cambier et al., 1979; Mendez et al., 1989; Caplan et al., 1990), depression (ventromedial or dorsolateral caudate, left more than right) (Mendez et al., 1989), and delayed-onset obsessive–compulsive disorder (compulsive skin scraping, forced counting, compulsive finger movements) (Williams et al., 1988; Croisile et al., 1989; Tonkonogy and Barreira, 1989). Caudate hemorrhage often presents with an acute confusional state including hallucinations (Pardal et al., 1985). Large, unilateral, isolated lesions of the caudate are often associated with mood or behavioral problems (86%: Bhatia and Marsden, 1994), depression, and speech disorder (left caudate: Cambier et al., 1979; Mehler, 1987; Croisile et al., 1989; Pedrazzi et al., 1990), word finding difficulty or frank aphasia, memory loss

(Stein et al., 1984; Caplan et al., 1990), anosognosia, hemineglect and ideatory per-severations (Cambier et al., 1979), and graphomania (Cambier et al., 1979).

Bilateral lesions (Richfield et al., 1987; Croisile et al., 1989; Mendez et al., 1989) were associated with bipolar alternating states of abulia, disinhibition, and agitation (Richfield et al., 1987; Mendez et al., 1989; Croisile et al., 1989; Caplan et al., 1990), emotional lability (Yasuda et al., 1995), apathy and anomia (Croisile et al., 1989), delayed-onset obsessive–compulsive disorder (Croisile et al., 1989), disinhibition (Cambier et al., 1979; Mendez et al., 1989), arithmomania (Penisson-Besnier et al., 1993), or bulimia (Cambier et al., 1979; Richfield et al., 1987).

Putamen

Isolated small lesions of the putamen rarely (5%: Bhatia and Marsden, 1994) present with behavior or mood disturbances. Speech abnormalities (dysarthria and aprosodia: Damasio et al., 1984), complex stereotypies (Maraganore and Marsden, 1990), obsessive–compulsive disorder (Maraganore and Marsden, 1990), and hallucinations (Laplane et al., 1992) have been reported.

Globus pallidus

Isolated lesions of the globus pallidus have presented when unilateral, when bilateral, as abulia (Ali-Chérif et al., 1984; Laplane et al., 1989), and obsessive–compulsive disorder (coprolalia, compulsive collecting, counting, turning a light on and off, timed scheduled activities, checking, and sentence repetition compulsion: Laplane et al., 1981; Pulst et al., 1983; Ali-Chérif et al., 1984; Laplane, 1989).

Subthalamic nucleus

Logorrhea has been reported in association with subthalamic nucleus lesions (Barat et al., 1978), as well as with agitation and akathisia (Carranza et al., 1989; Trillet et al., 1995).

Substantia nigra

Obsessive–compulsive disorder (checking compulsion) and bipolar disorder have been reported in an infarct involving substantia nigra, dentato-rubro-thalamic tract, and cerebellum (Kulisevsky et al., 1995; Lauterbach, 1996).

Mixed lesions

Lesions involving unilateral caudate and lenticulate nuclei (striatum) on the dominant side showed disturbance of speech (dysarthria, fluent, global aphasia, aspontaneity, anomia, deficits in comprehension, paraphasias, and hypophonia) (Damasio et al., 1984; Mehler, 1987; Ghika et al., 1991); on the nondominant side they were associated with anosognosia, visual memory deficit, motor impersistence, and hemineglect (Ghika et al., 1991). Bilateral caudate and lenticulate nuclei lesions presented abulia up to akinetic mutism and depression (Laplane et al., 1982, 1984, 1988a, 1989, 1992; Ali-Chérif et al., 1984; Williams et al., 1988; Asakura et al., 1989; Caplan et al., 1990; Desi et al., 1990; Trillet et al., 1990; Macucci et al., 1991; Wang, 1991; Lehembe and Graux, 1992; Hayashi et al., 1993; Mrabet et al., 1994; Alexander, 1995; Smadja et al., 1995); but compulsive counting (Laplane et al., 1984; Lehembe and Graux, 1992), typing (Williams et al., 1988), or compulsive stereotypic pseudo-obsessional activities like pedalling, pacing, thumb sucking, scratching, arythmomania, mastication, bruxism (Trillet et al., 1990), obsessive–compulsive disorder (Williams et al., 1988; Smadja et al., 1995), and, in striatal lacunar state, stercoral compulsion (Lehembe and Graux, 1992), arithmetic, language, and visuospatial task perseverations (Peatfield, 1987) were frequently associated stereotypies (Williams et al., 1988).

Lesions of the lenticulate nucleus rarely present with mood or behavioral symptoms (11%: Bhatia and Marsden, 1994). Rarely, in bilateral cases, abulia (Laplane et al., 1992), or obsessive–compulsive disorder (Laplane et al., 1989) has been reported.

Mood, cognitive, and behavioral manifestations in diseases of the basal ganglia

Parkinson's disease

Parkinson's disease (Parkinson, 1938) is a degenerative disease generally starting between the ages of 50 and 60 years – although earlier (young or early-onset forms) or later onset forms are well known – and is due to a progressive neuronal cell loss in the substantia nigra of the mesencephalon. The disease is associated with any combination of two or more of asymmetrical, dopa-responsive resting tremor, rigidity, and bradykinesia. A wide variety of mood, behavior, and cognitive disorders has been associated with parkinsonism. These include personality disorders, obsessive–compulsive disorder, depression, disorders of conduct, confusional states, drug-induced psychiatric disorders, and dementia.

Premorbid personality was studied in Parkinson's disease. Various descriptions of the presymptomatic personality traits of affected individuals were given, but these were not unanimously accepted. Patients are described by words that are often used to describe the used obsessive–compulsive personality, such as authority respectful, industrious, reliable, loyal, subordinate, dependent, morally rigid, virtuous, law abiding, truthworthy, respectful conformist, exemplary citizen, putting their home and family at the center of their lives, order and precision addicts, exacting, punctual, orderly, meticulous, perfectionist, methodical, perseverant, and bringing the problem to solution with thoroughness, no procrastination or delay. A limited range of emotional expression is also well recognized, due to overcontrol of internal and external compulsions, with consecutive withholding tendency, and an obsessive preoccupation with body image. Patients are described as introverted, cautious, reflective, less novelty seeking, less talkative, withdrawn, with depressed flat affect, frugal, abstinent, hypercontrolled, persistent, stoic, even-tempered, self-controlled, repressing aggressive behaviors and emotional moods, respectful conformists, not related to alcohol or smoke (for a review, see Hubble et al., 1993). Four types of personality were described:

1 well adjusted, stable, easy-going, calm and resilient,

2 submissive, dependent, easily upset,

3 restless, suspicious, worried, demanding, and depressed,

4 psychopathical.

Inflexibility, moral rigidity, introversion, and a tendency to depression were also mentioned. All these description show that there is an obsessional–compulsive-like personality in patients with Parkinson's disease. Frank obsessive–compulsive disorder, complex mannerisms and organized rituals have been reported in Parkinson's disease (Hollander et al., 1993), sometimes in association with L-dopa-induced fluctuations (Hoehn et al., 1960).

Mood disorders are also often reported. Depression, already recognized by Parkinson in 1817, who referred to patients as 'unhappy sufferers' and 'melancholy,' is a frequent finding (50–60%, with a range between 20% and 91% according to the authors' criteria: Huber et al., 1990; Starkstein et al., 1989; Cummings, 1993). Considered by a group of authors as a reaction to functional disability (Huber et al., 1990), depression has found to be significantly more prevalent in those with Parkinson's disease than in age-matched patients with a similar degree of handicap, such as paraplegics or orthopedic patients, and may be a presenting symptom before the handicap is significant. Attempts to correlate depression with progression of the disease, as assessed with the Hoehn and Yahr stage, showed that depression is most common in stage I, decreases in stage II, reappears in stage III–IV, and decreases again in stage V (Starkstein et al., 1990b). Only a weak association has been found with the severity of total disability scores (Vogel, 1982), but others did not find any correlation or subitems such as rigidity, akinesia, or tremor (Mayeux, 1990). Conflicting results were also found for the association of depression with the age of onset of Parkinson's disease: some authors did not find any correlation (Gotham et al., 1988), but others (Starkstein et al., 1989) found higher scores in young-onset patients. The depression of Parkinson's disease is atypical (Schiffer et al., 1988).

Attempts to correlate the side of predominant symptoms with depression showed conflicting results. No difference between right-sided or left-sided parkinsonism was reported in two studies (Barber et al., 1985; Blonder et al., 1989), but depression was five times more prevalent in left hemiparkinsonism, and left hemiparkinsonism was considered as a risk factor for depression. In Parkinson's disease, a widespread disruption is found in brain monoamines, which are all involved in the neurochemistry of depression. The loss of mesolimbic and mesocortical dopamine pathways is thought to be prevalent, together with involvement of paralimbic regions (OF and temporal), i.e., the orbito-frontal based ganglia-thalamic circuit and the basotemporal limbic circuit linking OF cortex and anterior temporal cortex via the uncinate fasciculus. However, norepinephrine and serotonin deficiencies are also decreased in Parkinson's disease, and SSRIs, tricyclics and ECT are effective in treating depression (Asnis, 1977).

Anxiety, anhedonia, and panic disorder are frequent (38%: Schiffer et al., 1988; Fleminger, 1991). PET studies in depressed parkinsonian patients showed bilateral decreased glucose metabolism in caudate and OF cortex (Mayberg et al., 1990). Patients with depression have a faster cognitive decline (Starkstein et al., 1989). Paroxysmal attacks of anxiety as well as affective symptoms such as sadness, despondency, anxiety, and irritability associated with L-dopa itself or its fluctuations are well documented (Hoehn et al., 1960), sometimes alternating with mania in 'mood' swings.' Tricyclic antidepressants are effective in the treatment of depression in Parkinson's disease, but not in treating the motor handicap, whereas L-dopa is highly efficient in treating motor symptoms but less effective at treating depression. ECT is efficient for both motor and depressive symptoms (Asnis, 1977).

Depression might be difficult to separate from apathy (Starkstein et al., 1992), which is found alone in 12% of patients with Parkinson's disease and in 30% associated with depression and bradyphrenia (Rogers et al., 1987), especially in the presence of akinesia, amimia, and the inherent loss of emotional motor expression of face, gestures, and prosody. As has been well known since its first description (Parkinson, 1938), parkinsonian patients have a major loss of spontaneous facial expression ('masked face'), which seems no to be correlated with either depression scores or the side of prevalent parkinsonian symptoms. Voluntary facial expression (Scott et al., 1984; Pitcairn et al., 1990) as well as facial expression perceptivity (Scott et al., 1984; Jacobs et al., 1995a) and prosody are also deficient in Parkinson's disease (Canter, 1963; Scott et al., 1984; Blonder et al., 1989), with monotone, monospeech, and monoloudness speech, and sometimes increased rate of speech, and difficulty in expressing anger and in prosodic comprehension (Cancelliere and Kertesz, 1990).

Early cognitive changes (for a summary, see Levin and Katzen, 1995) include impairment of language in nonlinguistic motor and emotional abilities, such as perseverations, intrusions, word and semantic fluency, shorter sentences, difficulties shifting between letter categories, silent hesitations at the beginning of sentences, increased number of open class optional phrases, fund of vocabulary, word retrieval, recitation of months backwards, difficulty in answering syntactically embedded questions, category alternation, and 'tip of the tongue' phenomena (Bayles, 1990). Other dysfunctions of emotional cognition include motor and sensory aprosodia, deficit in emotional facial expression and comprehension (Ekman and Friesen, 1971; Rinn, 1984; Blonder et al., 1989; Borod et al., 1986; Katsikis and Pilowsky, 1991; Jacobs et al., 1995a). A dysexecutive syndrome is well described in patients with early and late Parkinson's disease (for reviews, see Sagar et al., 1988a, 1988b; Taylor et al., 1996). Patients have problems in initiating behavior, shifting, changing or alternating sequences on a spontaneous uncued basis, temporal and spatial ordering of experience (Cooper et al., 1993), switching their attention to a previously irrelevant stimulus (perserveration of set), maintaining set once shifted, doing two things simultaneously, or dividing their attention between two different mental routines when executing two simple but different programs at the same time or bimanual tasks (Talland and Schwab, 1964; Cools et al., 1984). Patients rely more on external cues than on internal cues (Cooke et al., 1984), with a loss of flexibility in information processing, problem solving (Morris et al., 1988), stimulus-dependent or environmental cues, relying on prompting or priming (Cooke et al., 1978). These findings explain some of the handicaps in the activities of daily living (driving, walking with a cane, reading when walking etc.).

Deficits in visuospatial and visuomotor skills are a matter of controversy between studies, but difficulty in visuospatial analysis and synthesis, visual discrimination, recognition, attention and orientation, spatial planning, updating and memory, line orientation, facial recognition, personal space, and visuomotor integration have been described (Boller et al., 1984; Owen et al., 1992; Richards et al., 1993), especially in the presence of left-sided parkinsonism. When memory was studied, short-term memory, explicit memory, working memory, procedural learning, recall (improved by semantic cuing), backward digit span, difficulty in recall of recent items, and temporal order memory were found to be abnormal, as were attention and learning (El-Awar et al., 1987; Sagar et al., 1988a, 1988b; Taylor et al., 1990; Harrington et al., 1990; Mohr et al., 1991; Owen et al., 1992; Pillon et al., 1991, 1993, 1994). Longer cognitive processing time and an increased number of trials required are often observed during testing, with increased reaction times, slower decision making, poor temporal predictability (Pillon et al., 1991, 1993; Owen et al., 1992), and bradyphrenia (Rogers et al., 1987).

In late Parkinson's disease, subcortical dementia can be found in 20–30% of the patients, but others report up to 38–61%, mostly elderly patients over the age of 70 (for reviews, see Growdon et al., 1990; Dubois et al., 1990; Pillon et al., 1991; Mayeux et al., 1992). However, 'parkinsonian dementia' is highly heterogeneous and may cover several different pathological entities, including true endstage Parkinson's disease, diffuse Lewy body disease, additional vascular or Alzheimer pathology, depression, and effect of the medication. Classical parkinsonian dementia includes a variable mixture of deficits in attention, short-term and long-term explicit memory, spatial memory, declarative memory, implicit or procedural memory, abstract thinking, judgment, deficits in executive functions (planning, abstract thinking, shifting, performing two tasks simultaneously, difficulty in the ability to self-generate a response using internal control of information, with consecutive dependence on sensory cues, perseveration, decreased mental flexibility with difficulties in adaptation to novel, nonroutine expectations), visuospatial dysfunction, slowing of thinking process (bradyphrenia), and information processing.

Drug-induced psychiatric disorders are frequently found in Parkinson's disease, mostly due to dopaminergics and anticholinergics. Psychosis includes hallucinations (30%), illusions (28%), threatening or fighting visions (28%), delusions, paranoia, Capgras syndrome (3%) and delirium (Celesia and Barr, 1970), hypersexuality or aberrant sexual behavior (0.9–3%: Ballivet et al., 1973), frontal-like syndrome (Gotham et al., 1988), depression and chronic anxiety, panic attacks (38%: Cheifetz et al., 1970) or mania (1.5%), insomnia (28%), nightmares (6%), abnormal dreaming (5.7%), vivid dreaming (28%) and night terrors (6.8%), sometimes fluctuating like motor symptoms (mood swings) (Hoehn et al., 1960), and alteration of memory (Mohr et al., 1991). Obsessive–compulsive disorder has also been reported after L-dopa. Isolated nondrug-induced psychosis has been reported rarely (Celesia and Barr, 1970; Crow et al., 1976), as has bipolar mood disorder.

Other psychiatric manifestations of Parkinson's disease are excessive dependency, fearfulness, chronic anxiety, emotional lability, and mania. Clozapine is the best treatment for all these symptoms, alternatives being drugs such as olanzapine, risperidone, and quetiapine.

Parkinsonian syndromes

Striatonigral degeneration (Adams et al., 1961) is one of the clinical presentations of multiple system atrophy. Adult-onset (generally in the fifth decade), sporadic L-dopa-resistant or partially responding parkinsonian syndrome accompanied by one of the corticospinal signs, early autonomic failure, and cerebellar ataxia are part of the definition of this disease. Red flag signs have been mentioned by Quinn (1994). Dementia is absent. Psychiatric disorders have been poorly studied, but include depression, anxiety, and emotional lability (Feve et al., 1977; Fearnley and Lees, 1990; Robbins et al., 1992, 1994; Garcia-Campayo and Sanz-Carillo, 1994; Pillon et al., 1995). Loss of fluency is mentioned, but psychosis has never been described.

Pathologically, neuronal loss and oligodendroglial cytoplasmic inclusions are seen in the putamen, globus pallidus, and substantia nigra.

Progressive supranuclear palsy (Steele, et al., 1964) is a progressive degenerative disease characterized by axial rigidity, supranuclear gaze palsy, corticobulbar signs, autonomic dysfunction, and a frontal lobe-dominant type of cognitive dysfunction. Depression (Albert et al., 1974; Janati and Appel, 1984; Schneider and Chui, 1986; Litvan et al., 1996) is common and generally responds to tricyclic antidepressants. Apathy (91%), dysphoria (18%), and anxiety (18%) are commonly found (Pillon et al., 1994; Litvan et al., 1996); memory deficits, especially explicit memory (Litvan et al., 1989), changes in motor aspects of speech (Lebrun et al., 1986; Rosser and Hodges, 1994), and subcortical dementia are described (Albert et al., 1974; Kimura et al., 1981; Fisk et al., 1982; Sadler et al., 1984; D'Antona et al., 1988; Dubois et al., 1988; Pillon et al., 1991; Robbins et al., 1994), and other cognitive deficits such as memory loss, dysexecutive dysfunction, impaired calculation, abstract thinking, loss of insight, and slow cognitive processing. Emotional lability, aggressivity and psychosis have been described (Janati and Appel, 1984; Menza et al., 1995), as has obsessive–compulsive disorder (Destée et al., 1990). A major frontal syndrome with slowing of cognitive processes and environment dependency is often found (Kimura et al., 1981; Fisk et al., 1982; Cambier et al., 1985; Kish et al., 1985; Maher et al., 1985; Pillon et al., 1986, 1991; Dubois et al., 1988; Grafman et al., 1990; Robbins et al., 1994; Ghika et al., 1995). Psychosis has not been described.

PET studies in progressive supranuclear palsy have shown frontal lobe dysfunction (Grafman et al., 1990). Pathological studies have shown neurofibrillary tangles, gliosis, cell loss, granulovacuolar degeneration, and white matter changes in basal ganglia, including globus pallidus, subthalamic nucleus, red nucleus, substantia nigra, periaqueductal gray matter, pontine tegmentum, thalamus, and brain stem.

Mood disorders, obsessive–compulsive disorder, complex tics, and stereotypies have been described in Hallervorden–Spatz disease (Nardocci et al., 1994); progressive subcortical gliosis might be difficult to differentiate from that of progressive supranuclear palsy; and in Pick's disease, basal ganglia are also involved and might be responsible for some of the disinhibition syndrome (Kosaka et al., 1991; Akelaitis, 1994).

Encephalitis lethargica (epidemica) or postencephalitic parkinsonism

Encephalitis lethargica is a metencephalitis and diencephalitis of supposed viral origin, which presented as an epidemic in 1918–20 (von Economo, 1931). The acute phase of the disease was characterized by coma, stupor, somnolence, sleep disturbances – either hypersomnia or insomnia with agitation, sometimes alternating (Kirby and Davis, 1921) – oculomotor (oculogyric crises or mesencephalic syndromes) and limb paresis, extrapyramidal hypokinetic and hyperkinetic syndromes, sensory disturbances, autonomic dysfunction, and a large variety of psychiatric expression (for a summary, see Cheyette and Cummings, 1995). Pathologically, chronic inflammation, gliosis, and cell loss were found in mesencephalon, hypothalamus, subthalamus, pallidum, and striatum (Buzzard and Greenfield, 1919).

Survivors entered a postencephalitic phase with recovery, but more than 80% developed postencephalitic parkinsonism and various psychiatric disorders such as psychosis, mania, conduct disorders, depression, and obsessive–compulsive disorder (von Economo, 1931; for a summary, see Wimmer, 1924; Fairweather, 1947; Wohlfart et al., 1961; Cheyette and Cummings, 1995). A confusing number of psychiatric terms have been used to describe the mental disturbances accompanying or following epidemic encephalitis, including acute delirium, maniac delirium, afebrile mental confusion, amentia, mania, anxiety, depression, excitable depression, melancholia, emotional stupor, hebephrenia, catatonia, lucid catatonic stupor, paranoid state, grave delusional psychosis, fully elaborated psychosis, epileptico-maniac psychosis, Korsakoff's disease, hysterical attacks, psychoneurosis, manic–depressive insanity, dementia praecox, paranoiac state, and constitutional psychoses (Abrahamson, 1920; Kirby and Davis, 1921; Burger and Mayer-Gross, 1926). Psychiatric manifestations such as mood disorders like depression, mania, feelings of euphoria, bipolar syndromes, and emotional lability are noted, as well as anxiety in early or late phases (Kirby and Davis, 1921; Schilder and Dimitz, 1921; Naville, 1922; Hall, 1923; Steck, 1931). Disorders of impulse control were prominent (77%), with restlessness, nervousness, wandering, heterotypic change in personality, irritability, desire to tease, querulousness, uncontrolled outbursts of anger, scolding, use of abusive language, screaming, crying, stamping of feet, torrent of foul and gross language, talk in an odd, high-flown, silly manner, compulsive singing, dancing, spitting, nose picking, scratching, snapping fingers, chewing, letter writing, bathing, antisocial behavior with violence, attempts at murder, compulsive aggressive acts, arsonism, cruelty toward children or animals, truancy, vagrancy, propensity to destructiveness or self-injurious behavior, nocturnal excitement (jumping, noises, whirling, whistling, singing, shouting, getting in and out of bed, raving), smearing objects with feces and urine, singing, dancing, increased sexual drive, exhibitionism, paraphilias, micturition on surrounding persons or objects, jocularity or witzelsucht (Kirby and Davis, 1921; Naville, 1922; Wimmer, 1924; Steck, 1931), and confabulations (Hohman, 1921). Frank psychosis, delusion, hallucinations, and paranoia (Kirby and Davis, 1921; Hohman, 1921; Wimmer, 1924; Schilder, 1938) are also described, as are obsessive–compulsive disorder (Herrmann, 1922; Steck, 1931), psychomotor agitation, disorientation, confusion, vivid dreams, and delirium (Kirby and Davis, 1921). In addition, apathy, akinetic mutism, catatonia, catalepsy (Kirby and Davis, 1921; Naville, 1922; Hill, 1928), and bradyphrenia (40%: Naville, 1922; Schmidt, 1925; Steck, 1931) were also reported, as well as phobias and memory and attention deficits (Naville, 1922), and a Korsakoff-like syndrome (Kirby and Davis, 1921).

Von Economo (1931) noted a whole range of tics and compulsions in encephalitis lethargica, such as mimetic tics, clucking, hissing, fits of yelling, yawning, twitching of the eyelids and frontal muscle, tonic cramps of tongue or limbs, and tachypnea. Other motor phenomena were paralysis, tremor, chorea, stereotypies, parkinsonism (Naville, 1922; Steck, 1931; Fairweather, 1947), and Benedeck's klazomania (compulsory shouting and screaming for hours) (Benedeck, 1925; von Thurzo and Katona, 1927; Wohlfart et al., 1961).

No morphometric or blood flow or metabolic studies could be realized on these patients.

Gilles de la Tourette's syndrome

Tourette's syndrome (Gilles de la Tourette, 1885) is a disorder with onset between 2 and 21 years of age and a life-long waxing and waning course, including multiple tics (motor, sensory, psychic, and phonic tics) and sometimes other dyskinesias (dystonia, choreoathetosis, oculogyric-like movements), and complex cognitive and behavioral features which were recognized by Gilles de la Tourette; early works mention 'obsessions,' 'mental infantilism,' and 'obsessive–compulsive phenomena' (Creack and Guttman, 1935).

Obsessions and compulsions, such as touching things in a precise manner, putting objects in the right place, washing hands, checking and rechecking, counting, smelling things, compulsion to touch, vocalization, ripping off the closet doors, knocking holes in the wall, symmetry behavior, taking up/down objects, dressing–undressing, cleaning, measuring, switching lights or gas on and off, ranging, avoidance behavior, hoarding, preoccupations with sexual, religious, and aggressive content, repetitive rituals, are well described in patients and in up to 30–85% of probands of patients (first-degree relatives without tics but with obsessive–compulsive disorder or attention deficit hyperactivity disorder) with Tourette's syndrome. The distinction between complex motor tics and compulsive behaviors is often difficult or impossible to make in Tourette's syndrome. When they are severe enough, obsessions and compulsions meet the psychiatric criteria for obsessive–compulsive disorder (30–90%) (Gilles de la Tourette, 1885; Creack and Guttmann, 1935; Montgomery et al., 1982). 'Just right experience' (Leckman et al., 1995) is a frequent finding. Because of the high prevalence of obsessive–compulsive disorder in family members of those with Tourette's syndrome, the development of a lifetime history of tics in 59% of pure obsessive–compulsive disorder patients, and the impossibility of distinguishing between obsessive–compulsive symptoms of either condition, the possibility that some, at least, obsessive–compulsive disorder patients may have a minor form of Tourette's syndrome, or pleiotropic expression of this syndrome, has been raised.

Disorders of impulse control, with short temper, the ability to be easily angered or upset, temper tantrums, yells and screams, impulsive sexuality, exhibitionism (15%), self-destructiveness, antisocial behavior, aggression, anger, rage, or violence (61%), oppositional and confrontative or conduct behaviors, are common (Comings and Comings, 1988; Park et al., 1996). Coprophenomena (coprolalia (33%), copropraxia, and mental coprolalia), echophenomena (echolalia, echopraxia, and mental echolalia – sudden repetitive thoughts), paliphenomena (palilalia, palipraxia, mental palilalia), mental play (repetitive thoughts or images, sounds, words, number games, intended as pastime), ruminating, doubting, repetitive questioning, spelling words backward and forward (Comings and Comings, 1988) are often associated with various emotions (pleasant/unpleasant, fear, suffering, tension, 'just right' impression). Stereotypies can be found occasionally. Clomipramine, fluoxetine, and fluvoxamine may be useful.

Self-injurious and heteroinjurious or mutilative behaviors, and reckless behaviors are impulsive behaviors reported by Gilles de la Tourette (1885). Picking at sores, punching the abdomen, filing of teeth, head banging, tongue, lip, finger, and cheek biting, pummelling, punching, slapping of the head and chest, digging of the forefinger in the hollow of the cheek, eye damage, tooth extraction, pushing a pencil into the ear, putting the head or hand through windows, and scraping a leg against a hard surface can be found in up to 35–43% of patients (Woody and Eisenhauer, 1986).

Tics, like obsessions, are commonly preceded by a mental experience of motivational tension, and their expression is often followed by a sense of satisfaction. Often, sudden intrusion into consciousness of premonitory feelings or urges precedes both tics and compulsions that are relieved by the performance of the tic or by a need to perform it until it is felt to be 'just right' (Leckman et al., 1994).

Mood disorders such as depression, mood lability, bipolar disorder, anxiety, dysphoria, social phobia or phobias are frequent (Comings and Comings, 1988; Coffey et al., 1992; Kerbeshian et al., 1995), as are premonitory urges (Leckman et al., 1993). Anxiety is frequent in Tourette's syndrome (80%), as well as panic attacks (16%), social phobia, or simple but multiple (more than three) phobias (26%) (Comings and Comings, 1988). Benzodiazepines are useful here.

Learning disability and attention deficit hyperactivity disorder (54–75%) are common (Hagin et al., 1982; Comings and Comings, 1988; Matthews, 1988), and can precede the onset of tics in 40–50% of patients. Hyperactivity, inattention, and impulsivity are seen in most patients, especially children. A dysexecutive syndrome, as well as difficulty in tasks requiring sustained attention, and visuospatial deficits have been reported.

Frank psychosis has also been reported in up to 40% of patients (Comings and Comings, 1988).

Drug-induced psychiatric symptoms, especially with neuroleptics (especially dysphoria or school phobia) are often misdiagnosed.

Emotional and volitional influences can increase and decrease symptoms, in addition to the highly variable expression of the disease with spontaneous waxing and waning. Stress, anxiety, and depression increase tics, whereas concentration and volition can control them.

Quantitative MRI studies showed a statistically significant increase in ventricular volumes bilaterally, i.e., a lack of volumetric asymmetry with smaller left putamen, lenticular nucleus, and globus pallidus (Peterson et al., 1993; Singer et al., 1993; Hyde et al., 1995; Castellanos et al., 1996). Altered T2 relaxation time asymmetries have been shown in insular cortex, frontal white matter, putamen and caudate; shorter T2 times have been shown in right amygdala and red nucleus, and a 20% reduction in corpus callosum size (Peterson et al., 1994).

The pattern of Tourette's syndrome with blood flow and metabolic studies is a relative hypometabolism in caudal and lateral OF, insular, mesial temporal limbic cortices, parahippocampal and inferior insular, ventral striatum (accumbens, ventromedial caudate, and putamen), and midbrain, and relative hypermetabolism in superior sensorimotor cortex (SMA, lateral premotor, Rolandic); with obsessive–compulsive disorder, right frontal hypometabolism was found; when obsessive–compulsive disorder and tics were present, increased metabolism was found in the putamen when compared to obsessive–compulsive disorder alone. When attention deficit hyperactivity disorder was present, increased activity was described in OF cortex and inferior insula (Braun et al., 1995). Behavioral severity scores were related to OF and putaminal hypometabolism, but not with midbrain, ventral striatum, inferior insular cortex, parahippocampal gyrus, or sensorimotor cortex (Braun et al., 1995).

Autopsy studies have been largely deceptive, but clinical, pharmacological, metabolic, and blood flow studies suggest an underlying hyperactivity of frontal-striatal-limbic and paralimbic circuitry (Richardson, 1982; Devinski, 1983; Haber et al., 1986). Recently, some connection has been made between antineuronal antibodies against putamen and Tourette's syndrome (Singer et al., 1998). Postencephalitic tics, carbon monoxide intoxication, and drug-induced Tourette-like syndromes are also compatible with a lesion of the basal ganglia as a major player.

Increased activity of dopamine and norepinephrine and decreased serotonin are suspected in Tourette's syndrome. Clonidine can decrease both tics and obsessive–compulsive disorder, as can SSRIs such as fluoxetine. Refractory cases respond to psychosurgery (bilateral rostral intralaminar and medial nuclei of the thalamus).

Huntington's disease

Huntington's disease (Huntington, 1872) is an autosomal dominant disease, caused by an abnormal number of CAG triplets reduplication on chromosome 4q, manifested by choreiform movements, psychiatric symptoms, and progressive dementia (for a review, see Harper, 1996). In addition to motor and intellectual dysfunction, patients, as mentioned by Huntington, have emotional, psychiatric, and behavioral symptoms ('a tendency to insanity and sometimes to that form of insanity which leads to suicide is marked').

Inaugural psychiatric disorders, including anxiety, disorders of impulse control, and personality changes, are frequent in the early phase (20–80%), up to 20 years before chorea appears (Hamilton, 1908; Heathfield, 1967; Jason et al., 1988). This stage is generally followed by depression, mania, and psychosis, and late states are often characterized by apathy, abulia, and dementia.

Mood disorders, especially depression (30–44%) (Meggendorfer, 1923; for a review, see Harper, 1996), with 6–13% suicide risk (i.e., 8–20 times the normal prevalence), especially in the five to seven first years of disease, are frequent (Hamilton, 1908; Di Maio et al., 1993). Dysthymic disorders, especially dysphoria, are found in 5% of cases. PET studies on patients with Huntington's disease with depression showed decreased glucose metabolism in OF cortex, in addition to in the caudate, putamen, and cingulum, as seen in nondepressed patients (Kuwert et al., 1989; Mayberg et al., 1992). Antidepressant or ECT is helpful.

Mania or bipolar mood disorders are also reported (10%: Davenport, 1916; Taylor and Hansotia, 1983), with euphoria, hypomania, grandiose delusions, undue optimism, increased energy, logorrhea, and insomnia (10%). Carbamazepine, clonazepam, valproic acid, and lithium are helpful.

Disorders of impulse control are also frequent. Patients are described as difficult to live with, having temper bouts (30%), being irritable (50–58%), violent (5–10%), intolerant, inconstant, egoistic, aggressive (30–60%), labile and impulsive (15–20%), swearing, and being discourteous. Hypersexuality (10–25%), paraphilias (exhibitionism, rape, change in sexual preference, pedophilia) and marital infidelity, antisocial behavior (5%: stealing, prostitution, arsonism, homicides), but also automutilation, smoking or drinking compulsion, ravenous appetite, sometimes with burns on body parts because of smoking cigarettes to the extreme end, intolerance of changes in schedule or eating patterns, repetitive thoughts, becoming hostile or belligerent, and self-harm when compulsions are disrupted (King, 1985; Cummings and Cunningham, 1992; Watt and Seller, 1993; Rich and Ovsiew, 1994) have all been reported. Intermittent explosive disorder (31%) is frequent. Propranolol may be useful at this stage. PET studies show reduced glucose metabolism in ventrobasal striatum when behavioral symptoms occur (Kuwert et al., 1989).

Obsessive–compulsive disorder is uncommon in patients with Huntington's disease (Taylor and Hansotia, 1983; Cummings and Cunningham, 1992).

Psychosis (schizophrenic-like) (5–25%) can precede chorea by one to 35 years (Naef, 1917; Meggendorfer, 1923; Watt and Seler, 1993), especially paranoid delusions, visual and auditory hallucinations; bizarre somatic sensations are frequent. PET studies in patients with psychosis show reduced metabolism in anterior compared to posterior hemispheric structures (Kuwert et al., 1989).

Some degree of dysexecutive dysfunction is described in patients with Huntington's disease. They are more reliant on visual guidance and are impaired in using internally generated cues to guide movements, show poor performance on egocentric spatial processing, impaired set switching and planning difficulties, impaired acquisition of motor skills, and problems with sequences and organizational skills (Brouwers et al., 1984). They also have bradyphrenia, slowing of mental processes (Butters et al., 1978), reduced output on verbal fluency, and semantic difficulty (Smith et al., 1988). Visuospatial processing, visuospatial orientation, and constructional abilities are impaired (Brouwers et al., 1984). Immediate memory is preserved, but impaired recent memory and recall more than encoding and storage (Butters et al., 1978; Weingartner et al., 1979; Brandt, 1985) and short-term memory (30%), with some degree of retrograde or anterograde amnesia (28–50%), can be found (Caine et al., 1977; Aminoff et al., 1975; Albert et al., 1981; Beatty et al., 1988). Deficient procedural memory and deficits of attention and concentration are early findings. Performance at work is affected at an early stage, with loss of efficiency and interest, deficient abstraction, judgment and projection into the future and difficulties with calculation. Oral speech is also involved early (loss of fluency, dysarthria, perseverations, reduced lexical production, diminished level of syntactic complexity, reduced initiation of speech, short sentences, pauses between phrases, word-finding difficulties, but remarkably preserved comprehension and aprosody) (Kleist, 1922; Butters et al., 1978; Gordon and Iles, 1987; Podoll et al., 1988; Wallesh and Fehrenbach, 1988; Speedie et al., 1990). Handwriting (Podoll et al., 1988) is abnormal, with brisk, enlarged letters, arrests, slowing, omissions and perseverations. Emotional facial perception (Sprengelmeyer et al, 1996; Jacobs et al., 1995b) is also impaired.

'Subcortical dementia' (Wilson, 1912; Heathfield, 1967) was found in up to 15–95% of patients, with impairment of memory, judgment, insight, perseveration, disorientation, a dysexecutive syndrome, attentional deficits, and loss of motivation. Apathetic dementia has been described in late stages of the disease (Reyes and Gibbons, 1985), together with apathy, abulia, and mutism (48%) (Burns et al., 1990).

Pathologically, Huntington's disease is characterized by cell loss in the caudate nucleus and putamen, but also by less severe expression in the thalamus, claustrum globus pallidus, subthalamic nucleus, and cortex, but especially in the frontal lobe (Vonsattel et al., 1985).

Irritability and aggression can be treated with sertraline, bipolar mood disorders with lithium and butyrophenone, depression with tricyclics, monoamine oxidase inhibitors or SSRIs and ECT, and psychosis with clozapine, olanzapine, risperidone, or neuroleptics.

Basal ganglia calcification

Idiopathic basal ganglia calcification (Fahr, 1930) is a bilateral syndrome involving disturbances of movement (involuntary movements, parkinsonism) and psychiatric abnormalities.

Associated with extrapyramidal motor features such as dyskinesia and parkinsonism, with dementia and seizures, organic affective syndromes have been reported in this clinical entity: depression (37%) (Cummings et al., 1983; Francis and Freeman, 1984; Lauterback et al., 1994b), manic states (11%) (Trautner et al., 1988; Konig, 1989), bipolar disorders (20%), anxiety (Lauterbach et al., 1994b), psychosis (1.6%: hallucinations, delusions, thought disorders, agitation, paranoia) (Cummings et al., 1983; Francis and Freeman, 1984; Laplane et al., 1984; Trautner et al., 1988; Konig, 1989; Lauterbach et al., 1994b), forgetfulness, obsessive–compulsive disorder (1.6%) (Cummings et al., 1983; Trautner et al., 1988; König, 1989; Kotrla et al., 1994), dementia (Laplane et al., 1984; König, 1989), and hyperkinetic mutism (Inbody and Jankovic, 1986).

Pathologically, calcium deposits, cell loss, and gliosis are found in the globus pallidus, putamen, thalamus, dentate nucleus, cerebral and cerebellar white matter, concentrated in the walls of vessels and in the parenchyma surrounding them in both gray and white matter.

Wilson's disease

Wilson's disease (Wilson, 1912), or hepatolenticular degeneration, is an autosomal, recessive, inherited disorder of copper metabolism, generally starting between the ages of five and 35 years, involving movement disorders (parkinsonism, chorea, athetosis, tremor, tics, ataxia, dysarthria, drooling, or gait disturbances), emotional, cognitive and psychiatric symptoms, hepatic, ophthalmologic, hematologic, endocrine, cardiac, renal, metabolic, and osteoarticular manifestations.

Psychiatric symptoms are the presenting features in 14–20% of cases, but 50% (20–65%) will have psychiatric syndromes (Gysin and Cooke, 1950; Beard, 1959; Pandey et al., 1981; Dening, 1991; Akil et al., 1991). The most common psychiatric manifestations are personality changes, disorders of impulse control such as irritability and aggression (46%) (Tarter et al., 1987; Akil et al., 1991; Dening, 1991;

Kaul and McMahon, 1993; Rathun, 1996), offensive sexual behavior (Kaul and McMahon, 1993), aggressive impulsions, temper tantrums, anger, rage or anti-social behavior (50%) (Grunberger et al., 1967; Dening, 1991; Akil et al., 1991; Kaul and McMahon, 1993), alcohol abuse (Lhermitte and Muncie, 1930; Hawkins et al., 1987), incongruous behaviors, eating disorders (anorexia nervosa: Gwirstman et al., 1993), and sexual preoccupations (Akil et al., 1991). Cognitive impairment (attention, motivation, reading, and perception deficits), mental retardation, and poor school performance ranging from reading difficulty up to dementia (Wilson, 1912; Fisher, 1968) have been reported. Mood and affective disorders including anxiety, emotional lability, apathy, anhedonia, depression (20–30%), attempts at suicide (Lhermitte and Muncie, 1930; Walker, 1969; Pandey et al., 1981; Akil et al., 1991; Oder et al., 1991; Gwirstman et al., 1993), and mania (Wilson, 1912; Pandey et al., 1981), as well as psychosis or schizophrenic-like states (1%), delusions, hallucinations, schizotypal personality, withdrawal (Abély and Guyot, 1935; Gysin and Cooke, 1950; Beard, 1959; Walker, 1969; Dening, 1991), catatonia (Lisak, 1938; Akil et al., 1991; Davis and Borde, 1993), and confusional states (Inose, 1968) can occur.

Pathologically, lesions of Wilson's disease (cell loss and gliosis) are scattered in the putamen, and to a lesser degree in the globus pallidus, subthalamic nucleus, caudate, dentate nucleus, thalamus, frontal cortex, brainstem, hemispheric and cerebellar white matter.

Almost all symptoms can be reversible if treated early with copper-chelating agents such as penicillamine, zinc sulfate, BAL, trientine, or tetrathiomolybdate, or, in the late stage after hepatic transplantation. Some degree of personality changes, character or cognitive deficit may persist. Antidepressants may be useful; bouts of aggressivity may respond to propranolol.

Lesch–Nyhan syndrome, neuro(choreo)acanthocytosis, GM2 gangliosidosis, Cornelia de Lange syndrome

Lesch–Nyhan syndrome (Lesch and Nyhan, 1964) is a rare (1/10000 male births), inherited, recessive, X-linked complete deficiency of hypoxanthine-guanine phosphorybosyl-transferase with resulting overproduction of uric acid. Patients present in the first three months with nausea and vomiting, failure to thrive, arthritis, and nephropathy; then, around the first year, with choreoathetosis, rigidity, dystonic-athetoid dysphagia, dysarthria, mental retardation (IQ usually below 50), opisthotonic or extension spasms of the trunk, and occasional seizures; aggression and severe compulsive self-injurious behavior occur in 100% of the patients, between six months and 16 years, with substantial tissue loss around the mouth and on the palate, and amputation of the tongue and fingers, poking of the eyes and nose, and head banging (Lesch and Nyhan, 1964; Nyhan, 1976). A profound deficiency in dopamine in the striatum has been shown in metabolic studies, the mechanism of which is still unknown, but other neurotransmitters may be involved, such as norepinephrine, purine, serotonin, and GABA.

Neuroacanthocytosis or choreoacanthocytosis is a disorder presenting in the third or fourth decade with orofacial dyskinesias, vocalizations, chorea, and acanthocytes in 5–15% of the erythrocytes in the blood smear. Compulsive lip and finger biting, head banging, and echolalia are almost universal in this disease; obsessive–compulsive disorder, personality change, mood alterations and, rarely, psychosis have been described (Shear et al., 1971).

Adult GM2 gangliosidosis may present with psychosis (delusions, hallucinations) associated with dyskinesia (chorea, dystonia) and ataxia. On pathology, abnormal cells are present throughout the brain, but are more prominent in the basal ganglia (Streifler et al., 1989).

Cornelia de Lange syndrome is a disease with mental retardation, distinctive morphological and clinical features, which often present as self-mutilation (50%: self-scratching, biting of the fingers, lips, shoulders, knees, and head, and face slapping) (Bryson et al., 1971).

Hypoxic–ischemic, carbon monoxide, and other toxic diseases of the basal ganglia

Obsessive–compulsive disorder has been reported after perinatal anoxia (Weilberg et al., 1986), cardiac arrest (Durand et al., 1989; Trillet et al., 1990), carbon monoxide intoxication (Pulst et al., 1983), wasp sting (Laplane et al., 1981, Laplane et al., 1989), eclampsia (Grimshaw, 1964), manganese poisoning (compulsive singing, running, breaking things, dancing, chasing cars) (Schuler et al., 1957; Mena et al., 1967), cyanide intoxication (Grandas et al., 1989), disulfiram intoxication (Laplane et al., 1992), and familial paroxysmal kinesigenic choreoathetosis (Jan et al., 1995).

Stereotypies have been described with amphetamine abuse, L-dopa, and postencephalitic parkinsonism (see below).

Tourette-like syndrome is known to occur after amphetamine abuse, encephalitis, cardiopulmonary bypass, hypothermia (Singer et al., 1997), and carbon monoxide intoxication (Pulst et al., 1983).

Attention deficit hyperactivity disorder has been described after birth hypoxic injury (Lou et al., 1989), meningoencephalitis (Northan and Singer, 1991), lead poisoning, and head injury (Pulst et al., 1983; Singer et al., 1997).

Mania has been described after the use of cocaine (Kane and Taylor, 1963). A dysexecutive syndrome has been documented in MTPT parkinsonism.

Strokes involving basal ganglia

Mood disorders after stroke are well known (for a review, see Ghika-Schmid and Bogousslavsky, 1997). Depression, mania, and anxiety have been studied in relationship with the site of lesion (Gainotti, 1972; see Bogoùsslavsky, 1993, and Astrom, 1996, for reviews). Major depression has a prevalence of 8–21% after stroke, 23–34% in the first six months; anxiety without depression occurs in 20% of cases. Between 30% and 60% of patients have a clinically significant major or minor depression after stroke, mostly with left hemispheric strokes, especially anterior frontal lesions, independently of handedness and of whether the lesion was cortical or subcortical, but this is not accepted by all groups (see Robinson et al., 1983, 1984 and for reviews). Depression is more likely to occur when strokes involve the left frontal lobe and striatum (caudate and putamen), especially with pre-existing cortical atrophy (Starkstein et al., 1989), but the best predictor of depression is the proximity of the lesion to the left dorsolateral prefrontal cortico-subcortical region (Eastwood et al., 1989; Milhaud et al., 1994; Astrom, 1996). When the lesions were on the right side, posterior lesions were more associated with depression, but no mention of the basal ganglia was made (Starkstein et al., 1989). In contrast, damage to the right orbital cortex, striatum, thalamus, and subthalamic nucleus is associated with mania or bipolar mood disorder (Cummings and Mendez, 1984; Starkstein et al., 1987, 1988d, 1991; Bogousslavsky et al., 1988; Danel et al., 1991; McGilchrist et al., 1993; Lauterbach et al., 1994b; Fujikawa et al., 1995) and sometimes cheerfulness, but a few exceptions of bipolar post-stroke disorders with left striatal infarct are reported (Turecki et al., 1993). Mood disorders and especially emotional lability are well recognized in bilateral striatal, white matter, and stroke lesions, such as vascular dementia, Binswanger's disease, and lacunar strokes (Venna et al., 1988).

Abulia, apathy, loss of psychic self-activation, and akinetic mutism have been described in association with strokes (generally bilateral) at all levels of the fronto-subcortical circuit, including anterior cingulate gyrus, internal capsule, caudate, lenticular nucleus, pallidum, and thalamus (Laplane, 1990; Starkstein et al., 1993). Thus, studies in stroke generally support the association of depression with lesions interfering in the fronto-striatal or basal-limbic pathways; left anterior frontal lobe and striatum for depression; right frontal lobe, caudate, and thalamus for mania; and bilateral fronto-subcortical lesions for apathy or akinetic mutism (Cummings and Mendez, 1984; Robinson et al., 1984; Bogousslavsky, 1993; Ghika-Schmid and Bogousslavsky, 1997).

Obsessive–compulsive disorder and conduct disorders have been described as acute or delayed after caudate ischemic lesions (Fernandez-Pardal et al., 1985; Williams et al., 1988; Croisile et al., 1989; Tonkonogy and Barreira, 1989).

Delirium and agitation have been reported with ischemic or hemorrhagic lesions of the basal ganglia, especially the caudate nucleus (Weisberg, 1984; Pozzili et al., 1987; Caplan et al., 1990; Pedrazzi et al., 1990; Mrabet et al., 1994), and psychosis after right hemispheric lesions involving the striatum.

Complex stereotypies have been described after a right caudate infarct (Maraganore and Marsden, 1990).

Speech aphasic syndromes have been have been described after stroke involving left caudate or striatum (Cambier et al., 1979; Mehler, 1987; Croisile et al., 1989; Pedrazzi et al., 1990).

Subcortical dementia is a feature of lacunar state, with gait abnormalities, emotional lability, incontinence, and sometimes psychosis and delirium.

Tumors and trauma of basal ganglia

After trauma or tumors, mood disorders are well-known entities (Lishman, 1968; Lipsey et al., 1983; Binder, 1983). Mania has been associated with right hemispheric lesions at all levels of fronto-subcortical circuits, involving the frontal and temporal lobe (for reviews see Jorge et al., 1993a, 1993b), head of caudate (Starkstein et al., 1987, 1988a), thalamus (Cummings and Mendez, 1984; Starkstein et al., 1988d). Depression is frequent (Jorge et al., 1993a, 1993b).

Obsessive–compulsive disorder has been reported in up to 3.4% of patients after trauma (Hillbom, 1960; McKeon et al., 1984; Khana et al., 1985; Drummond and Gravestock, 1988; Jenike and Brandon, 1988).

Creutzfeldt–Jakob disease

Creutzfeldt–Jakob disease is a spongiform encephalopathy that can involve any region of the central nervous system. The presentation of the disease is highly variable, but the demential presentation is often associated with psychiatric manifestations such as personality changes, apathy, irritability, depression, psychosis, euphoria, or sexual disinhibition (for review, see Lopez et al., 1997). Obsessive–compulsive disorder and eating disorders have been reported recently (Lopez et al., 1997), with marked involvement of the basal ganglia on pathology.

Sydenham's chorea

Obsessive–compulsive disorder (Schilder, 1938; Freeman et al., 1965; Swedo et al., 1993, 1994), distractibility, and difficulty with concentration (Casey et al., 1994) are widely reported. Mood disorders are frequent (Freeman et al., 1965).

In Sydenham's chorea, perivascular infiltration and specific antibodies to the striatum have been described (Husby et al., 1976). MRI showed an abnormal signal in striatum, as did PET studies (Kienzle et al., 1991).

Dystonia

Dystonic syndromes are focal, segmental, or generalized dyskinesia associated with abnormal posture and movements. Bipolar disorders have been reported in idiopathic dystonia (Lauterbach et al., 1991, 1992), depression (20–80%) (Kraft, 1966; Tolosa, 1981; Jankovic and Ford, 1983; Diamond et al., 1984; Jahanshahi and Marsden, 1988; Bihari et al., 1992b), personality changes, and thought disorders (Kraft, 1966). Craniofacial dystonia seems to be more associated than limb dystonia (Grafman et al., 1991) with depression and obsessive–compulsive disorder (Tolosa, 1981; Jankovic and Ford, 1983; Cummings, 1985; Bihari, 1992a, 1992b).

Autopsy findings in focal and general dystonia have so far been inconclusive.

Tardive dyskinesias

Tardive dyskinesias are a very rich sample of all known hyperkinesias, including choreoatheosis, dystonia, tics, bucofacial and mandibular dyskinesia, tremor, and parkinsonian syndromes with focal or generalized expression, that arise in 15–25% of patients chronically treated with neuroleptic agents, but also with anticalcics, metoclopramide, and antihistamines. The pathogenesis is still unknown, but some alteration in dopamine receptor sensitivity and personal predisposing factors rather than the type of psychopathology are generally suggested (for a review, see Waddington, 1995). Some authors have suggested tardive pain syndromes, but also tardive psychosis and perhaps depression or mania that results from mesolimbic rather than nigrostriate pathways hypersensitivity (Chouinard and Jones, 1980; Weiner and Werner, 1982). Excess of cognitive dysfunction (attention, orientation, memory, perceptual or abstraction, dysexecutive, or global deficits) has been found in schizophrenics with tardive syndromes, but the interpretation is difficult because of the effect of medication (especially anticholinergic drugs) in these patients (for a review, see Waddington, 1995). Abnormal size of basal ganglia on quantitative MRI has been described (Elkashef et al., 1994).

PITANDs or PANDAS

Pediatric infection-triggered autoimmune neuropsychiatric disorders or pediatric autoimmune neuropsychiatric disorders associated with streptococcal infections is a recently defined entity sharing many features with Sydenham's chorea (Kurlan, 1998; Allen et al., 1995) that may be triggered by viruses or bacteria. Criteria for diagnosis are:

1 pediatric onset (between three years of age and the beginning of puberty);
2 the patient must have met diagnostic criteria for obsessive–compulsive disorder and/or tic disorder;
3 the onset is sudden, and there must be sudden, recurrent, clinically significant symptom exacerbations and remissions;
4 increased symptoms should not occur exclusively during stress or illness, should be pervasive, and of sufficient severity to suggest the need for treatment, and, if untreated, should last for at least four weeks before improvement is noted;

5 during obsessive–compulsive or tic exacerbation, neurological examination is
  normal (mild chorea accepted);
6 there must be evidence of antecedent or concomitant infection;
7 patients do not continue to have clinically significant symptoms between episodes of their obsessive–compulsive and/or tic disorder.

Plasmapheresis or immunoglobulin has been used. Antineuronal antibodies
(Swedo et al., 1994) or antileukocyte antibodies have been described.

Schizophrenia

Schizophrenia is a disease of unknown etiology. Neuropathologic and brain
imaging studies have produced evidence of brain abnormalities in limbic lobe,
basal ganglia, corpus callosum and septum pellucidum, thalamus, temporal lobe,
and cerebellum (Stevens, 1982).

The disorder of motility found in schizophrenia has received less attention
than the psychiatric symptoms. Abnormal gestures, involving fingers, arms, legs,
unusual facial expressions, such as mannerisms or other purposeful behavior performed in an unusual way, obsessive–compulsive disorder, bizarre gait and postures, and stereotypies (purposeless repetitive behaviors, repeated in an unvarying
way) are, however, generally present in association with delusion, hallucination,
thought and mood disturbances (Fenton and McGlashan, 1986). A poor prognosis
is generally associated when these are present (Yarden and Discipio, 1971). Negative
symptoms (impaired motivation, shallow affect, paucity of thought, social withdrawal, impairment of goal-directed behaviors, poor motivation, diminished work
capacity, psychic anergia, poor insight, diminished concern for personal hygiene,
overall restriction of spontaneity are similar to frontal lobe signs as well as other soft
signs. Positive symptoms include delusions and hallucinations. Cognitive impairment with dysexecutive dysfunction has been documented in schizophrenia, as has
obsessive–compulsive disorder in some patients and self-mutilation.

Basal ganglia dysfunction has been suspected in schizophrenia and psychosis by
several studies since the 1950s (Forstl et al., 1990; Beckson and Cummings, 1992;
Gray, 1994). Morphometric studies in schizophrenia showed mostly increased cortical atrophy and ventricular enlargement. Some found abnormalities in basal
ganglia (Davson, 1983; Harvey et al., 1991). A pathological study described
decreased volume of the internal segment of the globus pallidus on both right and
left sides (Bogerts et al., 1985; Woods et al., 1995) and smaller nucleus accumbens
and dorsomedial thalamic nucleus (Pakkenberg, 1990), but this was not found by
others (Rosenthal and Bigelow, 1972).

CT and MRI quantitative studies describe larger putamen and pallidum
(Heckers et al., 1991; Jernigan et al., 1991; Swayze et al., 1992; Elkashef et al., 1994),

caudate (Chakos et al., 1994), or no difference (Kelsoe et al., 1988; De Lisi et al., 1991), prolonged T2 times in left frontal white matter, left temporal cortex and white matter, and left lenticular nucleus (Williamson et al., 1992). Conflicting results are given for ventricular enlargement, cortical or temporal and corpus callosum atrophy, and volume loss in temporal lobe.

SPECT and PET metabolic studies showed conflicting results, either decreased striatal (caudate and putamen) and anterior thalamic metabolism in unmedicated schizophrenics (Sheppard et al., 1982; Early et al., 1987; Buchsbaum et al., 1992b; Siegel et al., 1993), or increased (Volkow et al., 1986; Early et al., 1987; Resnik et al., 1988), correlated with clinical response to neuroleptic treatment, especially in the ventral putamen, in the right more than the left (Szechtman et al., 1988; Buchsbaum et al., 1992a, 1992b). Abnormal, either increased or decreased, or normal metabolism in DLPF cortex and decreased metabolism in temporal, hippocampal, and limbic structures such as the cingulum have been reported.

Stereotactic surgery of movement disorders: pallidal and subthalamic functional neurosurgery

Unilateral pallidotomy in the treatment of Parkinson's disease can be followed by transient confusion, decrease in verbal fluency, and controversial changes in executive functions, whereas bilateral lesions can cause apathy, abulia, obsessive–compulsive disorder, environment dependency, changes in psychosocial and emotional control, decrease in verbal fluency, and executive dysfunction (Riordan et al., 1997; Soukup et al., 1997; Scott et al., 1998; Petrine et al., 1998; Trepanier et al., 1998; Ghika et al., 1999a, 1999b). Bilateral subthalamic or pallidal deep brain stimulation can induce depressive reaction (Bejjani et al., 1999; Ghika et al., 1999b), bipolar swings in mood (Ghika et al., 1999b), and laughter (Kumar et al., 1999), but generally no change in memory or executive functions (Ardouin et al., 1999).

Conclusion

The basal ganglia are part of the fronto-subcortical pathways processing the interface between internal drives and needs and the external world, with an overall activity of either facilitation or inhibition of cortical functions, gating, filtering, facilitating or inhibiting and focusing motor activity, moods, and behaviors to a specific context. Dysfunction of the basal ganglia at any level of the pathway can lead to similar behavioral, mood, or cognitive symptomatology. Dichotomic behavioral syndromes include hypokinetic, akinetic or hyperkinetic motor syndromes, apathy – emotional blunting – anhedonia or hyperactivity with attention deficit, disinihibition syndromes, disorders of impulse control or obsessive–compulsive behaviors, environment-dependency syndromes, and stereotyped behaviors. Binary mood and affective disorders encompass depression, apathy, and anhedonia to anxiety disorders and mania, as unipolar and bipolar disorders. Dichotomic expression of cognitive dysfunction varies from mental emptiness, bradyphrenia, dysexecutive, 'subcortical dementia' or apathetic dementia to flight of ideas, attentional deficit disorders, obsessional slowness, perseveration, mental automatism (echophenomena, paliphenomena, and coprophenomena, mental playing), and delirium, or even hallucinations and delusions of psychosis. A better understanding of the function of basal ganglia, together with that of limbic, paralimbic, and frontal structures, will probably be one of the revolutions of thinking psychiatry in the next century.

REFERENCES

Abély, P. and Guyot, P. (1935). Maladie de Wilson et troubles mentaux. *Ann Med Psychol* 93: 775–8.

Abrahamson, A. (1920). Mental disturbances in lethargic encephalitis. *J Nerv Ment Dis* 52: 193–200.

Adams, R.D., van Bogaert, L. and van de Eecken, H. (1961). Degenerescence nigrostriate and cerebello-nigrostriate. *Psychiatr Neurol* 142: 219–59.

Akelaitis, A.J. (1994). Atrophy of the basal ganglia in Pick's disease. *Arch Neurol Psychiatry* 51: 27–34.

Akil, M., Schwartz, J.A. and Dutchak, D. (1991). The psychiatric presentation of Wilson's disease. *J Neuropsychiatry Clin Neurosci* 3: 377–82.

Alarcon, R.D., Libb, J.W. and Boll, T.J. (1994). Neuropsychological testing in obsessive–compulsive disorder: a clinical review. *J Neuropsychiatry Clin Neurosci* 6: 217–18.

Albert, M.L., Feldman, R.G. and Wilis, A.L. (1974). The subcortical dementia of progressive supranuclear palsy. *J Neurol Neurosurg Psychiatry* 37: 121–30.

Albert, M.S., Butters, N. and Brandt, J. (1981). Development of remote memory loss in patients with Huntington's disease. *J Clin Neuropsychol* 3: 1–12.

Alexander, G.E., de Long, M. and Strick, P. (1986). Parallel organization of functionally segregated circuits linking the basal ganglia and cortex. *Annu Rev Neurosci* 9: 357–81.

Alexander, M.P. (1995). Reversal of chronic akinetic mutism after mesencephalic infarction with dopaminergic agents. *Neurology* 45 Suppl. 4, A330.

Ali-Chérif, A., Royere, M.L., Grosset, A. et al. (1984). Troubles du comportement et de l'activité mentale après intoxication oxycarbonée: lésions pallidales bilatérales. *Rev Neurol* 140: 401–5.

Allen, A.J., Leonard, H.I. and Swedo, S.E. (1995). Case study: a new infection-triggered, autoimmune subtype of pediatric OCD and Tourette's syndrome. *J Am Acad Child Adolesc Psychiatry* 34: 307–11.

Allison, R.S. (1966). Perseveration as a sign of diffuse and focal brain damage. *Br Med J* 2: 1027–32.

Altschuler, L.L., Curran, J.G., Hauser, P. et al. (1995). T2 hyperintensities in bipolar disorder: magnetic resonance imaging comparison and literature meta-analysis. *Am J Psychiatry* 152: 1139–44.

Ames, D., Cummings, J.L., Wirshing, W.C., Quinn, B. and Mahler, M. (1994). Repetitive and compulsive behavior in frontal lobe degenerations. *J Neuropsychiatry Clin Neurosci* 6: 100–13.

Aminoff, M.J., Marshall, J., Smith, E.M. and Wyke, M.A. (1975). Pattern of intellectual impairment in Huntington's chorea. *Psychol Med* 5: 169–72.

Andreasen, N.C. and Bardach, J. (1977). Dysmorphophobia: symptom or disease. *Am J Psychiatry* 134: 673–6.

Andreason, P.J., Altemus, M., Zametkin, A.J. et al. (1992). Regional cerebral glucose metabolism in bulimia nervosa. *Am J Psychiatry* 149: 1506–13.

Ardouin, C., Pillon, B., Pfeiffer, E. et al. (1999). Bilateral subthalamic or pallidal stimulation for Parkinson's disease affects neither memory nor executive functions: a consecutive series of 62 patients. *Ann Neurol* 46: 217–23.

Asakura, K., Mizuno, M. and Yasui, N. (1989). Clinical analysis of 24 cases of caudate hemorrhage. *Neurol Med Chir* 29: 1107–12.

Asnis, G. (1977). Parkinson's disease, depression and ECT. A review and case study. *Am J Psychiatry* 134: 191–4.

Astrom, M. (1996). Generalized anxiety disorder in stroke patients. A 3-year longitudinal study. *Stroke* 27: 270–5.

Aylward, E.H., Robert-Twilie, J.V., Barta, P.E. et al. (1994). Basal ganglia volumes and white matter hyperintensities in patients with bipolar disorder. *Am J Psychiatry* 151: 687–93.

Bach-y-Rita, G., Lion, J.R., Climent, C.E. and Ervin, F.R. (1971). Episodic dyscontrol: a study of 130 violent patients. *Am J Psychiatry* 127: 1473–8.

Ballivet, J., Marin, A. and Gisselmann, A. (1973). Aspects de l'hypersexualité observée chez les parkinsoniens lors du traitement par L-dopa. *Ann Med Psychol* 131: 515–22.

Barat, M., Mazaux, J.M., Bioulac, B. et al. (1978). Troubles du langage de type aphasique et lesions putamino-caudées: observation anatomo-clinique. *Rev Neurol* 139: 43–63.

Barber, J., Tomer, R., Srka, H. et al. (1985). Does unilateral dopamine deficit contribute to depression? *Psychiatry Res* 15: 17–24.

Baxter, L.R. Jr. (1994). Positron emission tomography studies of cerebral glucose metabolism in obsessive compulsive disorder. *J Clin Psychiatry* 55: 54–9.

Baxter, L.R. Jr, Phelps, M.E., Mazziotta, J.C. et al. (1985). Cerebral metabolic rates for glucose in mood disorders. Studies with positron emission tomography and fluorodeoxyglucose F 18. *Arch Gen Psychiatry*, 42: 441–7.

Bayles, K. (1990). Language and Parkinson's disease. *Alzheimer Dis Assoc Disord* 4: 171–80.

Beard, A.W. (1959). The association of hepatolenticular degeneration with schizophrenia. *Acta Psychiatr Neurol* 34: 411–28.

Beats, B., Levy, R. and Forst, H. (1991). Ventricular enlargement and caudate hyperintensity in elderly depressives. *Biol Psychiatry* 30: 452–8.

Beatty, W.W., Salmon, D.C., Buters, N., Heindel, W.C. and Granholm, E.L. (1988). Retrograde amnesia in patients with Alzheimer's disease and Huntington's disease. *Neurobiol aging* 9: 181–6.

Beckson, M. and Cummings, J.L. (1992). Psychosis in basal ganglia disorders. *Neuropsychiatry Neuropsychol Behav Neurol* 5: 126–31.

Behar, D., Rappoport, J.L., Berg, C.J. et al. (1984). Computerized tomography and neuropsychological test measures in adolescents with obsessive–compulsive disorders. *Am J Psychiatry* 141: 363–9.

Bejjani, B.P., Damier, P., Arnulf, I. et al. (1999). Transient acute depression induced by high frequency deep brain stimulation. *N Engl J Med* 19: 1476–80.

Benedeck, L. (1925). Zwangsmässiges Schreien in Anfällen als postencephalitische Hyperkinese. *Z Neurol Psychiatrie* 98: 17.

Benkelfat, C., Nordahl., T.E., Semple, W.E. et al. (1990). Local cerebral glucose metabolic rates in obsessive–compulsive disorder patients treated with clomipramine. *Arch Gen Psychiatry* 47: 840–8.

Benson, D.F. (1991). The role of frontal dysfunction in attention-deficit hyperactivity disorder. *J Child Neurol* 6 Suppl.: S9–S12.

Berthier, M.L., Kulisevsky, J., Gironell, A. and Fernandez-Benitez, J.A. (1996a). Poststroke bipolar affective disorder: clinical subtypes, concurrent movement disorders, and anatomical correlates. *J Neuropsychiatry Clin Neurosci* 8: 160–7.

Berthier, M.L., Kulisevsky, J., Gironell, A. and Heras, J.A. (1996b). Obsessive–compulsive disorder associated with brain lesions: clinical, phenomenology, cognitive function, and anatomic correlates. *Neurology* 47: 353–61.

Bhatia, K.P. and Marsden, C.D. (1994). The behavioral and motor consequences of focal lesions of the basal ganglia in man. *Brain* 117: 859–76.

Bihari, K., Hill, J.L. and Murphy, D.L. (1992a). Obsessive–compulsive characteristics in patients with idiopathic spasmodic torticollis. *Psychiatry Res* 42: 267–72.

Bihari, K., Pigott, T., Hill, J.L. and Murphy, D.L. (1992b). Blepharospasm and obsessive–compulsive disorder. *J Nerv Ment Dis* 180: 130–2.

Binder, R.L. (1983). Neurologically silent brain tumors in psychiatric hospital admissions: three cases and a review. *J Clin Psychiatry* 44: 94–7.

Blonder, L.X., Gur, R.E. and Gur, R.C. (1989). The effects of right and left parkinsonism on prosody. *Brain Lang* 36: 193–207.

Blumer, D. and Benson, D.F. (1975). Personality changes with frontal and temporal lobe lesions. In *Psychiatric Aspects of Neurologic Diseases*, ed. D.F. Benson and D. Blumer, pp. 497–522. New York: Grune and Stratton.

Bogerts, B., Meertz, E. and Schönfeldt-Bausch, R. (1985). Basal ganglia and limbic system pathology in schizophrenia. *Arch Gen Psychiatry* 42: 784–91.

Bogousslavsky, J. (1993). Troubles thymiques et accidents vasculaires cérébraux. *Rev Neuropsychol* 3: 257–69.

Bogousslavsky, J., Ferrazzini, M., Regli, F. et al. (1988). Manic delirium and frontal lobe syndrome with paramedian infarction of the right thalamus. *J Neurol Neurosurg Psychiatry* 51: 116–19.

Boller, F., Passafiume, D., Keefe, N.C. et al. (1984). Visuospatial impairment in Parkinson's disease: role of perceptual and motor factors. *Arch Neurol* 41: 485–90.

Borod, J., Koff, E., Perlman-Lorch, J. and Nicholas, M. (1986). The expression and perception of facial emotions in brain damaged patients. *Neuropsychologia* 24: 169–80.

Bradford, J. and Balmaceda, A. (1983). Shoplifting: is there a specific psychiatric syndrome? *Can J Psychiatry* 28: 248–54.

Brandt, J. (1985). Access to knowledge in the dementia of Huntington's disease. *Dev Neuropsychol* 1: 335–48.

Braun, A.R., Randolph, C., Stoetter, B. et al. (1995). The functional neuroanatomy of Tourette's syndrome: an FDG-PET study. II. Relationship between regional cerebral metabolism and associated behavioral and cognitive features of the illness. *Neuropsychopharmacology* 13: 151–68.

Breiter, H.C.R., Kwong, K.K., Baker, J.R. et al. (1996). Functional magnetic resonance imaging of symptom provocation in obsessive–compulsive disorder. *Arch Gen Psychiatry* 51: 663–4.

Brickner, R., Rosner, A. and Munro, R. (1940). Physiological aspects of the obsessive state. *Psychosom Med* 11: 369–83.

Brooks, D.J. (1995). The role of the basal ganglia in motor control: contributions from PET. *J Neurol Sci* 128: 1–13.

Brouwers, P., Cox, C., Martin, A., Chase, T.N. and Fedio, P. (1984). Differential perceptual–spatial impairment in Huntington's disease and Alzheimer's dementias. *Arch Neurol* 41: 1073–6.

Brown, J.W. (1967). Physiology and pathogenesis of emotional expression. *Brain Res* 5: 1–14.

Brunner, R.J., Kornhuber, H.H., Seemuller, E., Suger, G. and Wallesh, C.W. (1982). Basal ganglia participation in language pathology. *Brain Lang* 16: 281–99.

Bryson, N.S., Sakati, N., Nyhan, W.L. and Fish, C.H. (1971). Self-mutilative behavior in the Cornelia de Lange syndrome. *J Ment Defic Res* 76: 319–24.

Buchsbaum, M.S., Haier, R.J., Potkin, S.G. et al. (1992a). Fronto-striatal disorder of cerebral metabolism in never-medicated schizophrenics. *Arch Gen Psychiatry* 49: 974–82.

Buchsbaum, M., Potkin, S.G., Siegel, B. Jr, et al. (1992b). Striatal metabolic rate and clinical response to neuroleptic in schizophrenia. *Arch Gen Psychiatry*, 49: 966–74.

Buchsbaum, M.S., Wu, J. De Lisi, L.E. et al. (1986). Frontal cortex and basal ganglia metabolic rates assessed by position emission tomography with [18F] 2-deoxyglucose in affective illness. *J Affect Disord* 10: 137–52.

Buck, R. and Duffy, R.J. (1980). Nonverbal communication of affect in brain damaged patients. *Cortex* 16: 351–62.

Bürger, H. and Mayer-Gross, W. (1926). Schizophrene Psychosen bei Encephalitis lethargica. *Z Neurol Psychiatrie* 106: 438.

Burns, A., Folstein, S., Brandt, J. et al. (1990). Clinical assessment of irritability, aggression, and apathy in Huntington and Alzheimer's disease. *J Nerv Ment Dis* 178: 20–6.

Butters, N., Sax, D., Montgomery, K. et al. (1978a). Comparison of the neuropsychological deficits associated with early and advanced Huntington's disease. *Arch Neurol* 35: 585–9.

Butters, N., Tarlow, S., Cormat, L. et al. (1976). A comparison of the information processing deficits in patients with Huntington's disease and Korsakoff's syndrome. *Cortex* 12: 134–44.

Buzzard, E.F. and Greenfield, J.G. (1919). Lethargic encephalitis: its sequelae and morbid anatomy. *Brain* 42: 305–38.

Caine, E., Ebert, M. and Weingartner, H. (1977). An outline for the analysis of dementia: the memory disorder of Huntington's disease. *Neurology* 27: 1087–92.

Calabrese, G., Colombo, C., Bonfanti, A., Scotti, G. and Scarone, S. (1993). Caudate nucleus abnormalities in obsessive–compulsive disorder: measurements of MRI signal intensity. *Psychiatry Res* 50: 89–92.

Cambier, J., Elghozi, D. and Strube, E. (1979). Hemorrhagie de la tête du noyau caudé. *Rev Neurol* 13: 763–74.

Cambier, J., Masson, C., Bennamous, S. et al. (1988). La graphomaine. Activité graphique compulsive manifestation d'un fronto-calleux. *Rev Neurol* 144: 158–64.

Cambier, J., Masson, H., Viader, F., Limodier, J. and Strube, A. (1985). Le syndrome frontal de la maladie de Steele–Richardson–Olszewski. *Rev Neurol* 141: 528–36.

Cancelliere, A.E. and Kertesz, A. (1990). Lesion localization in acquired deficits of emotional expression and comprehension. *Brain Cogn* 13: 133–47.

Canter, G. (1963). Speech characteristics of patients with Parkinson's disease. Intensity, pitch, and duration. *J Speech Hear Disord* 29: 221–9.

Caplan, L.R., Schmahmann, J.D., Kase, C.S. et al. (1990). Caudate infarcts. *Arch Neurol* 47: 133–43.

Carranza, E., Rossitch, E. Jr and Martinez, J. (1989). Unilateral akathisia in a patient with AIDS and toxoplasmosis subthalamic abscess. *Neurology* 39: 449–50.

Casey, B.J., Vauss, Y.C. and Swedo, S.E. (1994). Cognitive functioning in Sydenham's chorea: part 1. Attentional functioning. *Dev Neuropsychol* 10: 75–88.

Castellanos, F.X., Giedd, J.N., Eckburg, P. et al. (1994). Quantitative morphology of the caudate nucleus in attention deficit and hyperactivity disorder. *Am J Psychiatry* 151: 1791–6.

Castellanos, F.X., Giedd, J.N., Hamburger, S.D., Marsh, W.L. and Rapoport, J.L. (1996). Brain morphometry in Tourette's syndrome: the influence of comorbid attention-deficity/hyperactivity disorder. *Neurology* 47: 1581–3.

Celesia, G.G. and Barr, A.N. (1970). Psychosis and other psychiatric manifestations of levodopa therapy. *Arch Neurol* 23: 193–200.

Chakos, M.H., Lieberman, J.A., Bilder, R.M. et al. (1994). Increase in caudate nuclei volumes of first-episode schizophrenic patients taking antipsychotic drugs. *Am J Psychiatry* 151: 1430–6.

Cheyette, S.R. and Cummings, J.L. (1995). Encephalitis lethargica: lessons for contemporary neuropsychiatry. *J Neuropsychiatry Clin Neurosci* 7: 125–34.

Cheifetz, D.I., Garron, D.C., Leavitt, F., Klawans, H.C. and Garwins, J.S. (1970). Emotional disturbance accompanying the treatment of parkinsonism with L-dopa. *Clin Pharmacol Ther* 12: 56–61.

Chouinard, G. and Jones, B.D. (1980). Neuroleptic-induced supersensitivity psychosis: clinical and pharmacologic characteristics. *Am J Psychiatry* 137: 16–21.

Chudler, E.H. and Dong, W.K. (1995). The role of the basal ganglia in nociception and pain. *Pain* 60: 3–38.

Coffey, B., Frazier, J. and Chen, S. (1992). Comorbidity, Tourette syndrome, and anxiety disorders. *Adv Neurol* 58: 95–104.

Coffey, C.E., Wilkinson, W.E., Weiner, R.D. et al. (1993). Quantitative cerebral anatomy in depression. A controlled magnetic resonance imaging study. *Arch Gen Psychiatry* 50: 7–16.

Coleman, E. (1990). The obsessive compulsive model for describing compulsive sexual behavior. *Am J Psychiatry Neurol* 2: 9–14.

Comings, D.E. and Comings, B.G. (1988). Tourette's syndrome and attention deficit disorder. In *Tourette's Syndrome and Tic Disorders: Clinical Understanding and Treatment*, ed. D.J. Cohen, R.D. Bruun and J.F. Leckman, pp. 119–35. New York: Wiley.

Cooke, J.D., Brown, J.D. and Brooks, V.B. (1978). Increased dependence on visual information for movement control in patients with Parkinson's disease. *Can J Neurol Sci* 5: 413–15.

Cools, A.R., van den Bercken, J.H.L., Horstink, M.W.L. et al. (1984). Cognitive and motor shifting aptitude disorder in Parkinsonism. *J Neurol Neurosurg Psychiatry* 47: 443–53.

Cooper, J.A., Sagar, H.J. and Sullivan, E.V. (1993). Short-term memory and temporal ordering in early Parkinson's disease: effects of disease chronicity and medication. *Neuropsychologia* 31: 933–49.

Coryell, W. (1981). Obsessive–compulsive disorder and primary unipolar depression: comparison of background, family history and mortality. *J Nerv Ment Dis* 164: 220–4.

Creack, M. and Guttman, E. (1935). Chorea, tics, and compulsive utterances. *J Ment Sci* 81: 834–9.

Croisile, B., Tourniaire, D., Confavreux, C., Trilet, M. and Amard, G. (1989). Bilateral damage to the head of the caudate nuclei. *Ann Neurol* 25: 313–14.

Crow, J.J., Johnstone, E.D. and McClelland, H.A. (1976). The coincidence of schizophrenia and parkinsonism: some neurochemical implications. *Psychiatr Med* 6: 227–33.

Cummings, J.L. (1985). Psychosomatic aspects of movement disorders. *Adv Psychosom, Med* 13: 111–32.

Cummings, J.L. (1993). Depression and Parkinson's disease: a review. *Am J Psychiatry* 4: 443–54.

Cummings, J.L. (1995). Anatomic and behavioral aspects of fronto-subcortical circuits. *Ann NY Acad Sci* 769: 1–13.

Cummings, J.L. and Cunningham, K. (1992). Obsessive–compulsive disorder in Huntington's disease. *Biol Psychiatry* 31: 263–70.

Cummings, J.L., Gosenfield, L.F., Houlihan, J.P. and McCaffay, T. (1983). Neuropsychiatric disturbances associated with idiopathic calcification of the basal ganglia. *Biol Psychol* 18: 591–601.

Cummings, J.L. and Mendez, M.F. (1984). Secondary mania with focal cerebrovascular lesions. *Am J Psychiatry* 141: 1084–7.

Damasio, H., Eslinger, P. and Adams, H.P. (1984). Aphasia following basal ganglia lesions: new evidence. *Semin Neurol* 4: 151–61.

Danel, T., Goudemand, M., Ghawche, F. et al. (1991). Mélancolie délirante et lacunes multiples des noyaux gris centraux. *Rev Neurol* 147: 60–2.

D'Antona, R., Baron, J.C., Samson, Y. et al. (1988). Subcortical dementia: frontal cortex hypometabolism detected by positron emission tomography with progressive supranuclear palsy. *Brain* 108: 785–9.

Davenport, C.B. (1916). Huntington's chorea in relation to heredity and eugenics. *Am J Insanity* 73: 195–222.

Davis, E.J. and Borde, M. (1993). Wilson's disease and catatonia. *Br J Psychiatry* 161: 256–9.

Davson, K. (1983). Schizophrenia-like psychoses associated with organic cerebral disorders: a review. *Psychiatr Dev* 1: 1–34.

De Lisi, L.E., Hoff, A.L., Schwartz, J.E. et al. (1991). Brain morphology in first-episode schizophrenic-like psychotic patients: a quantitative magnetic resonance imaging study. *Biol Psychiatry* 29: 159–75.

Demaret, A. (1973). Onychopagie, trichotillomanie et grooming. *Ann Med Psychol* 1: 235–42.

Dening, T.R. (1991). neuropsychiatry of Wilson's disease: a review. *Int J Psychiatr Med* 21: 135–48.

Denny Brown, D. (1962). *The Basal Ganglia and their Relation to Disorders of Movement.* Oxford: Oxford University Press.

Desi, M., Klein, J., Parman,Y., Seibel, N. and Segobia, R. (1990). Adynamia and repetitive behavior in a case of bilateral subcortical lesions. *J Neurol* 237 Suppl. 1: 38.

Destée, A., Gray, F., Parent, M. et al. (1990). Comportement compulsif d'allure obsessionnelle et paralysie supranucléaire progressive. *Rev Neurol* 146: 12–18.

Devinski, O. (1983). Neuroanatomy of Gilles de la Tourette's disease. *Arch Neurol* 40: 508–14.

Diamond, E.L., Trobe, J.D. and Behar, C.D. (1984). Psychological aspects of essential blepharospasm. *J Nerv Ment Dis* 172: 749–56.

Dide, M. and Guiraud, P. (1922). *Psychiatrie du Médecin Praticien.* Paris: Masson.

Diefendorf, A.R. (1912). Mental symptoms in acute chorea. *J Nerv Ment Dis* 39: 161–72.

Di Maio, L., Squiteri, F., Napolitano, G. et al. (1993). Suicide risk in Huntington's disease. *J Med Genet* 30: 293–5.

Drummond, L.M. and Gravestock, S. (1988). Delayed emergence of obsessive–compulsive neurosis following head injury: case report and review of its theoretical implications. *Br J Psychiatry* 153: 839–42.

Dubois, B., Pillon, B., Legault, F., Agid, Y. and Lhermitte, F. (1988). Slowing of cognitive processing in progressive supranuclear palsy. A comparison with Parkinson's disease. *Arch Neurol* 45: 1194–9.

Dubois, B., Pillon, B. and Sternic, N. (1990). Age-induced cognitive disturbances in Parkinson's disease. *Neurology* 40: 38–41.

Dupont, R.M., Jernigan, T.L., Heindel, W. et al. (1995). Magnetic resonance imaging and mood disorders. Localization of white matter and other subcortical abnormalities. *Arch Gen Psychiatry* 52: 747–55.

Durand, M.C., Vercken, J.B. and Goulon, M. (1989). Syndrome extrapyramidal après incompétence cardio-circulatoire. *Rev Neurol* 145: 398–400.

Early, T.S., Reiman, E.M., Raichle, M.E. and Spitznagel, E.L. (1987). Left globus pallidus abnormality in never-medicated patients with schizophrenia. *Science* 84: 561–3.

Eastwood, M.R., Rifat, S.L., Nobs, H. and Ruderman, J. (1989). Mood disorder following cerebrovascular accident. *Br J Psychiatry* 154: 195–200.

Ekman, P. and Friesen, W. (1971). Constants across cultures in the face and emotion. *J Pers Soc Psychol* 17: 124–9.

El-Awar, M., Becker, J.T., Hammond, K., Nebes, R.D. and Boller, F. (1987). Learning deficit in Parkinson's disease. *Arch Neurol* 44: 180–4.

Elkashef, A.M., Buchnan, R.W., Gellad, F., Munson, R.C. and Breier, A. (1994). Basal ganglia pathology in schizophrenia and tardive dyskinesia: an MRI quantitative study. *Am J Psychiatry* 151: 752–5.

Fahr, T. (1930). Idiopatische Verkalkung der Hirngefässe. *Centralbl Allg Pathol Anat L* 4: 129–33.

Fairweather, D.S. (1947). Psychiatric aspects of the post-encephalitic syndrome. *J Ment Sci* 93: 201–54.

Fearnley, J.M. and Lees, A.J. (1990). Striatonigral degeneration. A clinicopathological study. *Brain* 113: 1823–42.

Fenton, W.S. and McGlashan, T.H. (1986). The prognostic significance of obsessive–compulsive symptoms in schizophrenia. *Am J Psychiatry* 143: 437–41.

Fernandez-Pardal, M.M., Michel, F., Asconape, J. and Paradiso, G. (1985). Neurobehavioral symptoms in caudate hemorrhage: two cases. *Neurology* 1985; 35: 1806–7.

Feve, J.R., Mussini, J.M., Mathe, J.F. et al. (1977). Degenerscence striato-nigrique: étude clinique et anatomique d'un cas ayant réagi favorablement à la L-dopa. Rev Neurol 133: 271–8.

Figiel, G.S., Krishnan, K.R. and Doraiswamy, P.M. (1990). Subcortical structural changes in ECT-induced delirium. *J Geriatr Psychiatry Neurol* 3: 172–6.

Filipek, P.A., Semrud-Clikeman, M., Steingard, R.J. et al. (1987). Volumetric MRI analysis comparing subjects having attention-deficit hyperactivity disorder with normal controls. *Neurology* 48: 589–601.

Fisher, C.M. (1995). Abulia. In *Stroke Syndromes*, ed. J. Bogousslavsky and L. Capal, pp. 182–7. Cambridge: Cambridge University Press.

Fisher, G. (1968). Intellectual impairment in a patient with hepatolenticular degeneration (Wilson's disease). *J Ment Subnormal* 14: 91–5.

Fisk, J.D., Goodale, M.A., Burkhart, G. and Barnett, H.J.M. (1982). Progressive supranuclear palsy: the relationship between ocular motor dysfunction and psychological test performance. *Neurology* 32: 698–705.

Fleminger, S. (1991). Left-sided Parkinson's disease associated with greater anxiety and depression. *Psychol Med* 21: 629–38.

Flor-Henry, P. (1979). On certain aspects of localization of the cerebral systems regulating and determining emotions. *Biol Psychiatry* 14: 677–98.

Flor-Henry, P. (1990). Le syndrome obsessionel–compulsif: reflet d'un défaut de régulation fronto-caudée de l'hémisphère gauche? *Encéphale* 16: 325–9.

Ford, R.A. (1991). Neurobehavioral correlates of abnormal repetitive behavior. *Behav Neurol* 4: 113–19.

Forstl, H., Eden, S., Drumm, B. and Kohlmeyer, K. (1990). Psychotic symptoms in basal ganglia sclerosis. *Lancet* 335: 1193–4.

Francis, A. and Freeman, H. (1984). Psychiatric abnormality and brain calcification over four generations. *J Nerv Ment Dis* 172: 166–70.

Freeman, J., Aron, A., Collard, J. and MacKay, M. (1965). The emotional correlates of Sydenham's chorea. *Pediatrics* 35: 42–9.

Fromm, D., Holland, A.L., Swindel, C.S. and Reinmuth, O.M. (1985). Various consequences of subcortical stroke. *Arch Neurol* 42: 943–50.

Frosch, J. and Wortis, S. (1954). A contribution to the nosology of the impulse disorders. *Am J Psychiatry* 111: 133–8.

Fujikawa, T., Yamawaki, S. and Touhouda, Y. (1995). Silent cerebral infarctions in patients with late-onset mania. *Stroke* 26: 946–9.

Gainotti, G. (1972). Emotional behavior and hemispheric side of lesion. *Cortex* 8: 41–55.

Garber, H.J., Ananth, J.V., Chiu, L.C., Griswold, V.J. and Oldendorf, W.H. (1989). Nuclear magnetic resonance study of obsessive–compulsive disorders. *Am J Psychiatry* 146: 1001–5.

Garcia-Campayo, J.J. and Sanz-Carillo, C. (1994). Psychiatric onset of striatonigral degeneration. *Eur J Psychiatry* 8: 84–8.

Garcia Rill, E.E. (1986). The basal ganglia and the locomotor regions. *Brain Res* 396: 47–63.

George, M.S. (1994). Introduction: the emerging neuroanatomy of depression. *Psychiatr Ann* 24: 635–6.

George, M.S., Brewerton, T.D. and Cochrane, C.C. (1990). Trichotillomania and bulimia. *N Engl J Med* 322: 470–1.

Ghika, J., Bogousslavsky, J., Ghika-Schmid, F. and Regli, F. (1996). 'Echoing approval': a new speech disorder. *J Neurol* 243: 633–7.

Ghika, J., Bogousslavsky, J. and Regli, F. (1991). Infarcts in the territory of the lenticulostriate branches from the middle cerebral artery. Etiological factors and clinical features in 65 cases. *Arch Suisses Neurol Psychiatr* 142: 5–18.

Ghika, J., Tennis, M., Hoffmann, E. and Growdon, J.H. (1995). Environment-driven behaviors in progressive supranuclear palsy. *J Neurol Sci* 103: 104–11.

Ghika, J., Ghika-Schmid, F., Fankhauser, H. et al. (1999a). Bilateral contemporaneous postero-ventral pallidotomy for the treatment of Parkinson's disease: neuropsychological and neurological side effects. *J Neurosurg* 91: 313–21.

Ghika, J., Vingerhoets, F., Albanese, A. and Villemure, J.G. (1999b). Bipolar swings in mood in a patient with bilateral subthalamic deep brain stimulation (DBS) free of antiparkinsonian medication. *Parkinsonism Relat Dis.*, 5: S104.

Ghika-Schmid, F. and Bogousslavsky, J. (1997). Affective disorders following stroke. *Eur Neurol* 38: 75–81.

Gilles de la Tourette, G. (1885). Etude sur une affection nerveuse caractérisée par l'incoordination motrice accompagnée d'écholalie et de corpolalie. *Arch Neurol* 9: 19–42.

Goldberg, E. (1986). Varieties of perseveration: a comparison of two taxonomies. *J Clin Exp Neuropsychol* 8: 710–26.

Goldman, M.J. (1991). Kleptomania: making sense of the nonsensical. *Am J Psychiatry* 8: 986–96.

Goldstein, K. (1939). *The Organism: a Holistic Approach to Biology, derived from Pathological Data in Man.* New York: American Book.

Gordon, W.P. and Iles, J. (1987). Neurolinguistic characteristics of language production in Huntington's disease. A preliminary report. *Brain Lang* 31: 1–10.

Gotham, A.M., Brown, R.G. and Marsden, C.D. (1988). 'Frontal' cognitive function in patients with Parkinson's disease 'on' and 'off' levodopa. *Brain* 111: 299–321.

Graf, H. and Mallin, R. (1990). The syndrome of wrist cutter. *Am J Psychiatry* 124: 36–42.

Grafman, J., Cohen, L.G. and Hallett, M. (1991). Is focal hand dystonia associated with psychopathology? *Mov Disord* 6: 29–35.

Grafman, J., Litvan, I., Gomez, C. and Chase, T.N. (1990). Frontal lobe function in progressive supranuclear palsy. *Arch Neurol* 47: 553–8.

Grandas, F., Artiedo, J. and Obeso, J. (1989). Clinical and CT findings in a case of cyanide intoxication. *Mov Disord* 4: 188–93.

Gray, J.A. (1994). Modèle général du système limbique et des ganglions de la base: applications à la schizophrénie et aux comportements compulsifs d'allure obsessionnelle. *Rev Neurol* 150: 605–13.

Graybiel, A.M. (1990). Neurotransmitters and neuromodulators in the basal ganglia. *Trends Neurosci* 13: 244–54.

Graybiel, A.M. (1995). Building action repertoires: memory and learning functions of the basal ganglia. *Curr Opin Neurobiol* 5: 733–41.

Grimshaw, L. (1964). Obsessional disorder and neurological illness. *J Neurol Neurosurg Psychiatry* 27: 229–31.

Growdon, J.H., Corkin, S. and Rosen, T.J. (1990). Distinctive aspects of cognitive dysfunction in Parkinson's disease. *Adv Neurol* 53: 365–76.

Grünberger, J., Sluga, W.W. and Tschabitscher, H. (1967). Kriminelle Verhaltens-störungen bei Morbus Wilson. *Wien Z Nervenheilk* 24: 313–25.

Guirand, P. (1936). Analyse du symptôme stérétypie. *L'Encéphale* 31: 229–70.

Gwirstman, H.E., Prager, J. and Henkin, R. (1993). Case report of anorexia nervosa associated with Wilson's disease. *Int J Eat Disord* 13: 241–4.

Gysin, W.M. and Cooke, E.T. (1950). Unusual mental symptoms in a case of hepatolenticular degeneration. *Dis Nerv Syst* 28: 213–26.

Haber, S.N., Kowall, N.W., Vonsattel, J.P. et al. (1986). Gilles de la Tourette's syndrome. A postmortem neurological and immunohistochemical study. *J Neurol Sci* 75: 225–41.

Habib, M. and Poncet, M. (1988). Perte de l'élan vital, de l'intérêt et de l'activation (syndrome athymormique) au cours de lésions lacunaires des corps striés. *Rev Neurol* 144: 571–7.

Hagin, R.A., Beeccher, R., Pagano, G. et al. (1982). Effects of Tourette syndrome on learning. *Adv Neurol* 35: 323–30.

Hall, A.J. (1923). Encephalitis lethargica (epidemic encephalitis). *Lancet* 1: 731–40.

Hallopeau, X. (1889). Alopecia par grattage (trichomania ou trichotillomania). *Ann Derm Syphilol* 10: 440.

Hamilton, A.S. (1908). A report of 27 cases of chronic progressive chorea. *Am J Insanity* 64: 403–75.

Harper, P.S. (1996). *Huntington's disease*, 2nd edn. London: W.B. Saunders.

Harrington, L., Haaland, K.Y., Yeo, R.A. and Marder, E. (1990). Procedural memory in Parkinson's disease: impairment motor and motor visuo-spatial learning. *J Clin Exp Neuropsychol* 12: 325–39.

Harris, G.J., Hoehn-Saric, R., Lewis, R., Pearlson, G.D. and Streeter, C. (1994). Mapping SPECT cerebral perfusion abnormalities in obsessive–compulsive disorder. *Hum Brain Map* 2: 237–48.

Harvey, I., Ron, M.A., Murray, R. et al. (1991). MRI in schizophrenia: basal ganglia and white matter T1 times. *Psychol Med* 21: 587–98.

Haskovec, L. (1901). L'akathise. *Rev Neurol* 9: 1107–9.

Hauptmann, A. (1922). De 'Mangel and Antrieb' von innen gesehen. *Arch Psychiatry* 66: 615.

Hawkins, R.A., Mazziotta, J.C. and Phelps, M.E. (1987). Wilson's disease studied with FDG and positron emossion tomography. *Neurology* 37: 1707–1711.

Hay, J., Sachdev, P., Cummings, S. et al. (1993). Treatment of obsessive–compulsive disorder by psychosurgery. *Acta Psychiatr Scand* 87: 197–207.

Hayashi, R., Hayashi, K., Inoue, K. and Yanagisawa, N. (1993). A serial computerized tomographic study of the interval form of CO poisoning. *Eur Neurol* 33: 27–9.

Heathfield, K.W.G. (1967). Huntington's chorea. *Brain* 90: 203–32.

Heckers, S., Hensen, H., Heinsen, Y. and Beckmann, H . (1991). Cortex, white matter, and basal ganglia in schizophrenia: volumetric postmortem study. *Biol Psychiatry* 29: 556–66.

Heilman, K.M. (1994). Emotion and the brain. A distributed modular network mediating emotional experience. In *Neuropsychology*, ed. D. Zeidel, pp. 127–47. San Diego: Academic Press.

Herrmann, G. (1922). Zwangsdenken und andere Zwangserschienungen bei Erkrankung der striären System. *Monatschr Psych Neurol* 52: 324–44.

Hess, W.R. (1954). *Das Zwischenhim*, 2nd edn. Basel: Schwabe.

Hill, T.R. (1928). The problem of juvenile behavior disorders in chronic epidemic encephalitis. *J Neurol Psychopathol* 9: 1–10.

Hillbom, E. (1960). After effects of brain injuries. *Acta Psychiatr Neurol Scand* 142 Suppl.: 1–195.

Hoehn, M.M., Crowley, T.J. and Rutledge, C.O. (1960). Dopamine correlates of neurological and psychological status in untreated Parkinsonism. *Arch Psychiatr Nervenkr* 39: 941–51.

Hoehn-Saric, R. and Barksdale, V.C. (1983). Impulsiveness in obsessive–compulsive patients. *Br J Psychiatry* 143: 177–82.

Hoehn-Saric, R., Pearlson, G.D., Harris, G.J., Machlin, S.R. and Camargo, E.E. (1991). Effects of fluoxetine on regional cerebral blood flow in obsessive–compulsive patients. *Am J Psychiatry* 148: 1243–5.

Hoffnung, R., Aizenberg, D., Hermersh, H. et al. (1989). Religious compulsions and the spectrum concept of psychopathology. *Psychopathology* 22: 141–4.

Hohman, L.B. (1921). Epidemic encephalitis (lethargic encephalitis). *Arch Neurol Psychiatry* 6: 295–333.

Hollander, E., Cohen, I., Richards, M. et al. (1993). A pilot study of the neuropsychology of obsessive–compulsive disorder and Parkinson's disease: basal ganglia disorders. *J Neuropsychiatry Clin Neurosci* 5: 104–7.

Hollander, E. and Wong, C.M. (1995). Body dysmorphic disorder, pathological gambling, and sexual compulsions. *J Clin Psychiatry* 56, Suppl. 4: 7–12.

Holstege, G. (1992). The emotional motor system. *Eur J Morphol* 30: 67–79.

Hoogduin, C.A.L. (1986). On the diagnosis of obsessive–compulsive disorder. *Am J Psychother* 40: 36–51.

Hubble, J.P., Venkatesch, R., Hassanainen, R.E.S., Gray, C. and Koller, W.C. (1993). Personality and depression in Parkinson's disease. *J Nerv Ment Dis* 181: 657–62.

Huber, S.J., Friedenberg, D.L., Paulson, G.W., Shuttelworth, E.C. and Christy, J.A. (1990). The pattern of depressive symptoms varies with progression of Parkinson's disease. *J Neurol Neurosurg Psychiatry* 53: 275–8.

Hunter, R. and MacAlpine, I. (1963). *Three Hundred Years of Psychiatry*. Oxford: Oxford University Press.

Huntington, G. (1872). On chorea. *Med Surg Rep* 26: 217–231.

Husain, M.M., McDonald, W.M., Doraiswamy, P.M. et al. (1991). A magnetic resonance imaging study of putamen nuclei in major depression. *Psychiatry Res* 40: 95–9.

Husby, G., van de Rijn, I., Zabriskie, J., Abdin, Z. and Williams, R. (1976). Antibodies reacting with cytoplasm of subthalamic and caudate nuclei neurons in chorea and rheumatic fever. *J Exp Med* 114: 1094–110.

Hyde, T., Stacey, M., Coppola, R. et al. (1995). Cerebral morphometric abnormalities in Tourette's syndrome: a quantitative MRI study of monozygotic twins. *Neurology*, 45: 1176–82.

Hynd, G.W., Hern, K.L., Novey, E.S. et al. (1993). Attention deficit-hyperactivity disorder and asymmetry of the caudate nucleus. *J Child Neurol* 8: 339–47.

Inbody, S. and Jankovic, J. (1986). Hyperkinetic mutism: bilateral ballism and basal ganglia calcification. *Neurology* 36: 825–7.

Inose, T. (1968). Neuropsychiatric manifestations in Wilson's disease: attacks of disturbance of consciousness. *Birth Defects* 4: 74–6.

Izard, C.E. (1977). *Human Emotions.* New York: Plenum Press.

Jacobs, D.H., Shuren, J., Bowers, D. and Heilman, K.M. (1995a). Emotional facial imagery, perception, and expression in Parkinson's disease. *Neurology* 45: 1696–702.

Jacobs, D.H., Shuren, J. and Heilman, K.M. (1995b). Impaired perception of facial identity and facial affect in Huntington's disease. *Neurology* 45: 1217–18.

Jahanshahi, M. and Marsden, C.D. (1988). Personality in torticollis: a controlled study. *Psychol Med* 18: 375–87.

Jan, J.E., Freeman, R.D. and Good, W.V. (1995). Familial paroxysmal kinesigenic choreo-athetosis in a child with visual hallucinations and obsessive–compulsive behavior. *Dev Med Child Neurol* 37: 366–9.

Janati, A. and Appel, A.R. (1984). Psychiatric aspects of progressive supranuclear palsy. *J Nerv Ment Dis* 172: 85–9.

Jankovic, J. and Ford, J. (1983). Blepharospasm and orofacial–cervical dystonia: clinical and pharmacological findings in 100 patients. *Ann Neurol* 13: 402–11.

Jason, G.W., Pajurkowa, D.M., Sucherowsky, O. et al. (1988). Presymptomatic neuropsychological impairment in Huntington's disease. *Arch Neurol* 45: 769–73.

Jenike, M.A. (1992). Pharmacologic treatment of obsessive–compulsive disorders. *Psychiatry Clin N Am* 15: 895–920.

Jenike, M.A. and Brandon, A.D. (1988). Obsessive–compulsive disorder and head trauma: a rare association. *J Anxiety Disord* 2: 353–9.

Jernigan, T.L., Zisook, S., Heaton, R.K. et al. (1991). Magnetic resonance imaging abnormalities in lenticular nuclei and cerebral cortex in schizophrenia. *Arch Gen Psychiatry* 48: 881–90.

Jorge, R.E., Robinson, R.G., Arndt, S.V. et al. (1993a). Comparison between acute- and delayed-onset depression following traumatic brain injury. *J Neuropsychiatry Clin Neurosci* 5: 43–9.

Jorge, R.E., Robinson, R.G., Starkstein, S.E. et al. (1993b). Secondary mania following traumatic brain injury. *Am J Psychiatry* 150: 916–21.

Kahlbaum, K.L. (1973). *Catatonia.* Translated by Y. Levi and T. Priden Baltimore: Johns Hopkins University Press.

Kane, F.J. and Taylor, T.W. (1963). Mania associated with the use of INH and cocaine. *Am J Psychiatry* 119: 1098–9.

Katsikis, M. and Pilowsky, I. (1991). A controlled study of facial expression in Parkinson's disease and depression. *J Nerv Ment Dis* 179: 683–8.

Kaul, A. and McMahon, D. (1993). Wilson's disease and offending behavior – a case report. *Med Sci Law* 33: 353–8.

Kellner, C.H., Jolley, R.R., Holgate, R.C. et al. (1991). Brain MRI in obsessive–compulsive disorder. *Psychiatry Res* 36: 45–9.

Kelsoe, J.R., Cadet, J.L., Pickar, D. and Weiberger, D.R. (1988). Quantitative neuronatomy in schizophrenia: a controlled magnetic resonance imaging study. *Arch Gen Psychiatry* 45: 533–41.

Kerbeshian,J., Burd, L. and Klug, M.G. (1995). Comorbid Tourette's disorder and bipolar disorder: an etiologic perspective. *Am J Psychiatry* 152: 1646–51.

Khanna, S., Narayanan, H.S., Sharma, S.D. et al. (1985). Posttraumatic obsessive–compulsive disorder: a single case report. *Ind J Psychiatry* 27: 337–40.

Kienzle, G.D., Breger, R.K., Chun, R.W.M. et al. (1991). Sydenham's chorea: MR manifestations in two cases. *Am J Neuroradiol* 12: 73–6.

Kimura, D., Barnett, H.J.M. and Burkhart, G. (1981). The psychological test pattern in progressive supranuclear palsy. *Neuropsychologia* 19: 301–6.

Kimura, M. and Graybiel, A. (1995). Role of basal ganglia in sensorimotor association learning. In *Functions of the Cortico–Basal Ganglia Loop*, ed. M. Kimura and A.M. Graybiel, pp. 2–17. New York: Springer Verlag.

King, M. (1985). Alcohol abuse in Huntington's disease. *Psychol Med* 15: 815–19.

Kirby, G.H. and Davis, T.K. (1921). Psychiatric aspects of epidemic encephalitis. *Arch Neurol Psychiatry* 5: 491–551.

Kish, S.J., Chang, L.J., Mirchandai, I., Shannah, K. and Hornyckiewicks, O. (1985). Progressive supranuclear palsy: relationship between extrapyramidal disturbances, dementia and brain neurotransmitter markers. *Ann Neurol* 18: 530–6.

Kleist, K. (1922). Die psychomotrischen Störungen und ihr Verhäaltnis zu den Motilitätsstörungen bei Erkranken der Stammgangline. *Monatsschr Neurol Psychiatr* 52: 253–302.

Konig, P. (1989). Psychopathological alterations in cases of symmetrical basal ganglia sclerosis. *Biol Psychiatry* 25: 459–68.

Kosaka, K., Ikeda, K. and Kobayashi, K. et al. (1991). Striatopallidonigral degeneration in Pick's disease: a clincio-pathological study of 41 cases. *J Neurol* 238: 151–60.

Kotrla, K.J., Ardaman, M.F., Meyers, C.A., Novac, S. and Hayman, L.A. (1994). Unsuspected obsessive–compulsive disorder in a patient with bilateral striatopallidodentate mineralization. *Neuropsychiatry Neuropsychol Behav Neurol* 2: 130–5.

Kraft, I.A. (1966). A psychiatric study of two patients with dystonia musculorum deformans. *South Med J* 59: 284–8.

Krishnan, K.R., McDonald, W.M., Escalona, P.R. et al. (1992). Magnetic resonance imaging of the caudate nucleus in depression: preliminary observations. *Arch Gen Psychiatry* 49: 553–7.

Kulisevsky, J., Berthier, M.L. and Avila, A. (1995). Bipolar disorder and unilateral parkinsonism following a brainstem infarction. *Mov Disord* 10: 799–802.

Kumar, R., Krack, P., McViecker, A.M. and Benabid, A.L. (1999). Laughter induced by subthalamic brain stimulation in advanced Parkinson's disease. *Parkinsonism Relat Disord* 5: S107.

Kurlan, R. (1998). Tourette's syndrome and 'PANDAS'. Will the relation bear out? *Neurology* 50: 1530–4.

Kuwert, T., Lange, H.W., Langen, K.J. et al. (1989). Cerebral glucose consumption measured by

PET in patients with and without psychiatric symptoms of Huntington's disease. *Psychiatry Res* 29: 361–2.

Kuypers, H.G.J.M. (1982). A new look at the organization of the motor system. *Prog Brain Res* 57: 381–403.

Laplane, D. (1989). Transient feelings of compulsion caused by hemispheric lesions in three cases. *J Neurol Neurosurg Psychiatry* 52: 423.

Laplane, D. (1990). La perte d'auto-activation psychique. *Rev. Neurol* 146: 397–404.

Laplane, D. (1994). Obsessions et compulsions par lésions des noyaux gris centraux. *Rev Neurol* 150: 594–8.

Laplane, D., Attal, N., Sauron, B., de Billy, A. and Dubois, B. (1992). Lesions of basal ganglia due to disulfiram neurotoxicity. *J Neurol Neurosurg Psychiatry* 55: 925–9.

Laplane, D., Baulac, M., Pillon, B. and Panayotopoulos-Archimatsos, I. (1982). Perte de l'activation psychique. Activité compulsive d'allure obsessionnelle. Lésion lenticulaire bilatérale. *Rev Neurol* 138: 137–41.

Laplane, D., Baulac, M., Widlocher, D. and Dubois, B. (1984). Pure psychic akinesia with bilateral lesions of basal ganglia. *J Neurol Neurosurg Psychiatry* 47: 377–85.

Laplane, D., Bouillat, J., Baron, J.L., Pillon, B. and Beaulac, M. (1988a). Comportement compulsif d'allure obsessionnelle par lésion bilatérale des noyaux lenticulaires. Un nouveau cas. *Encéphale* 14: 27–32.

Laplane, D., Dubois, B., Pillon, B. and Baulac, M. (1988b). Perte d'activation psychique avec trouble obsessif–compulsif. *Rev Neurol* 144: 564–70.

Laplane, D., Levasseur, M., Pillon, B. et al. (1989). Obsessive–compulsive and other behavioral changes with bilateral basal ganglia lesions: a neuropsychological, magnetic resonance imaging and positron emission tomographic study. *Brain* 112: 699–725.

Laplane, D., Widlocher, D., Pillon, B., Baulac, M. and Binoux, F. (1981). Comportement compulsif d'allure obsessionnelle par nécrose circonscrite bilaterale pallido-striatale: encephalopathie par piqûre de guêpe. *Rev Neurol* 137: 269–76.

Larmande, P., Palisson, E., Saikali, I. et al. (1993). Disparition de l'akinésie dans une maladie de Parkinson au cours d'un accès maniaque. *Rev Neurol* 149: 557–8.

Lauterbach, E.C. (1996). Bipolar disorders, dystonia and compulsion after dysfunction of the cerebellum, dentatorubrothalamic tract, and substantia nigra. *Biol Psychiatry* 15: 726–30.

Lauterbach, E.C., Freeman, A., Spears, T.E. et al. (1991). Increased prevalence of affective disorders in dystonia does not correlate with motor disability. *Neurology* 41 Suppl. 1: 923.

Lauterbach, E.C., Price, S.T., Wilson, A.N., Kavali, C.M. and Jackson, J.G. (1994a). Post-stroke bipolar disorders: age and thalamus. *Biol Psychiatry* 35: 681.

Lauterbach, E.C., Spears, T.E., Prewett, M.J. et al. (1994b). Neuropsychiatric disorders, myoclonus, and dystonia in calcification of the basal ganglia. *Biol Psychiatry* 35: 345–57.

Lauterbach, E.C., Spears, T.E. and Price, S.T. (1992). Bipolar disorder in idiopathic dystonia: clinical features and possible neurobiology. *J Neuropsychiatry Clin Neurosci* 4: 435–9.

Lebrun, Y., Dereux, F. and Rousseau, J.J. (1986). Language and speech in a patient with a clinical diagnosis of progressive supranuclear palsy. *Brain Lang* 27: 247–56.

Leckman, J.F., Walker, D.E. and Cohen, D.J. (1993). Premonitory urges in Tourette's syndrome. *Am J Psychiatry* 150: 98–102.

Leckman, J.F., Walker, D.E., Goodman, W.K., Pauls, D.L. and Cohen, D.J. (1994). 'Just right' perceptions associated with compulsive behavior in Tourette's syndrome. *Am J Psychiatry* 151: 675–80.

LeDoux, J.D. (1993). Emotional memory systems in the brain. *Behav Brain Res* 58: 69–70.

Lehembe, P. and Graux, P. (1992). Athymormie, arithomanie ou compulsion stercorale et lacunes multiples des corps striés. *Ann Med Psychol* 150: 699–701.

Leonard, H.L., Lenane, M.C., Swedo, S.E., Rettew, D.C. and Rapoport, J.L. (1991). A double-blind comparison of clomipramine and desipramine treatment of severe onychophagia (nail biting). *Arch Gen Psychiatry* 48: 821–7.

Lesch,M. and Nyhan, W.L. (1964). A familial disorder of uric acid metabolism and central nervous system function. *Am J Med* 36: 561–70.

Lesieur, H., Blume, S. and Zoppa, R. (1986). Alcoholism, drug abuse and gambling. *Alcoholism* 10: 33–8.

Levin, B.E. and Katzen, H.L. (1995). Early cognitive changes and nondementing behavioral abnormalities in Parkinson's disease. In *Behavioral Neurology of Movement Disorders. Advances in Neurology*, Vol. 65, ed. W.J. Weiner and A.E. Lang, pp. 85–95. New York: Raven Press.

Levin, H.S., Madison, C.F., Bailey, C.B. et al. (1983). Mutism after closed head injury. *Arch Neurol* 40: 601–6.

Lhermitte, F. (1986). Human autonomy and the frontal lobes. Part II. Patient behavior in complex and social situations: the 'environmental dependency syndrome'. *Ann Neurol* 19: 335–43.

Lhermitte, J. and Muncie, W.S. (1930). Hepatolenticular degeneration: a report of three unusual cases. *Arch Neurol. Psychiatry* 23: 750–60.

Lilly, R., Cummings, J.L., Benson, D.F. et al. (1983). The human Klüver–Bucy syndrome. *Neurology* 33: 1141–5.

Lipsey, J.R., Robinson, R.G., Pearlson, G.D., Rao, K. and Price, T.R. (1983). Mood change following bilateral hemisphere brain injury. *Br J Psychiatry* 143: 266–91.

Lisak, A. (1938). Ein Fall von Wilson Pseudosklerose mit katatonem Symptomkomplex. *Schweiz Med Wschr* 19: 161–3.

Lishman, W.A. (1968). Brain damage in relation to psychiatric disability after head injury. *Br J Psychiatry* 114: 373–410.

Litvan, I., Grafman, J., Gomez, C. and Chase, T.N. (1989). Memory impairment in patients with progressive supranuclear palsy. *Arch Neurol* 46: 265–7.

Litvan, I., Mega, M.S., Cummings, J.I. and Fairbanks, L. (1996). Neuropsychiatric aspects of progressive supranuclear palsy. *Neurology* 47: 1184–9.

Livingston, K.E. (1977). Limbic system dysfunction induced by 'kindling': its significance for psychiatry. In *Nurosurgical Treatment in Psychiatry, Pain and Epilepsy*, ed. W.H. Sweet, S. Obrador and J.G. Martin-Rodriguez, pp. 63–75. Baltimore: University Park Press.

Lopez, O.L., Berthier, M.L., Backer, J.T. and Boller, F. (1997). Creutzfeldt–Jakob disease with features of obsessive–compulsive disorder and anorexia nervosa: the role of cortical–subcortical systems. *Neuropsychiatry Neuropsychol Behav Neurol* 10: 120–4.

Lou, H.C., Henricksen, L., Bruhn, P., Borner, H. and Nielsen, J.B. (1989). Striatal dysfunction in attention deficit and hyperkinetic disorder. *Arch Neurol* 46: 48–52.

Luria, A.R. (1978). *Les Fonctions Corticales Supérieures de l'Homme.* Paris: Presses Universitaires de France.

Luxenberg, J.S., Swedo, S.E., Flament, M.F. et al. (1988). Neuroanatomical abnormalities in obsessive–compulsive disorder detected with quantitative X-ray computed tomography. *Am J Psychiatry* 145: 1089–93.

Machlin, S.R., Harris, G.J., Pearlson, G.D. et al. (1991). Elevated medial-frontal cerebral blood flow in obsessive–compulsive patients: a SPECT study. *Am J Psychiatry* 148: 1240–2.

Macucci, M., Sitia, D., Mascalchi, M. et al. (1991). Athymormic syndrome: lacune bilaterali del neostriato. Studio clinico-radiologico di due casi. *Rev Neurol* 61: 47–50.

Maher, E.R., Smith, E.M. and Lees, A.J. (1985). Cognitive deficits in the Steele–Richardson–Olszewski syndrome (progressive supranuclear palsy). *J Neurol Neurosurg Psychiatry* 48: 1234–9.

Maraganore, D.M. and Marsden, C.D. (1990). Complex stereotypies following right caudate infarct: a case report. *J Neurol* 89 Suppl. 1: 237.

Marin, R.S. (1991). Apathy: a neuropsychiatric syndrome. *J Neuropsychiatry Clin Neurosci* 3: 243–54.

Martinez-Vila, E., Artieda, J. and Obeso, J. (1988). Micrographia secondary to lenticular hematoma. *J Neurol Neurosurg Psychiatry* 51: 1353.

Martinot, J.L., Allilaire, J.F., Mazoyer, B. et al. (1990). Obsessive–compulsive disorder: a clinical, neuropsychological, and positron emission tomography study. *Acta Psychiatr Scand* 82: 233–42.

Martuza, R.L., Chiocca, E.A., Jenike, M.A. et al. (1990). Stereotactic radiofrequency thermal cingulotomy for obsessive–compulsive disorder. *J Neuropsychiatry Clin Neurosci* 2: 331–6.

Mataro, M., Garcia Sanchez, C., Junque, C., Estevez-Gonzalez, A. and Pujol, J. (1997). Magnetic resonance imaging measurement of the caudate nucleus in adolescents with attention-deficit hyperactivity disorder and its relationship with neuropsychological and behavioral measures. *Arch Neurol* 54: 963–8.

Matthews, W.S. (1988). Attention deficits and learning disabilities in children with Tourette's syndrome. *Pediatr Ann* 17: 410–17.

Mayberg, H.S. (1994). Frontal lobe dysfunction in secondary depression. *J Neuropsychiatry Clin Neurosci* 6: 428–42.

Mayberg, H.S., Lewis, P.J., Regenold, W. and Wagner, H.N. (1994). Paralimbic hypoperfusion in unipolar depression. *J Nucl Med* 35: 929–34.

Mayberg, H.S., Starkstein, S.E., Peyser, C.E. et al. (1992). Paralimbic frontal lobe hypometabolism in depression associated with Huntington's disease. *Neurology* 42: 1791–7.

Mayberg, H.S., Starkstein, S.E., Sadzot, B. et al. (1990). Selective hypometabolism in the inferior frontal lobe in depressed patients with Parkinson's disease. *Ann Neurol* 28: 57–64.

Mayeux, R. (1990). Depression in the patient with Parkinson's disease. *J Clin Psychiatr* 51 Suppl.: 20–3.

Mayeux, R., Denaro, J., Hemenegildo, N. et al. (1992). A population-based investigation of Parkinson's disease with and without dementia. *Arch Neurol* 49: 492–7.

Mayeux, R., Stern, Y., Sano, M. et al. (1987). Clinical and biochemical correlates of bradyphrenia in Parkinson's disease. *Neurology* 37: 1130–4.

McGilchrist, I., Goldstein, L.H., Jadresic, D. and Fenwick, P. (1993). Thalamo-frontal psychosis. *Br J Psychiatry* 163: 113–15.

McGuire, P.K., Bench, C.D., Frith, C.D. et al. (1994). Functional anatomy of obsessive–compulsive phenomena. *Br J Psychiatry* 164: 459–68.

McKeon, J., McGuffin, P. and Robinson, P. (1984). Obsessive–compulsive neurosis following head injury: a report of four cases. *Br J Psychiatry* 144: 190–2.

Meggendorfer, F. (1923). Die psychischen Störungen bei der Huntingtonsche Chorea. Klinische und genealogische Untersuchngen. *Zeitschr, Neurol Psychiatrie* 87: 1–49.

Mehler, M.F. (1987). A novel disorder of linguistic expression following left caudate nucleus infarction. *Neurology* 37 Suppl. 1: 167.

Mena, I., Marin, O., Fuenzalida, S. and Cotzias, G.C. (1967). Chronic manganese poisoning. *Neurology* 17: 128–36.

Mendez, M.F., Adams, N.L. and Lewandowski, K.S. (1989). Neurobehavioral changes associated with caudate lesions. *Neurology* 39: 399–454.

Menza, M.A., Cocchiola, J. and Golbe, L. (1995). Psychiatric symptoms in progressive supranuclear palsy. *Psychosomatics* 36: 550–4.

Milhaud, D., Magnie, M.N., Roger, P.M. and Bedoucha, P. (1994). Infactus du noyau caudé ou infarctus striato-capsulaires antérierus? *Rev Neurol* 150: 286–91.

Minichiello, W.E., O'Sullivan, R.L., Osgood-Hynes, D. and Baer, L. (1994). Trichotillomania: clinical aspects and treatment strategies. *Harvard Rev Psychiatry* 1: 336–44.

Minski, L. (1933). Mental symptoms associated with 58 cases of cerebral tumors. *J Neurol Psychopathol* 13: 330–43.

Modell, J.G., Montz, M., Curtis, G.C. and Greden, J.F. (1989). Neurophysiologic dysfunction in basal ganglia/limbic striatal and thalamocortical circuits as a pathogenic mechanism of obsessive–compulsive disorders. *J Neuropsychiatry* 1: 27–36.

Modell, J.G., Mountz, J.M. and Beresford, T.P. (1990). Basal ganglia/limbic striatal and thalamocortical involvement in craving and loss of control in alcoholism. *J Neuropsychiatry Clin Neurosci* 2: 123–44.

Mohr, E., Juncos, J., Cox, C. et al. (1991). Selective deficits in cognition and memory in high functioning Parkinson's patients. *J Neurol Neurosurg Psychiatry* 54: 25–9.

Molina, V., Montz, R., Jimenez-Vicioso, A. and Carreras, J.L. (1995). Drug therapy and cerebral perfusion in obsessive–compulsive disorder. *J Nucl Med* 36: 2234–8.

Montgomery, M.A., Clayton, P.J. and Friedhoff, A.J. (1982). Psychiatric illness in Tourette syndrome patients and first degree relatives. In *Gilles de la Tourette syndrome*, ed. A.J. Friedhoff and T.N. Chase, pp. 335–59. New York: Raven Press.

Moran, E. (1970). Gambling as a form of dependence. *Br J Addiction* 64: 419–28.

Moreno, I., Saiz-Ruiz, J. and Lopez-Ibor, J.J. (1991). Serotonin and gambling dependence. *Hum Psychopharmacol* 6: S9–12.

Morgenson, G.J. (1987). Limbic–motor integration. *Prog Psychobiol Physiol Psychol* 12: 117–70.

Mori, E. and Yamadori, A. (1987). Acute confusional state and acute agitated delirium. *Arch Neurol* 44: 139–43.

Morris, R.G., Downes, J.J., Shahakian, B.J. et al. (1988). Planning and spatial working memory in Parkinson's disease. *J Neurol Neurosurg Psychiatry* 51: 757–66.

Mrabet, A., Mrad-Ben Hammouda, I., Abroug, Z., Smiri, W. and Haddad, A. (1994). Infarctus bilateral des noyaux caudés. *Rev Neurol* 150: 67–9.

Naef, M.E. (1917). Ueber Psychosen by Chorea. *Monatsschr Psychiatrie Neurol* 41: 65–88.

Nardocci, N., Rumi, V., Combi, M.L. et al. (1994). Complex tics, stereotypies, and compulsive behavior as clinical presentation of a juvenile progressive dystonia suggestive of Hallervorden–Spatz disease. *Mov Disord* 9: 369–71.

Nauta, W.H.J. (1986). A simplified perspective on the basal ganglia and their relation to the limbic system. Circuitous connections linking cerebral cortex, limbic system and corpus striatum. In *The Limbic System: Functional Organization and Clinical Disorders,* ed. B.K. Doane and K.E. Livingstone, pp. 43–54, 67–77. New York: Raven Press.

Naville, F. (1922). Etudes aur les complications et les séquelles mentales de l'encéphalite épidémique. La bradyphrénie. *Encéphale* 17: 369–75.

Nissenbaum, H., Quinn, N.P., Brown, R.G. et al. (1987). Mood swings associated with the 'on–off' phenomenon in Parkinson's disease. *Psychol Med* 17: 899–904.

Nordahl, T.E., Benkelfat, C., Sample, W.E. et al. (1989). Cerebral glucose metabolic rates in obsessive compulsive disorder. *Neuropsychopharmacology* 2: 23–8.

Northan, R.S. and Singer, H.S. (1991). Postencephalitic acquired Tourette-like syndrome in a child. *Neurology* 41: 592–3.

Nyhan, W.L. (1976). Behavior in the Lesch–Nyhan syndrome. *J Autism Schizophrenia* 6: 235–52.

Oder, W., Grimm, G., Kolleger, H. et al. (1991). Neurological and neuropsychiatric spectrum of Wilson's disease: a prospective study of 45 cases. *J Neurol* 238: 281–7.

O'Sullivan, R.L., Rauch, S.L., Breiter, H.C. et al. (1997). Reduced basal ganglia volumes in trichotillomania measured via morphometric magnetic resonance imaging. *Biol Psychiatry* 42: 39–45.

Owen, A.M., James, M., Leigh, P.N. et al. (1992). Fronto-striatal cognitive deficits at different stages of Parkinson's disease. *Brain* 115: 1727–51.

Pakkenberg, B. (1990). Pronounced reduction of total neuron number in mediodorsal thalamic nucleus and nucleus accumbens in schizophrenics. *Arch Gen Psychiatry* 47: 1023–8.

Pandey, R.S., Swamy, H.S., Sreenivas, K.N. and John, C.J. (1981). Depression in Wilson's disease. *Ind J Psychiatry* 23: 82–5.

Pardal, M.M.F., Micheli, F., Asonape, J. and Paradiso, G. (1985). Neurobehavioral symptoms in caudate hemorrhage: two cases. *Neurology* 35: 1806–7.

Parent, A. and Hazrati, L.N. (1995a). Functional anatomy of the basal ganglia. I. The cortico–basal ganglia–thalamocortical loop. *Brain Res Rev* 20: 91–127.

Parent, A. and Hazrati, L.N. (1995b). Functional anatomy of the basal ganglia. II. The place of the subthalamic nucleus and external pallidum in basal ganglia circuitry. *Brain Res Rev* 20: 128–54.

Park, K.S., Budman, C.L., Bruun, R.D. et al. (1996). Rage attacks in children and adolescents with Tourette's disorder. *Sci Proc Am Acad Child Adolesc Psychiatry* 12: 110–20.

Parkinson, J. (1938). An essay on the shaking palsy, 1817. *Med Classics* 2: 964–97.

Peatfield, R.C. (1987). Basal ganglia damage and subcortical dementia after possible insidious Coxsackie virus encephalitis. *Acta Neurol Scand* 76: 340–5.

Pedrazzi, P., Bogousslavsky, J. and Regli, F. (1990). Hématomes limités à al atête du noyau caudé. *Rev Neurol* 146: 726–38.

Penisson-Besnier, I., Le Gall, D. and Dubas, F. (1993). Comportement compulsif d'allure obsessionnelle (arithmomanie). Atrophie des noyaux caudés. *Rev Neurol* 148: 262–7.

Perani, D., Colombo, C., Bressi, A. et al. (1995). 18F FDG PET in obsessive–compulsive disorder: a clinical metabolic correlation study after treatment. *Br J Psychiatry* 166: 244–50.

Peterson, B.S., Gore, J.C., Riddle, M.A., Cohen, D.J. and Leckman, J.F. (1994). Abnormal magnetic resonance imaging T2 relaxation time asymmetries in Tourette's syndrome. *Psychiatry Res Neuroimaging* 55: 205–21.

Peterson, B.S., Riddle, M.A., Cohen, D.J. et al. (1993). Reduced basal ganglia volumes in Tourette's syndrome using three-dimensional reconstruction techniques from magnetic resonance images. *Neurology* 43: 941–9.

Petrine, K., Dogali, M., Fazzini, E. et al. (1998). Cognitive functioning after pallidotomy for refractory Parkinson's disease. *J Neurol Neurosurg Psychiatry* 65: 150–4.

Phillips, A.G. and Carr, G.D. (1987). Cognition and the basal ganglia: a possible substrate for procedural knowledge. *Can J Neurol Sci* 14: 381–5.

Pillon, B., Deweer, B., Agid, Y. and Dubois, B. (1993). Explicit memory in Alzheimer's, Huntington's and Parkinson's disease. *Arch Neurol* 50: 374–9.

Pillon, B., Deweer, B., Michon, A. et al. (1994). Are explicit memory disorders of progressive supranuclear palsy related to striato-frontal circuits? Comparisons with Alzheimer's, Parkinson's and Huntington's disease. *Neurology* 44: 1264–70.

Pillon, B., Dubois, B. and Agid, Y. (1991). Severity and specificity of cognitive impairment in Alzheimer's Huntington's, and Parkinson's disease and progressive supranuclear palsy. *Ann NY Acad Sci* 640: 224–7; *Neurology* 41: 634–43.

Pillon, B., Dubois, B., Lhermitte, F. and Agid, Y. ((1986). Heterogeneity of cognitive impairment in progressive supranuclear palsy, Parkinson's disease and Alzheimer's disease. *Neurology* 36: 1179–85.

Pillon, B., Govider-Khouja, N., Deveer, B. et al. (1995). Neuropsychological pattern of striato-nigral degeneration. Comparison with Parkinson's disease and progressive supranuclear palsy. *J. Neurol Neurosurg Psychiatry* 58: 174–9.

Pitcairn, T., Clemie, S., Gray, J. and Pentland, B. (1990). Non-verbal cues in the self-presentation of Parkinsonian patients. *Br J Clin Psychol* 29: 177–84.

Podoll, K., Caspary, P., Lange, H.W. and Noth, J. (1988). Language functions of Huntington's disease. *Brain* 111: 1475–503.

Pozzili, C., Passafiume, D., Bastianello, S., d'Antona, R. and Lenzi, G.L. (1987). Remote effects of caudate hemorrhage: a clinical and functional study. *Cortex* 23: 341–9.

Pulst, S.M., Walshe, T.M. and Romero, J.A. (1983). Carbon monoxide poisoning with features of Gilles de la Tourette's syndrome. *Arch Neurol* 40: 443–44.

Quinn, N. (1994). Multiple system atrophy. In *Movement Disorders 3*, ed. C.D. Mardsen and S. Fahn, pp. 262–81. London: Butterworth Heineman.

Rachman, S. (1974). Primary obsessional slowness. *Behav Res Ther* 12: 9–18.

Rafal, R.D., Posner, M.I., Walker, J.A. and Friedrich, F.J. (1984). Cognition and the basal ganglia: separating mental and motor components of performance in Parkinson's disease. *Brain* 107: 1083–94.

Rapoport, J.L. (1990). Obsessive–compulsive disorder and basal ganglia dysfunction. *Psychol Med* 20: 465–9.

Rasmussen, S.A. and Eisen, J.L. (1992). The epidemiology and clinical features of obsessive–compulsive disorder. *Psychiatr Clin N Am* 12: 743–58.

Rathun, J.K. (1996). Neuropsychological aspects of Wilson's disease. *Int J Neurosci* 85: 221–9.

Resnick, S.M., Gur, R.E., Alavi, A., Gur, R.C. and Reivich, M. (1988). Positron emission tomography and subcortical glucose metabolism in schizophrenia. *Psychiatr Res* 24: 1–11.

Reyes, M.G. and Gibbons, S.G. (1985). Dementia of the Alzheimer type and Huntington's disease. *Neurology* 35: 273–7.

Rich, S.S., and Ovsiew, F. (1994). Leuprolide acetate for exhibitionism in Huntington's disease. *Mov Disord* 9: 353–7.

Richards, M., Cote, L.J. and Stern, Y. (1993). The relationship between visuospatial ability and perceptual motor function in Parkinson's disease. *J Neurol Neurosurg Psychiatry* 56: 400–6.

Richardson, E.P. (1982). Neuropathological studies of Tourette's syndrome. In *Gilles de la Tourette's syndrome*, ed. A.J. Friedhoff and T.N. Chase, pp. 210–15. New York: Raven Press.

Richfield, E.D., Twyman, R. and Berent, S. (1987). Neurological syndrome following bilateral damage of the head of the caudate nuclei. *Ann Neurol* 22: 768–71.

Rinn, W. (1984). The neuropsychology of facial expression: a review of the neurological and psychological mechanisms for producing facial expressions. *Psychol Bull* 95: 52–77.

Riordan, H.J., Fleishman, L., Carool, K. and Roberts, D. (1997). Neurocognitive and psychological correlates of ventroposterolateral pallidotomy surgery in Parkinson's disease. *Neurosurg Focus* 2: 1–9.

Robbins, T.W., James, M., Lange, K.W. et al. (1992). Cognitive performances in multiple system atrophy. *Brain* 115: 275–91.

Robbins, T.W., Janes, M., Owen, A.M. et al. (1994). Cognitive deficits in progressive supranuclear palsy, Parkinson's disease and multiple system atrophy in tests sensitive to forntal lobe dysfunction. *J Neurol Neurosurg Psychiatry* 57: 79–88.

Robinson, R.G., Boston, J.D., Starkstein, S.E. and Price, T.R. (1988). Comparison of mania and depression after brain injury: causal factors. *Am J Psychiatry* 145: 172–8.

Robinson, R.G., Kubos, K.L., Starr, L.B., Rao, K. and Price, T.R. (1984). Mood disorders in stroke patients. Importance of location of lesion. *Brain* 107: 81–93.

Robinson, R.G. and Starkstein, S.E. (1990). Current research in affective disorders following stroke. *J Neuropsychiatry Res* 2: 1–14.

Robinson, R.G., Starr, L.B., Kubos, K.L. et al. (1983). A two-year longitudinal study of post-stroke mood disorders: findings during initial evaluation. *Stroke* 14: 736–41.

Robinson, D., Wu, H., Munne, R.A. et al. (1995). Reduced caudate nucleus volume in obsessive–compulsive disorder. *Arch Gen Psychiatry* 52: 393–8.

Rogers, D. (1985). The motor disorders of severe psychiatric illness: a conflict of paradigms. *Br J Psychiatry* 147: 221–32.

Rogers, D., Less, A.J., Smith, E., Trinkle, M. and Stern, G.M. (1987). Bradyphrenia in Parkinson's disease and psychomotor illness. *Brain* 145: 172–8.

Rosenthal, R. and Bigelow, L.B. (1972). Quantitative brain measurement in chronic schizophrenia. *Br J Psychiatry* 121: 259–64.

Ross, E.D., Homan, R. and Buck, R. (1994). Differential hemispheric lateralization of primary and social emotions. *Neuropsychiatry Neuropsychol Behav Neurol* 7: 1–19.

Ross, E.D. and Mesulam, M.M. (1979). Dominant language functions of the right hemisphere? Prosody and emotional gesturing. *Arch Neurol* 36: 144–8.

Ross, E.D. and Stewart, R.M. (1981). Akinetic mutism from hypothalamic damage: successful treatment with dopamine agonists. *Neurology* 31: 1435–9.

Rosser, A. and Hodges, J.R. (1994). Initial letter and semantic category fluency in Alzheimer's disease, Huntington's disease and progressive supranuclear palsy. *J Neurol Neurosurg Psychiatry* 57: 1389–94.

Rosvold, H.E. (1972). The frontal lobe system: cortical–subcortical interrelationships. *Acta Neurobiol Exp* 32: 439–60.

Rubin, R.T., Villanueva-Meyer, J., Ananth, J., Trajmar, P.G. and Mena, I. (1992). Regional xenon 133 cerebral blood flow and cerebral technetium 99m HMPAO uptake in unmedicated patients with obsessive–compulsive disorder and matched normal control subjects. Determination by high resolution single-photon emission computed tomography. *Arch Gen Psychiatry* 49: 695–702.

Sadler, J.Z., Kurtz, N.M. and Rush, A.J. (1984). Progressive supranuclear palsy presenting as pseudodementia. *Psychosomatics* 25: 713–714.

Sagar, H.J., Cohen, N.J., Sullivan, E.V., Corkin, S. and Growdon, J.H. (1988a). Remote memory function in Alzheimer's and Parkinson's disease. *Brain* 111: 185–206.

Sagar, H.J., Sullivan, E.V., Gabrielli, J.D.E., Corkin, S. and Growdon, J.H. (1988b). Temporal ordering and shift item memory in Parkinson's disease. *Brain* 111: 525–39.

Saint-Cyr, J.A., Taylor, A.E. and Lang, A.E. (1988). Procedural learning and neostriatal function in man. *Brain* 111: 941–59.

Saint-Cyr, J.A., Taylor, A.E. and Nicholson, K. (1995). Behavior and the basal ganglia. *Adv Neurol* 65: 1–28.

Sandson, J. and Albert, M.L. (1984). Varieties of perseveration. *Neuropsychologia* 22: 715–32.

Sandson, J. and Albert, M.L. (1987). Perseveration and behavioral neurology. *Neurology* 37: 1736–41.

Scarone, S., Colombo, C., Livian, S. et al. (1992). Increased right caudate nucleus size in obsessive–compulsive disorder: detection with magnetic resonance imaging. *Psychiatry Res* 45: 115–21.

Schalling, D., Asberg, M., Edman, G. et al. (1984). Impulsivity, nonconformity, and sensation seeking as related to biological markers for vulnerability. *Clin Neuropharmacol* 7 Suppl. 1: 746–7.

Schiffer, R.D., Durlan, R. and Rubin, A. (1988). Evidence for atypical depression in Parkinson's disease. *Am J Psychiatry* 145: 1020–2.

Schilder, P. (1928). Zur Kenntnis der Psychosen bei chronischen Encephalitis epidemica, nebst Bemerkungen uber die Beziehung organischer Strukturen zu der psychischen Vorgängen. *Z Neurol Psychiatrie* 118: 327–45.

Schilder, P. (1938). The organic background of obsessions and compulsions. *Am J Psychiatry* 94: 1397–416.

Schilder, P. and Dimitz, R. (1921). Ueber psychische Störungen bei Encephalitis epidemica. *Z Neurol Psychiatrie*, 68: 299.

Schmidt, M. (1925). Zur Feststellung der postencephalitischen Bradyphrenie. *Schweiz Med Wschr* 8: 72.

Schneider, J.S. (1984). Basal ganglia rôle in behavior: importance of sensory gating and its relevance to psychiatry. *Biol Psychiatry* 19: 1693–710.

Schneider, J.S. and Chui, H.L. (1986). Progressive supranuclear palsy manifesting with depressive features. *J Am Geriatr Soc* 34: 663–5.

Schuler, P., Oyanguren, H., Maturana, V. et al. (1957). Manganese poisoning. *Industrial Med Surg* 26: 167–73.

Scott, D.F. (1978). The problems of malicious fire raising. *Br J Hosp Med* 19: 259–63.

Scott, D.W. (1983). Alcohol and food abuse: some comparisons. *Br J Addict* 78: 339–49.

Scott, R., Gregory, H., Hines, N. et al. (1998). Neuropsychological, neurological and functional outcome following pallidotomy for Parkinson's disease: a consecutive series of eight simultaneous bilateral and twelve unilateral procedures. *Brain* 121: 659–75.

Scott, S., Carid, F. and Williams, B. (1984). Evidence for an apparent sensory speech disorder in Parkinson's disease. *J Neurol Neurosurg Psychiatry* 47: 840–3.

Shear, C.S., Nyhan, W.L., Kirman, B.H. and Stern, J. (1971). Self-mutilative behavior as a feature of the de Lange syndrome. *J Pediatr* 78: 506–9.

Sheppard, G., Gruzelier, J., Marchanda, R. et al. (1982). 15O positron emission tomographic scanning in predominantly never-treated acute schizophrenic patients. *Arch Gen Psychiatry* 39: 251–9.

Siegel, B. Jr. Buchsbaum, M.S., Bunney, W. Jr et al. (1993). Cortical–striatal thalamic circuits and brain glucose metabolic activity in 70 unmedicated male schizophrenic patients. *Am J Psychiatry* 150: 1325–36.

Singer, H.S., De la Cruz, P.S., Abrahms, M.T., Bean, S.C. and Reiss, A.L. (1997). A Tourette-like syndrome following cardiopulmonary bypass and hypothermia: MRI volumetric measurements. *Mov Disord* 12: 588–92.

Singer, H.S., Giuliano, J.D., Hansen, B.S. et al. (1998). Antibodies against human putamen in children with Tourette's syndrome. *Neurology* 50: 1618–24.

Singer, H.S., Reiss, A.L., Brown, J.E. et al. (1993). Volumetric MRI changes in basal ganglia of children with Tourette's syndrome. *Neurology* 43: 950–6.

Sivam, S.P. (1996). Dopamine, serotonin and tachykinin in self-injurious behavior. *Life Sci* 58: 2367–75.

Smadja, D., Cabre, P. and Vernant, J.C. (1995). Perte d'auto-activation psychique. Comportements compulsifs d'allure obsessionnelle. Abces toxoplasmique des noyaux gris centraux. *Rev Neurol* 151: 271–3.

Smith, S., Butters, N., White, R., Lyon, L. and Granholm, E. (1988). Priming semantic relations in patients with Huntington's disease. *Brain Lang* 33: 27–40.

Soukup, V.M., Ingram, F., Schiess, M.C. et al. (1997). Cognitive sequelae of unilateral posteroventral pallidotomy. *Arch Neurol* 54: 947–50.

Speedie, L.J., Brake, N., Folstein, S.E., Bowers, D. and Heilman, K.M. (1990). Comprehension of prosody in Huntington's disease. *J Neurol Neurosurg Psychiatry* 53: 607–10.

Spittle, B., Bragan, K. and James, B. (1976). Risk taking propensity, depression, and parasuicide. *Aust NZ J Psychiatry* 10: 269–73.

Sprengelmeyer, R., Young, A.W., Calder, A.J. et al. (1996). Loss of disgust. Perception of faces and emotions in Huntington's disease. *Brain* 119: 1647–65.

Stahl, S.M. (1988). Basal ganglia neuropharmacology and obsessive–compulsive disorder: the obsessive–compulsive disorder of basal ganglia dysfunction. *Psychopharmacol Bull* 24: 370–4.

Starkstein, S.E., Berthier, M.L., Bolduc, P.L., Preziosi, T.J. and Robinson, R.G. (1989). Depression in patients with early versus later onset of Parkinson's disease. *Neurology* 39: 1141–5.

Starkstein, S.E., Boston, J.D. and Robinson, R.G. (1988a). Mechanisms of mania after brain injury: 12 case reports and review of the literature. *J Nerv Ment Dis* 176: 87–100.

Starkstein, S.E., Brandt, J., Folstein, S. et al. (1988b). Neuropsychological and neuroradiological correlates in Huntington's disease. *J Neurol Neurosurg Psychiatry* 51: 1259–63.

Starkstein, S.E., Cohen, B.S., Fedoroff, J.P. et al. (1990a). Relationship between anxiety disorders and depressive disorders in patients with cerebrovascular injury. *Arch Gen Psychiatry* 47: 246–51.

Starkstein, S.E., Fedoroff, P., Berthier, M.L. and Robinson, R.G. (1991). Manic–depressive and pure manic status after brain lesions. *Biol Psychiatry* 29: 149–58.

Starkstein, S.E., Fedoroff, J.P., Price, T.R., Leiguarda, R. and Robinson, R.G. (1993). Apathy following cerebrovascular lesions. *Stroke* 24: 1625–30.

Starkstein, S.E., Mayberg, H.S., Preziosi, T.J. et al. (1992). Reliability, validity, and clinical correlates of apathy in Parkinson's disease. *J Neuropsychiatry Clin Neurosci* 4: 134–9.

Starkstein, S.E., Mran, T.H., Bowersox, J.A. et al. (1988c). Behavior abnormalities induced by frontal cortical and nucleus accumbens lesions. *Brain Res* 473: 74–80.

Starkstein, S.E., Pearlson, G.D., Boston, J.D. and Robinson, R.G. (1987). Mania after brain injury: a controlled study of causative factors. *Arch Neurol* 44: 1069–73.

Starkstein, S.E., Preziosi, T.J., Forrester, A.W. et al. (1990b). Specificity of affective and autonomic symptoms of depression in Parkinson's disease. *J Neurol Neurosurg Psychiatry* 53: 869–73.

Starkstein, S.E., Robinson, R.G. and Berther, M.L. (1988d). Differential mood changes following basal ganglia versus thalamic lesions. *Arch Neurol* 45: 725–30.

Steck, H. (1927). Les syndromes extrapyramidaux dans les maladies mentales *Arch Suisse Neurol Psychiatr* 20: 92.

Steck, H. (1931). Les syndromes mentaux postencephalitiques. *Schweiz Arch neurol Psychiatr* 27: 137–73.

Steele, J.C., Richardson, J.C. and Olszewski, J. (1964). Progressive supranuclear palsy. *Arch Neurol* 10: 333–59.

Stein, D.J., Hollander, E. and Liebowitz, M.R. (1993). Neurobiology of impulsivity and the impulse control disorders. *J Neuropsychiatry Clin Neurosci* 5: 9–17.

Stein, R.W., Kase, C.S., Hier, D.B. et al. (1984). Caudate hemorrhage. *Neurology* 34: 1549–54.

Stevens, J.R. (1982) Neuropathology of schizophrenia. *Arch Gen Psychiatry* 146: 1131–9.

Strakowski, S.M., Wilson, D.R., Tohen, M. et al. (1993). Structural brain abnormalities in first-episode mania. *Biol Psychiatry* 33: 602–9.

Streifler, J., Colomb, M. and Gadoth, N. (1989). Psychiatric features in adult GM2 gangliosidosis. *Br J Psychiatry* 155: 410–13.

Strub, R.L. (1989). Frontal lobe syndrome in a patient with bilateral globus pallidus lesions. *Arch Neurol* 46: 1024–7.

Stuss, D.T. and Benson, D.F. (1986). *The Frontal Lobes*, pp. 217–29, 429–54. New York: Raven Press.

Swayze, W.W., Andeasen, N.C., Alliger, R.J., Ehrhardt, J.C. and Yuh, W.T.C. (1992). Subcortical and temporal structures in affective disorder and schizophrenia: a magnetic resonance imaging study. *Biol Psychiatry* 31: 221–40.

Swedo, S.E. (1994). Sydenham's chorea: a model for childhood autoimmune neuropsychiatric disorders. *J Am Med Assoc* 272: 1788–91.

Swedo, S.E., Leonard, H.L. and Kiessling, L.S. (1994). Speculations on antineuronal antibody-mediated neuropsychiatric disorders of childhood. *Pediatrics* 93: 323–36.

Swedo, S.E., Leonard, H.L., Schapiro, M.B. et al. (1993). Sydenham's chorea: physical and psychological symptoms of St Vitus dance. *Pediatrics* 91: 706–13.

Swedo, S.E., Rapoport, J.L., Leonard, H.L. et al. (1991). Regional cerebral glucose metabolism of women with trichotillomania. *Arch Gen Psychiatry* 48: 828–33.

Szechtman, H., Nahmias, C., Garnett, E.S. et al. (1988). Effect of neuroleptics on altered cerebral glucose metabolism in schizophrenia. *Arch Gen Psychiatry* 45: 523–32.

Talland, G.A. and Schwab, S. (1964). Performance with multiple sets in Parkinson's disease. *Neuropsychologia* 2: 45–53.

Tarter, R.E., Switalia, J., Carra, J., Edwards, N. and van Thiel, D.H. (1987). Neuropsychological impairment associated with hepatolenticular degeneration (Wilson's disease) in the absence of overt encephalopathy. *Int J Neurosci* 23: 750–60.

Taylor, A.E., Saint-Cyr, J.A. and Lang, A.E. (1990). Subcognitive processing in the fronto-caudate 'complex loop' the role of the striatum. *J Alzheimer Dis Relat Disord* 13: 150–60.

Taylor, A.E., Saint-Cyr, J.A. and Lang, A.E. (1996). Frontal lobe dysfunction in Parkinson's disease. The cortical focus on neostriatal outflow. *Brain* 109: 845–83.

Taylor, H.G. and Hansotia, P. (1983). Neuropsychological testing of Huntington's patients: clues to progression. *J Nerv Ment Dis* 171: 492–6.

Tolosa, E.S. (1981). Clinical features of Meige's disease (idiopathic orofacial dystonia): a report of 17 cases. *Arch Neurol* 38: 147–51.

Tonkonogy, J. and Barreira, P. (1989). Obsessive–compulsive disorder and caudate–frontal lesion. *Neuropsychiatry Neuropsychol Behav Neurol* 2: 203–9.

Trautner, R.J., Cummings, J.L., Read, S.L. et al. (1988). Idiopathic basal ganglia calcification and organic mood disorder. *Am J Psychiatry* 145: 350–3.

Trepanier, L.P., Saint-Cyr, A., Lozano, A.M. and Lang, A.E. (1998). Neuropsychological consequences of posteroventral pallidotomy for the treatment of Parkinson's disease. *Neurology* 51: 207–15.

Trillet, M., Croisile, B., Tourniaire, D. and Schott, B. (1990). Perturbations de l'activité motrice volontaire et lésions des noyaux caudés. *Rev Neurol* 140: 338–44.

Trillet, M., Vighetto, A., Croisile, B., Charles, N. and Aimard, G. (1995). Hémiballisme avec libération thymo-affective et logorrhée par hématome du noyau sous-thalamique. *Rev Neurol* 151: 416–19.

Trzepacz, P.T., Scalabssi, R.J. and Van Thiel, D.H. (1989). Delirium: a subcortical phenomenon? *J Neuropsychiatry Clin Neurosci* 1: 283–90.

Turecki, G., de Mari, J. and Del Porto, J.A. (1993). Bipolar disorder following a left basal ganglia stroke. *Br J Psychiatry* 163: 690.

Valenstein, E. and Heilman, K.M. (1981). Unilateral hypokinesia and motor extinction. *Neurology* 31: 445–8.

Venna, N., Magocsi, S., Jay, M., Phull, B. and Ahmed, I. (1988). Reversible depression in Binswanger's disease. *J Clin Psychiatry* 49: 23–6.

Videbech, P. (1997). MRI findings in patients with affective disorder: a meta-analysis. *Acta Psychiatr Scand* 96: 157–68.

Vincent, A., Baruch, P., Pourcher, E. and Vincent, E.P. (1994). Implication des noyaux gris centraux dans le trouble obsessionnel compulsif: une revue. *Can J Psychiatry* 39: 545–50.

Vogel, H.P. (1982). Symptoms of depression in Parkinson's disease. *Pharmacopsychiatry* 15: 192–6.

Volkow, N.D., Brodie, J.D., Wolf, A.P. et al. (1986). Brain metabolism in patients with schizophrenia before and after acute neuroleptic administration. *J Neurol Neurosurg Psychiatry* 49: 1199–202.

Volow, M.R. (1985). Psychiatric aspects of blepharospasm. In *Blepharospasm. Advances in Ophthalmic Plastic and Reconstructive Surgery*, ed. S.L. Bosniak and B.C. Smith, pp. 163–74. New York: Pergamon Press.

von Economo, C. (1931). *Encephalitis Lethargica: its Sequelae and Treatment.* Translated by K.O. Newman. Oxford: Oxford University Press.

Vonsattel, J.P., Myers, R.H., Stevens, T.J. et al. (1985). Neuropathological classification of Huntington's disease. *J Neuropathol Exp Neurol* 44: 559–77.

von Thurzo, E. and Katona, T. (1927). Ueber die Benedecksche Klazomaia und die Souquesche Palilalie, als postenkepahlitische Hyperkinesien. *Dtsche Klin Wschr* 98: 278–84.

Waddington, J.L. (1995). Psychopathological and cognitive correlates of tardive dyskinesia in schizophrenia and other disorders treated with neuroleptic drugs. In *Behavioral Neurology of Movement Disorders*, ed. W.J. Weiner and A.E. Lang, pp. 211–29. *Advances in Neurology.* New York: Raven Press.

Walker, S. (1969). The psychiatric presentation of Wilson's disease with an etiologic explanation. Behav. *Neuropsychiatry* 1: 38–43.

Wallesh, C.W. and Fehrenbach, R.A. (1988). On the neurolinguistic nature of language abnormalities in Huntington's disease. *J Neurol Neurosurg Psychiatry* 51: 367–73.

Wang, P.Y. (1991). Neurobehavioral changes following caudate infarct: a case report with literature review. *Chunh Hua i Hsueh Tsa Chih* 47: 199–203.

Watt, D.C. and Seller, A.S. (1993). A clinico-genetic study of psychiatric disorder in Huntington's disease. *Psychol Med*, Monograph 23 Suppl.: 1–46.

Weilberg, J.B., Mesulam, M.M., Weintraub, S. et al. (1986). Focal striatal abnormalities in a patient with obsessive–compulsive disorder. *Arch Gen Psychiatry* 43: 114–24.

Weiner, W.J. and Werner, T.R. (1982). Mania-induced remission of tardive dyskinesia in manic–depressive illness. *Ann Neurol* 12: 229–30.

Weiner, W.J. and Lang, A.E. ed. (1995). *Behavioral Neurology of Movement Disorders, Advances in Neurology*, Vol. 65, pp. 85–95. New York: Raven Press.

Weingartner, H., Caine, E.D. and Ebert, M.H. (1979). Imagery, encoding, and retrieval of information from memory: some specific encoding-retrieval changes in Huntington's disease. *J Abnorm Psychol* 88: 52–8.

Weisberg, L.A. (1984). Caudate hemorrhage. *Arch Neurol* 41: 971–9.

White, J. (1940). Autonomic discharge from stimulation of the hypothalamus in man. *Res Nerv Ment Dis* 20, 854–63.

Wickham, A.E. and Read, J.V. (1987). Lithium for the control of aggressive and self-mutilating behavior. *Int Clin Psychopharmacol* 2: 181–90.

Williams, A.C., Owen, C. and Heath, D.A. (1988). A compulsive movement disorder with cavitation of caudate nucleus. *J Neurol Neurosurg Psychiatry* 51: 447–8.

Williamson, P., Pelz, D., Merskey, H. et al. (1992). Frontal, temporal, and striatal proton relaxation times in schizophrenic patients and normal comparison subjects. *Am J Psychiatry* 149: 549–51.

Wilson, S.A.K. (1912). Progressive lenticular degeneration: a familial nervous system disease associated with cirrhosis of the liver. *Brain* 34: 295–509.

Wilson, S.A.K. (1925). The Croonian lectures on some disorders of motility and muscle tone with special reference to the corpus striatum. *Lancet* 2: 1–10, 53–62, 169–78, 215–19, 268–76.

Wilson, S.A.K. (1927). The tics and allied conditions. *J Neurol Psych* 8: 93–109.

Wimmer, A. (1924). *Chronic Encephalitis.* London: Heinemann.

Winchel, R.M. and Stanley, M. (1991). Self-injurious behavior: a review of the behavior and biology of self-mutilation. *Am J Psychiatry* 148: 306–71.

Winslow, J.T. and Insel, T.R. (1990). Neurobiology of obsessive–compulsive disorder: a possible role for serotonin. *J Clin Psychiatry* 51 (Suppl.): 36–43.

Wohlfart, G., Ingvar, D.H. and Hellberg, A.M. (1961). Compulsory shouting (Benedek's 'klazomania') associated with oculogyric spasms in chronic epidemic encephalitis. *Acta Psychiatr Scand* 36: 369–77.

Woods, B.T., Brennan, S., Yurgelun Todd, D., Panzarino, P. (1995). MRI abnormalities in major psychiatric disorders: an exploratory comparative study. *J Neuropsychiatry Clin Neurosci* 7: 918–22.

Woody, R.C. and Eisenhauer, G. (1986). Tooth extraction as a form of self-mutilation in Tourette's disorder. *South Med J* 79: 1466.

Yamadori, A., Mori, E., Tabuchi, M., Kudo, Y. and Mitani, Y. (1986). Hypergraphia: a right hemispheric syndrome. *J Neurol Neurosurg Psychiatry* 49: 1160–4.

Yarden, P.E. and Discipio, W.J. (1971). Abnormal movements and prognosis in schizophrenia. *Am J Psychiatry* 128: 317–23.

Yasuda, K., Kondo, T., Hiraizumi, Y., Fujii, H. and Yamasaki, M. (1995). A case of focal encephalitis with psychological symptoms similar to chorea minor. *No To Hatatsu* 27: 239–44.

Zametkin, A.J., Liebenhauer, L.L., Fitzgeral, G.A. et al. (1993). Brain metabolism in teenagers with attention-deficit hyperactivity disorder. *Arch Gen Psychiatry* 50: 333–40.

Zitterl, W., Wimberger, D., Demal, U., Hofer, E. and Lenz, G. (1994). Kernspintomographiesche Befunde bei der Zwangserkrankung. *Nervenarzt* 65: 619–22.

Zohar, J., Insel, T., Foa, E. et al. (1989). Physiological and psychological changes during in vivo exposure and imaginal flooding of obsessive–compulsive disorder patients. *Arch Gen Psychiatry* 46: 505–10.

7

Mania and manic-like disorders

Sergio E. Starkstein and Facundo Manes

Introduction

In 1888, Leonore Welt, a German psychiatrist, suggested for the first time an association between focal cerebral lesions and manic-like behaviors. She described the case of a patient with a change in character, expressed by restlessness, euphoria, overtalkativeness, and a lowering of ethical and moral standards, after bilateral damage to the orbitofrontal cortex. In the same year, Jastrowitz (1888) reported elated behavior, pressured speech, and obscene language in a series of patients with frontal lobe tumors.

Surgical brain procedures were also reported to produce manic behaviors. Reitman (1946) reported hyperactivity, euphoria, and disinhibited behaviors in a group of patients treated with orbitofrontal leukotomy, whereas in a comprehensive study of cognitive and emotional complications of frontal surgery, Rylander (1939) described euphoria, hyperactivity, and hypersexuality as frequent behavioral sequelae.

On the other hand, manic disorders after focal brain lesions have been reported only recently. Jampala and Abrams (1983) reported two patients who developed manic behaviors after left and right fronto-temporal lesions respectively, and Cummings and Mendez (1984) reported two patients with manic behaviors after right thalamic lesions. Milder cases of disinhibited behavior have been recently reported. Gorman and Cummings (1992) reported hypersexuality in two patients with septal injury, and Regard and Landis (1997) described a nondisabling form of hyperphagia, with a specific preference for fine food (which they termed the 'gourmand syndrome'), with most patients having right anterior lesions. Taken together, the above descriptions suggest that either partial or full-blown disinhibition syndromes may result from focal brain lesions.

This chapter examines methodological issues, clinical characteristics, and anatomical correlates of manic behaviors after focal brain damage. Based on the above, a mechanism for this interesting behavioral phenomenon is proposed.

Table 7.1. Diagnostic criteria for manic episode (adapted from DSM-IV)

A	Distinct period of abnormally and persistently elevated, expansive or irritable mood, lasting at least one week (or any duration if hospitalization is necessary)
B	During the period of mood disturbance, three (or more) of the following symptoms have persisted (four if the mood is only irritable) and have been present to a significant degree:
(1)	Inflated self-esteem or grandiosity
(2)	Decreased need for sleep (e.g., feels rested after only 3 hours of sleep)
(3)	More talkative than usual or pressure to keep talking
(4)	Flight of ideas or subjective experience that thoughts are racing
(5)	Distractibility (i.e., attention too easily drawn to unimportant or irrelevant external stimuli)
(6)	Increase in goal-directed activity (either socially, at work or school, or sexually)
(7)	Excessive involvement in pleasurable activities that have a high potential for painful consequences (e.g., engaging in unrestrained buying sprees, sexual indiscretions, or foolish business investments)

Methodological issues

In a recent publication, Starkstein and Robinson (1997) discussed important methodological considerations concerning the diagnosis of manic-like disorders in patients with brain lesions, and we will briefly summarize the most relevant points.

Manic-like behaviors have been ascribed different terms within neurological and psychiatric fields. Thus, the neurological literature includes terms such as the 'frontal lobe syndrome,' 'pseudopsychopathic syndrome,' 'disinhibition syndrome,' and 'acquired sociopathy.' One important limitation is that none of these terms has been syndromically defined, and whether they refer to independent or overlapping syndromes has not been empirically determined.

The psychiatric literature also includes a varied terminology for manic-like behaviors. Krauthammer and Klerman (1978) used the term 'secondary mania' to refer to a manic syndrome occurring in the context of organic factors. The DSM-IV (APA, 1994) offers three different entries which may fit the phenomenon of manic-like behaviors after brain injury. The criteria for a Manic Episode (Table 7.1) may be used provided the patient meets the qualifiers 'due to a general medical condition,' and whenever 'the mood disturbance is judged to be the direct physiological consequence' of a medical illness. One obvious limitation of these criteria is the difficulty of establishing whether or not a medical illness is physiologically related to the mood disturbance. Another related DSM-IV entry is 'Personality change due to a general medical condition,' which may be further classified into disinhibited or aggressive types (i.e., whenever the predominant feature is aggressive or disinhibited behavior). Limitations for using these criteria include both difficulties in determining the role of the medical condition in the etiology of the personality change, and the lack of more specific criteria to define disinhibition or aggressiveness. Another related DSM-IV entry is 'Impulse-control disorders not elsewhere classified,' and, more specifically, the 'intermittent explosive disorder,' although this diagnosis is excluded when produced by a general medical condition.

In their earlier studies, Starkstein and Robinson (1997) have used the DSM-III-R criteria for a 'manic episode' because these criteria were the most detailed and specific, but kept Krauthammer and Klerman's (1978) term 'secondary mania' to separate these patients from those with 'primary mania' (i.e., a manic episode in the absence of known brain damage). It is important to note that the term 'Manic episode due to a general medical condition' was not available.

In conclusion, whereas manic-like behaviors after brain damage are a well-known condition, the terminology for this disorder varies widely, and specific criteria have not been developed. Future studies should examine the full spectrum of behavioral symptoms in patients with a manic-like disorder after brain injury, and validate a specific set of criteria.

Epidemiology

Few studies have empirically examined the prevalence of secondary mania after brain lesions, which may vary depending on the type of brain injury. Thus, whereas Robinson et al. (1988) found a prevalence of 1% of manic patients among a consecutive series of more than 300 patients with acute stroke lesions, Jorge et al. (1993) found a prevalence of secondary mania of 9% in a study that included a consecutive series of 66 patients with acute traumatic brain injuries. This discrepancy may be explained by the higher prevalence of lesions involving basotemporal and orbitofrontal cortices in traumatic brain injury patients as compared to stroke patients. The relevance of lesion location for the production of secondary mania is discussed below.

Phenomenology

In a study that included 11 patients with mania after brain lesions and 25 patients with primary mania, Starkstein, Boston and Robinson (1988a) found that both groups had a similar prevalence of manic symptoms, such as elation, pressured speech, flight of ideas, grandiose delusions, insomnia, hallucinations, and paranoid delusions (Fig. 7.1). However, whether patients with secondary mania had disinhibition symptoms beyond those included in DSM-IV has not been specifically examined.

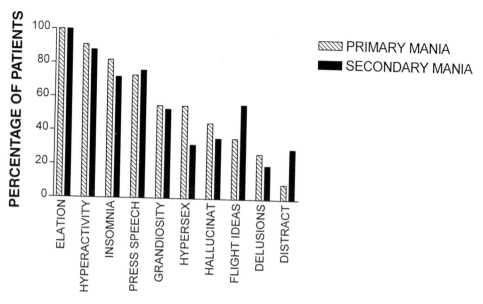

Fig. 7.1   The prevalence of manic symptoms in patients with either primary or secondary mania.

In a recent study (Walzer, Chemerinski and Starkstein, 1998), we designed a dis-inhibition scale that includes 32 items and is divided into five main areas (motor, sensitive, affective, instinctive, and cognitive). We examined the validity of this scale in a group of 13 demented patients and ten age-comparable normal controls. We found that demented patients had significantly higher disinhibition scores than the control group (mean $\pm$ SD $= 16 \pm 11$ vs. 4 ± 11, respectively, $p < 0.01$), and there were significant correlations between the disinhibition scale scores and scores of irritability ($r = 0.70$, $p < 0.05$), apathy ($r = 0.70$, $p < 0.05$), and agitation ($r = 0.80$, $p < 0.05$).

In conclusion, whereas the phenomenology of secondary mania is similar to the symptoms shown by patients with primary mania, this may result from diagnostic restrictions, and newer scales may allow a more comprehensive description of dis-inhibition syndromes produced by focal brain lesions.

Demographic and psychiatric correlates of secondary mania

Starkstein et al. (1987) examined the presence of demographic and clinical cor-relates of secondary mania in a study that included 11 patients with mania after brain lesions (secondary mania group), 11 patients with similar brain lesions but no mania (lesion control group), 25 patients with mania but no brain lesions (primary mania), and 11 normal controls. There were no significant between-group differences in relevant demographic factors such as age, education, and socioeconomic status. Moreover, there were no significant differences in the prevalence of neurological deficits among patients with brain lesions with or without mania. The only relevant finding was that patients with secondary mania had significantly more severe subcortical brain atrophy (as measured by the bifrontal and third ventricle to brain ratios) compared to brain-injured patients without mania. Another important finding was that patients with secondary mania and a positive family history of psychiatric disorder had significantly less subcortical atrophy than patients with secondary mania and a negative family history of affective disorders. Strakowski et al. (1993) examined the presence of subcortical atrophy using magnetic resonance imaging (MRI) in patients with first-episode mania and age-comparable normal controls. They reported significantly larger third-ventricular volumes in the mania group compared to the controls. Taken together, these findings suggest that subcortical atrophy may constitute a relevant risk factor for the production of manic episodes. Manic episodes may occur spontaneously after being triggered by as yet unknown mechanisms, or may occur after injuries to a specific brain location.

A role for genetic factors in the mechanism of secondary mania was reported by Robinson et al. (1988), who compared demographic and psychiatric differences between patients who developed mania ($n = 17$), depression ($n = 31$), or no mood disorder ($n = 28$) after a brain lesion. They found a significantly higher frequency of positive family (but not personal) history of affective disorders in patients with secondary mania as compared to the other two groups.

In conclusion, both a genetic burden for affective disorders and subcortical brain atrophy probably predating the brain lesion may be independent risk factors for secondary mania.

Lesion location and secondary mania

Whereas a specific relationship between manic behaviors and lesion location was suggested more than 100 years ago, most cases with secondary mania have been reported as single cases or in small groups, and controlled studies appeared only recently.

A review of most cases of secondary mania reported in the literature was carried out by Starkstein et al. (1988a), who also included 12 additional new cases. Six of those 12 patients had tumors, four had strokes, and two had traumatic brain injuries. Five patients had frontal lobe lesions (primarily involving the orbitofrontal area), three patients had inferior temporal lesions, three patients had subcortical diencephalic lesions, and one patient had a frontal head trauma with cerebellar signs. The lesion was restricted to the right hemisphere in seven patients, four patients had midline or bilateral lesions, and only one patient had a lesion restricted to the left hemisphere. Of the 19 patients gleaned from the literature, diencephalic lesions were present in nine, temporal lobe lesions in four, a frontal lobe lesion in two, and the remaining patients had more widespread brain damage.

In one of the first controlled studies to examine neuropathological factors involved in secondary mania, Robinson et al. (1988) assessed consecutive patients with diagnoses of secondary mania ($n = 17$), post-stroke major depression ($n = 31$), or no mood disturbance after brain injury ($n = 28$). There were no significant between-group differences in demographic characteristics, time from brain lesion to the onset of the affective disorder, frequencies of neurological focal deficits, and lesion volumes. On the other hand, 71% of the patients with secondary mania had right hemisphere lesions, whereas 61% of the post-stroke depressed patients had left hemisphere damage ($X^2 = 14.8$, df $= 1$, $p < 0.0001$). Lesion location was also different: whereas most patients with secondary mania had lesions involving ventral and diencephalic brain areas, patients with post-stroke depression had more widely distributed lesions. Moreover, although a few depressed patients had right hemisphere lesions, there was no overlap of the right hemisphere lesions associated with mania and those associated with major depression. Based on these and previous findings, Robinson et al. (1988) suggested that secondary mania may require both a lesion restricted to specific right hemisphere regions and either a genetic loading for affective disorder or a pre-existing subcortical atrophy. The relatively rare coexistence of these factors may account for the low prevalence of secondary mania. Robinson et al. also pointed out that the significant association with right hemisphere lesions and the relatively late age of onset of the affective disorder argue against the interpretation of secondary mania as just the occurrence of an affective disorder in coincidence with brain injury.

In a subsequent study, Starkstein et al. (1990b) presented a new consecutive series of eight patients who developed a manic episode after brain injury. Five patients had cortical lesions (four with damage to the right basotemporal region, and one with bilateral damage to the orbitofrontal area), whereas the remaining three patients had subcortical lesions (white matter of the right frontal lobe, right anterior limb of the internal capsule, and right head of the caudate). An 18-fluorodeoxyglucose positron emission tomography study was carried out in all three patients with subcortical lesions, and showed a significant metabolic asymmetry (right side < left side) in the lateral basotemporal area (remote from the brain lesion) for all three patients. There were two important implications for this study: firstly, it confirmed the importance of lesion location (orbitofrontal and basotemporal areas) and lesion side (right hemisphere) in the production of secondary mania, and secondly, it demonstrated that lesions outside the basotemporal region may produce secondary mania through a remote metabolic effect (diaschisis).

Starkstein et al. (1990a) examined the long-term prognosis of secondary mania, and whether some patients may develop a bipolar (manic–depressive) syndrome after focal brain lesions. They divided a series of 19 patients with secondary mania into a manic–depressive group (who met DSM-III-R criteria for both a Manic episode followed or preceded by Organic mood syndrome, depressed), and a mania-only group (who met criteria for a Manic episode, not followed or preceded by depression). Seven of the 19 patients had a bipolar manic–depressive syndrome, whereas the remaining 12 patients had mania only. There were no significant between-group differences in demographic variables or neurological focal signs. Six of the seven manic–depressed patients had right hemisphere lesions involving subcortical structures (head of the caudate and thalamus), whereas nine of the 12 mania-only patients had cortical lesions (restricted to the right hemisphere in eight cases) (Fig. 7.2). This different prevalence of cortical and subcortical lesions was statistically significant (Fisher test $p < 0.005$). Additionally, patients with mania-only also showed significantly larger lesions but less cognitive impairment than depressed–manic patients (Fig. 7.3).

The question now arising is why some patients develop secondary manic–depression, while others develop secondary mania only? Starkstein et al. (1988a) suggested that secondary mania may result from release of limbic and hypothalamic structures from orbitofrontal and basotemporal control. On the other hand, the higher prevalence of subcortical lesions in manic–depressive patients and the fact that these lesions may produce widespread hypometabolic deficits even in contralateral brain areas (i.e., crossed-hemisphere and crossed-cerebellar diaschisis) suggest a different mechanism for the manic–depressive syndrome. Thus, depression may result from diaschisis involving left frontal areas, and mania may develop at a later stage, when the remote metabolic deficits are restricted to the orbitofrontal and/or basotemporal regions of the right hemisphere.

Further support for the presence of right basotemporal dysfunction in the mechanism of mania is found in a study that examined brain metabolic changes in patients with primary (i.e., no known brain injury) mania (Migliorelli et al., 1993). Five patients with primary mania and seven age-comparable normal controls were assessed with HMPAO-single photon emission tomography (SPECT). Manic patients were assessed while in the manic stage, and there were two important findings. First, manic patients showed a significantly lower blood perfusion in the right basal temporal cortex as compared to the control group. Second, there were two significant asymmetries within the manic group: a left–right asymmetry (which resulted from a significantly lower blood flow in the right vs. left temporal area), and a ventral dorsal asymmetry (which resulted from a significantly lower basal vs. dorsal right temporal blood flow).

In conclusion, existing studies suggest that about one-third of patients with

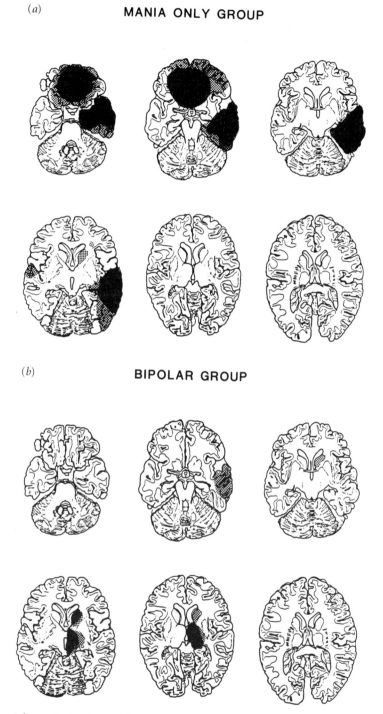

Fig. 7.2   Schematic drawings of lesion location for patients with (a) mania after brain injury (mania-only group), and (b) both mania and depression (bipolar group).

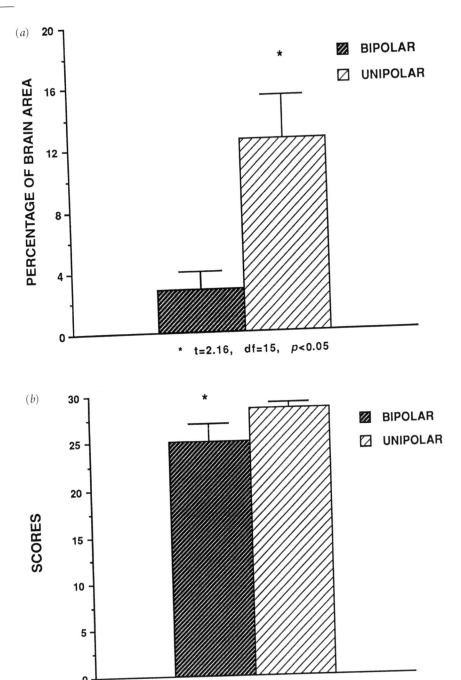

Fig. 7.3   Patients with a bipolar syndrome after brain injury had significantly smaller lesions (a) and significantly lower Mini Mental State Examination scores (b) than patients with mania only.

secondary mania have a prior episode of depression. Whereas most patients with a bipolar manic–depressive syndrome had subcortical lesions (mainly involving the right head of the caudate or right thalamus), most patients with pure mania had cortical lesions (primarily involving orbitofrontal and basotemporal regions of the right hemisphere).

Mechanism of secondary mania

Whereas the ultimate mechanism of secondary mania remains unknown, findings from different studies converge upon the critical role of ventral brain areas in the regulation of behaviors. Welt (1888) suggested that injuries to the medial orbital surface of the frontal lobes may produce a disinhibition syndrome. Other reports further supported this clinico-pathological association, and it was Kleist (1937) who first suggested a dissociation between dorsal and ventral frontal areas in the regulation of emotions. He posited that the frontal convexity is associated with psychomotor and intellectual activities, and lesions to this area may produce a lack of motor and psychiatric initiative. On the other hand, Kleist considered area 11 within the orbitofrontal cortex to be related to personal and social ego, and area 47 to be related to mood and emotional sensations. He further suggested that lesions to this area would induce euphoria, puerility, and moral insanity. In 1939, Klüver and Bucy observed that monkeys with a bitemporal lobectomy not only developed hypersexuality, but also explored the environment ('as if the animal were acting under the influence of some compulsive or irresistible impulse'). They used the term 'lack of inhibition' for these behaviors, and suggested that the temporal lobes may constitute an inhibitory structure, so that temporal lesions could produce release symptoms such as logorrhea, echolalia, and echopraxia. In 1972, Goldar and Outes suggested that the orbitofrontal–basotemporal complex (connected through the uncinate fasciculus) might exert a tonic inhibitory control over the amygdala. By releasing this tonic inhibition, lesions in the ventral brain cortex could produce emotional disinhibition. They further suggested that the loss of frontolimbic connections may release emotions from intellectual control, which may produce the cluster of symptoms that characterize secondary mania.

In their 1988 article, Starkstein et al. (1988a) suggested that secondary mania may result from disruption of septal, hypothalamic, thalamic, and mesencephalic areas connected to the frontal lobes. The orbitofrontal cortex is one of the main limbic output channels and the only cortical structure with direct connections to subcortical areas that regulate autonomic, instinctive, affective, locomotor, and endocrine functions. They speculated that lesions to the orbitofrontal–basotemporal cortex or any of their efferent pathways may result in either partial or full-blown manic behaviors. Starkstein et al. (1988a) linked the significant association between secondary mania and lesion lateralization to asymmetric behavioral responses to focal brain lesions found in rodents. Robinson (1979) demonstrated that right (but not left) frontal cortical lesions produce locomotor hyperactivity. Subsequently, Starkstein et al. (1988b) reported a significant correlation between higher locomotor activity produced by right frontal suction lesions and more severe norepinephrine depletions within the contralateral and ipsilateral cerebral cortex and nucleus ceruleus, as well as a significant bilateral increment in dopaminergic turnover in the nucleus accumbens. A similar lateralized behavior was found after right (but not left) electrolytic lesions of the nucleus accumbens (Starkstein et al., 1988b). Mayberg et al. (1988) demonstrated similar asymmetric biogenic amine pathways in humans. Taken together, these studies suggest that in both rats and humans there is an asymmetrical biochemical response to brain damage depending on whether the right or left hemisphere is injured.

Recent neuroanatomical findings allowed a further elaboration of the mechanism of secondary mania. Based on Sanides' (1969) hypothesis of a dual origin of the cerebral cortex (both the orbitofrontal and basotemporal cortices deriving from the archicortex; and limbic, prefrontal dorsolateral, and visual, somatosensory, and motor cortices evolving from the archicortex), Petrides and Pandya (1994) described important connecting pathways within paleocortical regions (e.g., between orbitofrontal, insular, inferior parietal, and basotemporal cortical areas), as well as between paleocortical and archicortical regions (e.g., between orbitofrontal and frontal dorsal regions, inferior and superior parietal regions, and inferior temporal – subserving central vision – and dorsal temporo-occipital cortices – subserving peripheral vision).

Goldar (1993) suggested that the architectonic pattern of brain development may result in functional differentiation of dorsal and ventral brain areas. Whereas dorsal areas related to visuospatial functions, somatosensation, and spatial memory are connected to dorsal prefrontal areas, ventral brain areas related to central vision and biographical memory project to ventral fronto–temporal areas.

Subcortical structures may also play an important role in the regulation of emotions, and show a similar pattern of connections to paleocortical and archicortical areas as demonstrated by cortical regions. The ventral or limbic striatum, which includes the nucleus accumbens and the fundus striati, receives afferents from both the amygdala and the anterior temporal cortex, and may participate in inhibitory processes through projections to preoptico-hypothalamic and nigrostriatal neurons (Somogyi et al., 1981). Inhibition may be the result of a reduced dopaminergic tone in the dorsal or motor striatum (primarily the putamen). Moreover, the subcallosum–tapetum system may contain an inhibitory pathway of ventral neocortical fibers directed to the caudate nucleus. The substantia innominata, which receives fibers from the orbito-insular-temporopolar cortices and sends widespread projections to the dorsal neocortex, constitutes the midpoint of a pathway that extends from the ventral to the dorsal cortex (Kievit and Kuypers, 1975). There is also an indirect pathway through the medial pulvinar thalamic nucleus, which is connected to both the ventral and dorsal neocortices and the limbic cortex (Mauguiere and Baleydier, 1986).

Based on contextual cues (converging from polymodal association areas) and object–reward associative memories (converging from the dorsomedial thalamic nucleus), paleocortically derived regions may regulate the release of behaviors produced in dorsal brain areas (Goldar, 1993). In a recent review, Starkstein and Robinson (1997) speculated that basotemporal and orbitofrontal cortices share important connections that may underlie the association between frontal-related volitional and psychomotor behaviors, and limbic-related emotional and instinctive drive. Thus, different behaviors may be disinhibited after disruption of specific ventral–dorsal pathways: lesions to the ventromedial prefrontal cortex or its efferent pathways from the striatum may produce motor disinhibition; release of the hypothalamus, amygdala, and brainstem biogenic amine nuclei from orbitofrontal tonic control may produce instinctive disinhibition; release of dorsal temporal–parietal regions from tonic basotemporal control may produce intellectual and sensory disinhibition; and release of paralimbic areas from paleocortical tonic control may result in emotional disinhibition.

In conclusion, motor, sensory, affective, intellectual, and instinctive disinhibition may result from damage to specific brain areas. Prospective studies and case reports have demonstrated that most patients with secondary mania have orbitofrontal and/or basotemporal dysfunction. Brain asymmetries may also play an important role in the production of disinhibited behaviors. The production of secondary mania may require both a lesion in a specific brain area (such as the orbitofrontal and basotemporal cortices) as well as involvement of the right hemisphere.

Treatment of secondary mania

Given the low prevalence of secondary mania, formal treatment studies are difficult to carry out. In a single case study, Bakchine et al. (1989) reported that clonidine was useful in the treatment of a 44-year-old woman with a manic-like state after bilateral orbitofrontal and right temporo-parietal contusions. On the other hand, levodopa and carbamazepine were not useful. Most patients with secondary mania reported in the literature were treated with drugs frequently used among patients with primary mania, such as neuroleptics, anticonvulsants, and lithium, as well as electroconvulsive therapy (Starkstein et al., 1990a). However, whether the usefulness of these treatment modalities is similar for patients with secondary mania as compared to patients with primary mania remains to be empirically established.

Conclusions

Manic behaviors may follow focal brain lesions. Whereas the prevalence of secondary mania among stroke patients is low, it increases significantly in patients with traumatic brain injury. Predisposing factors to secondary mania are either a genetic liability to the disease, or atrophy in frontal and diencephalic regions, probably predating the brain damage. Lesion location has a critical role in the mechanism of secondary mania: most patients reported in the literature had lesions involving ventral brain areas (mainly orbitofrontal and basotemporal cortices). Dysfunction of these heteromodal ventral brain regions may release archicortical brain areas, which may result in disinhibited behaviors. Whereas patients with secondary mania are usually treated with medications with proven efficacy in primary mania, the most effective treatment modality remains to be determined.

Acknowledgments

This chapter was partially supported by grants from the Raul Carrea Institute of Neurological Research (SES), the Fundación Perez Companc (SES), and the following NIH grants: MH 52879 and 53592 (FM).

REFERENCES

APA (1994). *Diagnostic and Statistical Manual of Mental Disorders*, 4th edn. Washington, DC: American Psychiatric Press.

Bakchine, S., Lacomblez, L., Benoit, N. and Lhermitte, F. (1989). Manic-like state after orbitofrontal and right temporoparietal injury: efficacy of clonidine. *Neurology* 39: 777–81.

Cummings, J.L. and Mendez, M.F. (1984). Secondary mania with focal cerebrovascular lesions. *Am J Psychiatry* 141: 1084–7.

Goldar, J.C. (1993). *Anatomia de La Mente*. Buenos Aires: Salerno.

Goldar, J.C. and Outes, D.L. (1972). Fisiopatología de la desinhibición instintiva. *Acta Psiq Psicol Amer Lat* 18: 177–85.

Gorman, D.G. and Cummings, J.L. (1992). Hypersexuality following septal injury. *Arch Neurol* 49: 308–10.

Jampala, V.C. and Abrams, R. (1983). Mania secondary to left and right hemisphere damage. *Am J Psychiatry* 140: 1197–9.

Jastrowitz, M. (1888). Beitrage zur Lokalisation im Grosshirn und uber deren praktische Verwerthung. *Dtsch Med Wochnschr* 14: 81–3.

Jorge, R.E., Robinson, R.G., Starkstein, S.E. et al. (1993). Secondary mania following traumatic brain injury. *Am J Psychiatry* 150: 916–21.

Kievit, L. and Kuypers, M.G.J.M. (1975). Basal forebrain and hypothalamic connections to frontal and temporal cortex in the rhesus monkey. *Science* 187: 660–2.

Kleist, K. (1937). Bericht über die Gehirnpathologie in ihrer Bedeutung für Neurologie und Psychiatrie. *Z Ges Neurol Psychiat* 158: 159–93.

Klüver, M. and Bucy, P. (1939). Preliminary analysis of functions of the temporal lobes in monkeys. *Arch Neurol Psychiatry* 42: 979–1000.

Krauthammer, C. and Klerman, G.L. (1978). Secondary mania: manic syndromes associated with antecedent physical illness or drugs. *Arch Gen Psychiatry* 35: 1333–9.

Mauguiere, F. and Baleydier, C. (1986). Place du thalamus dans le réseau d'interconnexions entre les cortex associatifs et limbiques chez le singe. *Rev Neurol* 142: 406–17.

Mayberg, M.S., Robinson, R.G., Wong, D.F. et al. (1988). PET imaging of cortical S2 serotonin receptors after stroke: lateralized changes and relationship to depression. *Am J Psychiatry*, 145: 937–43.

Migliorelli, R., Starkstein, S.E., Teson, A. et al. (1993). SPECT findings in patients with primary mania. *J Neuropsychiatry Clin Neurosci* 5: 379–83.

Petrides, M. and Pandya, D.N. (1994). Comparative architectonic analysis of the human and macaque frontal cortex. In *Handbook of Neuropsychology*, ed. J. Grafman and F. Boller, pp. 17–59. Amsterdam: Elsevier Science Publishers.

Regard, M. and Landis, T. (1997). 'Gourmand syndrome': eating passion associated with right anterior lesions. *Neurology* 48: 1185–90.

Reitman, F. (1946). Orbital cortex syndrome following leucotomy. *Am J Psychiatry* 103: 238–46.

Robinson, R.G. (1979). Differential behavioral and biochemical effects of right and left hemispheric cerebral infarction in the rat. *Science* 205: 707–10.

Robinson, R.G., Boston, J.D., Starkstein, S.E. and Price, T.R. (1988). Comparison of mania with depression following brain injury: causal factors. *Am J Psychiatry* 145: 172–8.

Rylander, G. (1939). *Personality Changes after Operations on the Frontal Lobes*. Oxford: Oxford University Press.

Sanides, F. (1969). Comparative architectonics of the neocortex of mammals and their evolutionary interpretation. *Ann N Y Acad Sci* 167: 404–23.

Somogyi, P., Bolam, J.P., Totterdell, S. and Smith, A.D. (1981). Monosynaptic input from the nucleus accumbens–ventral striatum region to retrogradely labelled nigrostriate neurons. *Brain Res* 217: 245–63.

Starkstein, S.E., Boston, J.D. and Robinson, R.G. (1988a). Mechanisms of mania after brain injury: 12 case reports and review of the literature. *J Nerv Ment Dis* 176: 87–100.

Starkstein, S.E., Fedoroff, P., Berthier, M.L. and Robinson, R.G. (1990a). Manic–depressive and pure manic states after brain lesions. *Biol Psychiatry* 29: 149–58.

Starkstein, S.E., Mayberg, H.S., Berthier, M.L. et al. (1990b). Mania after brain injury: neuroradiological and metabolic findings. *Ann Neurol* 27: 652–9.

Starkstein, S.E., Moran, T.H., Bowersox, J.A. and Robinson, R.G. (1988b). Behavioral abnormalities induced by frontal cortical and nucleus accumbens lesions. *Brain Res* 473: 74–80.

Starkstein, S.E., Pearlson, G.D., Boston, J.D. and Robinson, R.G. (1987). Mania after brain injury: a controlled study of causative factors. *Arch Neurol* 44: 1069–73.

Starkstein, S.E. and Robinson, R.G. (1997). Mechanism of disinhibition after brain lesions. *J Nerv Ment Dis* 185: 108–14.

Strakowski, S.M., Wilson, D.R., Tohen, M. et al. (1993). Structural brain abnormalities in first-episode mania. *Biol Psychiatry* 33: 602–9.

Walzer, T., Chemerinski, E. and Starkstein, S.E. (1998). The disinhibition syndrome in Alzheimer's disease: validation of a scale. Presented at the 10th Congress of the Alzheimer Disease International, Amsterdam.

Welt, L. (1888). Uber Charakterveränderungen der Menschen infolge von Läsionen des Stirnhirm. *Deutsch Arch Klin Med* 42: 339–90.

8

Behavioral and emotional changes after focal frontal lobe damage

Paul J. Eslinger and Laszlo Geder

Introduction

Historical and contemporary accounts of focal lesions affecting the frontal lobe have emphasized significant changes in personality and behavior but often minimal findings on clinical neurological, neuropsychological, and psychiatric examinations. Diagnosis and management of frontal lobe syndromes, particularly those involving the prefrontal cortex, encompass an unusually broad range of signs and symptoms. The underlying mechanisms of these syndromes are not yet clear, due to the complex organizational features of prefrontal cortex as well as its mediation of a broad range of variation in human adaptive behavior.

Neuropsychological studies have suggested a pivotal role for this cortical region in executive functions and in the regulation of cognition, emotion, and behavior. These appear to be two essential processes characterizing the neural networks involving prefrontal cortex. When attention, memory, goal-directed behaviors, emotions, and social interaction are no longer regulated by the knowledge systems and operational features of executive functions, the result is a wide range of over-regulated, under-regulated, and erratically regulated processes producing symptoms that are diverse and disabling, yet at times surprisingly subtle and discounted by the untrained examiner. This is not to say that the prefrontal cortex is the sole mediator of such processes, as numerous studies have indicated that similar signs and symptoms can be associated with other sites of cerebral damage, including the basal ganglia, thalamus and certain nonfrontal cortical regions (Cummings, 1993; Eslinger and Grattan, 1993; Bogousslavsky, 1994; Mega and Cummings, 1994). Rather, the prefrontal cortex participates in multiple cortical–cortical and cortical–subcortical neural networks that have high integrative demands in cognitive and emotional domains.

The role of the prefrontal cortex in cognitive aspects of behavior has been widely recognized, including processes such as object and spatial working memory, planning, and strategic problem solving. Its role in emotional aspects of behavior, previously subsumed under the rubric of personality, has recently engendered renewed interest, as understanding of emotional processes has yielded better experimental tasks and measures for animal and human studies. With these developments, it has become clear that prefrontal cortex is a kind of melting pot for diverse influences on behavior and psychological processes, including cognitive, experiential, emotional and social–environmental. Optimally, the result can be a marvellous amplification of expertise and adaptation that permits individuals to accomplish goals they thought not possible, and to engage productively in many different facets of human experience throughout their life. Conversely, distortions and disruptions to adaptation can occur, leading to emotional imbalance, social impairment, and self-destructive patterns of behavior. Therefore, the understanding of this cerebral region, its interactions with other structures, its relation to patterns of behavior, and options for managing its dysfunction remain important areas of investigation.

This chapter is organized to address organizational and clinical aspects of the frontal lobe, including diagnosis and management of behavioral and emotional changes associated with focal frontal lobe damage. Sections focus on the neural and behavioral organization of the frontal lobe, common disease processes, illustrative clinical cases, frontal networks related to emotional processing, recovery of function, and treatment options after frontal damage.

Neural and behavioral organization of the frontal lobe

To uncover organizational features and operational properties of the frontal lobe, it is possible to draw upon both animal model and human subject data. Animal model studies include anatomical connections and neuronal responses to stimulus/task conditions, while human studies include functional brain imaging in normal individuals and experimental analysis of clinical cases with well-defined, focal frontal lesions. The following is intended to highlight findings from such studies to inform a working model of frontal lobe organization, emphasizing the prefrontal cortex and its interactions with other neural regions, but this is far from a comprehensive review. The reader is referred to recent books and special journal issues for more detailed discussions (e.g., Stuss and Benson, 1986; Uylings et al., 1990; Levin et al., 1991; Eslinger and Grattan, 1991; Grafman, 1995a; Krasnegor, Lyon and Goldman-Rakic, 1997).

Anatomic and physiologic observations in animal models

To mediate executive and regulatory aspects of behavior, the frontal lobes must be in a position to receive and evaluate diverse neural information about the organism, the environment, prior experiences, and expectancies in order to formulate and maintain appropriate goals that guide behavior. There must also be efferent pathways that influence perceptual, memory, and knowledge systems and, importantly, the motor system for preparation, implementation, and modification of responses. Such data have been derived from a large body of studies including those of Pandya and Kuypers (1969), Porrino, Crane and Goldman-Rakic (1981), Mesulam and Mufson (1982), Goldman-Rakic (1987), Barbas and Pandya (1989, 1991), Alexander, Crutcher and DeLong (1990), Fuster (1991), Goldman-Rakic and Friedman (1991), Cummings (1993), Ray and Price (1993) Barbas (1995), Grafman (1995b), Sirigu et al. (1995), Price, Carmichael and Drevets (1996), Dias, Robbins and Roberts (1996), and Watanabe (1996).

That the frontal lobe, particularly the prefrontal cortex, is organized to mediate such processes is suggested by the following.

- The cytoarchitecture of the prefrontal cortex is heterogeneous and includes diverse laminar organization, encompassing both neocortical (six-layer) and limbic (three to four layer) tissue features. Such organization may reflect architectonic stages and evolutionary trends of developmental complexity. Furthermore, physiological frameworks are present for both neocortical processing (such as temporary and long-term memory storage as well as associative mechanisms for decision-making) and limbic system processing (such as learning and emotions).

- Patterns of connectional anatomy indicate that prefrontal cortex is interconnected with cortical areas that have similar laminar organization. Thus, the auditory association cortices give rise to multiple projections to prefrontal cortex, with earlier association areas, for example, targeting certain prefrontal neurons, while later association areas target other prefrontal neurons. Similar patterns are observed from visual and somatosensory cortices as well. Therefore, a single, final projection pathway from a particular modal association region is apparently not as adaptive as waves of input reflecting different levels of associative analysis. The cumulative result is that prefrontal cortices receive diverse multimodal information that is well differentiated through keen sensory–perceptual processes linked with long-term memory or knowledge systems devoted to stimulus feature, spatial, language, and other domains.

- The prefrontal cortices are interconnected with several limbic and paralimbic system structures implicated in memory and emotion, including the amygdala, hippocampus, dorsomedial nucleus of the thalamus, temporal polar cortex, insula and anterior cingulate gyrus. The limbic areas of the prefrontal cortex, particularly the orbital and inferior mesial frontal regions, receive the strongest projections. Therefore, physiological and anatomical characteristics of prefrontal cortex suggest that convergent processing of cognitive and emotional streams of information is probable.

- Cortical and subcortical structures involved in somatic, visceral, autonomic, and hormonal mediation are interconnected with the prefrontal cortices, along with pathways to motor system structures of the basal ganglia, thalamus, and cortex. Therefore, the prefrontal cortices are in a position not only to monitor but also to influence such processes and effect specific actions and behavioral responses.

- The frontal lobe is interconnected with subcortical structures (particularly the basal ganglia via frontal–striatal projections, the thalamus via reciprocal projections, and limbic system nuclei such as the amygdala, septum, and dorsomedial nucleus of the thalamus via reciprocal connections) that operate in concert with frontal mechanisms and, when damaged, can cause frontal cortex-type impairments such as disinhibition, perseveration, disorganization, loss of initiation, emotional changes, inattention, and hemispatial neglect. Therefore, frontal–subcortical networks are an important extension to frontal cortex models.

- Neurons in the dorsolateral prefrontal cortex respond selectively to changing stimulus information that is needed for problem-solving and delayed responding (i.e., working memory). Such cells not only remain active during a delay interval when no stimulus is present, but also activate in coordination with certain interconnected subcortical structures such as the thalamus and hippocampus. Both dorsolateral and orbital prefrontal regions participate in such processes, providing response guidance for spatial/object processes as well as emotional/reward processes, and probably monitor and record the outcome of goal-directed behaviors.

- As with other neocortical regions, the prefrontal cortices have the capacity to store short-term and long-term information that is necessary in specific, temporary circumstances (e.g., working memory) and knowledge associated with a plethora of long-term goals that must be achieved in a step-by-step process over extended periods of time and that guide many daily behaviors. The time frame and detail of such knowledge are much broader and more complex than current concepts of working memory, and are probably related to mental models of events, actions, and goals that can span many years.

- Neurobehavioral studies of patients with focal lesions to the prefrontal cortices indicate that it is in the real-life handling of changing circumstances, long-term goals, and particularly social–emotional interactions that the impairments associated with frontal lobe lesions can be most effectively detected and surveyed. Impairments can include disorganization, loss of initiative, motivation and emotional expression, hypomania, irritability, euphoria, disinhibition and impulsivity, distractibility, perseveration, obsessive behaviors, apathy, poor memory, loss of insight and of discourse processing.

Many recent reports have described involvement of the prefrontal cortex in diverse cognitive operations that can be implemented during brain imaging studies of positron emission tomography (PET) and functional magnetic resonance imaging (fMRI). These innovative techniques have disclosed a similar wide range of cognitive processes that can entail activation of prefrontal cortex. Examples include deductive reasoning (Goel et al., 1998), interpretation of figurative aspects of language (Bottini et al., 1994), memory (Tulving et al., 1994), diverse working memory tasks in children and adults (e.g. Petrides et al., 1993; Jonides et al., 1993; Casey et al., 1995; Gold et al., 1996; Ungerleider et al., 1998), planning (Owen et al., 1996), language comprehension (Binder, 1997), verbal fluency (Paulesu et al., 1997), and semantic maps (Spitzer et al., 1998).

Specialized frontal regions and their damage in humans

From the available animal model studies and clinical studies of patients with focal frontal lobe disease, it has been possible to identify specialized regions that have distinctive anatomical, physiological, and clinical–behavioral characteristics. These particular profiles help define the functional organization of the frontal lobe. Seven specialized regions are described here: (1) the primary motor and lateral premotor cortices; (2) the superior mesial cortices; (3) the inferior mesial cortices; (4) the basal forebrain; (5) the orbito-frontal cortices; (6) the deep white matter pathways subjacent and adjacent to the frontal horns; and (7) the dorsolateral prefrontal cortices.

The anatomical characteristics of these regions are summarized in Table 8.1 and span motor, premotor, limbic, paralimbic, and prefrontal neural systems as well as deep white matter pathways. These regions are distinctive in terms of their structure–function correlations. Clinical impairments that can be associated with each region are summarized in Table 8.2 and as follows.

- The *primary motor and premotor cortices* are involved in the mediation of motor planning, programmed execution of movement, and coordination with sensory–perceptual systems. Input from prefrontal cortices, basal ganglia, and thalamus informs these areas of complex sensory–perceptual processing and decision-making choices that activate options and initiation of movement. Contralateral limb and facial weakness results from damage to primary cortex, according to homonuclear representation. Apraxia results from premotor cortex damage, including melokinetic and oral. Damage to the frontal operculum (areas 44, 45) on the left produces a nonfluent (Broca's) aphasia, whereas homotypic injury may disrupt emotional intonation of speech (aprosodia).
- The *superior mesial frontal region* is comprised of the supplementary motor area and anterior cingulate gyrus. These structures project to the basal ganglia and are interconnected with primary motor cortex, pons, and limbic system structures such as the anterior nucleus of the thalamus. Bilateral damage to superior mesial frontal structures from stroke, head trauma, and parsagittal tumors can cause profound disruption of initiation, motivation, and emotional processing, leading to akinesia and mutism. Unilateral lesions can also cause loss of spontaneous

Table 8.1. Anatomical features of specialized lobe regions

	Motor/lateral premotor	Superior mesial	Inferior mesial	Basal forebrain	Orbital	Deep white matter	Dorsolateral
Brodmann's cytoarchitectonic areas	4, 6 (lateral)	24, 6 (mesial)	25, 32, 14	–	10, 11, 12, 13, 14	–	8, 9, 10, 11, 43, 46, 47
Prominent anatomical landmarks	Central sulcus Precentral gyrus Broca's area (left)	Anterior cingulate gyrus Supplementary motor area	Subcallosal gyrus Mesial gyrus rectus	Septal nuclei Precommissural fornix Nucleus accumbens Substantia innominata Diagonal band of Broca	Gyrus rectus Olfactory tracts Orbital gyri	Rostral and lateral to frontal horns	Frontal gyri • inferior • medial • superior Frontal pole
Neural systems	Motor Premotor	Premotor Limbic	Paralimbic Prefrontal	Limbic	Paralimbic Prefrontal	Fronto-striatal Fronto-thalamic Fronto-limbic pathways	Prefrontal

Table 8.2. Prominent impairments associated with damage to specific frontal lobe regions

Motor/lateral premotor	Superior mesial	Inferior mesial	Frontal lobe regions		Orbital	Deep white matter	Dorsolateral
			Basal forebrain				
Hemiparesis	Akinesia/bradykinesia	Disinhibition	Amnesia		Personality change	Personality change	Disorganized thinking and behavior
Apraxia	Mutism	Lack of motivation	Confabulations		Impulsive actions	Poor empathy	Impaired working memory
Dysarthria	Apathy	Utilization behavior	Reduced motivation		Poor social judgment	Reduced emotions	Perseveration
Nonfluent asphasia (left)	Loss of motivation	Altered emotional processing			Reduced empathy	Irritability	Cognitive rigidity
Aprosodia (right)	Apraxia	Altered self-regulation			Lack of goal-directed behavior		Poor planning
	Alien hand				Altered self-regulation		Intentional disorders
	Grasp reflex				Environmental dependency		Impulsive responding
	Altered self-regulation						Inattention
	Intentional disorders						Stimulus-boundedness
							Lack of empathy
							Poor self-regulation
							Right
							Left hemispatial neglect
							Poor spatial cognition
							Left
							Transcortical motor aphasia

behavior, emotional expression, and initiation, but recovery is generally quicker and more complete than with bilateral lesions. The superior mesial frontal region also regulates certain aspects of intentional behavior, skilled motor behaviors, and response flexibility.

- The *inferior mesial frontal cortices* comprise a region whose functional significance is evolving. This region has strong connections with the limbic system, particularly the amygdala, and it probably plays an important role in emotional processing. It has been implicated in depression and bipolar disorder, and is often damaged along with the basal forebrain (i.e., from anterior communicating artery aneurysm) or the orbito-frontal cortex (e.g., meningioma). Isolated injury is rare, but has been associated with memory changes, spatial–temporal confusion, disinhibition, and possibly environmental dependency with utilization behavior.

- The *basal forebrain* includes several allied subcortical structures that are heavily limbic related and interconnect with amygdala, hippocampus, and ventral striatum. Damage is most often from ruptured anterior communicating artery aneurysms and may be limited to this region or more widespread and involve inferior medial and orbito-frontal cortices as well as basal ganglia. Memory impairment, confabulations, and motivational changes can occur.

- The *orbito-frontal* region is perhaps best known for its association with personality changes, disinhibition, and autonomic processing. It is strongly interconnected with limbic system structures, sensory association cortices, and dorsolateral prefrontal cortex as well as with autonomic/visceral centers in the hypothalamus and brainstem. It is likely to be a high convergence area for sensory–perceptual and emotion-related processing. Neuronal activation patterns suggest that outcome-based contingencies to behavior (e.g., reward, punishment) may be represented in orbito-frontal cortex, with more recent human studies suggesting that orbital damage significantly alters a patient's anticipation of future consequences of behaviors. Hence, impulsive actions and poor social judgment can be prominent deficits despite the lack of change in intellect, memory, perception, and language. Interpersonal behaviors are further marred by reduced empathy and related capacities to appreciate the situation and emotional experiences of others.

- *Deep white matter pathways* of the frontal lobe, subjacent and laterally adjacent to the frontal horns, may be particularly important because of their connections to other structures. The region includes frontal–limbic pathways (including the uncinate fasciculus) that involve the amygdala, temporal polar cortex, and anterior insula; frontal–striatal pathways that involve multiple prefrontal circuits through the head of the caudate (Alexander, Crutcher and DeLong, 1990; Cummings, 1993); and reciprocal frontal–thalamic pathways that involve anterior (VA and VL), and dorsomedial (DM) nuclei. Disconnection of some or all of these projection systems can occur after ischemic stroke in the rostral branches of the middle cerebral artery, traumatic brain injury, or rupture of anterior communicating artery aneurysms. The result can be a marked alteration in patients' emotional experience and expression, with irritability and reduced empathy.

• The *dorsolateral prefrontal cortex* has been subjected to close scientific scrutiny and appears to mediate a diversity of highly cognitive processes related to goal-directed achievements, organization and cognitive implementation of plans, coordination of attentional capacities, working memory, and cognitive aspects of relating to and understanding others. It receives and reciprocates very extensive projections from association cortices of the temporal, parietal, and occipital lobes, the orbital and inferior mesial frontal cortices, as well as the hippocampus and thalamus. It projects strongly to the basal ganglia as part of the cortico-striatal system.

Diseases causing focal frontal lesions

There are numerous diseases that can affect the frontal lobe. Whereas several occur within its anatomic borders, others extend to or emanate from adjacent cortical and subcortical structures. Among the more common causes of focal frontal lobe damage are the following:

• Ischemic and hemorrhagic infarctions of the anterior cerebral artery and more rostral branches of the middle cerebral artery.
• Rupture of anterior communicating artery aneurysms, usually with subsequent clipping to minimize hemorrhage.
• Arteriovenous malformations at cortical and subcortical levels, which can become hemorrhagic and require surgical resection.
• Tumors of benign and malignant nature.
• Traumatic brain injury from acceleration–deceleration forces, projectiles, and blunt forces causing diffuse axonal injury as well as localized contusions, lacerations, and hemorrhagic lesions, primarily to frontal and temporal lobe structures.
• Multiple sclerosis with demyelinating plaques in rostral white matter regions.
• Mass effects of hydrocephalus, including normal pressure hydrocephalus.
• Necrotic lesions in the mesial and orbital regions of the frontal lobe from herpes simplex encephalitis.
• Atypical forms of degenerative dementias affecting the frontal lobes, including Pick's disease, frontal lobe dementia, and frontal–temporal dementias.

Importantly, the physiological, anatomical, and chemical characteristics of each disease differ, causing variations in pathophysiology and clinical presentation. Some of the many variables are *momentum* of the lesion (e.g., slow-growing tumor, sudden occlusion of a vessel), the *anatomical location* (e.g., cortex, white matter, unilateral vs. bilateral, orbital vs. dorsolateral, single vs. multiple locations), *physiology* (e.g., epileptogenic, edematous), *occupation of space* (e.g., mass effect, shift), and cumulative effects of these variables. Furthermore, pathophysiology occurs within the context of each person's pattern of cerebral organization (e.g., language dominance), comorbid conditions, and neural response to disease. Therefore, heterogeneity in pathophysiology and in the functions subserved by the frontal lobes leads to an array of possible clinical presentations and subsequent patterns of impairment.

Illustrative cases of focal frontal damage

Right frontal lesion from head trauma causing executive function impairment in vocational activities

A 43-year-old, right-handed woman suffered head injury with loss of consciousness, skull and facial fractures when her vehicle collided with an oncoming truck. Brain computed tomography (CT) scan revealed right frontal contusion and small subdural hematoma. The woman was amnestic for the accident and suffered a two-week period of post-traumatic amnesia, being unable to recognize her friends. She returned to work as a secretary three months after the accident and reported in retrospect that she quickly became exhausted from trying to discharge her usual job responsibilities. She encountered numerous problems, such as forgetting how to sign on to the computer, difficulty keeping track of information, and being disorganized. Despite using extensive notes and doubling her efforts, she was eventually downgraded in her position to clerk and was assigned routine tasks such as copying, mail delivery, and filing. She came to our attention almost five years after the accident because she was about to lose the clerk position. Clinical neurological examination at that time was intact, but brain MRI scan showed a focal right frontal encephalomalacia in white matter, extending to lateral prefrontal cortex and to orbital cortex, essentially undercutting these cortical regions (Fig. 8.1).

Neurobehavioral examination revealed a pleasant woman with mild disinhibition, anxiety, and disorganization. She described having constantly to push herself through daily activities, and excessive worry about daily matters because they took so much effort and organization. She did not appear clinically depressed, but acknowledged more frequent mood swings, reduced motivation, and variable sleep due to anxiety about her problems.

Neuropsychological testing revealed impairments in working memory, set-shifting behaviors, mastering of sequential tasks, and spatial memory. When learning new material, she showed inefficiency and interference effects (e.g., significant disruption caused by introducing a second word list after learning the first one),

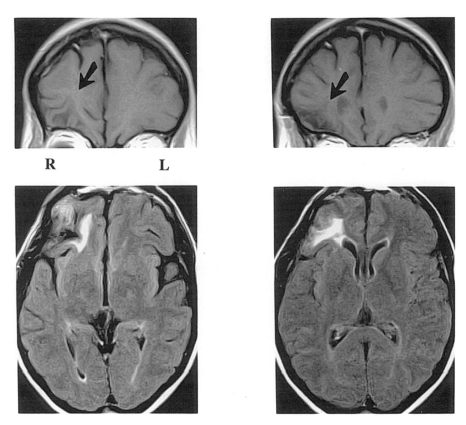

R   L

Fig. 8.1   Brain MRI scan demonstrating residual right prefrontal lobe lesion from traumatic brain injury. The upper images are T1 coronal sections showing orbital frontal damage. The lower images are T2 axial cuts showing orbital frontal cortex and white matter changes. The patient exhibited impairments in working memory, attentional regulation, and emotional processing.

which clearly limited her performance. Divided attention tasks (e.g., dichotic listening) were also confusing. However, parameters of general intelligence, orientation, basic attention, speech and language, visual, auditory, and tactile perceptual abilities, and motor function were all within normal limits.

In summary, despite clear improvements following the head injury five years previously, this patient continued to suffer noticeable effects of right frontal lobe traumatic lesion. The disorganizing effects of impaired working memory, sequencing behaviors, flexible thinking, and attentional regulation have caused her to lose her job as a secretary and barely hold onto a clerk-level position. Emotionally, she has experienced increased anxiety and mild depression. Fortunately, she has not shown disruptive behaviors or social misconduct, and in fact can be socially engaging and friendly. Her home life has been stable, and she has successfully engaged in

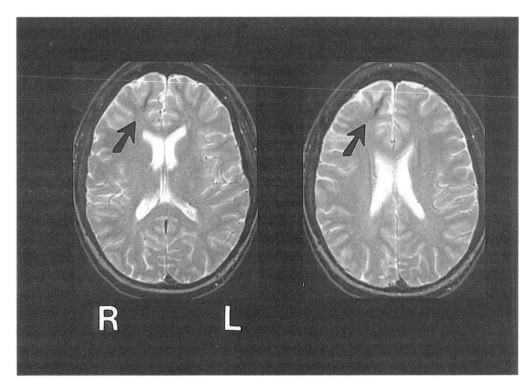

Fig. 8.2   Brain MRI scan showing residual scarring in prefrontal cortex from traumatic brain injury, associated with hypomanic behaviors in the chronic recovery phase.

part-time work helping older people in a local retirement community. In addition to psychotherapeutic work centered around head injury, adjustment, and emotional issues, the major focus of services was vocationally oriented, and concerned locating a more effective match between her abilities and work demands. At the present time, she is thriving in a receptionist position, possibly because of the strong environmental cuing and well-defined routines.

Frontal lesion from head trauma causing hypomania

A 35-year-old, right-handed woman suffered trauma-induced frontal lobe lesion from a motor vehicle accident seven years before presentation (see Fig. 8.2 for her brain MRI scan). Her primary complaint was difficulty maintaining a job. Interview and examination revealed a disinhibited young woman with pressured speech and hypomanic behaviors. Prior to her accident, she was an energetic person who had completed a college education and worked as a lending analyst, beginning a career in finance. After her accident, she held various jobs without success, each lasting usually two to three months before disorganization, frustration, and distractibility stymied her productivity. Interestingly, her job interviews were highly positive, with the impression of an energetic and enthusiastic employee. However, this impression gradually faded as interpersonal difficulties and erratic job performance became evident. Outside occupational areas, she experienced as much difficulty, with substance abuse, promiscuity, unstable relationships, and altercations with authority figures. Despite above-average intelligence and memory, deficits in executive functions were evident on neuropsychological testing, as might be predicted from her recent history. Certain improvements have been possible though. Treatment with Depakote (divalproex sodium) 250 mg t.i.d. has helped her racing thoughts, distractibility, and disinhibition. With clearer rational thoughts, she can cognitively self-regulate her excessive behaviors to some degree. In addition, a low-stimulus living environment, a well-structured job in one of her natural interests (care of horses at a local farm), and continuing behavioral–cognitive therapy have supported the highest adaptation and independent functioning since her accident.

Bilateral frontal lesion from explosion causing pervasive executive impairments

A 60-year-old, right-handed man underwent bifrontal craniotomy and debridement after an accidental explosion during pipe inspection that caused skull fracture, frontal lacerations, and hemorrhage (see Fig. 8.3 for his brain MRI scan). In the early rehabilitation stages, examination revealed a prominent amnesic syndrome along with executive function impairments that severely limited regulation of his attention, working memory, planning, problem-solving abilities, and self-monitoring capacities. Perseveration, disinhibition, and distractibility were evident, as was a new religious preoccupation that has become so pervasive that every conversation quickly becomes a recitation of recurring religious themes, regardless of questions asked, social context, and redirection. Because of motivational loss, bromocriptine treatment (5 mg b.i.d.) was used for a substantial period of time with beneficial effects. Over three years of recovery, significant improvements have been observed, but a highly structured schedule of family care and respite care continues to be necessary for his safety, daily activities, and socialization. The man's attentional regulation and memory have improved, but executive function impairments have remained. Left to his own devices, he becomes distracted, disorganized, and shows minimal motivation for goal-directed activities. There have been no signs of depression, but rather an indifferent attitude with occasional disinhibition in speech and behavior. However, the patient shows a remarkable sensitivity to the plight and illnesses of others, regularly attending church activities and visiting a nursing care facility where he enjoys socializing with residents.

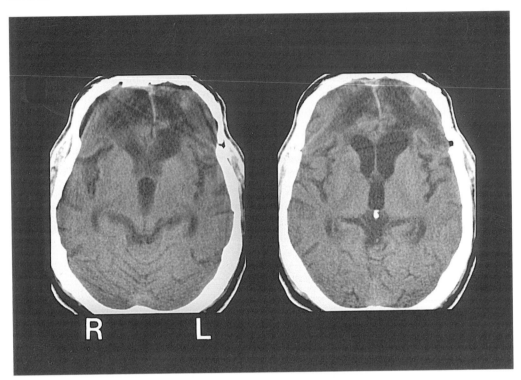

Fig. 8.3   Brain MRI scan showing extensive bilateral frontal lobe damage from a penetrating head injury requiring debridement. Severe executive function impairments continue to persist three years later.

Aneurysms causing focal frontal lobe lesion with memory and motivational changes

A 56-year-old, right-handed woman was surgically treated for a ruptured left pericallosal aneurysm (1995) and ruptured anterior communicating artery aneurysm (1997), the latter of which brought her to our attention. Following correction of the left pericallosal aneurysm (a distal branch of the anterior cerebral artery), hemorrhagic infarction affecting the medial frontal lobe caused personality change. This was described as reduced yet labile emotional expression, loss of motivation in work and leisure activities, and disinhibition in social discourse. Following rupture and surgical correction of the anterior communicating artery, forgetfulness and slower reading became evident. Results of a brain scan are shown in Fig. 8.4.

Neuropsychological examination revealed an alert and pleasant woman who was responsive to questions yet quite unsure of her response. Clear deficits were observed in measures of working memory, set-shifting, cognitive flexibility, and memory retrieval (recognition memory was intact, as were other cognitive parameters). The areas of greatest concern for this woman were her memory retrieval difficulties, lack of motivation, and lack of emotional intensity with family

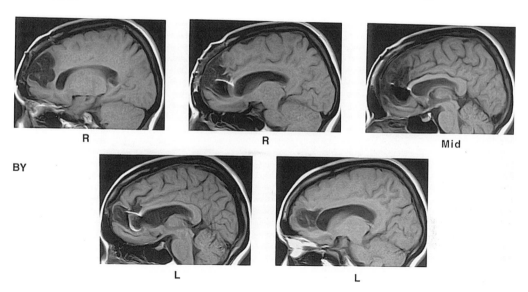

R   R   Mid

BY

L   L

Fig. 8.4   Brain MRI scan with sagittal views revealing bilateral mesial frontal damage from ruptured aneurysms. Changes in both motivation and memory were evident.

members. Memory difficulties were addressed by compensatory, self-cueing strategies geared to her part-time work (as a receptionist at a college fitness center) and other daily chores. A trial of bromocriptine 2.5 mg b.i.d., a postsynaptic dopamine agonist, was also undertaken, with the result of gradual improvement in her motivation and emotional responsiveness.

Prefrontal arteriovenous malformation with resection associated with developmental executive function impairments

At seven years of age, this right-handed boy with no neurologic history developed vomiting, seizures, and loss of consciousness, leading to discovery of right frontal intraparenchymal hemorrhage and diagnosis of a deep right frontal arteriovenous malformation requiring surgical treatment. There was no history of developmental, cognitive, or behavioral difficulties, and standardized academic testing just two months prior to symptoms showed all areas to be ≥75th percentile. The arteriovenous malformation was quite deep but successfully resected, and the boy has continued to recover and thrive. Brain MRI scan two years after hemorrhage (Fig. 8.5) revealed a focal area of hypodensity in the right dorsolateral prefrontal region. This involved predominantly Brodman's areas 9, 10, and 46 as well as 44, 45, and 47, including deep white matter and extending minimally into premotor cortex (area 6) and anterior insula.

The patient has been studied for four years after the hemorrhage. He has had exellent neurological outcome, with no motor, sensory, cranial nerve defects, or

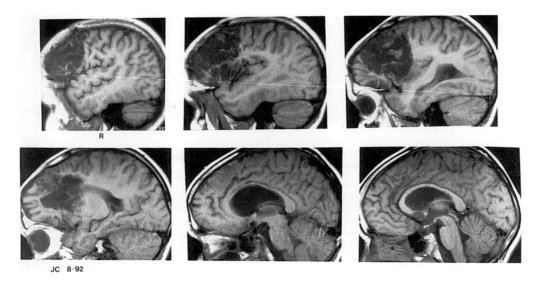

JC 8·92

Fig. 8.5   Chronic brain MRI scan of a 7-year-old boy demonstrating residual right dorsolateral
prefrontal cortex lesion, extending to the insula and deep white matter, after surgical
treatment of hemorrhagic arteriovenous malformation. Both acute and chronic effects on
social behavior and executive functions have resulted.

seizures. However, cognitive, behavioral, and social–emotional changes were
evident. A left hemispatial neglect with constructional apraxia and spatial planning
difficulties occurred. Spatial working memory impairment also posed problems, as
the patient could not keep track, for example, of offensive and defensive ends of a
basketball court; however, the coach did discover that simply shouting 'offense'
and 'defense' as the team went up and down the court solved the confusion.
Behaviorally, the boy was fidgety, distractible, and impulsive. He could not complete multistep tasks without persistent cueing. Socially, he appeared to regress,
preferring younger playmates and solitary activities.

Since these initial effects, the patient has shown continuing gains. The hemispatial neglect resolved, constructional praxis and spatial planning have improved,
but working memory limitations remain in multistep activities and judging
amounts of time. Measured intelligence and academic levels have remained above
average, but adjustments at school were necessary, with support services similar to
those provided for children with attentional deficit/hyperactivity disorder. Detailed
evaluation of age-appropriate executive functions shows disproportionate difficulties in the following areas: spatial working memory tasks such as delayed spatial
responding and delayed alternation (verbal working memory was normal),
complex spatial planning (e.g., Tower of Hanoi tasks), attentional control/inhibi-
tion, visual processing speed, cognitive flexibility (particularly spatially oriented

tasks, but performance on the Wisconsin Card Sorting Test was normal), organization of verbal learning (organizational strategies were poor), and social discourse (disorganization and simplified narratives caused a greater listener burden for others).

As the patient enters early adolescence, social issues are becoming more of a concern, but have not been problematic in the 7–11-year-old period. These new concerns involve understanding the intentions of others based on their comments, understanding group dynamics, and anticipating social circumstances. The patient interprets social interactions in quite literal ways. However, because his verbal processing is well above average, compensatory strategies that utilize verbal mediation (such as rules of conduct) may become increasingly important for mid-adolescent adjustment.

The findings from this case and other childhood frontal lesion cases (see Eslinger, Biddle and Grattan, 1997, for review) have supported the following conclusions about developmental prefrontal processes:

- School, daily living, and social–emotional difficulties can be related to altered maturation of executive functions and not basic cognitive deficiencies in intelligence, memory, or perception. The excutive function domains affected can include working memory, spatial planning, attentional control/inhibition, processing speed, cognitive flexibility, organization and efficiency of learning, and discourse. An acquired form of attention deficit/hyperactivity disorder may be evident.
- Social–emotional maturation can be affected by early prefrontal damage, becoming most evident in adolescence, sometimes several years after cerebral damage, suggesting that a delayed *arrest* of social maturation can occur.
- Childhood-onset prefrontal damage can cause certain types of early deficits also observed in adults (e.g., left hemispatial neglect), suggesting a key role for prefrontal system in developing cognitive and behavioral processes. Certain of these deficits appear to recover quickly, whereas others gradually emerge and progressively worsen over time, especially as more complex demands occur in educational, vocational, and social–emotional spheres.

Ischemic stroke affecting deep frontal pathways and social–emotional behavior

A 49-year-old college-educated man suffered a right middle cerebral artery ischemic stroke affecting the deep white matter pathways of the frontal lobe as well as portions of the insula and temporal lobe (Fig. 8.6). As a result, he developed a predominant change in personality, particularly in emotional processing, social behavior, and interactive decision-making. His cognitive changes were minimal and neurologic symptoms were mild, with left-sided weakness and a feeling of

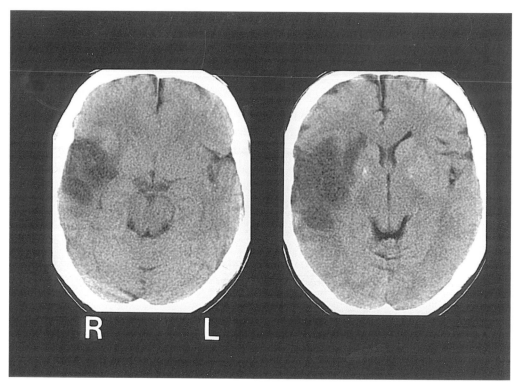

Fig. 8.6   Brain CT scan showing a right middle cerebral artery stroke affecting deep white matter pathways of the frontal lobe, as well as portions of the premotor and motor cortex, anterior insula, and temporal lobe. The frontal white matter lesion may have disrupted limbic, basal ganglia, and thalamic projection systems. Prominent social–emotional changes were associated with this lesion.

coldness in his left upper extremity. However, great distress was reported by his family, including his spouse of 25 years and three children, who noted that the patient had complete loss of emotional animation, social spontaneity, and empathy. Prosody of voice and facial expressions showed little to no emotional inflections. Interactive decision-making and interpersonal dynamics were awkward because of the patient's new insensitivity to others' feelings, intentions, and emotional comments of humor, sarcasm, and items of personal importance. The patient failed to understand his family's concerns. He denied depression, showed no vegetative changes, and was content to seek few social interactions, despite the fact that he successfully returned to work as a systems accountant. His family interpreted his behavior as intentional lack of interest and insensitivity, because he expresses what is on his mind without the grace, humor, and consideration he showed before his stroke.

Interventions focused around three goals. First, treatment with Prozac led to some improvement in the man's spontaneous emotional expressions, but he continued to articulate quite clearly that he felt few emotions and furthermore had little need to feel emotions. Increasing Prozac to 40 mg q.d. had no added effect. Reducing Prozac dosage and adding a low-dose of amitriptyline (50 mg q.h.s.) led to further improvement in emotional expressiveness and reduction of the cold sensations he experienced in his left upper extremity. Second, as a highly intelligent and even insightful person (e.g., he readily acknowledged his emotional changes but was not concerned about them), individual psychotherapy addressed his perception and understanding of his family's distress at losing the 'emotional' side of him. After he came to understand this more clearly, behavioral changes began to occur. His discussions and interactions with family members increased. He initiated questions about their everyday activities. This occurred despite the fact that he continued to report few emotional states or needs. His compensatory emotional behaviors appeared to be a response to his family's need for such behaviors rather than a natural expression from him. Finally, family therapy focused on the family members' need to recognize and understand their 'emotional loss' despite the fact the patient was otherwise functioning at his prestroke baseline.

The personality change in this patient can probably be related to his acquired inability to experience emotional states, to express himself emotionally, and to utilize emotional processing to understand and relate to others (i.e., a primary defect in empathy). From another perspective, the patient's attribution of salience or meaningfulness, conveyed through emotional processing, appeared to be minimal. In a small series of case comparisons, we previously described a characteristic anatomic difference between favorable and unfavorable recovery outcomes in patients with frontal lobe lesions (Grattan and Eslinger, 1991). In particular, unfavorable outcome was associated with damage to the periventricular region of the left or right frontal lobe, specifically the deep white matter pathways rostral and lateral to the frontal horn, including frontal–limbic and frontal–striatal pathways (see Fig. 8.8 in the section on Recovery and treatment options after frontal lobe lesion). These were the frontal areas that remained after 'subtracting' the locations of other unilateral frontal lesions that did not cause such effects. Damage to the anterior insula also occurred in these cases. Because of its involvement in autonomic regulation, damage to the insula may be an important structural component of this syndrome.

Anterior cerebral artery ischemic stroke causing akinesia and mutism

A 34-year-old man developed severe headache, nausea, and lethargy, prompting evaluation and leading to a diagnosis of subarachnoid hemorrhage from anterior cerebral artery aneurysm. Clipping was successfully completed, but postoperative vasospasm led to bilateral infarction of the anterior cerebral arteries (Fig. 8.7). The

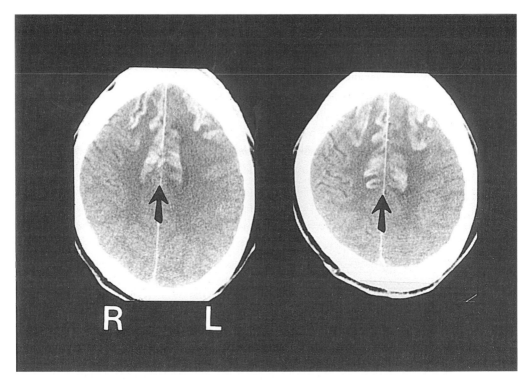

Fig. 8.7   Brain CT scan of a patient with profound akinesia and mutism. The lesion involved bilateral structures of the mesial frontal lobe including the anterior cingulate and supplementary motor area.

lesion involved inferior and superior aspects of the mesial frontal lobe, including the anterior cingulate and supplementary motor area. Examination revealed an alert patient with minimal responsiveness. He did not initiate speech or other spontaneous behaviors, but occasionally offered brief, correct verbal responses, which lasted for one to two queries, and then lapsed into nonresponsiveness. After a few minutes and a change of topics, he again would verbally respond briefly. When shown the Cookie Theft picture of the Boston Diagnostic Aphasia Exam, he responded 'She's washing the cookie mess.' On different occasions, he could complete three simple written calculations, copy simple geometric designs, and identify the faces of recent presidents before he discontinued responding and became quietly vigilant to events around him. Neurological examination indicated that he could move his upper extremities with purpose and without weakness. He was paraparetic with hyperreflexia in the lower extremities. He was treated with bromocriptine, gradually increasing the dosage to 7.5 mg b.i.d. This appeared to accelerate his improvement, with gains in fluency of speech, initiation, and safety judgment. Responses to greetings, questions, and commands improved to 50%

consistency. He continued with rehabilitation services, transitioning to outpatient care, and continued with bromocriptine treatment.

Frontal networks related to emotional processing

In reviewing the historic and recent human case studies of the remarkable and puzzling effects of focal prefrontal cortex damage, we observed that depression has not been an evident concern. The cases of Phineas Gage (Harlowe, 1848, 1868), Joe A (Brickner, 1936), KM (Hebb, 1945; Hebb and Penfield, 1940), JP (Ackerly and Benton, 1948; Ackerly, 1964; Benton, 1991a), EVR (Eslinger and Damasio, 1985), GK and MH (Price et al., 1990); PL (Marlowe, 1992), DT (Eslinger, Grattan and Damasio, 1992), as well as those of JC and MJ (Eslinger et al., 1997) have *not* been notable for depressive behaviors or symptoms. On the contrary, several of these individuals were better known for their gregariousness, bravado, euphoria, and ready initiation in social contexts, albeit poorly regulated and disinhibited. However, these subjects constitute a select sample, and whether such observations have minimized the extent of emotional impairments in frontal lobe lesion patients can reasonably be questioned. Indeed, recent studies suggest that release changes such as disinhibition, and hypomania may be only one side of the coin, as depression has also been reported as a consequence of stroke, trauma, and tumors affecting the frontal lobe.

Cerebral tumors

A recent study of early postoperative mood changes after cerebral tumors in 141 patients (Irle et al., 1994) indicated that negative mood was most evident after ventral-frontal and temporal-parietal tumors. Lesions of the ventral-frontal group involved orbital prefrontal cortex (areas 10, 11, 12, 13) as well as inferior mesial frontal structures (e.g., areas 24, 25, 32), and some dorsolateral regions (e.g., areas 9, 45, 46). Lesions of the temporal-parietal group damaged posterior, multimodal association cortices (e.g., heteromeral regions such as areas 20, 21, and 22 in the temporal lobe and areas 39 and 40 in the parietal lobe), but also extended to limbic/paralimbic structures such as the amygdala, hippocampus, and insula. These patients reported that in the ten-day postoperative period, they experienced more of an increase in fatigue, irritability/anger, and anxiety/depression than other tumor groups. Although right, left, and bilateral hemisphere lesion groups did not show overall differences in emotional measures, right posterior lesion subjects had significantly worse mood states than anterior lesion subjects and left posterior lesion subjects. Interestingly, type of tumor, lesion size, edema, and degree of mass effect did not contribute statistically to differences in mood state. However, female patients reported more negative mood symptoms than males, particularly in the ventral-frontal and parietal-temporal groups. In contrast, all other groups reported an improvement in mood following surgical treatment, including those with motor cortex tumors, medial temporal tumors, and large frontal-temporal-parietal tumors. The investigators emphasized that it may be a combination of damage to heteromeral association cortices in the frontal or temporal-parietal regions together with limbic-paralimbic structural involvement that cause the most negative mood effects in the early recovery phase after the surgical treatment of cerebral tumors. Follow-up studies should disclose long-term patterns and overall outcome.

Stroke

Cerebrovascular disease causes lesions of the prefrontal cortex and white matter that are frequently different from those associated with traumatic brain injury (TBI) and tumor. Unlike tumor, the onset is sudden and dependent upon the particular branches of the anterior and middle cerebral arteries that are occluded. Unlike TBI, accompanying diffuse effects such as axonal injury are not a concern. Unlike both tumor and TBI, cerebrovascular damage to orbital and polar prefrontal regions is infrequent, whereas damage to lateral and mesial prefrontal structures is more common. Therefore, these and other factors contribute to somewhat different behavioral and mood presentations, prompting a different set of diagnostic and treatment issues.

Some of the most comprehensive survey work in assessing the frequency, characteristics, and long-term outcome of mood after stroke has come from Robinson and colleagues (see Robinson, 1997, for review). In recent years, the initial conclusion that depression is more frequent as small lesions in the hemisphere moved anteriorly and lesions in the right hemisphere moved posteriorly (Robinson et al., 1984) has been further elaborated, as follows.

- Women reported more symptoms of depression up to two years post-stroke (Schultz et al., 1997).
- Lesions involving the left prefrontal cortex or left basal ganglia caused most frequent depression (9/12 cases with depressive disorder), followed by right hemisphere lesions (5/17 cases with depressive disorder) (Morris et al., 1996b). The authors did not differentiate prefrontal from basal ganglia lesion cases.
- Comparison of cases with new-onset cerebrovascular disease ($n=193$) showed no specific anatomic associations with depression, except among those with comparable small-sized lesions in whom left hemisphere stroke caused more frequent depression (31%) than right hemisphere stroke (16%) (Morris et al., 1996a).
- Depression at two months after stroke was found to be associated with slower

recovery 14 months later in cognitive screening, functional status, and deterioration over time, but no difference in recovery of activities of daily living (Morris, Raphael and Robinson, 1992).

- The association of left anterior lesions with major depression held for subjects with typical occipital-frontal asymmetry on brain CT scan, but not for subjects with reversed cerebral asymmetry (Starkstein et al., 1991).
- Among subjects with right hemisphere stroke ($n=93$), 18% developed major depression, 12% developed minor depression, 20% showed unduly cheerful behavior, and 50% showed no mood changes. Right stroke subjects with major depression had a higher frequency of parietal lobe lesion and family history of psychiatric disorder. Undue cheerfulness was associated predominantly with right frontal opercular lesions (Starkstein et al., 1989).
- PET studies of post-stroke patients have suggested that right stroke is associated with an increase in serotonin receptor binding, while left stroke does not show such an increase. Among left stroke patients, lower serotonin receptor binding is associated with more severe depression.

Frontal lobe imaging with depressed and bipolar disorder patients

A different approach to the study of mood disorders and frontal lobe mechanisms has been to investigate the functional brain activity of well-defined psychiatric groups with PET. Drevets et al. (1997) identified drug-free patients meeting the criteria for the bipolar disorder–depressed phase and who also had a parent or sibling with probable or definite bipolar disorder. Brain imaging analysis compared the bipolar–depressed group with controls. Results indicated that the subgenual prefrontal cortex showed the largest absolute difference in mean blood flow, with a 7.7% decrement. This region is described as agranular frontal cortex, subjacent to the genu of the corpus callosum and part of the rostral extent of anterior cingulate gyrus. Reduced cerebral glucose metabolism confirmed this abnormality in another sample of bipolar–depressed subjects relative to controls, with a 16.3% decrease in mean normalized metabolism and an 18.5% decrease in mean blood flow. Similar decrements were also evident with a sample of familial pure depression, but this region was actually more active in a small group of bipolar patients in the manic phase. Finally, anatomic measurements from MRI revealed that left subgenual frontal gray matter volume was reduced by 39% in bipolar subjects and by 48% in unipolar depression subjects compared to controls. No differences were evident in right subgenual cortex or other portions of the anterior cingulate gyrus. This anatomic region has been associated with emotional behavior, given its prominent connections with the amygdala, other limbic system structures and diverse medial frontal areas mediating autonomic functions and limbic processing.

Recent animal model studies of emotion-related frontal networks

There is a strong interrelationship between limbic system and prefrontal cortex processing. In posterior orbital and mesial prefrontal regions in particular, there are identified limbic and paralimbic structures as well as pathways from other limbic system structures (Barbas 1995; Price et al., 1996). Recent animal model research has identified both limbic-related cortical trends in the prefrontal cortex and distinctive orbital and medial-orbital networks with strong limbic system influences.

Barbas (1995; Barbas and Pandya, 1989, 1991) has described two major trends in prefrontal cortex development that appear to emanate from frontal limbic tissue. These are labelled as *basoventral* and *mediodorsal*. The basoventral trend arises from the agranular limbic cortex of the posterior orbitofrontal region and gradually increases in cell layers and definition as it spreads rostrally and laterally (through granular cortical areas 13, 14, 12, 11, and 10) onto the lateral prefrontal surface to the inferior bank of the arcuate sulcus, including ventral areas 46 and 8. The progressive architectonic stages within the mediodorsal prefrontal trend emanate from the agranular medial limbic cortex around the genu of the corpus callosum. The stages spread rostral-medially to the frontal pole and then culminate in the dorsal bank of the arcuate sulcus, to areas 46 and 8. In both architectonic trends, there is gradual laminar development and differentiation from three-layer limbic cortex to six-layer prefrontal cortical areas with the most distinctive laminar borders (areas 46 and 8). Barbas also suggests that this organizational framework is reflected in the patterns of cortical–cortical projections of the prefrontal cortex. Specifically, prefrontal areas appear to be interconnected with other cortical regions of similar laminar definition. Thus, inputs from auditory association cortices, for example, arrive in multiple pathways to different prefrontal regions, possibly underlying parallel processing for different purposes. Such parallel cortical–cortical pathways might include mediation of working memory, establishing the intention of others (e.g., theory of mind processing), problem-solving, and regulating divided and modality specific attentional pools.

Based upon other connectional anatomy studies in the nonhuman primate, Price et al. (1996) have identified distinctive *orbital* and *medial-orbital* prefrontal networks. The orbital network comprises most of the orbitofrontal cortex (including areas 10, 11, 12, 13, and 14). The authors suggest it is organized to provide mechanisms for the convergence of several unimodal sensory inputs including olfaction, taste, somatosensory, visual, and visceral. These projections arrive initially in posterior and lateral orbitofrontal regions (areas 13, 12 and adjacent rostral-inferior insula), then converge in more central orbitofrontal cortex (areas 13 and 11). The latter are interconnected with the medial orbitofrontal cortex where there is substantial limbic system input. The orbital network, therefore, may be in a position to receive and integrate sensory processing with limbic system processing, particularly when stimulus items have specific reinforcement contingencies. In contrast, the medial-orbital network proposed by Price and colleagues has intense projections with other medial prefrontal areas (including areas 24, 32, 10, 25, and 14) and appears to be distinct from the orbital network since few labelled cells from tract-tracing experiments appear in orbitofrontal cortices. The medial-orbital network is also interconnected with structures different from the orbital network, including multimodal integration areas of the superior temporal sulcus and the cingulate gyrus. Both networks receive projections from the amygdala, with the most intense pathways reaching the posterior and medial orbitofrontal cortex. Finally, these regions participate in a larger neural network that includes interconnections with the dorsomedial nucleus of the thalamus, the amygdala, ventral striatum, and ventral pallidum, where limbic and neocortical influences on motor behaviors can occur.

Given such well-formulated networks involving orbitofrontal cortices, their functional significance can be further illuminated by physiological recording studies. Rolls and colleagues (e.g., Thorpe, Rolls and Maddison, 1983; Wilson and Rolls, 1990; Rolls, 1990) have described some functional properties of single orbito-frontal neurons in the alert monkey. These data indicate that orbito-frontal neurons may reflect the motivational significance of stimuli in ways that are more selective and flexible than noncortical areas of the basal forebrain and hypothalamus, which can also activate with rewards of food and juice. Two-thirds of the orbito-frontal neurons recorded were selective in responding to specific food items and to specific aversive stimuli such as hypertonic saline presented through visual and gustatory modalities. Response latencies of cells were consistent with projections from modal association cortices. Interestingly, several cells also showed selective bimodal responding, such as the same cell activating to the sight of a banana and independently to the taste of banana, suggesting some potential for cross-modal recognition and matching of stimuli. In addition to sensory coding, orbito-frontal neurons appear to encode representational knowledge such as the reward value or motivational significance of stimuli. *Conditional orbito-frontal neurons* responded differentially to stimuli depending upon reward value in a go/no go discrimination task. In the front arm of the task, subjects readily learned that one of the two stimuli signalled a flavorful liquid reward, whereas the other signaled a mildly aversive liquid. When the reward contingency was then reversed, conditional orbito-frontal neurons quickly began activating to the other stimulus, which now signalled reward. Since the sensory coding aspects of the task obviously remained the same and could not explain the difference, such neurons nonetheless 'showed clear dependence on the reward value of the stimuli' (Thorpe et al., 1983). However, the complexity of such processing in orbito-frontal neurons was even greater, as there was an interaction between initial selectivity of sensory coding and reward contingencies. That is, orbito-frontal neurons responded to stimuli that sig- nalled reward only when they also responded selectively to the sensory features of the stimuli in the first place. These complex features of physiological activity could not be accounted for solely by sensory properties of the stimuli or by the reinforce- ment contingencies alone. Rather, the data suggest that orbito-frontal neurons are involved in the mediation of representational knowledge that has the capacity to guide behavioral responses, i.e., working memory. However, in contrast to what has been demonstrated for sensory and spatial aspects of working memory in dorso- lateral neurons of the nonhuman primate (e.g., Goldman-Rakic, 1987; Fuster, 1991; Wilson et al., 1993), the guidance of behavior via orbito-frontal systems may include specific and changing stimulus–reward associations that the organism must record, bear in mind, and activate when faced with behavior choices (i.e., emotion-related working memory). Finally, certain orbito-frontal neurons were found in these studies to activate selectively around the time the choice was being made to respond or not to respond.

Human emotional processing after frontal lobe lesion

Although the aforementioned data are preliminary and require much greater elab- oration, they raise the possibility of understanding how some of the functions involving orbito-frontal and inferior mesial frontal cortices may affect motivational and social–emotional aspects of human behavior when cerebral damage occurs to these regions. The erroneous coding of specific stimulus-reinforcement contingen- cies could easily alter the motivational forces that drive goal-directed behavior, but in more abstract and complex ways than a food or liquid reward. What a person gains, for example, from productive vocational behaviors are secondary rewards (e.g., money) that can bring safety, shelter, food, leisure activities, care of family, etc. Identifying, encoding, and implementing those select stimulus–response actions that earn such reward constitute a demanding and immense process that encompasses tremendous variance and potential for change as well. Erratic encod- ing of those specific stimuli and their representations that guide what needs to be done when, would seem disabling enough, but additional erratic encoding of their changing reinforcement contingencies would further exacerbate the problem, and may be part of the reason that many frontal-damaged patients (particularly orbito- frontal damage) cannot benefit from insight-oriented therapy and instructions that clearly lay out the significant stimuli and their reinforcement contingencies.

Empirical support for some of these notions has been provided through the his- toric case of Phineas Gage (Harlowe, 1848, 1868; Stuss, Gow and Hetherington, 1992; Damasio et al., 1994), the case studies of EVR (Eslinger and Damasio, 1985; Damasio, Tranel and Damasio, 1991), DT (Eslinger et al., 1992), and other ventral frontal lesion cases (Grafman et al., 1986; Rolls et al., 1994). Rolls et al. (1994) recently described a study in which patients with ventral frontal and nonfrontal lesions had first to learn a straightforward stimulus–reward association and then alter their response when the reinforcement contingencies changed. After subjects acquired 90% correct recognition of one of two simple visual patterns on a computer monitor, the relation between stimulus patterns and their consequences (either correct or incorrect choice) was reversed or extinguished. In the reversal task, the other visual pattern now signalled a correct choice, while in the extinction task neither pattern was correct and the subject needed simply to advance to the next trial. Subjects with ventral frontal lesions from diverse etiologies performed more poorly than other brain-damaged subjects, despite the fact that they detected a change in the reinforcement contingencies. Significant correlations were obtained between reversal and extinction task scores and a questionnaire that surveyed problematic behaviors such as disinhibition, social difficulties, lack of initiative, perseveration, and other impairments associated with frontal damage ($r = 0.69$, $p < 0.01$ for reversal; and $r = 0.61$, $p < 0.023$ for extinction). No correlations were evident for verbal IQ or paired associate learning. Interestingly, three of the ventral frontal damage subjects with reversal and/or extinction impairment were also tested with the Tower of London task and found to be normal. This task, which requires planning and well-organized problem solving, has been associated most frequently with dorsolateral prefrontal cortex function. Two patients from the brain-injured control group had dorsolateral prefrontal lesions, and both showed the opposite dissociation from the ventral frontal-damaged subjects: impaired Tower of London score but normal reversal and extinction scores.

In a series of studies, Damasio and colleagues have investigated cognitive and psychophysiological aspects of decision-making in patients with ventromedial prefrontal lesions (Damasio et al., 1991; Bechara et al., 1994, 1996). The patients targeted for study had lesions affecting orbital and inferior mesial prefrontal regions. Emphasis was placed on assessing the capacities of patients to show selective autonomic activation to photos depicting emotion-laden stimuli (e.g., scenes of disaster, mutilation, and nudity) and to a card-sorting task that resulted in monetary profits and losses according to the patient's choices. Autonomic activation was measured via electrodermal skin conductance responses. When patients with ventromedial prefrontal lesions passively viewed the pictures, they failed to generate normal skin conductance responses despite intact autonomic activation to orienting stimuli. This was in striking contrast to normal control and brain-damaged control samples (the latter with lesions to premotor, temporal, parietal, and occipital cortices). When ventromedial prefrontal lesion subjects were required to respond verbally to each picture with a description or impression, significant autonomic activation was observed. Autonomic activation was not observed when patients verbally responded to intermixed photos of neutral objects. The pattern of findings was interpreted as consistent with the decision-making impairments of these patients, particularly in personal and social contexts. Such impairments, not apparent via standard neuropsychological tests, were related to defective activation of somatic states and altered autonomic regulation caused by ventromedial prefrontal lesions, a neural region positioned not to only receive extensive projections relevant to visceral, somatic, and sensory processing, but also to influence efferent autonomic centers (Nauta, 1971; Neafsey, 1990). Further studies have extended these findings to an experimental decision-making task in which patients with ventromedial prefrontal lesions failed to adjust their choices according to future consequences or longer-term outcome, whether positive or negative. It was the more immediate consequences that guided their actions. Interestingly, during the task, these patients also failed to develop anticipatory skin conductance responses to card choices that generally signalled more monetary loss or negative consequences over time, even though an individual card may lead lead to an initial gain in assets. Since patients responded autonomically to initial gains and losses, they showed neural evidence of recognition of positive and negative consequences, but apparently could not utilize such experience to anticipate overall outcome of their choices.

Emotion recognition and expression after frontal lobe lesion

Recognition of emotional facial expressions is a key perceptual process in understanding the emotional intent and emotional states of others, and hence essential for gauging how best to respond to others. Available studies suggest an important role of the right cerebral hemisphere in emotional perception processes, whether in face or voice recognition (DeKosky et al., 1980; Blonder, Bowers and Heilman, 1991; see review by Borod, 1992). In a recent study comparing patients with left or right cerebral lesions on an emotional face perception task, Adolphs et al. (1996) required subjects to judge 39 photographical expressions according to each of six emotions: happy, sad, disgusted, angry, afraid, and surprised. Results indicated that only patients with *right* cerebral lesions showed difficulties, particularly those whose lesions involved the inferior parietal cortex and the infracalcarine cortex. Although all patients accurately identified happy facial expressions, recognition of negative emotions was more difficult, with recognition of fearful expressions being most impaired, followed by anger and sadness. These findings are consistent with the larger literature suggesting a dominant role for the right hemisphere in the perception of emotional facial expressions independent of any deficits in non-emotional facial perception. Data have not suggested a specific or disproportionate role for the prefrontal cortex in such tasks, with the exception of the recent study by Hornak, Rolls and Wade (1996). These investigators reported that acquired lesions, predominantly to the ventral frontal lobe from stroke, head injury, and colloid cyst with acute hydrocephalus, resulted in defective perceptual discrimination of facial emotional expressions (i.e., nine of 12 subjects impaired). The scores were significantly more impaired than those of nonventral frontal brain-damaged and normal control samples. Furthermore, significant relationships were found between facial expression score and inventories of subjective emotional change and social behavior. Similar, though less striking, findings have been reported with the perception of emotional intonations of speech (i.e., prosody). With regard to subjective emotional experience, which has usually been probed only for symptoms of depression, the ventral and medial prefrontal regions may mediate important aspects of emotional experience, suggested not only by the anatomical data indicating strong amygdala and other limbic projections to these areas (e.g. Barbas, 1995; Price et al., 1996), but also by PET data indicating differential activation of these prefrontal regions with emotional states (Lane et al., 1997).

Studies and observations of emotional expression after frontal cortex damage have indicated a mixed picture. As with other aspects of behavior after frontal damage, impairments will be variable because of altered regulation. These can include overactive (e.g., hypomanic, aggressive, hypersexual, and disinhibited expression, obsessive–compulsive behaviors) as well as erratic and underactive (e.g., lability, blunted affect, akinetic-mutism, apathy) forms of emotional expression and emotional experience. Both spontaneous and posed forms of emotional expression can be reduced in frequency, intensity, and accuracy (Damasio and Van Hoesen, 1983; Weddell, Miller and Trevarthen, 1990; Borod, 1992). This obtains for facial, vocal, and gestural aspects of emotional communication. Interestingly, there may be an important interaction to consider in such research; namely, individual differences in emotional reactivity and right–left frontal lobe activation patterns. Davidson and colleagues have suggested that the frontal lobe may be a major neural substrate influencing emotional reactivity. Specifically, asymmetries in baseline or resting levels of right–left frontal electrophysiological activity may indicate very different temperament patterns. Individuals with predominant left frontal activation have been described as experiencing more intense positive affect and less intense negative affect to positive and negative emotional stimuli, respectively. Individuals with predominant right frontal activation show the reverse pattern of emotional reactivity (e.g., Davidson, 1984; Wheeler, Davidson and Tomarken, 1993). These emotional reactivity patterns have also been correlated to approach-avoidance tendencies, and are viewed as contributing causes rather than sole determinants of emotional responses. Such differences may be important for neural models of cerebral damage and emotion, whether poststroke depression studies, emotional expression, or related-emotion processing.

Alterations in empathy as a core deficit after frontal lobe lesions

How a person relates to others within his or her family, community, school/occupational setting, and other situations that bring people together provides the foundation for diverse relationships that serve many personal and societal purposes. Empathy has been conceptualized as a *binding force* among people, vital to many types of relationships and interpersonal behaviors, and hence an adaptive mechanism for understanding others and sharing common experiences (Eslinger, 1998). Given that frontal lobe syndromes are often characterized by profound disturbances in how people relate to others, the investigation of empathy and related processes may be a fruitful approach to the social impairments associated with frontal lobe damage.

Historically, empathy has been described primarily in emotional terms; that is, sharing of emotional experiences with others and sensitivity to the emotional experiences of others. More recent accounts, though, have also identified cognitive processes contributing to empathy such as role-taking and perspective-taking. Such cognitive–empathic processes are separate from sharing of emotional experiences, and probably rely upon complex forms of thinking that lead to an understanding of what others experience (i.e., theory of mind processes). From a neuropsychological perspective, empathic processes entail not only complex mental models of human experience but also capacities to consider such experiences within different contexts and from different vantage points, i.e., cognitive flexibility. Generating different possibilities to a problem or question, shifting a response pattern to an alternative approach, and adjusting to changing environmental contingencies are examples of the flexibility of cognition that have been associated with prefrontal networks. Hence, emphatic processes may well be intertwined with executive functions such as cognitive flexibility and similarly affected by damage to prefrontal networks.

We examined these possibilities in a series of studies. Initially, we found that 56% of a diverse neurologic sample generated self-report scores on a standardized empathy inventory (Hogan, 1969) that were greater than two standard deviations below the mean (Grattan and Eslinger, 1989). The results were similar whether generated from self-report of patients or patient ratings by family members. Significant correlations in the 0.5–0.6 range were evident between empathy scores and measures of cognitive flexibility, suggesting a similar effect of cerebral injury on both types of processes.

In a separate study, patients with focal frontal lobe lesions were investigated. The results varied according to the specific location of the frontal injury (Grattan et al., 1994). Dorsolateral prefrontal lesions resulted in correlated changes in empathy and cognitive flexibility tasks such as Wisconsin Card Sorting Test. Findings were statistically significant for the left dorsolateral prefrontal lesion sample ($r=0.76$–0.81), with the right dorsolateral prefrontal lesion sample showing a similar pattern (i.e., lowered empathy and lowered flexibility scores), but insignificant correlation. The alterations in these scores, therefore, varied in similar fashion and raised the possibility that cognitive inflexibility may limit the capacity for empathic processing. In contrast, the orbito-frontal lesion sample was lowest in empathy scores, but showed unimpaired cognitive flexibility scores. Such dissociation suggests that impairments other than cognitive flexibility may contribute to empathic changes. Alternatives could include autonomic regulation changes that inform decision-making and behavioral responses (e.g., somatic marker model of Damasio et al., 1991), and impaired learning of shifting contingencies related to positive and negative consequences for actions (Rolls et al., 1994).

Although patients with nonfrontal cerebral lesions also reported a change in empathy ratings, this appeared to follow a different course and to be related to different causes. These patients were adept at recognizing and reporting such changes soon after their cerebral injury and remained steady in their scores over six months. Patients with prefrontal lesions initially rated themselves as unchanged, although family members quickly recognized empathic alterations. During six-month follow-up studies though, the prefrontal lesion patients reported a steep drop in empathy levels, well below the nonfrontal group. This delayed pattern of awareness was evident in subjects with moderate closed head injury as well. Item analysis of the inventory suggested that nonfrontal lesion patients experienced lower social self-confidence. However, the six-month drop in empathy scores for the prefrontal lesion subjects was related more to their preference for routine, structured, and predictable situations. Interestingly, those prefrontal lesion patients with normal ratings of empathy showed more favorable social and vocational outcomes up to two to four years later.

Early frontal lesions can also influence the development and maturation of empathic capacities, as shown in cases DT and MJ (Eslinger et al., 1992, 1997). DT is a woman who suffered left prefrontal lesion at the age of seven and was studied at 33 years of age; MJ is a man who suffered right prefrontal lesion at the age of three and has been studied up to 18 years of age. Both have shown marked insensitivity to the emotional experiences of others and difficulties in implementing reciprocal actions that benefit others despite normal range of general intelligence, memory, perception, and language.

Although data relating empathic processing to neural systems are still preliminary, a model is beginning to emerge which suggests that the prefrontal cortex is a critical substrate for the development, elaboration, and regulation of empathy (Eslinger, 1998). Orbito-frontal cortices may be particularly necessary for mediating emotional aspects of empathy, including the autonomic activation and visceral–somatic states that underlie emotional responsiveness and sensitivity. The prominent connections of the orbito-frontal cortex with the amygdala and other limbic as well as autonomic-related centers might permit such processing. Dorsolateral prefrontal cortices, in contrast, may provide the neural substrate for the integration of cognitive aspects of empathy. This region has been associated with cognitive flexibility and the manipulation of variables and circumstances in relation to antecedents, personal experiences, and possible outcomes, which all contribute to understanding the experiences and situations of others. Since orbital and dorsolateral prefrontal cortices are interconnected, integration and even shifting control by both systems may be possible for different kinds of interpersonal relationships and social adaptation.

Recovery after frontal lobe lesion and treatment options

There is a substantial role for health providers in supporting patients recovering from frontal lobe damage. Rehabilitation services necessarily involve a multidisciplinary treatment plan, beginning with the comprehensive assessment of neurological, neuropsychological and everyday functional abilities of patients.

Few studies have tracked the short-term and long-term outcomes of patients with focal frontal lesions. This is particularly important since the underlying deficits may not be as apparent as hemiplegia, aphasia or amnesia, for which physical, occupational, and speech therapy services can be clearly directed and justified. However, these common modes of therapy may not be able effectively to address motivational, emotional, executive, and interpersonal difficulties as readily as more instrumental impairments associated with frontal injuries. Therefore, neurologists, neuropsychologists, and neuropsychiatrists have important roles in detecting and uncovering deficits that may not be readily apparent, yet are critical to treatment plans and outcome. Such investigations are leading to emerging guidelines for neurorehabilitation, which are briefly summarized below.

Predictors of favorable/unfavorable outcome

In a preliminary case-control study of unilateral frontal lesion patients with favorable versus unfavorable outcome, it was possible to identify several variables that differentiated such patients in the chronic recovery phase, two to four years post-stroke (Grattan and Eslinger, 1991). Favorable outcome was defined by objective criteria (i.e., return to 75% levels of work [hours/week], social–familial activities [contacts/week], and functional independence measure [FIM score]), and by subjective criteria (i.e., report by patient and at least one family member indicating positive postlesion personality, social, emotional, and cognitive adjustment). Data were obtained from medical as well as neuropsychological records and repeated interviews. Subjects were recruited from a consecutive series of frontal lesion cases, with favorable outcome subjects meeting both objective and subjective criteria. Furthermore, patients from each group ($n = 3$) were matched on the basis of age, sex, education, marital status, premorbid occupational level, severity of acute neurologic deficit, neurorehabilitation services, and level of residual disability.

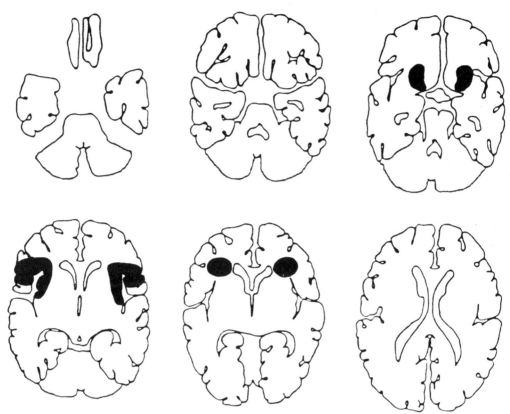

Fig. 8.8   Brain template depicting areas of damage in a small sample of patients who had unfavorable outcome after frontal lobe lesions. Damage to deep white pathways subjacent and adjacent to the frontal horns (affecting frontal-limbic as well as frontal-striatal and frontal thalamic pathways), the frontal operculum, and the anterior insula differentiated these patients from those with a favorable outcome pattern.

Results indicated that variables related to lesion site, cognitive flexibility, empathy level, and premorbid personality tendencies separated the outcome samples, as follows.

Lesion site

Favorable outcome was associated with lesions that *spared* deep white matter pathways, the frontal operculum, and extension of lesion to the anterior insula and basal ganglia. Through a transparency overlay method utilizing a standardized lesion localization procedure (Damasio and Damasio, 1989), the anatomic lesions of the favorable outcome sample were spatially subtracted from the lesion locations for the unfavorable outcome sample. The results were lesion areas that were unique to the unfavorable outcome sample (Fig. 8.8).

Damage subjacent and laterally adjacent to the frontal horns was evident in all unfavorable outcome subjects. Such lesions appeared to disrupt frontal-limbic circuitry, particularly involving paralimbic orbito-frontal cortex, ventral striatum and basal forebrain, amygdala, and temporal polar cortex. These structures have been implicated in regulatory processes related to emotion, autonomic responsiveness, motivation, and social–affiliative behavior. In addition, frontal-striatal and frontal-thalamic projections related to executive functions and cognitive–emotional integration also appeared to be affected. Damage to the basal ganglia (particularly the head of the caudate) in certain of the unfavorable outcome cases probably contributed to further disruption of frontal-striatal processes. The other sites of damage, the frontal operculum and anterior insula, have been associated with emotional and autonomic alterations that may compromise adaptation and recovery as well. Frontal operculum lesion has been correlated with impairment of emotional intonation of speech and undue cheerfulness (Starkstein et al., 1989). Anterior insula damage occurred in two of the three unfavorable outcome subjects. This region has been anatomically aligned with orbito-frontal and temporal polar cortices as a paralimbic network devoted to motivational, prosocial, and emotional processes (e.g., Mesulam and Mufson, 1982; Lane et al., 1997). However, whether damage to all of these structures is necessary to produce unfavorable outcome is unclear. Possibly, graded effects are associated with more limited unilateral lesions. However, the distinctive character of these structures involves emotional processing, motivation, and social–affiliative processes, which may be the reasons they are critically important for adaptation and adjustment.

Cognitive flexibility

Though memory impairment was present, it was equivalent in both samples (as were average levels of general intelligence, visual perception, and language). What distinguished the two samples were measures of cognitive flexibility which depended upon shifting of response set, working memory, and generating alternative possibilities. The unfavorable outcome sample, as might be predicted, was impaired in the Wisconsin Card Sorting Test and Alternate Uses Test, whereas the favorable outcome sample was not. Favorable outcome subjects were more creative in rearranging work responsibilities, pursuing recreation, and participating in social activities.

Empathy levels

Normal scores on a reliable and valid self-report measure of empathy were found in the favorable outcome subjects but not in the unfavorable outcome subjects. These scores correlated with the tone and texture of how frontal lesion subjects related to family members, coworkers, and friends. Normal range of empathy scores was associated with social adjustment, continuation of supportive relationships, and a positive attitude from others. Low empathy levels were associated with hostile treatment of others, marital strain, social withdrawal, and resentment from others.

Premorbid personality

Favorable outcome subjects were reported to be more agreeable, flexible, and sensitive to interpersonal concerns than unfavorable outcome subjects whose premorbid personality descriptors included 'controlling,' 'antagonistic,' and 'rigid.' In general, personality changes were reported to be a combination of exaggerated preexisting characteristics and new features not previously observed.

Although these analyses need to incorporate more empirical measures and to be completed in a larger sample of frontal and nonfrontal lesion subjects, the preliminary findings suggest that specific anatomic, cognitive, social–emotional, and premorbid personality factors contribute to prognosis and rehabilitation outcome. Many questions remain. For example, are there decisive roles for protective psychological factors, social–environmental supports, and nontraditional therapeutic resources (e.g., music therapy, recreational therapy) in the recovery from frontal lobe damage? Are the influences of younger age, degree of neuropsychological impairment, vocational history, and neurological deficit similar to those reported for penetrating and traumatic brain injury (e.g., Schwab et al., 1993; Dikmen et al., 1994)? Assessment methods, therefore, might consider these diverse variables in rehabilitation planning, therapies, family education, and outcome measurement.

Drug interventions

Medications are becoming an increasingly important part of rehabilitation for frontal lobe injuries. Perhaps the most novel development in this area has been the use of dopamine agonists because of the importance of ascending dopaminergic projections to diverse parts of the frontal lobe. The well-known nigrostriatal portion of the pathways enriches the basal ganglia with dopamine, while the mesocorticolimbic portion gives rise to projections to phylogenetically older cortical derivatives (e.g., olfactory, tubercle, amygdala, septal nuclei, and pyriform cortex) and to neocortical structures (e.g., Fallon, 1988; Gaspar et al., 1989; Cortes et al., 1989). Furthermore, projections of the mesoneocortical component have been shown to be involved in complex cognitive functions associated with prefrontal cortex (e.g., Sawaguchi and Goldman-Rakic, 1994).

Previous studies have reported that bromocriptine treatment might be helpful to the recovery from nonfluent aphasia and hemispatial neglect following lesions which involved frontal-parietal and frontal-temporal-parietal regions (Fleet et al., 1987; Gupta and McCoch, 1992). We were interested in establishing through a pilot study whether bromocriptine treatment would foster recovery from other frontal lobe impairments. A clinical rating scale was formulated to include indicators of certain prefrontal functions (e.g., goal-directed behavior, appreciation of social nuances) and certain mesial frontal functions (e.g., affect, verbal responsiveness, and purposeful voluntary movements). Subjects were postacute patients admitted to the neurorehabilitation unit with profound deficits (often with varying degrees of akinesia, bradykinesia, blunted affect, and mutism) from focal frontal lesions due to cerebrovascular disease or from frontal and multiple cerebral lesions due to traumatic brain injury or multiple strokes (see Eslinger, Grattan and Geder, 1995, for further details). Bromocriptine dosage began at 5 mg q.d. for six days, followed by increase to 10 mg q.d. for 14–22 days, than 15 mg q.d. for the rest of the treatment period. Patients otherwise participated in as many treatment services as they could tolerate, involving cognitive–behavioral, physical, occupational, speech, and recreational therapies. The results indicated substantial improvements in prefrontal and mesial frontal functions, with five of seven patients reaching maximum ratings. The strongest effects were observed for initiation behaviors, affect, and voluntary movements, often with resolution of akinesia and mutism. An important limitation of this study was the lack of a double-blind, placebo-controlled design, which is needed to establish clearly the efficacy of this intervention. We did observe that one patient temporarily discontinued on bromocriptine suffered a decline in goal-directed and social behaviors until the drug treatment was restored. Another piece of suggestive evidence comes from informal clinical trials of bromocriptine in chronic outpatients who present with lingering motivational and initiation difficulties (e.g., cases 3 and 4 described earlier in the chapter). These patients and their families have reported beneficial effects up to three years after frontal injury. Therefore, further studies with appropriate controls, outcome measures, and other dopamine agonist agents are warranted.

Other medication options to consider for patients with frontal damage include selective serotonin reuptake inhibitors and tricyclic agents for depression, as well as anticonvulsants such as Depakote (divalproex sodium) or Tegretol (carbamazepine) for hypomania. Data supporting the specificity and efficacy of these agents for diverse aspects of frontal syndromes are still developing. What appears most clear, though is that medications will play an increasingly important role in neuro-rehabilitation planning, complementary to social–environmental, restorative, and compensatory treatment efforts.

Social–environmental and cognitive–behavioral interventions

Because of the varied and complex nature of impairments associated with frontal damage, rehabilitation must address not only the self-awareness and self-regulation aspects of each patient, but also the many points of their interaction with complex environments and social–emotional contexts. Therapeutically, this is a tall order, which requires increasing involvement of family members and significant others (e.g., vocational, recreational, community) in the long-term management of frontal impairments. Cicerone and Giacino (1992) have described several different levels of treatment with focal frontal lesions. Specifically, varying degrees of *environmental modifications, behavioral management,* and *cognitive self-management training* can be applied to individual cases depending upon the severity of impairment. Obviously, the need for such interventions is predicated upon thorough assessment through formal examinations and observational methods during the rehabilitation phase. Those patients with the most impaired executive functions typically require a high degree of environmental modification and behavioral management. The goals of these interventions are to decrease and simplify the demands environments place on impaired patients, to provide direct and consistent feedback on patients' behavior, and to provide the cues necessary to foster adaptive behavioral responses. These approaches essentially alter factors external to the patient, in order to provide the environmental supports to elicit and sustain adaptive responses (Mateer, 1997).

Patients with less severe executive impairments can participate in a broader range of executive strategy training that strives to restore executive-type cognitive processes or encourage compensatory processes that aid executive functions. Options include training patients in attention skills and verbal mediation strategies, self-prediction for anticipatory behavior deficits, self-instruction for planning and prospective memory deficits, and self-monitoring for error recognition and utilization, particularly in multistep tasks (see Cicerone and Giacino, 1992, and Mateer, 1997, for further details of training paradigms and measurement of behavior change). The key to long-term improvement and maintenance of gains is the involvement of family members in understanding these interventions, monitoring the patient's progress in everyday situations, and recognizing how strategies and skills might be modified to a particular goal or activity for that patient.

Interventions for social–emotional and interpersonal deficits are equally challenging to articulate, evaluate, and develop into treatment models. In our experience, there are important roles for individual psychotherapeutic methods and for group/interactional methods. The effectiveness of individual psychotherapy depends a good deal on the nature of the relationship between patient and therapist, but also on the creativeness of the therapist in modifying treatment methods according to the cognitive–emotional impairments of the patient. For example, the case 3 illustration described earlier in the chapter depicted a man with pervasive executive impairments after bilateral prefrontal injuries, who required very strong interventions centered around environmental modification and behavior management. Such interventions can engender resistance from patients and even aggressive outbursts. These concerns have been managed in part through ongoing individual and family psychotherapy, providing the patient with a forum for voicing resentment and frustration, and developing the communication channels for a larger choice in his services and activities. This mechanism also provides options for addressing social–emotional issues that develop, particularly lack of empathy, unawareness of effects of one's behavior on others, and compensating for difficulties in perceiving the emotional intent of others based on their facial expressions and prosody.

Group interactional formats also provide important means of addressing social–emotional impairments. Music therapy, recreational therapies (including not only social events but also horseback riding and domestic pets), and social support groups all have some potential to improve patients' psychological adjustment and outcome after frontal injuries. In particular, music therapy and support group formats have led to increased levels of emotional empathy and decreased depression in brain-injured patients (Eslinger, 1998).

Conclusion

While the consequences of focal frontal lobe damage remain puzzling and problematic in many respects, there has been tremendous progress in deciphering the organization of the frontal lobe, many of its common clinical presentations, and even certain aspects of its rehabilitation. In addition to its well-known role in cognition and self-regulation of behavior, the frontal lobe is intimately involved in emotional processing, perhaps mediating the integration of cognitive and emotional streams of processing that underlie personality, interpersonal behavior, empathy, motivation, and overall adaptation. The interrelationship of prefrontal networks with other cortical association areas, the basal ganglia, thalamus, and the limbic system is both intricate and precise, suggesting that a complete model of frontal cortex organization and function really requires an understanding of the whole brain. While this may be an elusive goal at the moment, there are increasingly clear models of prefrontal networks that guide current clinical decision-making and management of impairments. These rely upon distinctions among dorsolateral, orbital, mesial, and other specialized areas of frontal lobe as well as diverse frontal-subcortical circuits. Current interventions draw largely upon selective medications, environmental modifications, cognitive–behavioral therapies, and family education in providing a comprehensive rehabilitation program after frontal lobe injuries. Further studies are needed, particularly with regard to influences on long-term outcome and specific intervention effects.

REFERENCES

Ackerly, S.S. (1964). A case of paranatal bilateral frontal lobe defect observed for thirty years. In *The Frontal Granular Cortex and Behavior*, ed. J.M. Warren and K. Albert, pp. 192–218. New York: McGraw-Hill.

Ackerly, S.S. and Benton, A.L. (1948). Report of a case of bilateral frontal lobe defect. *Proc Assn Res Nerv Ment Dis* 27: 479–504.

Adolphs, R., Damasio, H., Tranel, D. and Damasio, A.R. (1996). Cortical systems for the recognition of emotion in facial expressions. *J Neurosci* 16: 7678–87.

Alexander, G.E., Crutcher, M.D. and DeLong, M.R. (1990). Basal ganglia–thalamocortical circuits: parallel substrates for motor, oculomotor, 'prefrontal' and 'limbic' functions. *Prog Brain Res* 85: 119–46.

Barbas, H. (1995). Anatomic basis of cognitive–emotional interactions in the primate prefrontal cortex. *Neurosci Biobehav Rev* 19: 499–510.

Barbas, H. and Pandya, D.N. (1989). Architecture and intrinsic connections of the prefrontal cortex in the rhesus monkey. *J Comp Neurol* 286: 353–75.

Barbas, H. and Pandya, D.N. (1991). Patterns of connections of the prefrontal cortex in the rhesus monkey associated with cortical architecture. In *Frontal Lobe Function and Dysfunction*, ed. H.S. Levin, H.M. Eisenberg and A.L. Benton, pp. 35–58. New York: Oxford University Press.

Bechara, A., Damasio, A.R., Damasio, H. and Anderson, S.W. (1994). Insensitivity to future consequences following damage to human prefrontal cortex. *Cognition* 50: 7–15.

Bechara, A., Tranel, D., Damasio, H. and Damasio, A.R. (1996). Failure to respond autonomically to anticipated future outcome following damage to prefrontal cortex. *Cereb Cortex* 6: 215–25.

Benton, A.L. (1991a). Prefrontal injury and behavior in children. *Dev Neuropsychol* 7: 276–81.

Benton, A.L. (1991b). The prefrontal region: its early history. In *Frontal Lobe Function and Dysfunction*, ed. H.S. Levin, H.M. Eisenberg and A.L. Benton, pp. 3–32. New York: Oxford University Press.

Binder, J.R. (1997). Neuroanatomy of language processing studied with functional MRI. *Clin Neurosci* 4: 87–94.

Blonder, L.X., Bowers, D. and Heilman, K.M. (1991). The role of the right hemisphere in emotional communication. *Brain* 114: 1115–27.

Bogousslavsky, J. (1994). Frontal stroke syndromes. *Eur Neurol* 34: 306–15.

Borod, J.C. (1992). Interhemispheric and intrahemispheric control of emotion. A focus on unilateral brain damage. *J Consult Clin Psychol* 60: 339–48.

Bottini, G., Corcoran, R., Sterzi, R. et al. (1994). The role of the right hemisphere in the interpretation of figurative aspects of language. A positron emission tomography activation study. *Brain* 117: 1241–53.

Brickner, R.M. (1936). *The Intellectual Functions of the Frontal Lobes: Study Based upon Observation of a Man after Partial Bilateral Frontal Lobotomy*. MacMillan: New York.

Casey, B.J., Cohen, J.D., Jezzard, P. et al. (1995). Activation of prefrontal cortex in children during a nonspatial working memory task with functional MRI. *Neuroimage* 2: 221–9.

Cicerone, K.D. and Giacino, J.T. (1992). Remediation of executive function deficits after traumatic brain injury. *NeuroRehabilitation* 2: 12–22.

Cortes, R., Gueye, B., Pazos, A. and Palacios, J.M. (1989). Dopamine receptors in human brain: autoradiographic distribution of the D1 sites. *Neuroscience* 28: 263–78.

Cummings, J.L. (1993). Frontal–subcortical circuits and human behavior. *Arch Neurol* 50: 873–80.

Damasio, A.R., Tranel, D. and Damasio, H.C. (1991). Somatic markers and the guidance of behavior: theory and preliminary testing. In *Frontal Lobe Function and Dysfunction*, ed. H.S. Levin, H.M. Eisenberg and A.L. Benton, pp. 217–29. New York: Oxford University Press.

Damasio, A.R. and Van Hoesen, G.W. (1983). Emotional disturbances associated with focal lesions of the limbic frontal lobe. In *Neuropsychology of Human Emotion*, ed. K.M. Heilman and P. Satz, pp. 86–110. New York: Guilford Press.

Damasio, H. and Damasio, A.R. (1989). *Lesion Localization in Neuropsychology*. New York: Oxford University Press.

Damasio, H., Grabowsky, T., Frank, R., Galarirda, A.M. and Damasio, A.R. (1994). The return of Phineas Gage: clues about the brain from the skull of a famous patient. *Science* 264: 1102–5.

Davidson, R.J. (1984). Affect, cognition, and hemisphere specialization. In *Cognition and Behavior*, ed. C.E. Izard, J. Kagan and R. Zajonc, pp. 320–65. New York: Cambridge University Press.

DeKosky, S.T., Hielman, K.M., Bowers, D. and Valenstein, E. (1980). Recognition and discrimination of emotional faces and pictures. *Brain Lang* 9: 206–14.

Dias, R., Robbins, T.W. and Roberts, A.C. (1996). Dissociation in prefrontal cortex of the affective and attentional shifts. *Nature* 380: 69–72.

Dikmen, S.S., Temkin, N.R., Machamer, J.E. et al. (1994). Employment following traumatic brain injuries. *Arch Neurol* 51: 177–86.

Drevets, W.C., Price, J.L., Simpson, J.R. Jr et al. (1997). Subgenual prefrontal cortex abnormalities in mood disorders. *Nature* 386: 824–7.

Eslinger, P.J. (1998). Neurological and neuropsychological bases of empathy. *Eur Neruol* 39: 193–9.

Eslinger, P.J., Biddle, K.R. and Grattan, L.M. (1997). Cognitive and social development in children with prefrontal cortex lesions. In *Development of the Prefrontal Cortex: Evolution, Neurobiology, and Behavior*, ed. N.A. Krasnegor, G.R. Lyon and P.S. Goldman-Rakic, pp. 295–335. Baltimore: Paul H. Brookes Publishing Co., Inc.

Eslinger, P.J. and Damasio, A.R. (1985). Severe disturbance of higher cognition after bilateral frontal lobe ablation: patient EVR. *Neurology* 49: 764–9.

Eslinger, P.J. and Grattan, L.M. (eds.) (1991). Developmental consequences of early frontal lobe damage. Special issue. *Dev Neuropsyhol* 7: 257–419.

Eslinger, P.J. and Grattan, L.M. (1993). Frontal lobe and frontal–striatal substrates for different forms of human cognitive flexibility. *Neuropsycholigia* 31: 17–28.

Eslinger, P.J., Grattan, L.M. and Damasio, A.R. (1992). Developmental consequences of childhood frontal lobe damage. *Arch Neurol* 49: 764–9.

Eslinger, P.J., Grattan, L.M. and Geder, L. (1995). Impact of frontal lobe lesions on rehabilitation and recovery from acute brain injury. *NeuroRehabilitation* 5: 161–82.

Fallon, J.H. (1988). Topographic organization of ascending dopaminergic projections. *Ann NY Acad Sci* 537: 1–9.

Fleet, W.S.H., Valenstein, E., Watson, R.T. and Heilman, K.M. (1987). Dopamine agonist therapy for neglect in humans. *Neurology* 37: 1765–70.

Fuster, J.M. (1991). Role of the prefrontal cortex in delay tasks: evidence from reversible lesion and unit recording in monkey. In *Frontal Lobe Function and Dysfunction*, ed. H.S. Levin, H.M. Eisenberg and A.L. Benton, pp. 66–71. New York: Oxford University Press.

Gaspar, P., Berger, B., Febvret, A., Vigny, A. and Henry, J.P. (1989). Catecholamine innervation of the human cerebral cortex as revealed by comparative immunohistochemistry of tyrosine hydroxylase and dopamine-beta-hydroxylase. *J Comp Neurol* 279: 249–71.

Goel, V., Gold, B., Kapur, S. and Houle, S. (1998). Neuroanatomical correlates of human reasoning. *J Cogn Neurosci* 10: 293–302.

Gold, J.M., Berman, K.F., Randolph, C. et al. (1996). PET validation of a novel prefrontal task: delayed response alternation. *Neuropsychology* 10: 3–10.

Goldman-Rakic, P.S. (1987). Circuitry of primate prefrontal cortex and regulation of behavior by representational memory. In *Handbook of Physiology, the Nervous System V*, ed. V.B. Mountcastle, pp. 373–417. New York: Raven Press.

Goldman-Rakic, P.S. and Friedman, H.R. (1991). The circuitry of working memory revealed by anatomy and metabolic imaging. In *Frontal Lobe Function and Dysfunction*, ed. H.S. Levin, H.M. Eisenberg and A.L. Benton, pp. 72–91. New York: Oxford University Press.

Grafman, J. (ed.) (1995a). Structure and function of the human prefrontal cortex. *Ann NY Acad Sci* 769: 1–411.

Grafman, J. (1995b). Similarities and distinctions among current models of prefrontal cortical functions. *Ann NY Acad Sci* 769: 337–68.

Grafman, J., Vance, S.C., Weingartner, H., Salazar, A.M. and Amin, D. (1986). The effects of lateralized frontal lesions on mood regulation. *Brain* 109: 1127–48.

Grattan, L.M. and Eslinger, P.J. (1989). Higher cognition and social behavior: changes in cognitive flexibility and empathy after cerebral lesions. *Neuropsychology* 3: 175–85.

Grattan, L.M., Bloomer, R.H., Archambault, F.X. and Eslinger, P.J. (1994). Cognitive flexibility and empathy after frontal lobe lesion. *Neuropsychiatry Neuropsychol Behav Neurol* 7: 251–9.

Grattan, L.M. and Eslinger, P.J. (1991). Characteristics of favorable recovery from frontal lobe damage. *Neurology* 41: 266.

Gupta, S.R. and McCoch, A.G. (1992). Bromocriptine treatment of non-fluent aphasia. *Arch Phys Med Rehabil* 73: 373–6.

Harlowe, J.M. (1848). Passage of an iron bar through the head. *Boston Med Surg J* 39: 389–93.

Harlowe, J.M. (1868). Recovery from passage of an iron bar through the head. *Pub Mass Med Soc* 2: 327–47.

Hebb, D.O. (1945). Man's frontal lobes: a critical review. *Arch Neurol Psychiatry* 54: 10–24.

Hebb, D.O. and Penfield, W. (1940). Human behavior after extensive bilateral removal from the frontal lobes. *Arch Neurol Psychiatry* 44: 421–38.

Hogan, R. (1969). Development of an empathy scale. *J Consult Clin Psychol* 33: 307–16.

Hornak, J., Rolls, E.T. and Wade, D. (1996). Face and voice expression identification in patients with emotional and behavioral changes following ventral frontal lobe damage. *Neuropsychologia* 34: 247–61.

Irle, E., Pepe, M., Wowra, B. and Kunze, S. (1994). Mood changes after surgery for tumors of the cerebral cortex. *Arch Neurol* 51: 164–74.

Jonides, J., Smith, E.E., Koeppe, R.A. et al. (1993). Spatial working memory in humans as revealed by PET. *Nature* 363: 623–5.

Krasnegor, N.A., Lyon, G.R. and Goldman-Rakic, P.S. (eds.) (1997). *Development of the Prefrontal Cortex, Evolution, Neurobiology, and Behavior.* Baltimore: Paul H. Brookes.

Lane, R.D., Reiman, E.M., Ahern, G.L. et al. (1997). Neuroanatomical correlates of happiness, sadness, and disgust. *Am J Psychiatry* 154: 926–33.

Levin, H.S., Eisenberg, H.M. and Benton, A.L. (eds.) (1991). *Frontal Lobe Function and Dysfunction.* New York: Oxford University Press.

Marlowe, W. (1992). The impact of right prefrontal lesion on the developing brain. *Brain Cogn* 20: 205–13.

Mateer, C.A. (1997). Rehabilitation of individuals with frontal lobe impairments. In *Neuropsychological Rehabilitation: Fundamentals, Innovations and Directions*, ed. J. Leon-Carrion, pp. 285–300. Debray Beach, FL: GR/St Lucia Press.

Mega, M.S. and Cummings, J.L. (1994). Frontal–subcortical circuits and neuropsychiatric disorders. *Neuropsychiatry Clin Neurosci* 6: 358–70.

Mesulam, M.-M. and Mufson, E.J. (1982). Insula of the old world monkey. I. Architectonics in the insulo–orbito–temporal component of the paralimbic brain. *J Comp Neurol* 212: 1–22.

Morris, P.L.P., Raphael, B. and Robinson, R.G. (1992). Clinical depression is associated with impaired recovery from stroke. *Med J Aust* 157: 239–42.

Morris, P.L., Robinson, R.G., deCarvalho, M.L. et al. (1996a). Lesion characteristics and depressed mood in the stroke data bank study. *J Neuropsychiatry Clin Neurosci* 8: 153–9.

Morris, P.L., Robinson, R.G., Raphael, B. and Hopwood, M.J. (1996b). Lesion location and post-stroke depression. *J Neuropsychiatry Clin Neurosci* 8: 399–403.

Nauta, W.J.H. (1971). The problem of the frontal lobe: a reinterpretation. *J Psychiatr Res* 8: 167–87.

Neafsey, E.J. (1990). Prefrontal cortical control of the autonomic nervous system: anatomical and physiological observations. *Prog Brain Res* 85: 147–65.

Owen, A.M., Doyon, J., Petrides, M. and Evans, A.C. (1996). Planning and spatial working memory: a positron emission tomography study in humans. *Eur J Neurosci* 8: 353–64.

Pandya, D.N. and Kuypers, H.G.J.M. (1969). Cortico–cortical connections in the rhesus monkey. *Brain Res* 13: 13–36.

Paulesu, E., Goldaire, B., Scifo, P. et al. (1997). Functional heterogeneity of left inferior frontal cortex as revealed by fMRI. *Neuroreport* 8: 2011–117.

Petrides, M., Alivisates, B., Meyer, E. and Evans, A.C. (1993). Functional activation of the human frontal cortex during the performance of verbal working memory tasks. *Proc Natl Acad Sci USA* 90: 878–82.

Porrino, L.J., Crane, A.M. and Goldman-Rakic, P.S. (1981). Direct and indirect pathways from the amygdala to the frontal lobe in the rhesus monkey. *J Comp Neurol* 198: 121–36.

Price, B.H., Daffner, K.R., Stowe, R.M. and Mesulam, M.M. (1990). The compartmental learning disabilities of early frontal lobe damage. *Brain* 113: 1383–93.

Price, J.L., Carmichael, S.T. and Drevets, W.C. (1996). Networks related to the orbital and medial prefrontal cortex; a substrate for emotional behavior? *Prog Brain Res* 107: 523–36.

Ray, J.P. and Price, J.L. (1993). The organization of projections from the mediodorsal nucleus of the thalamus to orbital and medial prefrontal cortex in macaque monkeys. *J Comp Neurol* 337: 1–31.

Robinson, R.G. (1997). Neuropsychiatric consequences of stroke. *Annu Rev Med* 48: 217–29.

Robinson, R.G., Kubos, K.L., Starr, L.B., Rao, K. and Price, T.R. (1984). Mood disorders in stroke patients. Importance of location of lesion. *Brain* 107: 81–93.

Rolls, E.T. (1990). A theory of emotion, and its application to understanding the neural basis of emotion. *Cognition Emotion* 4: 161–90.

Rolls, E.T., Hornak, J., Wade, D. and McGrath, J. (1994). Emotion-related learning in patients with social and emotional changes associated with frontal lobe damage. *J Neurol Neurosurg Psychiatry* 57: 1518–24.

Sawaguchi, T. and Goldman-Rakic, P.S. (1994). The role of DI-dopamine in working memory: local injection of dopamine antagonists into the prefrontal cortex of rhesus monkeys performing an oculomotor delayed-response task. *J Neurophysiol* 71: 515–28.

Schultz, S.K., Castillo, C.S., Kosier, J.T. and Robinson, R.G. (1997). Generalized anxiety and depression. Assessment over 2 years after stroke. *Am J Geriatr Psychiatry* 5: 229–37.

Schwab, K., Grafman, J., Salazar, A.M. and Kraft, J. (1993). Residual impairments and work status 15 years after penetrating head injury: report from the Vietnam Head Injury Study. *Neurology* 43: 95–103.

Sirigu, A., Zalla, T., Pillon, J., Grafman, J., Agid, Y. and Dubois, B. (1995). Selective impairments in managerial knowledge following prefrontal cortex damage. *Cortex* 31: 301–16.

Spitzer, M., Kischka, U., Guckel, F. et al. (1998). Functional magnetic resonance imaging of category-specific cortical activation: evidence for semantic maps. *Cognit Brain Res* 6: 309–19.

Starkstein, S.E., Robinson, R.G., Honig, M.A. et al. (1989). Mood changes after right hemisphere lesions. *Br J Psychiatry* 155: 79–85.

Starkstein, S.E., Gryer, J.B., Berthier,M.L. (1991). Depression after stroke. The importance of cerebral hemisphere asymmetries. *J Neuropsychiatry Clin Neurosci* 3: 276–85.

Stuss, D. and Benson, D.F. (1986). *The Frontal Lobes*. New York: Raven Press.

Stuss, D.T., Gow, C.A. and Hetherington, C.R. (1992). 'No longer Gage': frontal lobe dysfunction and emotional changes. *J Consult Clin Psychol* 60: 349–59.

Thorpe, S.J., Rolls, E.T. and Maddison, S. (1983). Neuronal activity in the orbitofrontal cortex of the behaving monkey. *Exp Brain Res* 49: 93–115.

Tulving, E., Kapur, S., Craik, F.I.M. et al. (1994). Hemisphere encoding/retrieval symmetry in episodic memory; positron emission tomography findings. *Proc Natl Acad Sci USA* 91: 2016–20.

Ungerleider, L.G., Courtney, S.M. and Haxbry, J.V. (1998). A neural system for human visual working memory. *Proc Natl Acad Sci USA* 95: 883–90.

Uylings, H.B.M., van Eden, C.G., DeBruin, J.P.C., Corner, M.A. and Feenstra, M.G.P. (eds.)

(1990). The prefrontal cortex: its structure, function and pathology. *Prog Brain Res* 85: 3–574.

Watanabe, M. (1996). Reward expectancy in primate prefrontal neurons. *Nature* 382: 629–32.

Weddell, R.A., Miller, J.D. and Trevarthen, C. (1990). Voluntary emotional facial expression in patients with focal cerebral lesions. *Neuropsychologia* 28: 49–60.

Wheeler, R.E., Davidson, R.J. and Tomarken, A.J. (1993). Frontal lesion asymmetry and emotional reactivity: a biological substrate of affective style. *Psychophysiology* 30: 82–9.

Wilson, F.A.W., O'Scalaidhe, S.P. and Goldman-Rakic, P.S. (1993). Dissociation of object and spatial processing domains in primate prefrontal cortex. *Science* 260: 1955–8.

Wilson, F.A. and Rolls, E.T. (1990). Neuronal responses related to the novelty and familiarity of visual stimuli in the substantia innominata, diagonal band of Broca and periventricular region of the primate basal forebrain. *Exp Brain Res* 80: 104–20.

9

Disorders of motivation

Michel Habib

Introduction

During the last 20 years or so, several reports (mainly in the French-speaking neurological literature) have dealt with the description of profound behavioral and personality changes occurring abruptly following small focal brain lesions in the basal ganglia regions, and presenting as isolated disturbances in motivation and action.

Such disturbances have been variously named 'loss of psychic self-activation,' 'pure psychic akinesia,' or 'athymhormic syndrome.' At present, about 20 such cases of specific motivational disorders due to focal subcortical lesions have been reported in some detail (Table 9.1). In all of these cases, the authors have empha-sized the fact that these disorders of personality and affect arose in subjects without any previous psychiatric disorder, and entailed dramatic behavioral changes, dis-proportionate to cognitive involvement, which remained, if at all, quite moderate. Beyond their clinical interest, these observations have also contributed toward deepening our knowledge of the role of subcortical brain structures in a previously almost unexplored area of brain/mind relationships.

The purposes of this chapter are: (1) to summarize the clinical features of these observations and to show that, collectively, these features may comprise a distinct neurobehavioral syndrome; (2) to provide arguments suggesting that this syn-drome results from the disruption of a specific brain system and to delineate, on the basis of radio-anatomical/behavioral correlations, the structural organization of this brain system; and (3) to propose a tentative neuroanatomical and psycho-dynamic model of human motivation.

Clinical descriptions of isolated motivational disorders following focal brain damage

Overview of clinical concepts and terminology

This chapter deals with a group of behavioral disorders that have been variably termed in the early neurological literature as 'placidity' or 'abulia,' and that were

Table 9.1. Isolated disturbances of motivation and action in focal basal ganglia lesions

Authors	Number of cases	Age (years)	Lesion site	Lesion type
Laplane et al. (1981, 1982, 1984, 1989)	8	53	Pallido-striatal, bilateral	Wasp sting
		23	Pallidal, bilateral	CO
		59	Pallidal, bilateral	CO
		52	Pallido-striatal, bilateral	Disulfiram intoxication
		27	Pallidal, bilateral	Anoxic
		?	Pallido-striatal, bilateral	Anoxic
		31	Pallidal, bilateral	CO
		22	Pallidal, bilateral	CO
Ali Chérif et al. (1984)	2	39	Pallidal, bilateral	CO
		18	Pallidal, bilateral	CO
Habib and Poncet (1988)	2	64	Caudate, bilateral	Ischemic (lacunes)
		60	Caudate bilateral	Ischemic (lacunes)
Strub (1989)	1	60	Pallidal, bilateral	Ischemic/anoxic
Trillet et al. (1990)	3	54	Caudate, bilateral	Ischemic hemorrhage
		56	Caudate, bilateral	Ischemic
		59	Caudate, bilateral	Ischemic
Luauté et al. (1990)	1	27	Left caudate	Ischemic
Danel et al. (1991)	1	72	Caudate, bilateral	Ischemic (lacunes)
Milandre et al. (1995)	1	51	Right caudate, Left pallidum	Ischemic (Moya-Moya)
Bellmann and Assal (1996)	1	68	Left caudate, Right pallidum	Ischemic

often considered as a milder form of akinetic mutism. This position, which was dominant in classical neurological writings, has probably obscured the real nature of these disorders and of their anatomical substrate, the only suggested pathophysiology being an interruption of fronto-thalamic connections. One interesting approach, however, has been the endeavor of some psychiatrists to group under the term 'apathy' certain behavioral traits shared by both psychiatric and neurological patients. Marin (1990) thus defined apathy as 'absence or lack of feeling, emotions, interest, or concern,' and proposed that it 'refers primarily to lack of motivation,' clearly suggesting that human motivation, as one aspect of the emotional life, may be the object of clinical investigation. However, this author made no attempt at defining its neural substrate.

Isolated motivational disturbance following pallidal lesions

Apart from these marginal mentions in the classical neurological literature, the first complete analysis of such behavioral changes was made by Laplane and colleagues from Paris, who, in 1981 and 1982, successively reported on two patients having sustained small bilateral lesions of the basal ganglia (the first being due to a wasp sting, the other to carbon monoxide poisoning). At this time, magnetic resonance imaging (MRI) not yet being available, pallidal involvement was only suspected on computerized tomography (CT) scan, and the exact location of deep brain damage was difficult to ascertain. In both cases, however, the clinical features were quite similar, yielding a singular picture of major motor and behavioral inertia and loss of spontaneous mental activity. Laplane et al. mainly focused on a compulsive behavior, mimicking obsessive–compulsive disorder, also present in the same patients (e.g., one of them considered it an 'absolute necessity' to count until reaching a multiple of nine). In fact, such behavior later proved not to be relevant to the diagnosis.

In their first patient, these authors described a total motor inactivity without motor weakness, and 'mental emptiness,' i.e., absence of spontaneous mental activity, without anxiety or particular suffering, and with otherwise surprisingly intact intellectual capabilities. Discussing the co-occurrence of loss of physical and psychic activity, and chiefly emphasizing the fact that motor as well as intellectual aptitudes were spared, Laplane et al. (1981) hypothesized an impairment of a so-called 'auto-activation system for psychic, intellectual and affective life.' According to this view, the basal ganglia would play a dual role in motor and psychic activity in such a way that impairment of this system would suspend spontaneous action as well as mental activity, possibly giving rise to compulsive behaviors. In their subsequent paper, Laplane et al. (1982) reported a similar case due to carbon monoxide intoxication. Here again, the patient was totally inactive but acted properly on external command, and displayed 'pseudo-compulsive' symptoms. In this case, CT scan data were more convincing, showing bilateral pallidal hyodensities, leading the authors to postulate a hitherto unsuspected role for the globus pallidus in psychic self-activation mechanisms. Laplane also pointed out some similarities between this syndrome and various psychiatric conditions such as severe depressive states, obsessive–compulsive disorders, and certain forms of schizophrenia.

Shortly after these papers were published, Ali Chérif and colleagues (1984), in Marseille, extended Laplane's findings to three new cases of pallidal lesions due to carbon monoxide intoxication, and focused their description on the comportmental and mental changes in their patients, thus providing a confirmation of the role of the globus pallidus in these aspects of mental functioning. The following is a summary of one of these observations.

Case PA

This 20-year-old woman was first examined in 1982 in the neurological ward, one year after accidental carbon monoxide poisoning. Having received hyperbaric oxygenotherapy, she had no motor sequelae but was referred for persisting behavioral disorders. Her mother mainly reported a profound loss of initiative and spontaneous activity. The patient stayed motionless in an armchair all day long and only acted on external stimulation. However, when she was prompted to do something, she would comply willingly and act quite normally. Furthermore, she manifested no desire, no complaint, and no care about the future. Her mother also noticed a striking loss of food preferences and a total absence of sexual desire. When asked about the content of her own thoughts, especially during extended periods of inactivity, the patient claimed she had none, suggesting a state of total mental emptiness similar to that reported in Laplane's patients. Also, at this stage of her illness, a pseudo-obsessive behavior was present, with a compulsive tendency to tidy up and to collect useless objects. As an illustration of the intensity of her apathy, the authors report two very significant anecdotal episodes. One day her father had taken her to town; he left her alone, 1 kilometer away from home, and asked her to walk around and then get back home. Four hours later, worried that she had not come back, her father returned to the same place and found her motionless, sitting on a bench close to where he had left her. In another instance she had been left in a shady place on the beach; her parents found her two hours later at the very same place, but in hot sun, lying on her back, motionless but awake, with heavy sunburn.

Neuropsychological evaluation showed subnormal general intellectual performances (Weschler Adult Intelligence Scale IQ: 87, with no verbal/performance dissociation). Copy of the Rey-Osterreith figure was correct, verbal fluency was within normal limits (18 animal names/min), in contrast with very poor spontaneous expression. However, she answered questions properly and was able to report normally recent or remote events. Formal memory testing showed preserved learning abilities (memory quotient, Wechsler Memory Scale: 102).

A CT scan performed at this time showed two symmetrical hypodensities projecting on the internal part of the globus pallidus. Seven years later, a brain MRI confirmed the exclusive pallidal topography of lesions (Fig. 9.1). The woman was re-examined at this time, i.e., eight years after her accident. The clinical picture was very similar: totally inactive, she would not get up in the morning, nor wash or dress unless prompted by her parents. She still manifested no desire, her only motivation being to watch television. She slept more than 12 hours per day. Besides a total absence of search for pleasure, she appeared indifferent to her mother's problems or affects. In particular, she showed no apparent reaction to her father's death. However, formal cognitive performances had significantly dropped, probably due to long-lasting absence of intellectual activity or training.

It must be noted that in neither Laplane's nor Ali Chérif's reports was any mention made of the terms 'motivation' or 'motivational disorder'. Instead, both authors emphasized the motor component of the syndrome, insisting on the fact

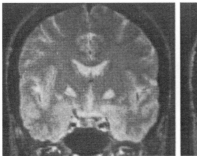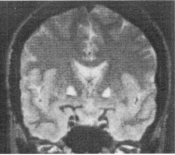

Fig. 9.1   Case PA: T2-weighted brain MRI in coronal slices showing bilateral, symmetrical
hyperintensities involving selectively the internal pallidal nuclei.

that patients were spontaneously inactive and inert but that adequate activity might
be obtained from external demands or stimulations, thus pointing out the contrast
between impaired 'self-activation' and intact 'hetero-activation' of behavior. Both
authors noticed the conspicuous similarity between the motor and mental components of the syndrome, whereby the deficit seemed to affect both activities inas-
much as they are self-initiated. As will be seen later, this suggests a common
mechanism underlying both action and thought generation, or at least that their
impairments represent two separate manifestations of the same impaired process.

Another aspect already pointed out by Ali Chérif and only marginally alluded to
by Laplane, and which may be of considerable importance, is the usual coexistence
of impairment in still another domain of mental life, i.e., affect and emotion:
'Affectivity is equally impaired, at least in the domain of expression of affects, and
this "grande indifférence affective" is regularly pointed out by the patient's relatives'
(Ali Chérif et al., 1984). In fact, in this author's experience, it is clear that there exists
a purely emotional component to the syndrome, distinct from and probably
upstream to its most obvious and directly observable behavioral expression. In the
author's opinion, it is in this aspect that the pathophysiological crux of the syndrome lies, as discussed below.

Motivational disturbances in caudate lesions

Observations of such a behavioral syndrome following pallidal lesions raise two
separate questions from the point of view of anatomoclinical relationships. First, it
is not clear, from these reports, whether or not the pallidal lesions are the sole cause
of the syndrome, because other lesions at the microscopic level may also coexist,
due to an anoxic or toxic mechanism of brain damage possibly responsible for more
diffuse neuronal involvement. Although the internal globus pallidus is known to be
especially vulnerable to carbon monoxide toxicity, it may not be the sole site of

lesions (Uchino et al., 1994; Tom et al., 1996; Silver et al., 1996). Second, one may wonder about the exact nature of the role played by the globus pallidus. The observation, a few years later, of a similar clinical picture occurring with caudate lesions provided preliminary answers to these questions.

The author's group (Habib and Poncet, 1988) and others (Trillet et al., 1990) have reported the occurrence of very similar behavioral changes in several patients with focal ischemic lesions bilaterally involving the region of the head of the caudate nuclei.

Case FM

A 64-year-old retired police officer was hospitalized for 'recent and abrupt behavioral change.' Over the two or three weeks prior to admission, he had become, according to his spouse, totally apathetic, inactive, and prostrate. His medical history was unremarkable except for occasional bouts of elevated blood pressure, which had never justified continuous antihypertensive medication, and a few episodes of angor pectoris. On admission, he was clearly hypokinetic, with decreased spontaneous movements, facial amimia, and Parkinson-like gait. Neurological examination was otherwise normal, except for a moderate limb stiffness. An electroencephalogram (EEG) showed mild, nonspecific, diffuse slowing and a CT scan was interpreted as normal for the patient's age. His general behavior (Table 2) was characterized by a dramatic decrease in spontaneous activity. Totally abulic, he had no projects, showed no evidence of needs, wills, or desires. His activities were dramatically reduced and he spent his time in a stereotyped manner: he would wake up late in the morning, would not wash unless urged to do so, but meekly complied as soon as his wife asked him to. Then he would sit in his armchair, from which he would not move spontaneously. His main activity was watching television, but he never asked for it. He showed an obvious lack of concern for relatives as well as for his own condition. When questioned about his mood, he reported no sadness or anxiety. Also noteworthy was a loss of appetite (he never asked for food, even if left more than 24 hours without eating) and food preferences (he would eat with the same apparent satisfaction dishes he had or had not liked before). Finally, each time he was questioned about the content of his mind, he reported a striking absence of thoughts or spontaneous mental activity. Contrasting with these massive behavioral changes, cognitive functions seemed relatively spared. On bedside examination, he appeared fully conscious and well oriented. Neuropsychological evaluation (Table 9.2) was within normal limits, except for tests exploring frontal lobe function.

A T2-weighted spin-echo brain MRI scan (Fig. 9.2) showed multiple small zones of hyperintensity consistent with the definition of lacunes, located bilaterally in the basal ganglia regions. A single-photon emission tomography (SPET) with Tc99-HMPAO showed a relative bilateral hypoperfusion in the basal ganglia regions without significant modification of cortical – especially frontal – blood flow.

More recently, we have observed a very similar hypertensive patient (case BT, Table 9.2 and Fig. 9.3) with profound motivational impairment and relatively

Table 9.2. Cognitive performances in three cases of multiple lacunar infarcts of the caudate nuclei and adjacent white matter (see text and Figs. 9.2, 9.3 and 9.5)

	Case FM	Case BT	Case CJ
Global intellectual functioning			
MMS	27	30	30
Others	PM 38: IQ = 105	WAIS total IQ = 105 PIQ = 103, VIQ = 106	PM 38: IQ = 110
Language	No aphasia	Few naming errors; dysprosodia	Normal
Verbal fluency (animals)/2 min	9	17	27, then 26
Verbal fluency (letter P)/2 min	6	3	14, then 4
Discourse abilities	Poor spontaneous discourse; constant stimulation needed	Defective organization of discourse	Normal
Attention	Trail-making test: normal	Trail-making test: 1 error Stroop test: 19 color interferences/100 stimuli	Trail-making test and Stroop test: no errors but longer time needed
Memory[a] *(Wechsler Memory Scale)*			
Quotient	104	103	103
Digit span	8 (10.2 ± 1.92)	9 (10.36 ± 1.68)	10 (10.12)
Logical memory	7.5 (8.25 ± 3.32)	11 (10,15)	6.5 (9.81 ± 4.39)
Visual memory	10 (7,51)	12 (10.67)	11 (9.98)
Paired associates	13 (12.89)	15.5 (16.27 ± 2.23)	17.5 (15.61)
Memory (others)	Episodic memory: normal if cued	Rey auditory verbal learning: 9/15 5th trial; 10/15 delayed recall	Rey auditory verbal learning: 9/15 5th trial; 5/15 delayed recall
Visuo-spatial abilities	Rey figure copy: good apprehension, slowed execution	Rey figure, copy: normal in 4mn30	Rey complex figure: normal
Wisconsin card-sorting test	3 categories	0 categories	6 categories, 2 perseverations, then 5 categories, 5 perseverations
'Frontal' tests			
Alternating graphic sequences	Normal	Normal	Impaired
Motor gestural series	Impaired	Normal	Normal

Notes:
[a] First assessment: July 1990; second assessment: September 1990. Unless indicated, values from second assessment. Patients performance (normal ± SD).
CO, carbon monoxide; PM, Progressive Matrices; WAIS, Wechsler Adult Intelligence Scale; PIQ, Performance Intellectual Quotient; VIQ, Verbal Intellectual Quotient; MMS, Mini Mental Status examination.

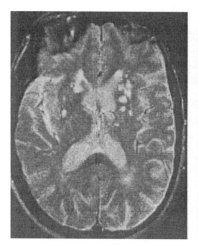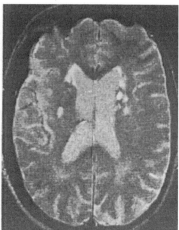

Fig. 9.2   Case FM: T2-weighted brain MRI showing multiple bilateral hyperintensities suggesting lacunar infarcts in the region of the caudate head.

spared cognitive functioning (except for frontal executive functions, which were significantly impaired, in particular on the Stroop and Wisconsin Card Sorting tests). As in the above-reported case, the patient was totally abulic, whereas neurological examination was strictly normal. In this case, behavioral changes had appeared quite abruptly following a brief left hemiparetic episode, suggesting a determinant role of the right caudate lesion. As shown in Fig. 9.3, lesions here, although also meeting the criteria for lacunes, were significantly larger than in the previous case.

The observation of dramatic loss of motivated behavior in cases of caudate infarcts has two important implications. First, it ascertains the direct relationship between these lesions and the observed mental changes, since in this case, unlike in pallidal cases, there is little reason to suspect associated microscopic damage. Second, it confirms that the same syndrome can occur after bilateral damage at two separate levels in the basal ganglia, pallidal and caudate, suggesting that these two structures are functionally linked in a unique network whose role is crucial for the organization of motivated behavior.

Other instances of motivational disturbances in subcortical lesions

Following the initial observations, several case reports have confirmed that caudate lesions may specifically alter motivated behavior. Trillet et al. (1990) reported three cases with persistent apathy, flattened affect, and lack of interest and initiative following bilateral deep infarcts involving the head of the caudate nuclei and adjacent anterior limb of the internal capsule. The authors discussed the function of the caudate nuclei in spontaneous motor activity as a regulator of prefrontal cortex

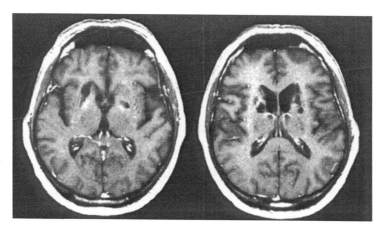

Fig. 9.3   Case BT: brain MRI showing bilateral ischemic lesions involving the caudate head and surrounding white matter. The frontal lobes appear intact.

activity. Bilateral, nonvascular involvement of the caudate occurs in Huntington's disease, in which similar behavioral changes, in association with global cognitive impairment, have been reported, even in the early stages of the disease (Caine et al., 1978). Moreover, several general reviews have reported apathy or abulia as a relatively frequent occurrence following caudate, generally bilateral, lesions (Caplan et al., 1990; Cummings, 1993; Bhatia and Marsden, 1994). These studies, however, did not provide detailed discussion of the underlying mechanisms. In their review of 240 cases of basal ganglia lesions, Bhatia and Marsden observed that abulia is the most frequent behavioral disorder (13%, i.e., 30 patients), and report that, among these 30 patients, lesions involved the caudate nucleus in 70% of the cases. However, this figure may only reflect the higher frequency of caudate lesions because lesions of the globus pallidus (the only other lesional site at the origin of apathetic behavior in this series) are much less frequent.

Paramedian mesencephalo-diencephalic infarcts have also been reported to give rise to apathetic and unmotivated behavior (Katz, Alexander and Mandell, 1987; Bogousslavsky et al., 1991). In the latter case, a brain metabolic exploration with single-photon emission computerized tomography demonstrated a decrease in frontal blood flow, unlike in our cases of caudate lesions. Actually, disturbances of action and motivation are often present in cases of bilateral medial thalamic lesions, but interpretation of behavioral changes is generally obscured by the co-occurrence of severe memory and cognitive impairment.

Motivational disorders in frontal lesions

In frontal lobe lesions, apathy, loss of interest, and apragmatism are classical elements of the so-called frontal syndrome, classically after lesions involving the dorsolateral part of the lobes (Blumer and Benson, 1975). According to Damasio (1985), however, such symptoms are more likely to be the consequence of damage to the mesial aspect of the lobes. Changes in personality following psychosurgery (leucotomies, cingulotomies) have often been described as a lack of emotional expression, decreased interest and drive, and impoverishment of affective life (Stuss and Benson, 1983, 1986; Damasio and Van Hoesen, 1983). The presence of the underlying psychiatric illness, however, renders an interpretation difficult.

Eslinger and Damasio (1985) have reported the detailed case study of a patient (EVR) with bilateral postsurgical destruction of the mesial and orbital parts of the frontal lobes. Whereas intellectual functioning was normal, even on tests of executive functions, massive behavioral changes were present, some of them being very similar to those of our patients: '. . . EVR was not motivated for action. He seemed not to have available programs of action capable of driving him to motion . . . There was no evidence that an internal, automatic program was ready to propel him into the routine daily activities of self-care and feeding . . .' The authors proposed that these behavioral abnormalities could be due to the loss of connections between dorsolateral frontal cortex, which was intact, and limbic structures.

Laplane et al. (1988) reported a case of bilateral frontal traumatic lesions involving exclusively the periventricular white matter, with a very similar clinical picture associating loss of interest, lack of goals and motivation, and mental emptiness. As in the previously reported cases, there was a considerable contrast between almost normal neuropsychological functioning and profound behavioral changes.

Neuroanatomical correlates of human motivation

Fronto-subcortical connections

The similarity of the syndrome reported after subcortical lesions to certain aspects of the frontal syndrome, as well as the constant association of impairment on tests sensitive to frontal lobe dysfunction, may lead to the conclusion that the subcortical abulic syndrome described here is due to some indirect effect of the basal ganglia (and/or adjacent white matter) lesion on the normal functioning of the frontal cortex. Based on the results of positron emission tomography studies in bipallidal patients, Laplane (1990) suggests that 'loss of self-activation' observed in pallidal lesions results from a mechanism of deactivation of the frontal cortex, since patients in their series had (moderate) frontal hypoperfusion (Laplane et al., 1989). The role played by the basal ganglia would then be considered tantamount to that of a nonspecific activation system. Habib and Poncet (1988; see also Habib, 1995; Habib and Galaburda, 1998) have proposed a radically different interpretation on the basis of anatomical studies of fronto-subcortical circuits.

According to current neuroanatomical modelling of the connections between

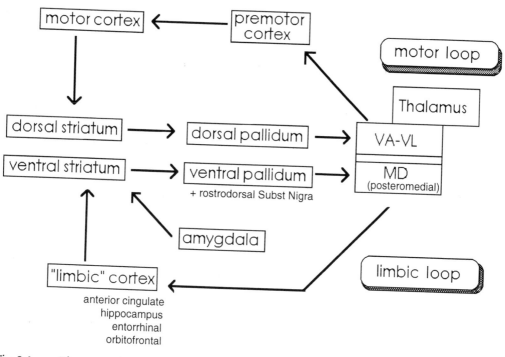

Fig. 9.4   Diagrammatic representation of the two cortical–subcortical loops. (Adapted from Nauta, 1986, and Alexander et al., 1986.) Abulic symptoms may result from lesions at any point of the limbic loop (see text).

the basal ganglia and frontal cortex (as recently summarized by Cummings, 1993), it is now generally accepted that cortico-subcortical connections are organized in several loops functioning in parallel, each presumably subserving a specific function. Alexander et al. (Alexander, DeLong and Strick, 1986, Alexander, Crutcher and DeLong, 1990) described five parallel cortico-subcortical loops originating from and terminating in different parts of the frontal cortex. One of these circuits, mainly originating in anterior cingulate cortex, encompasses the ventral striatum, the ventral part of the globus pallidus, and the posteromedial medial–dorsal nucleus of the thalamus, and projects back again to the anterior cingulate (Fig. 9.4). This circuit, connecting cortical and subcortical components of the limbic system, is very similar to the 'limbic loop' postulated by Nauta (1986) to be involved in motivational and emotional control in the rat. There is now enough converging evidence to consider the limbic (or ventral) striatopallidum as an 'interface between motivation and action' (Mogenson, Jones and Yim, 1980) or as the site of 'conversion of motivational processes into behavioral output' (Apicella et al., 1991). Such conceptions are logically derived from the observation that the limbic striatopallidum is ideally situated to subserve this role, because it receives afferents from the amygdala, involved in the emotional labelling of sensory stimuli, and from the hippocampal formation, supposed to compare incoming information with past experience, and projects to the rest of the basal ganglia mass, involved in initiating and organizing motor acts (Salamone, 1994; Schultz, 1995).

Experimental evidence

Such a role in converting affective information into motivated acts was first suggested from the classical self-stimulation experiments in rats, and various subsequent manipulations of this model have shown a major participation of the ventral striatum, recipient of dopaminergic afferents, in such behavior. For instance, direct infusion of dopaminergic agents in the nucleus accumbens, the main part of the limbic striatum in rodents, considerably alters the animal's approach behaviors (Ikemoto and Panksepp, 1996), whereas rats allowed to self-stimulate with autoinjections of amphetamines in the accumbens develop a strong tendency to autostimulate. Various other interventions in the dopamine system within the accumbens have shown alterations of stimulating effects of rewarding stimuli on the animal's behavior (Everitt and Robbins, 1992). The most convincing results, however, are those obtained from unit recordings in monkeys. Rolls and colleagues (see Rolls, 1994) recorded a large number of neurons in the limbic striatum and showed that they can react to such various conditions as novel stimuli, various previously reinforced visual stimuli, or even cues announcing the beginning of the task. Data concerning the role of the globus pallidus are more sparse, but recent work has implicated pallidal neurons in reward mechanisms (McAlonan, Robbins and Everitt, 1993; Panagis et al., 1995).

Toward a unified neuroanatomical interpretation of motivational disorders following basal ganglia lesions

Finally, the well-documented demonstration of a circuit centered on the basal ganglia, probably involved in the 'process of converting motivation into action,' suggests that the above-mentioned human abulic syndromes may result from bilateral disruption (at various levels) of this circuit.

The purest form of the syndrome would be completed after damage to the limbic striatopallidum. Worthy of note is that in primates, the limbic (mainly cingulate) afferents to the striatum, unlike those in rodents, are not restricted to its ventral part – the accumbens nucleus – but are represented on a broader part of the caudate itself, along a strip extending rostrocaudally on the mesial aspect of the nucleus (Selemon and Goldman-Rakic, 1985). This could explain the occurrence of the abulic syndrome in humans, with caudate lesions apparently sparing the more ventrally located accumbens nucleus (see Figs. 9.2 and 9.3).

The syndrome may also result from disconnection of the limbic striatopallidum from mesial frontal structures (for instance in lesions damaging the short cingulo-caudate fibers, running close to the frontal horn of the lateral ventricle) or from lesions situated at the output side of the system (i.e., paramedian 'limbic' nuclei of the thalamus and thalamocortical afferents). Although structures at different levels of the system may have functional specificities, they all share a common implication in motivational processes, in such a way that bilateral damage at either point of the loop would produce apathetic and abulic behavior.

A plausible argument in favor of this view is provided by observations in which the same syndrome results from asymmetrical lesions of this circuit.

Case CJ

A 48-year-old man, who had been receiving antidepressant treatment for two years, was referred in July 1990 for neuropsychological evaluation by his psychiatrist. Over a period of eight years prior to admission, he had sustained several unexplained, brief syncopal episodes, for which repeated cardiovascular evaluations had yielded negative results. A CT scan performed in 1986 was normal. Depressive symptoms, including suicidal ideas, feelings of incompetence, sadness, and sleeping disorders, had appeared in 1988, and proved to be totally resistant to antidepressant drugs. More recently, he also complained of memory difficulties and decreased motivation, which were ascribed to depression. However, a follow-up CT scan showed a right hemisphere hypodensity suggestive of an old ischemic infarct involving the head of the caudate nucleus. At this time, neurological examination was normal. Neuropsychological evaluation was unremarkable, except for some difficulties in temporal indexation of autobiographical events.

In August 1990, he sustained a new syncopal episode, followed by a two-day confusional state. He was examined again in September 1990. At this time, his mental status was totally modified: he no longer felt depressed, and his wife reported profound behavioral changes, describing his new behavior as childish, without any initiative, doing nothing at home unless prompted by someone. He also showed unusual indifference toward his relatives, and did not demonstrate any tenderness toward his spouse. Finally, he reported that he was able to stay several minutes without thinking when inactive. Neurological examination was still normal, but neuropsychological evaluation showed some abnormalities not present two months earlier, especially on tests of arithmetical reasoning, logical memory of the Wechsler Memory Scale, verbal fluency, and alternating graphomotor sequences. An MRI brain scan performed at this time (Fig. 9.5) disclosed new ischemic changes in the left hemisphere, consisting in several hyperintense signals located at the border between the territories of the anterior and middle cerebral arteries. A SPECT with Tc99-HMPAO demonstrated a deep area of decreased perfusion in the right basal ganglia region.

Eight years later, the man's clinical status is unchanged: he has become totally dependent, completely inactive, and affectively indifferent. Perfectly aware of his own personality changes, he claims not to suffer from these changes, but only regrets having to impose them on his wife and children.

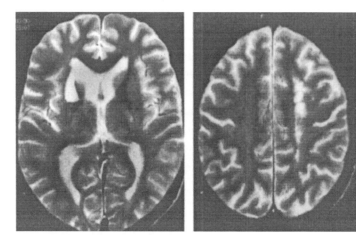

Fig. 9.5   Case CJ: T2-weighted brain MRI showing asymmetrical involvement of the fronto-striatal loop. In the right hemisphere, a triangular infarct involves the caudate nucleus (left picture), whereas in the left hemisphere, coalescent lacunar infarcts disconnect the cingulate gyrus from subjacent basal ganglia (right).

Not only a convincing piece of evidence in favor of the striatal–limbic disconnection theory, this observation also illustrates the complex relationship between abulia and depression, as discussed in the last section of this chapter.

The 'athymhormic syndrome:' a proposed interpretation and underlying mechanism

As mentioned above, observations of motivational disorders, although not necessarily identified as such, have already been reported in the classical neurological literature. Adams and Victor (1985: 388), under the term 'apathy,' referred to 'a quantitative reduction of all activities,' not unlike akinetic mutism, and ascribed both conditions to the impairment of a 'centrencephalic-cortical energetic mechanism.' They furthermore proposed to isolate, among this group, patients designed as 'hypobulic,' showing a lesser degree of the same defect, with 'apathy, indifference, loss of interest and shallowness of thinking.' Miller Fisher (1983) prefers the term 'abulia minor,' considering the syndrome, here again, as a minimal form of akinetic mutism. Actually, neither the terms apathy or abulia, nor that of loss of self-activation are totally satisfactory because they do not account for the underlying mechanism linking the different facets of the syndrome. In particular, if the most obvious changes concern the domain of action, it is highly probable that the primary dysfunction is located upstream to the action itself, at the level of emotional processes.

Pathology of action: only a surface symptom

Patients are massively inert, spending their days in a stereotyped manner, staying inactive in the same place for hours, with their eyes open. This inertia is coupled with a striking passivity. One of the author's patients would stay motionless and mute for several minutes in front of the examiner – who remained deliberately silent – without asking any question or showing the slightest manifestation of impatience. This profound inertia, however, appears as a mere surface manifestation, covering a subjacent, probably affective, disturbance. Patients demonstrate a more or less total indifference to life events that would normally provoke an emotional response, positive or negative. When reminded of memorable personal or familial episodes, such as the loss of a loved one, or of dramatic social events, inappropriately flat emotional expression may be observed. Patients report their own experience of such situations 'with coldness and purely verbally' (Ali Chérif et al., 1984). Some of them report that they no longer feel the physical and mental modifications they used to experience in emotional situations. Others seem more specifically unable to express their feelings. The relatives of one patient (Habib and Poncet, 1988) said that 'although he seemed happy, for instance, in the presence of his grand-children, he did not show any affective manifestation either on their arrival or their leaving, never asking to see them again.' Patients are able to recall which activities, occupations or hobbies they were formerly interested in, but claim that they are not bothered by their indifference and that they do not miss these past experiences.

More than a mere affective indifference, it seems as though stimuli had lost their reinforcing value. One patient's wife reported: 'Formerly, he liked money very much and always had some with him; he loved touching it. Now, he is totally disinterested. He does not ask about his business, his house under construction, his dog. He has lost every kind of passion, for cars, for outings.' This heavy smoker had not stopped smoking but smoked less than before. Interestingly, he reported he no longer felt the sensation of frustration he used to feel when he was short of cigarettes.

Finally, the apparent affective indifference may, in fact, be better characterized by the loss of a spontaneous tendency to gain immediate satisfaction of primary needs, i.e., absence of desire rather than absence of emotion. To paraphrase a recently proposed dichotomy, the primary disturbance may be one of 'wanting' rather than one of 'liking' (Berridge, 1996), but large variations may exist depending on individuals and, probably, also depending on lesional topography. Berridge suggests that 'liking' involves the ventral pallidum, whereas 'wanting' would rely more heavily on dopaminergic mechanisms in the accumbens nucleus. Although the clinical pictures in pallidal and caudate cases do not appear to differ significantly, it remains possible that pallidal lesions result in a more pervasive emotional deficit, much akin to that observed in cases of hypoemotionality due to destruction or disconnection of temporal–limbic structures (Habib, 1986).

From affect to motivation: 'athymhormia' as a striatal–limbic disconnection syndrome

Such a close relation between lack of activity and emotional blunting is strongly reminiscent of the behavior of a subtype of schizophrenic patients with negative symptoms (often referred to as type II schizophrenia). In fact, more than 70 years ago, French psychiatrists (Dide and Guiraud, 1922) coined the term *athymhormie* to refer to those characteristics of behavior and affect of schizophrenic patients, namely 'loss of interest, affect and *elan vital*,' thus pointing to the two components they considered as central to the syndrome, from the two Greek roots: ορμη (which means impulse, drive, or *elan*) and θυμος (mood, affect). Moreover, these authors, in a quite premonitory discussion, ascribed these mental functions to archaic brain structures situated in the depth of the hemispheres (see Guiraud, 1956).

We have proposed the use of the term 'athymhormic syndrome,' rather than abulia or apathy, to describe the behavior of our brain-damaged patients, not only to point out the similarity to some psychiatric disorders, but mainly because it stresses the dual nature of the syndrome (i.e., both the hormic component contained in abulia and the thymic component contained in apathy). The interface between these two aspects may best describe the concept of motivation.

Conceiving the disorder as a fundamental defect in converting past or present emotional experience into an actual action, it appears that an account in terms of 'loss of self-activation' becomes clearly insufficient. Instead, one must rather conceive the relevant mechanism as supported by a brain system interfacing, on one hand, systems apt to analyze, maintain in long-term memory, and retrieve the affective value of a given stimulus or contextual cue (a process presumably subserved by the amygdala–hippocampus system), and, on the other hand, systems in charge of controlling movement initiation, mental activity, and emotional expression, possibly represented in various parts of the basal ganglia, as separate fronto-subcortical loops.

Figure 9.6 summarizes a tentative model of brain mechanisms subserving motivation in humans. In the light of theories derived from animal research, motivation may appear as the behavioral consequence of processes leading to establishing an association between a stimulus and its affective significance for the animal, i.e., the potentially rewarding nature of the stimulus (Apicella et al., 1991; Rolls, 1995). Not unlike classical Pavlovian conditioning, repetition of such associations over time would result in some kind of conditioning, which determines goal-directed behaviors. The distinction is usually made, among these stimuli, between primary rewards, whose motivational value is innately determined for the species, and whose role is to restore homeostatic balance, and secondary reinforcers, which

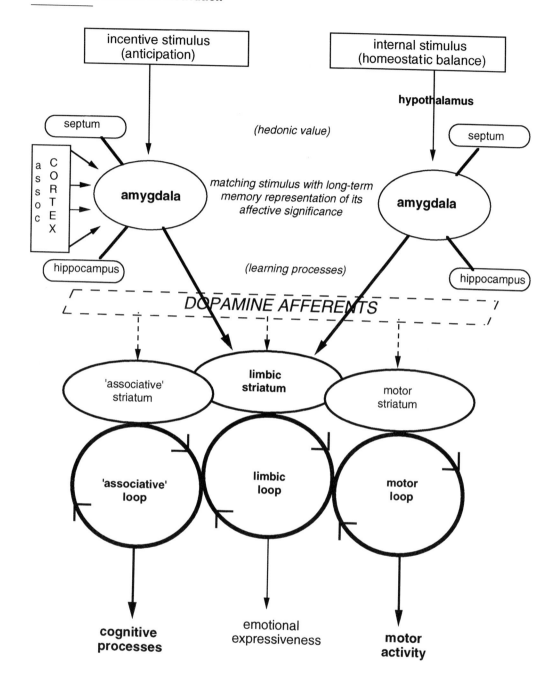

behavioral level

Fig. 9.6   A proposed anatomical–functional model of human motivation.

acquire their motivational value by repeated association with primary reinforcers. In the latter group, one may consider anticipation as the key process, since the animal must possess some kind of mental representation of the result of its action. Obviously, the situation may be much more complex in humans, because most of our behaviors may depend on more or less conscious actualization of the goal to be reached, but the basic mechanisms may be fundamentally similar.

From an anatomical point of view, there is strong evidence that the amygdala is the structural site of association between stimulus and reward (Rolls, 1986, 1995). The strong projections from amygdala to the limbic striatum and connections between limbic and motor parts of the striatum suggest for the limbic striato-pallidum the role of converting affective representations contained in the amygdala into motor programs: supplied with dopamine by specific dopamine afferents, the limbic part of the striatum would represent the driving center of the three main fronto-striatal loops functioning as three articulated gears turning together. Continuous functioning of the motor and associative loops would be dependent on the functioning of the limbic loop, with 'energy' being provided by their respective dopaminergic input. Each loop possesses a specific output (motor acts for the motor loop, emotional expression for the limbic loop, and spontateous mental activity for the associative loop), accounting for the three main symptoms of the athymhormic syndrome. According to this representation, damage to the limbic loop, while leaving intact the other two, would result in impaired spontaneous cognitive and motor activity, giving rise to the characteristic symptoms of athymhormia: lack of spontaneous action (but intact motor functioning) and poverty of spontaneous thinking (but relatively preserved intellectual capacities). This model provides a plausible explanation for the curious association between loss of motor and mental activity, as well as their reversibility upon external stimulation. According to the model, however, blunting of emotional expression would be, unlike the other two symptoms, a nonreversible phenomenon, but this does not preclude the possible preservation of emotional experience itself.

Final diagnostic considerations

Athymhormia is not rare in neurological practice

The conditions of patients described in the previous sections of this chapter correspond to extreme forms of the syndrome. Such a dissociation between behavioral changes and intact cognition is obviously not a common observation. In the author's experience, milder forms of the same syndrome may be recognized much more frequently in neurological practice. One common instance of such milder forms is that of lacunar syndromes. Hypertensive patients, especially those with 'unstable' hypertension, presenting with episodic bouts of elevated blood pressure, are especially prone to develop multiple subcortical lacunes in the more distal territory of perforating arterioles (Habib et al., 1991). After several years of evolution, cognitive symptoms may arise, classically with phases of rapid evolution alternating with plateaus, ultimately evolving toward a highly disabling picture of vascular dementia. In addition to this cognitive decline, proportional to the diffusion of lesions throughout the hemispheres' (especially frontal) white matter, behavioral symptoms are invariably present to some extent, resulting in a more or less complete form of athymhormia. The relative proportion of cognitive versus behavioral impairment is closely related to the distribution of lacunar lesions, as best demonstrated on T2-weighted MRI images, and to whether or not the basal ganglia, especially the caudate head, are involved. In milder cases, symptoms of apathy and indifference are often misinterpreted as depressive reactions to cognitive decline (see below).

Another instance in which athymhormic symptoms may be underdiagnosed is that of sequelae from craniocerebral trauma. In this case, patients may be much more disabled by their behavioral than cognitive impairment, so that the resulting handicap may be erroneously ascribed to premorbid psychological fragility, a common error which may have dramatic consequences in forensic practice. In our experience, a crucial element to the diagnosis is provided when sequelar lesions are demonstrated on brain imaging to involve the periventricular white matter fibers bilaterally, thus interrupting the limbic–striatal connections.

Athymhormia and its relations to dementia

Basal ganglia lesions, whatever their causes and mechanisms, may by themselves produce diffuse cognitive impairment, a condition referred to as subcortical dementia. In addition to a vascular origin, subcortical dementia may also result from etiological processes as varied as degeneration, infections, inflammatory processes, or tumors. Among these, two conditions particularly have been reported as giving rise to prominent associated behavioral changes: von Economo postencephalitis parkinsonism (Naville, 1922) and progressive supranuclear palsy. Although resulting from very different mechanisms, the lesions are topographically similar, predominantly involving upper brainstem structures, responsible for both cognitive symptoms (bradyphrenia and dementia without aphasia, agnosia or apraxia but with frontal-like impairment) and behavioral changes, with apathy, inertia, and indifference (Darvesh and Freedman, 1996). In one case of progressive supranuclear palsy, Destée et al. (1990) have related the prominent athymhormic symptoms to the particularly severe lesions observed postmortem in the globus pallidus.

In cortical dementias, the most frequent being Alzheimer's disease, changes in personality and affect are often reported, and their observation is especially useful for diagnosis when present early in the course of the illness. Because the basal ganglia are relatively spared in Alzheimer's disease, one may suspect that athymhormia symptoms are due to cortical or basal frontal involvement. Recently, however, the severity of apathy has been related to the importance of leukoaraiosis on brain imaging (Starkstein et al., 1997). One important point concerning Alzheimer's disease is that symptoms of lack of motivation and action are often reversed by new cholinergic medication requiring specific evaluation with *ad hoc* batteries (Habib, 1995; Marin, 1990, 1991).

Finally, although behavioral changes are classical components of the syndrome of dementia, athymhormia must be differentiated from dementia, because it can occur without cognitive impairment. However, the presence of even mild athymhormic symptoms in association with signs of cognitive decline suggests the involvement of the limbic part of fronto-subcortical circuits and thus focuses the search for an etiology toward pathological conditions likely to damage these regions.

Athymhormia and depression

The last issue to be considered in this chapter is of major clinical relevance: how to differentiate athymhormia from depression? Indeed, apathy, lack of goals and perspective are all common symptoms in depressive disorders. In the most severe forms of the pure motivational disorders referred to in the previous sections, the issue is probably less crucial because the patient's examination fails to disclose any sign of sadness or negative thoughts. Instead, patients are more or less – sometimes dramatically – indifferent to any environmental event as well as to their own condition. Moreover, the mental emptiness demonstrated in these patients is diametrically opposite to the classical negative 'rumination' of depressed patients. It is thus of primary importance to investigate specifically the actual content of patients' spontaneous thoughts to reach the appropriate diagnosis.

In less severe cases, however, the evidence for emotional indifference is less observable, and close scrutiny may often fail to disclose a characteristic mental emptiness. In such cases, a depressive mood may be prominent and the clinical picture may be indistinguishable from authentic depression. This was the case for the patient reported above (case CJ) where the component of inertia and adynamism was, at the beginning, not accompanied by significant blunting of affect, so that negative mood could arise, probably as a 'normal' reaction to his own behavioral changes and incompetence. However, the whole clinical picture was observed following the subsequent vascular episode, probably because of the bilateralization of limbic-striatal disconnection.

Conclusion

Apathy, abulia, loss of self-activation, and athymhormia constitute a unique syndrome whose components are well defined and which can be identified and measured for the purpose of therapeutic evaluation (Marin, 1990, 1991; Habib, 1995). Plausible hypotheses concerning its brain substrate as well as the pathophysiological link between its components are now available. The concepts thus developed through the observation of the most severe cases can be applied with reasonable confidence to a much wider array of clinical observations, including similar symptoms occurring in such diverse conditions as vascular or degenerative dementias and brain traumatic injuries. The close relationship between radiological evidence of damage along a specific brain circuit and a specific set of clinical symptoms is of major diagnostic importance in neurological practice.

Finally, the analogy between the motivation defects following focal brain lesions and those observed in certain schizophrenic patients is consistent with hypotheses emphasizing dysfunction of the limbic-striatal connections in schizophrenia (Swerdlow and Koob, 1987).

REFERENCES

Adams, R.D. and Victor, M. (1985). *Principles of Neurology*, 3rd edn. New York: McGraw-Hill.

Alexander, G.E., Crutcher, M.D. and DeLong, M.R. (1990). Basal ganglia–thalamocortical circuits: parallel substrates for motor, oculomotor, 'prefrontal' and 'limbic' function. *Prog Brain Res* 85: 119–46.

Alexander, G.E., DeLong, M.R. and Strick, P.L. (1986). Parallel organization of functionally segregated circuits linking basal ganglia and cortex. *Ann Rev Neurosci* 9: 357–81.

Ali Chérif, A., Royère, M.L., Gosset, A. et al. (1984). Troubles du comportement et de l'activité mentale après intoxication oxy-carbonée. Lésions pallidales bilatérales. *Rev Neurol* 140: 401–5.

Apicella, P., Ljundberg, T., Scarnati, E. and Schultz, W. (1991). Responses to reward in monkey dorsal and ventral striatum. *Exp Brain Res* 85: 491–500.

Bellmann, A. and Assal, G. (1996). Les multiples propos d'une athymhormique. *Rev Neuropsychol* 6(1): 101–20.

Berridge K.C. (1996). Food reward: brain substrates of wanting and liking. *Neurosci Biobehav Rev* 20(1): 1–25.

Bhatia, K.P. and Marsden, D. (1994). The behavioural and motor consequences of focal lesions of the basal ganglia in man. *Brain* 117: 859–76.

Blumer, D. and Benson, D.F. (1975). Personality changes with frontal and temporal lobe lesions. In *Psychiatric Aspects of Neurologic Disease*, Vol I, ed. D.F. Benson and D. Blumer, pp. 151–70. New York: Grune & Stratton.

Bogousslavsky, J., Regli, F., Delaloye, B. et al. (1991). Loss of psychic self-activation with bithalamic infarction: neurobehavioural, CT, MRI and SPECT correlates. *Acta Neurol Scand* 83: 309–16.

Caine, E.D., Hunt, R.D., Weingartner, H. and Ebert, M.H. (1978). Huntington's dementia. Clinical and neuropsychological features. *Arch Gen Psychiatry* 35: 377–84.

Caplan, L.R., Schmahmann, J.D., Kase, C.S. et al. (1990). Caudate infarcts. *Arch Neurol* 47: 133–43.

Cummings, J.L. (1993). Frontal–subcortical circuits and human behavior. *Arch Neurol* 50: 873–80.

Damasio, A.R. (1985). The frontal lobes. In *Clinical Neuropschology*, ed. K.M. Heilman and E. Valenstein. New York: Oxford University Press.

Damasio, A.R. and Van Hoesen, G.W. (1983). Emotional disturbances associated with focal lesions of the limbic frontal lobe. In *Neuropsychology of Human Emotion*, ed. K.M. Heilman and P. Satz. New York, London: The Guilford Press.

Danel, T., Goudemand, M., Ghawche, F. et al. (1991). Mélancholie délirante et lacunes multiples des noyaux gris centraux. *Rev Neurol* 147: 60–2.

Darvesh, S. and Freedman, M. (1996). Subcortical dementia: a neurobehavioral approach. *Brain Cogn* 31(2): 230–49.

Destée, A., Gray, F., Parent, M. et al. (1990). Comportement compulsif d'allure obsessionnelle et paralysie supranucléaire progressive. *Rev Neurol* 146: 12–18.

Dide, M. and Guiraud, P. (1922). *Psychiatrie du Médecin Praticien.* Masson: Paris.

Eslinger, P.J. and Damasio, A.R. (1985). Severe disturbance of higher cognition after bilateral frontal lobe ablation: patient EVR. *Neurology* 35: 1731–41.

Everitt, B.J. and Robbins, T.W. (1992). Amygdala–ventral striatal interactions and reward-related processes. In *The Amygdala*, ed. J.P. Aggleton, pp. 401–30. Chichester: Wiley.

Fisher, C.M. (1983). Abulia minor versus agitated behavior. *Clin Neurosurg* 31: 9–31.

Guiraud, P. (1956). *Psychiatrie Clinique.* Paris: Le François.

Habib, M. (1986). Visual hypoemotionality and prosopagnosia associated with right temporal lobe isolation. *Neuropsychologia* 24: 577–82.

Habib, M. (1995). Troubles de l'action et de la motivation en neurologie: proposition d'une échelle d'évaluation. *L'Encéphale* 21: 563–70.

Habib, M. and Galaburda, A.M. (1998). Disorders of movement and action in limbic lesions. In: *Disorders of Movement in Psychiatry and Neurology*, 2nd edn, ed. A.B. Joseph. Cambridge, MA: Blackwell.

Habib, M. and Poncet, M. (1988). Perte de l'élan vital, de l'intérêt et de l'affectivité (syndrome athymhormique) au cours de lésions lacunaires des corps striés. *Rev Neurol* 144: 571–7.

Habib, R., Royère, M.L., Habib, G. et al. (1991). Modifications de la personnalité et hypertension artérielle: le syndrome athymhormique. *Arch Mal Coeur* 84: 1225–30.

Ikemoto, S. and Panksepp, J. (1996). Dissociations between appetitive and consummatory responses by pharmacological manipulations of reward-relevant brain regions. *Behav Neurosci* 110(2): 331–45.

Katz, D.I., Alexander, M.P. and Mandell, A.M. (1987). Dementia following strokes in the mesencephalon and diencephalon. *Arch Neurol* 44: 1127–33.

Laplane, D. (1990). La perte d'auto-activation psychique. *Revue Neurol (Paris)* 146: 397–404.

Laplane, D., Baulac, M., Pillon, B. and Panayotopoulou-Achimastos, I. (1982). Perte de l'auto-activation psychique. Activité compulsive d'allure obsessionnelle. Lésion lenticulaire bilatérale. *Rev Neurol* 138: 137–41.

Laplane, D., Baulac, M., Widlöcher, D. and Dubois, B. (1984). Pure psychic akinesia with bilateral lesions of basal ganglia. *J Neurol Neurosurg Psychiatry* 47: 377–85.

Laplane, D., Dubois, B., Pillon, B. and Baulac, M. (1988). Perte d'autoactivation psychique et activité mentale stéréotypée par lésion frontale. Rapports avec le trouble obsessivo-compulsif. *Rev Neurol (Paris)* 144: 564–70.

Laplane, D., Levasseur, M., Pillon, B. et al. (1989). Obsessive–compulsive and other behavioral changes with bilateral basal ganglia lesions. *Brain* 112: 699–725.

Laplane, D., Widlocher, D., Pillon, B., Baulac, M. and Binox, F. (1981). Comportement compulsif d'allure obsessionnelle par nécrose circonscrite bilatérale pallido-striatale. Encéphalopathie par piqure de guêpe. *Rev Neurol* 137: 269–76.

Luauté, J.P., Bidault, E. and Sanabria, E. (1990). État athymhormique après accident vasculaire cérébral du post-partum. Apport de l'imagerie cérébrale. Société Médico-Psychologique. Séance du 22 janvier 1990, pp. 532–8.

Marin, R.S. (1990). Differential diagnosis and classification of apathy. *Am J Psychiatry* 147: 22–30.

Marin, R.S. (1991). Apathy: a neuropsychiatric syndrome. *J Neuropsychiatry Clin Neurosci* 3: 243–54.

McAlonan, G.M., Robbins, T.W. and Everitt, B.J. (1993). Effects of medial dorsal thalamic and ventral pallidal lesions on the acquisition of a conditioned place preference: further evidence for the involvement of the ventral striatopallidal system in reward-related processes. *Neuroscience* 52(3): 605–20.

Milandre, L., Habib, M., Royere, M.L., Gouirand, R. and Khalil, R. (1995). Syndrome athymhormique par infarctus striato-capsulaire bilatéral. Maladie de Moya-Moya de l'adulte. *Rev Neurol* 151: 383–7.

Mogenson, G.J., Jones, D.L. and Yim, C.J. (1980). From motivation to action: functional interface between the limbic system and the motor system. *Progr Neurobiol* 14: 69–97.

Nauta, W.J.H. (1986). Circuitous connections linking cerebral cortex, limbic system, and corpus striatum. In *The Limbic System: Functional Organization and Clinical Disorders*, ed. B.K. Doane and K.E. Livingston, pp. 43–54. New York: Raven Press.

Naville, F. (1922). Études sur les complications et les séquelles mentales de l'encéphalite épidémique. La bradyphrénie. *Encéphale* 17: 369–75.

Panagis, G., Miliaressis, E., Anagnostakis, Y. and Spyraki, C. (1995). Ventral pallidum self-stimulation: a moveable electrode mapping study. *Behav Brain Res* 68(2): 165–72.

Rolls, E.T. (1986). Neural systems involved in emotion in primates. In: *Emotion: Theory, Research, and Experience*, ed. R. Plutchik and H. Kellerman, pp. 125–43. London: Academic Press.

Rolls, E.T. (1994). Neurophysiologie et fonctions cognitives du striatum. *Rev Neurol (Paris)* 150: 648–60.

Rolls, E.T. (1995). A theory of emotion and consciousness, and its application to understanding the neural basis of emotion. In: *The Cognitive Neurosciences*, ed. M.S. Gazzaniga, pp. 1091–106. Cambridge, MA: MIT Press.

Salamone, J.D. (1994). The involvement of nucleus accumbens dopamine in appetitive and aversive motivation. *Behav Brain Res* 61(2): 117–33.

Schultz, W. (1995). The primate basal ganglia: between the intention and outcome of action. In *Functions of the Cortico-Basal Ganglia Loop*, ed. M. Kimura and A.M. Graybiel. Tokyo: Springer.

Selemon, L.D. and Goldman-Rakic, P.S. (1985). Longitudinal topography and interdigitation of corticostriatal projections in the Rhesus monkey. *J Neurosci* 5: 776–94.

Silver, D.A., Cross, M., Fox, B. and Paxton, R.M. (1996). Computer tomography of the brain in acute carbon monoxide poisoning. *Clin Radiol* 51(7): 480–3.

Starkstein, S.E., Sabe, L., Vazquez, S. et al. (1997). Neuropsychological, psychiatric, and cerebral perfusion correlates of leukoaraiosis in Alzheimer's disease. *Neurol Neurosurg Psychiatry* 63(1): 66–73.

Strub, L.R. (1989). Frontal lobe syndrome in a patient with bilateral globus pallidus lesions. *Arch Neurol* 46: 1024–7.

Stuss, D.T. and Benson, D.F. (1983). Emotional concomitants of psychosurgery. In: *Neuropsychology of Human Emotion*, ed. K.M. Heilman and P. Satz. New York, London: The Guilford Press.

Stuss, D.T. and Benson, D.F. (1986). *The Frontal Lobes*. New York: Raven Press.

Swerdlow, N.R. and Koob, G.F. (1987). Dopamine, schizophrenia, mania, and depression: toward a unified hypothesis of cortico-striato-pallido-thalamic function. *Behav Brain Sci* 10: 197–245.

Tom, T., Abedon, S., Clark, R.I. and Wong, W. (1996). Neuroimaging characteristics in carbon monoxide toxicity. *J Neuroimaging* 6(3): 161–6.

Trillet, M., Croisile, B., Tourniaire, D. and Schott, B. (1990). Disorders of voluntary motor activity and lesions of caudate nuclei. *Rev Neurol (Paris)* 146: 338–44.

Uchino, A., Hasuo, K., Shida, K. et al. (1994). MRI of the brain in chronic carbon monoxide poisoning. *Neuroradiology* 36(5): 399–401.

10

Thalamic behavioral syndromes

Atsushi Yamadori

Introduction

The thalamus has been regarded as the primary ganglion of the brain and its importance is well recognized. It has complicated bidirectional and sometimes unidirectional connections with the cortical structures of the cerebral hemispheres, cerebellum, hypothalamus, and many brainstem nuclear structures. Almost all incoming information passes through the thalamus before finally arriving at its cortical destination. Most of the outgoing fibers from the cortex also send direct or indirect messages to the thalamus. Because the thalamus is buried deep in the brain and its nuclei are packed in such a compact mass, definition of clinical symptomatology caused by a specific nuclear lesion has been difficult. Even with today's neuroimaging technology, the symptomatology of each thalamic nucleus remains obscure, especially in the sphere of higher cognitive functions.

Anatomy

Before going into the details of clinical symptomatology, any confusion caused by the different terminology used in the literature should be clarified. In the literature different terminology appears. For instance, the terms mediodorsal nucleus (MD) and dorsomedial nucleus are used interchangeably. It is all the more confusing when the abbreviation MD is used together with the descriptive name of dorsomedial nucleus. In the official Latin terminological system (*Nomina Anatomica*), the general attribute comes immediately after the word nucleus, followed by the more restrictive attribute such as 'nucleus medialis dorsalis (MD).' In this chapter, the terminology of Carpenter's (1991: pp. 255–83) *Core Text of Neuroanatomy*, fourth edition is employed. According to this textbook, thalamic nuclei are divided into ten main groups (Table 10.1).

A more simple summary was presented by Nauta and Feirtag (1986): the lateral geniculate body (LGB), medial geniculate body (MGB) and ventral posterior nucleus (VP) belong to the specific sensory nuclei. They receive sensory

Table 10.1. Classification of thalamic nuclei

---

1. Anterior nuclear group (AN*)
    Anteroventral nucleus (AV)
    Anterodorsal nucleus (AD)
    Anteromedial nucleus (AM)
2. Mediodorsal nucleus (MD)
    Magnocellular portion (MDmc)
    Parvicellular portion (MDpc)
    Paralaminar portion (MDpl)
3. Midline nuclei
4. Intralaminar nuclei
    Centromedian nucleus (CM)
    Parafascicular nucleus (PF)
    Rostral intralaminar nuclei
        Paracentral nucleus (PCN)
        Central lateral nucleus (CL)
        Central medial nucleus
5. Lateral nuclear group
    Lateral dorsal nucleus (LD)
    Lateral posterior nucleus (LP)
    Pulvinar
6. Ventral nuclear mass
    Ventral anterior nucleus (VA)
        Magnocellular part (VAmc)
        Parvicellular part (VApc)
    Ventral lateral nucleus (VL)
        Pars oralis (VLo)
        Pars caudalis (VLc)
    Ventral posterior nucleus (VP)
        Ventral posterolateral nucleus (VPL)
        Ventral posteromedial nucleus (VPM)
        Ventral posterior inferior nucleus (VPI)
7. Posterior thalamic nuclear group (PO)
8. Medial geniculate body (MGB)
9. Lateral geniculate body (LGB)
10. Thalamic reticular nucleus (RN)

Note:
*AN: author's abbreviation.
Source: From Carpenter, M.B. (1991). *Core Text of Neuroanatomy*, 4th edn. Baltimore: Williams and Wilkins.

information from the periphery and send it into the sensory field of the neocortex. The ventral anterior nucleus (VA) and ventral lateral nucleus (VL) belong to the secondary relay nuclei. They receive information from the globus pallidus and cerebellum, and project it toward the motor cortex and its vicinity. MD and the lateral nuclear group are the association nuclei. MD receives inputs from the amygdala and has bilateral connections with the frontal association cortex. The lateral nuclei receive inputs from the superior colliculus and have bilateral connections with the parieto-occipito-temporal association cortex. The anterior nucleus (AN) participates in the Papez circuit and receives inputs from the mamillary body and has bilateral connections with the cingulate gyrus. Finally, the intralaminar and midline nuclei belong to the nonspecific nuclei. They receive inputs from the motor cortex, cerebellum, and reticular formation and project diffusely to the neocortex, ignoring functional boundaries.

A more theoretical summary was presented by Yakovlew (1969) for clinicians, based on developmental–cytoarchitectorial studies. Here, the thalamus is viewed as a structure consisting of three evolutionally as well as functionally different systems. The midline, intralaminar, and reticular nuclei are the reticulate components of the thalamus, which appear in the second embryonal months and have close relations with the entocortex of the hemispheres. The ventral caudal nuclear group (VPM, VPL, CM, LGB, and MGB) and rostral nuclear group (VA, AV, AD, AM, LD, and MDpc) appear later during the third and fourth fetal months, and have close relations with the heterotypical neocortex. Yakovlew grouped them as the heterotypical nuclei of the paramedian zone of the thalamus. The pulvinar and lateral posterior nucleus (LP) make up the homotypical nuclei of the dorsolateral and posterior zone of the thalamus. They develop late and project to the homotypical ectocortex of the posterior association areas.

Major symptoms

In the following section, symptoms that have been observed after thalamic damages are discussed in terms of: (1) attention, (2) wakefulness, (3) cognition, (4) mood and affect, and (5) behavioral disorder. Of course, these parameters are not independent of each other, and tend to merge or overlap. Therefore, it should be understood that this is simply an effort to emphasize the conspicuous aspect of the symptoms so far described.

Disorders of attention

A typical thalamic dysfunction often manifests itself as attentional difficulty. Especially with lesions involving the bilateral median and paramedian areas, a confusional state is very common. Even after the somnolent state is cleared, patients' attention remains limited in extent and duration. An irrelevant stimulus would easily disturb ongoing cognitive processes, leading to incoherent comprehension of the environment. Poor attention would also lead to memorizing difficulty and disorientation for time, place, and personal events. This state may be induced by a unilateral right-sided lesion (Friedman, 1985), although the author speculated a possible presence of unidentified lesion in the contralateral thalamus. If inattention is combined with hallucination or illusion, a delirious state would ensue. In rare instances, a unilateral right thalamic lesion is enough to induce delirium (Bogousslavsky, Regli and Uske, 1988).

A less severe disturbance of attention and concentration coupled with increased distractibility would produce secondary amnesic syndrome (Mennemeier et al., 1992). Aphasia usually observed with left thalamic lesions is often tinged with confusion, making the neuropsychological evaluation very difficult. The state is called aphasic delirium (Mohr, 1983).

Spatial (directional) attention disorders have also been described. A right medial thalamic lesion would cause left unilateral spatial neglect (Watson and Heilman, 1979; Watson, Valenstein and Heilman, 1981; Motomura et al., 1986), or motor neglect (Watson and Heilman, 1979; Watson et al., 1981; Laplane, Baulac and Carydakis, 1986). A left medial lesion would cause a contralateral motor neglect characterized by underutilization, abnormal placement, and poor withdrawal from pain (Bogousslavsky, Regli and Assal, 1986).

Disorders of sleep–wakefulness

Hypersomnia, defined as excessive daytime sleepiness or prolonged sleep, or both, is very characteristic of bilateral thalamic midline or paramedian lesions (Castaigne et al., 1981; Gentilini, De Renzi and Crisi, 1987; Bogousslavsky et al., 1988). Some patients would sleep more than 16 hours a day (Bassetti et al., 1996). Their REM stage remains intact, but night-time slow-wave sleep is conspicuously reduced (Bassetti et al., 1996).

An opposite state is also produced by thalamic lesions. Rare familial cases of insomnia, i.e., fatal familial insomnia, first described in 1986, develop a progressive insomnia and other vegetative signs such as dysautonomia (Lugaresi et al., 1986). The disease progressively and selectively destroys the anterior ventral and mediodorsal thalamic nuclei. Patients with fatal familial insomnia show an early reduction in sleep spindles and K complexes, and a drastic reduction in total sleep time. With progression of the disease, NREM sleep is completely abolished and only brief residual periods or REM sleep persist (Sforza et al., 1995). In these patients, barbiturates and benzodiazepine failed to produce EEG sleep patterns.

Disorders of cognition

Language, visuospatial ability, memory, and other cognitive disorders are often encountered following selective thalamic damage.

Most authors agree that left-sided thalamic damage produces language disturbance. Relatively fluent speech output, with substitution of one word for another and with spoken language sometimes deteriorating into incomprehensible jargon, comprehension that is less impaired than the type of language output would normally indicate, and relatively preserved repetition constitute a typical pattern (Crosson, 1985). When symptoms are mild, a more circumscribed symptom complex, characterized by disturbances of verbal fluency, word finding, and confrontation naming, may be observed (Mori, Yamadori and Mitani, 1986). The author experienced the case of a patient with a left thalamic infarct showed a severe anomia without comprehension difficulty. Another case showed severe perseveration errors on confrontation naming.

Visuospatial and visuoperceptual disorders may be observed with thalamic lesions of either side. Not only a right thalamic lesion tends to produce visuospatial disability without language disturbance (Vilkki, 1978; Graff-Radford et al., 1984; Bogousslavsky et al., 1986; Stuss et al., 1988), but also a left-sided lesion may produce visuospatial disorders in the early stage (Graff-Radford et al., 1984, 1985).

Amnesic syndrome is much more frequently encountered than linguistic or visuospatial disorders. Although many cases of thalamic amnesia are contaminated with confusion, confabulation, disorientation or low vigilance, a pure amnesia characterized by severely disturbed recent memory (anterograde amnesia), and disturbed retrograde amnesia, against the background of relatively well-preserved immediate memory and nonmemory dependent cognitive function, has been reported. Severe amnesia is usually a result of bilateral thalamic lesions (Victor, Adams and Collins, 1971; Mills and Swanson, 1978; Graff-Radford et al., 1990). A unilateral lesion may reflect lateralized hemispheric function. Thus, a thalamic lesion often produces memorizing difficulty, a left lesion especially for verbal material (Speedie and Heilman, 1982; Mori et al., 1986), and a right lesion for nonverbal material (Speedie and Heilman, 1983). Figure 10.1 shows a typical left thalamic lesion producing a selective memory difficulty for verbal material.

It has to be emphasized that there are many exceptions to this rule. A left unilateral lesion may be responsible for global anterograde amnesia involving both verbal and nonverbal memory (Graff-Radford et al., 1984; von Cramon, Hebel and Schuri, 1985; Hirono et al., 1987). Thalamic amnesia due to bilateral lesions often shows an extended retrograde amnesia, but in rare cases virtually no retrograde amnesia was observed (Winocur et al., 1984; Catsman-Berrevoets and von Harskamp, 1988).

Bilateral thalamic lesions often result in generalized intellectual decline. This

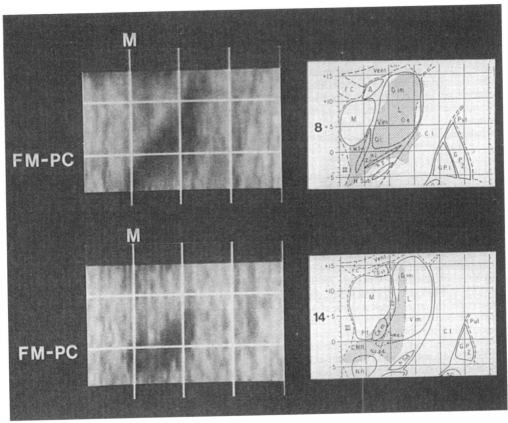

Fig. 10.1   A case of a left thalamic infarction with a disturbance of verbal memory. Two illustrative images of coronal CT scans of 2 mm section perpendicular to FM–PC (Foramen Monroe–posterior commissure) line are shown on the left, and corresponding atlases of Andrew and Watkins are shown on the right. M = midline; numbers represent the distance (mm) from the FM. (From Mori et al., 1986, by courtesy of the publisher.)

so-called thalamic dementia has been observed in cases of thalamic tumor (Smyth and Stern, 1938; Partlow et al., 1992) as well as of infarction (Castaigne et al., 1966). A well-studied case with bilateral paramedian thalamic infarction showed amnesia, striking slowness in the rate of information processing, absence of apraxia, agnosia and true aphasia, average IQ with impairment in the use of acquired knowledge, breakdown in organization of new or complex material, striking inertia and apathy, coupled with lack of concern and a jovial attitude (Stuss et al., 1988). According to the authors' opinion, this type of thalamic dementia can be summarized as a combination of subcortical dementia (Albert, Feldman and Willis, 1974) and diencephalic amnesia.

A similar case, characterized by an impairment of complex executive behaviors mimicking frontal lobe dysfunction, was reported after a left paramedian thalamic infarction that involved the dorsomedial nucleus and neighboring nuclei and fibers (Sandson et al., 1991). Impairment of working memory was described in cases of fatal familial insomnia (Gallassi et al., 1996).

Disorders of mood and affect

In the course of paramedian thalamic damage, apathy is often encountered in conjunction with lack of motor drive or dementia (Mills and Swanson, 1978; Castaigne et al., 1981). Typical patients show no emotional reaction and remain unconcerned about things happening around them, even when they are of personal importance. This symptom should be separated, at least in concept, from aspontaneity or dementia because apathy is a disturbance in the domain of affect and emotion. Sometimes apathy is mixed with irritability (Gentilini et al., 1987).

Euphoria may also emerge after bilateral mediodorsal nuclei damage (Graff-Radford et al., 1984; Gentilini et al., 1987; Stuss et al., 1988). It is often accompanied by attentional and/or cognitive impairment. An outright manic state coupled with confusion was reported in a case of a right paramedian thalamic lesion (Bogousslavsky et al., 1988). Two of 12 cases of secondary mania after brain injury had a thalamo-capsular stroke (Starkstein, Boston and Robinson, 1988).

As for depression, a patient with bilateral paramedian thalamic lesions was reported to have fallen into a depressive state after a phase of abnormal irritability, requiring admission to a psychiatric ward and amitriptyline treatment (Gentilini et al., 1987). Right unilateral paramedian thalamic damage was also attributed as a cause of depression (Baumgartner, Landis and Regard, 1992). Two cases with left dorsolateral thalamic lesions were reported to have shown minor depression (Starkstein et al., 1988).

Disorders of behavior

Thalamic lesions may produce hypoactive as well as hyperactive behavioral change. An extreme state of generalized hypoactivity is known as akinetic mutism. It is characterized by reduced responsiveness to the environment in the absence of gross alteration of sensory motor function. A typical patient is seen lying in bed, immobile but not paralyzed, somnolent but not in coma, quiet but not speechless, occasionally open-eyed and seemingly alert, yet hardly reacting to any stimuli except perhaps very painful ones (Segarra, 1970).

Hyperkinetic or hyperactive state is also observed. Patients' behavior is disinhibited, and may be extremely inappropriate: one patient urinated on the floor without embarrassment (Friedman, 1985). A case with bilateral medial thalamic and midbrain infarcts (Fig. 10.2) showed a dramatic and persistent personality change characterized by childish behavior and euphoria (Fukatsu et al., 1997). The

(a)   (b)

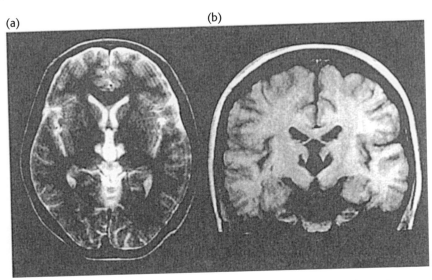

Fig. 10.2   A case of bilateral paramedian thalamic infarcts. The patient showed a dramatic personality change characterized by childish behavior and euphoria. The figure shows axial (left) and coronal (right) T2-weighted MR images. Lesions involved the dorsomedial nuclei and the central nuclei as well as the internal medullary lamina bilaterally. (From Fukatsu et al., 1997, by courtesy of the publisher.)

patient's responses to an examiner's questions were always playful, and inappropriate to a certain degree (Ganser's syndrome).

A similar case was all the more striking because the patient's behavioral change occurred without associated cognitive and memory decline, as evidenced by his Wechsler Memory Scale (WMS) quotient of 124. The patient was jocular, talkative, and playful; he talked and played like a child (Hirayama, Muroi and Yamamoto, 1997).

Hyperphagia or bulimia was observed in four of eight patients with bilateral paramedian thalamic infarcts (Gentilini et al., 1987). A typical patient ate and drank voraciously and indiscriminately, without becoming satiated. A bilateral thalamic glioma also produced hyperphagia (Partlow et al., 1992).

Behavioral changes limited to a particular domain have also been described, such as Lhermitte's utilization behavior (Eslinger et al., 1991; Hashimoto, Yoshida and Tanaka, 1995) or 'compulsive pre-sleep' behavior in which the patient assumed a sleeping posture all the time (Catsman-Berrevoets and van Harskamp, 1988).

Anatomoclinical correlation

'Nonspecific' thalamic system

The reticular nuclei of the thalamus, i.e., midline, intralaminar, and reticular nuclei, have intimate connections with the reticular formation of the brainstem. These nuclei have 'reticulate' (Yakovlew, 1969) structure and are phylogenetically continuous with the brainstem reticular formation caudally and with the midline structure of the old part of the cerebrum or entocortex, i.e., the olfactory cortex, hippocampus, and septal areas, rostrally (Yakovlew, 1969). They also project diffusely to the neocortex through the externally situated reticular nucleus.

Physiologically, this axial system of reticulate cells has been established as the core structure of the so-called reticular activating system (French, 1967). It is composed of ascending and descending activating systems. The ascending system arouses an organism in response to a relevant stimulus, and the descending system prepares the organism for a necessary response by setting it to an appropriate alerting posture. If the stimulus is biologically relevant, the animal maintains its attention on it, while recruiting necessary cortical areas for further analysis.

The thalamic nonspecific nuclei are not just a relay station to the cortex; they have intricate connections within the thalamus. One of the two major ascending fibers from the mesencephalic reticular formation projects to the intralaminar and dorsolateral thalamic fields (dorsal route), and the other runs ventrally and laterally through the subthalamus and hypothalamus, then swings ventral to the thalamic reticular nuclei (Scheibel and Scheibel, 1966, quoted from Brodal, 1981).

When this system is damaged in the midbrain, irreversible coma is the outcome. When it is disconnected at the junction between the mesencephalic reticular formation and the thalamic 'nonspecific' nuclei, somnolent type of akinetic mutism is induced (Segarra, 1970). The patient is not in sleep but lacking activating stimuli, locked into an extreme state of adynamia.

When the nonspecific nuclei are destroyed bilaterally, a global confusional state would be expected (Partlow et al., 1992). In some instances, a unilateral right thalamic lesion might be enough for global confusion (Friedman, 1985). A left-sided lesion producing amnesia or aphasia may have a component of attentional difficulty (Mohr, 1983; Mennemeier et al., 1992).

Unilateral spatial neglect and unilateral motor neglect associated with thalamic lesions do not essentially differ in their symptomatology from neglect reported as a result of hemispheric lesions. Watson et al. (1981) hypothesized a wide and elaborate network for directional attention that connects the mesencephalic reticular formation and the nonspecific nucleus of the thalamus, especially the intralaminar CM–PF complex, on the one hand, and the prefrontal–inferior parietal–anterior cingulate system on the other. According to their theory, if any part of this ipsilateral circuit is broken, contralateral hemi-inattention, which would be global or modality specific, would be expected.

The central gray network

Lugaresi (1992) proposed a concept of a 'central gray network,' which is constituted of the limbic cortex, ventral striatum (the nucleus accumbens and medium-celled portion of the olfactory tubercle), 'visceral' thalamus (AN and MD), hypothalamus, and brainstem reticular formation. This network was postulated as the basis for endocrine homeostasis and restorative body processes, to which the rhythmic activity of sleep–wakefulness belongs. The emphasis on the role of the thalamus for hypnogenesis is unique, since most of the experimental researchers have identified neural substrates for hypnogenesis outside the thalamus, such as the nucleus basalis (Steriade, 1992; Silberzweig et al., 1995).

The hypothesis was based on findings that highly selective degenerative damage affecting AN and MD in humans led to intractible insomnia and dysautonomia. According to this hypothesis, intrinsic and diffuse thalamic neuronal loss itself is undoubtedly a cause of insomnia.

A recent study of thalamic hypersomnia also suggests an important role of MD nucleus for sleep regulation (Bassetti et al., 1996). It is curious that lesions in the same location can lead to insomnia in one situation and to hypersomnia in the other. A difference in the speed of disease progress or type of lesion distribution may be an explanation (Bassetti et al., 1996).

Fatal familial insomnia patients cannot sleep, and show impairment of attention and vigilance from the early stage of the disease (Gallassi et al., 1996). Likewise, some patients with medial thalamic damage seem to develop confusion that is not necessarily accompanied by somnolent tendency (Smyth and Stern, 1938; Bogousslavsky et al., 1988; Partlow et al., 1992). These facts suggest that tonic attention may be modulated by the coordinated action of the 'nonspecific' (midline and intralaminar) and 'central gray' (AN-MD) systems, because damage to either system would lead to attentional disturbance.

Prefrontal connections

The dorsolateral prefrontal cortex (DLPC) has rich connections with the medial part of the parvicellular portion of the ventral anterior nucleus (VApc) and the parvicellular part of the mediodorsal nucleus (MDpc). This connection is both directly bilateral and via multiple nuclei passing through the caudate, dorsomedial globus pallidus, and substantia nigra (Alexander, Crutcher and DeLong, 1990). These interconnections are shown in Fig. 10.3.

Destruction of this network by a thalamic lesion would result in syndromes

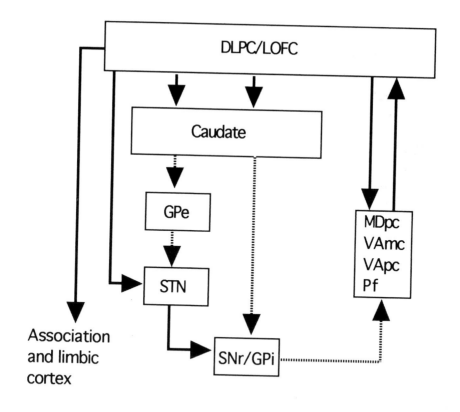

 inhibitory neuron

—— excitatory neuron

Fig. 10.3   Schema of basal ganglia-thalamocortical circuits. Dorsolateral and lateral orbital prefrontal connections with the thalamus. (Redrawn from Alexander et al., 1990, by courtesy of Elsevier Science Publishers.) DLPC, dorsolateral prefrontal cortex; LOFC, lateral orbitofrontal cortex; STN, subthalamic nucleus; Gpe, external segment of the globus pallidus; Gpi, internal segment of the globus pallidus; SNr, substantia nigra; MDpc, medialis dorsalis pars parvocellularis; Vamc, ventralis anterioris pars magnocellularis; Vapc, ventralis anterioris pars parvocellularis; Pf, parafascicularis.

similar to those produced by dorsolateral prefrontal lobe lesions such as executive difficulty (Sandson et al., 1991) or impairment of working memory (Gallassi et al., 1996).

The lateral orbitofrontal cortex (LOFC), on the other hand, has rich connections with the magnocellular portion of MD (MDmc) and the median portion of the magnocellular portion of VA (VAmc). Again, these connections are both directly bilateral and via the ventromedian caudate, globus pallidus, and substantia nigra. Dysfunction of this system was suggested as a possible basis for obsessive–compulsive behavior (Alexander et al., 1990). Compulsive presleep behavior of a thalamic origin (Catsman-Berrevoets and van Harskamp, 1988) may be explained in this context.

Medial orbitofrontal connections

Parts of MDmc receive multisynaptic inputs from the medial orbital frontal cortex (MOFC) and anterior cingulate area (ACA) via the ventral striatum and ventral pallidus. The nucleus then feeds back to the ACA/MOFC, completing a circuit (Fig. 10.4; Alexander et al., 1990). The thalamus is also closely connected with the subcortical septo-hypothalamo-mesencephalic limbic region.

Feeling, mood, and emotion are intimately related with a dysfunction of this distributed medial orbital–medial thalamo-cingulate system. Recent studies emphasized the importance of right hemisphere damage in the emergence of secondary mania, and left hemisphere damage in the emergence of depression (Sackeim et al., 1982; Starkstein et al., 1988). Whether this theory of affect lateralization can be applied to the thalamus is yet to be studied. Incidentally, a patient with severe depression had a right paramedian thalamic lesion (Baumgartner et al., 1992), while a patient with euphoric mania also had lesions in the right paramedian area (Bogousslavsky et al., 1988).

Apathy, a frequent thalamic symptom, may be an outcome of damage to this ACA-MDmc circuit (Cummings, 1993).

The orbitofrontal–thalamic circuit may also have a role in cognitive processes. Thus, the nonamnesic behavior of a patient with thalamic dementia that mimicked subcortical type of dementia was attributed to a dysfunction of this circuit (Stuss et al., 1988).

Hippocampo-amygdala connections

Probably the best understood thalamic circuit involving the thalamic nuclei is the Papez's circuit, which is composed of the hippocampus, fornix, mamillary body, mamillothalamic tract, AN and cingulate gyrus. The circuit has been strongly implicated in memory function (Valenstein et al., 1987; McMackin et al., 1995). As for thalamic parts of the circuit, there have been case reports of amnesia involving mamillothalamic tract (von Cramon et al., 1985) or AN (Clarke et al., 1994) supporting this thesis.

On the other hand, there are data suggesting a strong relation between damage of MD and disturbance of memory (Victor et al., 1971; Speedie and Heilman, 1982; Bogousslavsky et al., 1988). MD has rich connections with the amygdala. Based on this fact, the circuit involving the amygdala and MD has been proposed as a

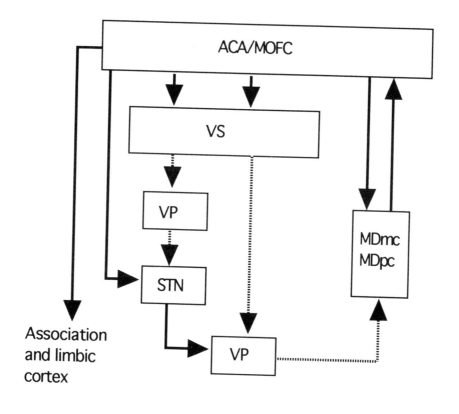

inhibitory neuron

excitatory neuron

Fig. 10.4   Schema of basal ganglia-thalamocortical circuits. Anterior cingulate and medial orbitofrontal connections with the thalamus. (Redrawn from Alexander et al., 1990, by courtesy of Elsevier Science Publishers.) ACA, anterior cingulate areas; MOFC, medial orbitofrontal cortex; VS, ventral striatum or limbic striatum. The nucleus accumbens and the medium-celled portion of the olfactory tubercle; VP, ventral pallidum; STN, subthalamic nucleus; MDmc, medialis dorsalis pars magnocellularis; MDpc, medialis dorsalis pars parvocellularis.

candidate for episodic memory (Mishkin, 1982). Because AN, mamillothalamic tract, and MD are positioned so close to each other, it is not yet entirely clear which system is more contributory for thalamic amnesia. It may be that both systems contribute to memory, and damage involving both systems may exaggerate amnesic syndrome (Mishkin, 1982; Stuss et al., 1988; Graff-Radford et al., 1990). Anatomically, a specific component of the ventro-amygdalo-fugal pathway is situated lateral but immediately adjacent to the mamillothalamic tract (Graff-Radford et al., 1990).

Other cortical connections

The pulvinar has rich reciprocal innervation with the parieto-occipito-temporal association cortex. This anatomical fact led to speculation that thalamic aphasia is principally caused by left pulvinar damage (Ojeman, Fedio and Van Buren, 1968; Van Boren and Borke, 1969; Ojeman and Ward, 1971). Thalamic aphasia is often transient and, when it is severe, often fluctuates. This clinical observation is consistent with a hypothesis deduced from stimulation data that indicate that thalamic language disturbance may be due to some types of alerting or vigilance dysfunction related specifically to language (Ojeman, 1976).

Damage to the left VL may also cause a language disturbance (Bell, 1968; Ojeman and Ward, 1971). VL contains *en passage* fibers relating to the centrum medianum and DM. It is assumed that damage not of VL neurons per se, which are principally connected with areas 4 and 6 but of these fibers causes language disturbances (Ojeman and Ward, 1971).

Anomia and deficient verbal fluency often coexist with anterograde verbal amnesia, indicating a possible thalamic role in the interaction of memory and language (Ojeman, 1976).

A possible relation of complex visual pattern perception and right VL was suggested from the VL thalamotomy experience (Vilkki, 1978). A possible involvement of the pulvinar of either side in cognitive functions tapped by such tests as Similarities or Wisconsin Card Sorting was also speculated (Wallesche et al., 1983).

General cerebrothalamic interaction

Almost all the patients with behavioral change reported in the literature or observed personally have paramedian lesions, be it unilateral or bilateral.

Patients with akinetic mutism have been shown, without exception, to have bilateral ventrocaudal thalamic–rostral mesencephalic lesions, which are strategically placed to cut off activating upstream information of the mesencephalic reticular-formation feeding into the thalamic nonspecific nuclei (Segarra, 1970). Without activating stimuli, patients would lose the impetus for action and speech and stay immobile and mute.

Hyperactive state of childish behavior seems to be a reflection of underlying mood change. The patient quoted earlier had bilateral paramedian lesions damaging the orbitofrontal-thalamo-cingulate network. However, euphoria does not necessarily lead to childish behavior; some decline of social judgment must have been an additional factor for the behavior shown.

Bulimic behavior has also been shown to result from bilateral paramedian lesions (Gentilini et al., 1987). This may have been related to adjacent putative hypothalamic lesions or release of intact hypothalamic functions, although these possibilities were not discussed by the authors.

Utilization behavior was described as identical to behavior reported following frontal lobe lesions, indicating damage of the bilateral medial orbitofrontal-MDmc circuit at the MD level (Eslinger et al., 1991; Hashimoto et al., 1995). The compulsive nature of the described 'presleep' behavior suggests a dysfunction of the lateral orbitofrontal-MDmc/VAmc circuit (Alexander et al., 1990).

This brief review makes it clear that the thalamus is the hub of the various neuronal activities. Almost all information converges on this small area and also diverges from here. Penfield (1972) was probably correct in stating that the diencephalon constitutes the principal structure of the 'centrencephalic' integrating system. A more detailed neurobehavioral description of thalamic symptoms is greatly needed, which will further enhance our understanding of how the complex neuronal networks are integrated at the thalamic level.

Schizophrenia and thalamus

Recently, an interesting hypothesis has been proposed concerning the pathogenesis of schizophrenia. Magnetic resonance imaging volumetric studies performed on a large number of schizophrenic patients found that the thalamus is conspicuously smaller in schizophrenics than in control subjects (Andreasen et al., 1994; Flaum et al., 1995). A positron emission tomography study reported activation of the bilateral thalamus in schizophrenic patients who had been experiencing active auditory hallucinations (Silberzweig et al., 1995).

Based on these and other studies, Andreasen emphasized the importance of thalamic dysfunction as one of many possible causes of schizophrenia. Because the thalamus is considered to play a major role in gating and filtering information, she argues that these thalamic abnormalities may lead to dysfunction of input evaluation, causing schizophrenia. In this theory, the thalamus is considered to be an important member of the distributed cognitive system that includes the prefrontal cortex (dorsolateral, orbital, and medial), basal ganglia, anterior cingulate, posterior association cortices, and the cerebellum (Andreasen, 1997).

Acknowledgments

Preparation of this manuscript was partly supported by grants-in-aid (08279103) for science research from the Ministry of Education, Science and Culture in Japan, and by a 'Research for the Future' program (JSP-RFTF 97L00202) from the Japan Society for the Promotion of Science.

REFERENCES

Albert, M.L., Feldman, R.G. and Willis, A.L. (1974). The 'subcortical dementia' of progressive supranuclear palsy. *J Neurol Neurosurg Psychiatry* 37: 173–80.

Alexander, G.E., Crutcher, M.D. and DeLong, M.R. (1990). Basal ganglia–thalamocortical circuits: parallel substrates for motor, oculomotor, 'prefrontal' and 'limbic' functions. In *Progress in Brain Research*, Vol. 85, ed. H.B.M. Uylings, C.G. Van Eden, J.P.C. De Bruin, M.A. Corner and M.G.P. Feenstra, pp. 119–46. Amsterdam: Elsevier Science Publishers.

Andreasen, N.C. (1997). The role of the thalamus in schizophrenia. A review. *Can J Psychiatry* 42: 27–33.

Andreasen, N.C., Arndt, S., Swayze, V. II et al. (1994). Thalamic abnormalities in schizophrenia visualized through magnetic resonance image averaging. *Science* 266: 294–8.

Bassetti, C., Mathis, J., Gugger, M., Lövblad, K.O. and Hess, C.W. (1996). Hypersomnia following paramedian thalamic stroke: a report of 12 patients. *Ann Neurol* 39: 471–80.

Baumgartner, R.W., Landis, T. and Regard, M. (1992). Relapsing depression in paramedian thalamic infarctions. *Behav Neurol* 5: 129–32.

Bell, D.S. (1968). Speech functions of the thalamus inferred from the effects of thalamotomy. *Brain* 91: 619–38.

Bogousslavsky, J., Regli, F. and Assal, G. (1986). The syndrome of unilateral tuberothalamic artery territory infarction. *Stroke* 17: 434–41.

Bogousslavsky, J., Regli, F. and Uske, A. (1988). Thalamic infarcts: clinical syndromes, etiology, and prognosis. *Neurology* 38: 837–48.

Brodal, A. (1981). The reticular formation and some related nuclei. In *Neurological Anatomy in Relation to Clinical Medicine*, 3rd edn, pp. 394–447. New York: Oxford University Press.

Carpenter, M.B. (1991). The diencephalon. In *Core Text of Neuroanatomy*, 4th edn, pp. 250–96. Baltimore: Williams and Wilkins.

Castaigne, P., Buge, A., Cambier, J. et al. (1966). Démence thalamique d'origine vasculaire par ramollissement bilatéral, limité au territoire du pédicule rétromamillaire. A propos de deux observations anatomo-cliniques. *Rev Neurol* 114: 89–107.

Castaigne, P., Lhermitte, F., Buge, A. et al. (1981). Paramedian thalamic and midbrain infarcts: clinical and neuropathological study. *Ann Neurol* 10: 127–48.

Catsman-Berrevoets, C.E. and von Harskamp, F. (1988). Compulsive pre-sleep behavior and apathy due to bilateral thalamic stroke: response to bromocriptine. *Neurology* 38: 647–9.

Clarke, S., Assal, G., Bogousslavsky, J. et al. (1994). Pure amnesia after unilateral left polar thalamic infarct. *J Neurol Neurosurg Psychiatry* 57: 27–34.

Crosson, B. (1985). Subcortical functions in language: a working model. *Brain Lang* 25: 257–92.

Cummings, J.L. (1993). Frontal–subcortical circuits and human behavior. *Arch Neurol* 50: 873–80.

Eslinger, P.J., Warner, G.C., Grattan, L.M. and Easton, J.D. (1991). 'Frontal lobe' utilization behavior associated with paramedian thalamic infarction. *Neurology* 41: 450–2.

Flaum, M., Swayze, V.W. 2nd, O'Leary, D.S. et al. (1995). Effects of diagnosis, laterality, and gender on brain morphology in schizophrenia. *Am J Psychiatry* 152: 704–14.

French, J.D. (1967). The reticular formation. *Sci Am* 196: 54–60.

Friedman, J.H. (1985). Syndrome of diffuse encephalopathy due to nondominant thalamic infarction. *Neurology* 35: 1524–6.

Fukatsu, R., Fujii, T., Yamadori, A., Nagasawa, H. and Sakurai, Y. (1997). Persisting childish behavior after bilateral thalamic infarcts. *Eur Neurol* 37: 230–5.

Gallassi, R., Morreale, A., Montagna, P. et al. (1996). Fatal familial insomnia: behavioral and cognitive features. *Neurology* 46: 935–9.

Gentilini, M., De Renzi, E. and Crisi, G. (1987). Bilateral paramedian thalamic artery infarcts: report of eight cases. *J Neurol Neurosurg Psychiatry* 50: 900–9.

Graff-Radford, N.R., Damasio, H., Yamada, T., Eslinger, P.J. and Damasio, A.R. (1985). Nonhemorrhagic thalamic infarction. Clinical, neuropsychological, and electrophysiological findings in four anatomical groups defined by computerized tomography. *Brain* 108: 485–516.

Graff-Radford, N.R., Eslinger, P.J., Damasio, A.R. and Yamada, T. (1984). Nonhemorrhagic infarction of the thalamus: behavioral, anatomic, and physiologic correlates. *Neurology* 34: 14–23.

Graff-Radford, N.R., Tranel, D., Van Hoesen, G.W. and Brandt, J.P. (1990). Diencephalic amnesia. *Brain* 113: 1–25.

Hashimoto, R., Yoshida, M. and Tanaka, Y. (1995). Utilization behavior after right thalamic infarction. *Eur Neurol* 35: 58–62.

Hirayama, K., Muroi, A. and Yamamoto, T. (1997). Childish behavior and disappearance of stuttering after bilateral paramedian thalamic infarction. *Clin Neuropsychol (Proc Tohoku Neuropsychol Conf)* 7: 61–6. (In Japanese.)

Hirono, N., Yamadori, A., Miyai, I., Kitahara, Y. and Fujita, M. (1987). A case of left thalamic infarction developing verbal and visual memory disturbance with mild aphasia. *Clin Neurol (Tokyo)* 27: 1170–9.

Laplane, D., Baulac, M. and Carydakis, C. (1986). Négligence motrice d'origine thalamique. *Rev Neurol* 142: 375–9.

Lugaresi, E. (1992). The thalamus and insomnia. *Neurology* 42 (Suppl. 6): 28–33.

Lugaresi, E., Medori, R., Montagna, P. et al. (1986). Fatal familial insomnia and dysautonomia with selective degeneration of thalamic nuclei. *N Engl J Med* 315: 997–1003.

McMackin, D., Cockburn, J., Anslow, P. and Gaffan, D. (1995). Correlation of fornix damage with memory impairment in six cases of colloid cyst removal. *Acta Neurochir* 135: 12–18.

Mennemeier, M., Fennell, E., Valenstein, E. and Heilman, K.M. (1992). Contributions of the left intralaminar and medial thalamic nuclei to memory. *Arch Neurol* 49: 1050–8.

Mills, R.P. and Swanson, P.D. (1978). Vertical oculomotor apraxia and memory loss. *Ann Neurol* 4: 149–53.

Mishkin, M. (1982). A memory system in the monkey. *Philos Trans R Soc Lond B*, 298: 85–95.

Mohr, J.P. (1983). Thalamic lesions and syndromes. In *Localization in Neuropsychology*, ed. A. Kertesz, pp. 269–93. New York: Academic Press.

Mori, E., Yamadori, A. and Mitani, Y. (1986). Left thalamic infarction and disturbance of verbal memory: a clinicopathological study with a new method of computed tomographic stereotaxic lesion localization. *Ann Neurol* 20: 671–6.

Motomura, N., Yamadori, A., Mori, E. et al. (1986). Unilateral spatial neglect due to hemorrhage in the thalamic region. *Acta Neurol Scand* 74: 190–4.

Nauta, W.J.H. and Feirtag, M. (1986). *Fundamental Neuroanatomy*. New York: Freeman WH and Company.

Ojeman, G.A. (1976). Subcortical language mechanisms. In *Studies in Neurolinguistics*, Vol. 1, ed. H. Whitaker and H.A. Whitaker, pp. 103–38. New York: Academic Press.

Ojeman, G.A., Fedio, P. and Van Buren, J.M. (1968). Anomia from pulvinar and subcortical parietal stimulation. *Brain* 91: 99–116.

Ojeman, G.A. and Ward, A.A. (1971). Speech representation in ventrolateral thalamus. *Brain* 94: 669–80.

Partlow, G.D., del Carpio-O'Donovan, R., Melanson, D. and Peters, T.M. (1992). Bilateral thalamic glioma: review of eight cases with personality change and mental deterioration. *Am J Neuroradiol* 13: 1225–30.

Penfield, W. (1972). The electrode, the brain and the mind. *Z Neurol* 201: 297–309.

Sackeim, H.A., Greenberg, M.S., Weiman, A.L. et al. (1982). Hemispheric asymmetry in the expression of positive and negative emotions. Neurologic evidence. *Arch Neurol* 39: 210–18.

Sandson, T.A., Daffner, K.R., Carvalho, P.A. and Mesulam, M-M. (1991). Frontal lobe dysfunction following infarction of the left-sided medial thalamus. *Arch Neurol* 48: 1300–3.

Segarra, J.M. (1970). Cerebral vascular disease and behavior. 1. The syndrome of the mesencephalic artery (basilar artery bifurcation). *Arch Neurol* 22: 408–18.

Sforza, E., Montagna, P., Tinuper, P. et al. (1995). Sleep–wake cycle abnormalities in fatal familial insomnia. Evidence of the role of the thalamus in sleep regulation. *Electroencephalogr Clin Neurophysiol* 94: 398–405.

Silberzweig, D.A., Stern, E., Frith, C. et al. (1995). A functional neuroanatomy of hallucinations in schizophrenia. *Nature* 378: 176–9.

Smyth, G.E. and Stern, K. (1938). Tumors of the thalamus – a clinico-pathological study. *Brain* 61: 339–74.

Speedie, L.J. and Heilman, K.M. (1982). Amnesic disturbance following infarction of the left dorsomedial nucleus. *Neuropsychologia* 20: 597–604.

Speedie, L.J. and Heilman, K.M. (1983). Anterograde memory deficits for visuospatial material after infarction of the right thalamus. *Arch Neurol* 40: 183–6.

Starkstein, S.E., Boston, J.D. and Robinson, R.G. (1988). Mechanisms of mania after brain injury. *J Nerv Ment Dis* 176: 87–100.

Steriade, M. (1992). Basic mechanisms of sleep generation. *Neurology* 42 (Suppl. 6): 9–18.

Stuss, D.T., Guberman, A., Nelson, R. and Larochelle, S. (1988). The neuropsychology of paramedian thalamic infarction. *Brain Cogn* 8: 348–78.

Valenstein, E., Bowers, d., Verfaellie, M. et al. (1987). Retrosplenial amnesia. *Brain* 110: 1631–46.

Van Buren, J.M. and Borke, R.C. (1969). Alteration in speech and the pulvinar. A serial section study of cerebrothalamic relationships in cases of acquired speech disorders. *Brain* 92: 255–84.

Victor, M., Adams, R. and Collins, G.H. (1971). *Wernicke–Korsakoff's Syndrome*. Philadelphia: FA Davis.

Vilkki, J. (1978). Effects of thalamic lesions on complex perception and memory. *Neuropsychologia* 16: 427–37.

von Cramon, D.Y., Hebel, N. and Schuri, U. (1985). A contribution to the anatomical basis of thalamic amnesia. *Brain* 108: 993–1008.

Wallesche, C.W., Kornhuber, H.H., Kunz, T. and Brunner, R.J. (1983). Neuropsychological deficits associated with small unilateral thalamic lesions. *Brain* 106: 141–52.

Watson, R.T. and Heilman, K.M. (1979). Thalamic neglect. *Neurology* 29: 690–4.

Watson, R.T., Valenstein, E.V. and Heilman, K.M. (1981). Thalamic neglect. Possible role of the medial thalamus and nucleus reticularis in behavior. *Archives of Neurology* 38: 501–6.

Winocur, G., Oxbury, S., Roberts, R., Agnetti, V. and Davis, C. (1984). Amnesia in a patient with bilateral lesions to the thalamus. *Neuropsychologia* 22: 123–43.

Yakovlew, P.I. (1969). Localization of lesions of the thalamus. In *Bing's Local diagnosis in Neurological Diseases*, 15th edn, ed. W. Haymaker, pp. 441–64. St Louis: C.V. Mosby.

11

Obsessive–compulsive disorders in association with focal brain lesions

Frédérique Etcharry-Bouyx and Frédéric Dubas

Introduction

In earlier centuries, obsessive–compulsive disorder (OCD) symptomatology was considered to be indicative of demonic possession. Janet (1903) was the first to attempt to describe the phenomenon of OCD without reliance on supernatural forces. Freud saw obsessions as manifestations of repressed sexual and aggressive impulses. Because themes of aggression and dirt or contamination are common in OCD, this led to the speculation that disturbance during the anal sadistic phase plays a role. The conception of a relationship between OCD and cerebral lesions began with the lethargic encephalitis observations from von Economo (1931; see also Jellife, 1929). The anatomical data made it possible to establish the importance of basal ganglia lesions compared to cortical lesions. It was not until much later that this concept was integrated, in particular with the first modern case report of OCD after bipallidal lesions (Laplane et al., 1981).

Since then, more recent studies have suggested a neurological etiology with basal ganglia and frontal lobe pathology as reported in many neuroimaging studies (Baxter et al., 1990; Baxter, 1992; Insel, 1992a) or in cases of acquired obsessive–compulsive disorder (A-OCD). Detailed reports of cases with focal brain lesions may contribute to the understanding of the pathogenesis of OCD.

The aim of this chapter is to describe OCD in association with focal brain lesions, which is one of the best examples of a psychopathological organic disorder that may mimic a classical psychiatric syndrome.

The clinical variants are described first, and then the different etiologies and anatomic correlates that relate them to the functional physiopathology. The final part of the chapter deals with therapeutic issues.

Clinical aspects

Obsessive–compulsive disorder encompasses a broad range of symptoms that include various intrusive thoughts, preoccupations, rituals, and diverse motor behaviors. A definition of OCD was given by the DSM IV (American Psychiatric Association, 1994):

Obsessions are recurrent and persistent thoughts, impulses or images that are experienced, as intrusive and inappropriate and that cause marked anxiety or distress. The person attempts to ignore, suppress or neutralize them with some other thought or action. Compulsions are repetitive behaviors or mental acts that the person feels driven to perform in response to an obsession, or according to rules that must be applied rigidly. The behaviors or mental acts are aimed at preventing or reducing distress.

To assess the nature and severity of obsession and compulsion, some scales are available. Frequenty used, the Yale–Brown Obsessive Compulsive Scale (Y-BOCS) (Goodman et al., 1989) is a clinician-rated scale, designed to remedy the problems of other scales by providing a specific measure of severity of symptoms (Table 11.1). Ten items are selected, each of them rated (on a five-point scale) from 0 (least symptomatic) to 4 (most symptomatic). The total score ranges from 0 to 40, and a severity scale may be measured with subtotals for severity of obsessions (item 1 to 5) and compulsions (item 6 to 10). Concurrently, a symptom checklist is established. It includes 50 different types of obsessions and compulsions divided into 15 categories according to their behavioral expression or thematic content. In a recent study (Leckman et al., 1997) an identical set of four symptom dimensions emerged. The authors analyzed 13 items of obsessions and compulsions in the four-symptom checklist and determined factors with a statistical analysis, in two independent groups of patients ($n = 306$). The first symptom dimension concerned aggressive, sexual, and religious obsessions with checking compulsions. The second symptom dimension combined compulsions of ordering–arranging, counting, and repeating rituals with obsessions of symmetry. A third symptom dimension paired washing and cleaning compulsions with contamination obsessions. Finally, hoarding obsessions were highly correlated with hoarding behaviors and other collecting compulsions.

A second, less utilized, scale is a self-rated scale that quantifies the range of obsessional thoughts and compulsive behaviors. The Leyton Obsessional Inventory (LOI) contains 69 questions as well as assessing the degree of resistance to symptoms and interference with the patient's life. Müller et al. (1997) used the Maudsley Obsessive Compulsive Inventory (MOCI), a self-report scale for obsessive–compulsive symptoms. It consists of 30 items and allows the determination of four subscales. The short version of the Hambourg Obsessive Compulsive Inventory (HZI-K), consisting of 72 items on six different dimensions, is also used. The Y-BOCS scale is frequently used because it was not constructed as a symptom inventory, unlike the LOI or the MOCI, and thus it is not biased in favor of particular types of obsessions and compulsions.

Table 11.1. Yale–Brown Obsessive–Compulsive Scale

	None	Mild	Moderate	Severe	Extreme
1. Time spent on obsessions	0	1	2	3	4
2. Interference from obsessions	0	1	2	3	4
3. Distress of obsessions	0	1	2	3	4
4. Resistance	Definitely resists				Completely yields
	0	1	2	3	4
5. Control over obsessions	Complete control	Much control	Moderate control	Little control	No control
	0	1	2	3	4
6. Time spent on compulsions	0	1	2	3	4
7. Interference from compulsions	0	1	2	3	4
8. Distress from compulsions	0	1	2	3	4
9. Resistance	Definitely resists				Completely yields
	0	1	2	3	4
10. Control over compulsions	Complete control	Much control	Moderate control	Little control	No control
	0	1	2	3	4

Obsessive–compulsive symptoms are reported after a period varying from days to years following cerebral lesions, often with a progressive worsening over time in the initial phase. Laplane et al. (1981) described obsessions and compulsions two years after an encephalopathy and four months after hypoxia in another case (1989). The parkinsonian patient of Daniele et al. (1997) developed obsessions some days after a putaminal infarct, and compulsions two months later. Paunovic (1984) described obsessions ten months after an infarct of the left anterior frontal lobe. After head injuries, the period is variable: within the first month for three cases of Kant, Smith-Seemiller and Duffy (1996), after 24 hours for four patients of McKeon, McGuffin and Robinson (1984). Khanna et al. (1985) reported a patient who developed obsessions and compulsions three years after his head injury. The repetitive behaviors began within four years of frontal lobe degenerations and Ames et al. (1994) found the prevalence to be strikingly high (78%).

Generally, in contrast to idiopathic obsessive–compulsive disorder (I-OCD), patients with A-OCD are older. Demographic information on these patients is dependent on the causal disease, but generally they have no familial history of obsessive–compulsive symptoms. In a recent study, Berthier et al. (1996) compared two groups of idiopathic and acquired OCD. The groups consisted of a consecutive series of I-OCD ($n=25$) and A-OCD ($n=13$). There were no statistically significant differences in sex ($X^2=3.2$, df$=2$, $p=$NS), age ($F=0,11$, df$=2$, $p=$NS), and years of education ($F=0,88$, df$=2$, $p=$NS).

A phenomenologic comparison of obsessive–compulsive symptoms of patients was performed. The total scale, frequency, and clinical features were compared using the Y-BOCS. There were no significant differences between groups in most symptoms. However, patients with I-OCD had more frequent hoarding and somatic obsessions, as well as ordering/arranging and hoarding/saving compulsions, compared to those with A-OCD. The symptom severity was similar in the two groups.

The neurological examination was abnormal in eight of the 13 A-OCD patients and only in three of 13 I-OCD patients (Berthier et al., 1996), but not all the patients were examined. Laplane et al. (1989), in a report of eight cases of A-OCD, found relatively few neurological physical signs (only three patients had an abnormal neurological examination). In general, when they exist, symptoms are hemiparesis or extrapyramidal signs (Tables 11.2 and 11.3). Thus, neither a normal or an abnormal neurological examination allows the nature of obsessions or compulsions, i.e., acquired or idiopathic, to be confirmed.

In the study of Berthier et al. (1996), neuropsychological examination was performed for the two groups, and a normal control (NC) group was examined with a battery of neuropsychological tests especially selected to cover a wide range of cognition deficits. This battery included tests of general intelligence (Wechsler Adult Intelligence Scale, WAIS), attention span (Wechsler Adult Intelligence Scale digit span), verbal and nonverbal memory (Wechsler Memory Scale, WMS), word retrieval (Boston Naming Test), verbal fluency, visuospatial function (WAIS block design), and cognitive set-shifting abilities (Trail Making Test, TMT, the Money's Road Map Test, MRMT, and the Wisconsin Card Sorting Test, WCST). Statistical differences between the A-OCD and NC group remained highly significant in all but one (TMT A) cognitive test. A comparison with a group of I-OCD patients showed that both groups had a relatively similar pattern of neuropsychological deficits affecting attention, intelligence, memory, language, and executive functions. On the other hand, statistical differences between the I-OCD and NC groups remained highly significant only for verbal intelligence quotient score ($p<0.05$), logical memory subtest of the WMS ($p<0.05$), and MRMT ($p<0.01$). In I-OCD, some authors have reported specific cognitive deficits in tests sensitive to frontal lobe dysfunction (Veale et al., 1996; Tallis, 1997), whereas Abbruzzese, Ferri and Scarone (1995) described normal performance on the WCST.

Single case studies or studies of patient groups with similar lesion locations have reported various neuropsychological deficits (Tables 11.1 and 11.2). The eight patients of Laplane et al. (1989) had sustained bilateral necrosis of globus pallidus.

Table 11.2. Obsessive–compulsive disorder with basal ganglia lesions

First author/year	Etiologies	Sex/age (years)	Premorbid personality delay	Neurological examination	Abnormal behaviors	Neuropsychological deficits	Treatment	Lesions
Laplane (1981)	Encephalopathy	M/41	No/2 years	Choreic	Mental counting, compulsions to switch on/off light, psychic akinesia	Fluency, retention, learning memory	Clomipramine	Bilateral globus pallidus, rostral putamen, right head caudate
Laplane (1982)	CO	M/25	No/uk		Counting, psychic akinesia	Memory		Bipallidal
Ali-Cherif (1984)	CO Case 1	M/39	No/uk	Normal	Coprolalia compulsive, psychic akinesia	Logic memory		Bipallidal
	CO Case 2	F/18	uk/uk	Normal	Ordering, collecting, psychic akinesia	Normal		Bipallidal
Laplane (1984)	CO	M/23	No/uk	Akinesia	Counting, psychic akinesia	Memory, verbal fluency		Internal part of the lentiform nucleus
	CO	M/59	uk/uk	Rigidity	Psychic akinesia	Verbal fluencey (Russian)		Internal part of the lentiform nucleus
Laplane (1988a)	CO	F/31	Psychopathy obsession/uk		Steretoped verbal rituals, word counting, watching hours	Memory, fluency, WCST	Clembuterol	Anterior part of pallidum/PET: frontal medial, L frontal, R striatal
Ward (1988)	Infarct	F/62	uk/uk		urge to shake her right arm			L basal ganglia, R superior, cerebellar peduncle
Williams (1988)	Infarct	F/48	uk/uk	Normal	Compulsive hand movements	Intellectual function		Caudate bilateral, R putamen
Croisile (1989)	Infarct	F/56	uk/uk	Normal	Chewing, skin scraping, counting	Fluency		Bilateral head caudate, putamen; SPECT bilateral frontal hypoperfusion
Durand (1989)	Cerebral anoxia	F/43	No/uk	Parkinsonism	Compulsive knitting	Efficiency intelligence, verbal learning		Internal bilateral in pallidum and putamen/PET normal
Laplane (1989)	Cerebral anoxia Case 5	M/27	No/uk		Schedule her tasks			Bilateral lentiform nuclei/PET bilateral striatal, L lateral frontal
	Hypoxia Case 6	M/uk	uk/4 months		Turn on/off light, counting, recite alphabet	Learning, verbal fluency, attention		Bilateral lentiform/PET R striatal

Reference	Etiology	Sex/Age	CO/duration	Neurological signs	OC symptoms	Neuropsychology	Treatment	Neuroimaging
Tonkonogy (1989)	Degenerative	F/36	No/uk	Normal	Hand washing, thoughts of contamination, cleanliness, compulsive eating	Efficiency intelligence		Bilateral caudate atrophy – frontal atrophy
Weilburg (1989)	Infarct (neonatal)	M/24	uk/uk		Repetitive intrusive thoughts, obsessive thoughts of cleanliness, checking rituals, hand washing, showering	IQ, naming, word list, Stroop		L caudate, L putamen
Wyszynski (1989)	Choreoacantho-cystosis	F/39	No	Palilalia Choreiform movements	Compulsion to bite lips, tongue, fingers, humming, vocalization	Intelligence retrieval, memory attention	Diphenhydramine	Caudate atrophy
Desi (1990)	Infarct	F/38	uk/uk	uk	Repetitive behavior, apragmatism	Verbal fluency, attention		Bilateral medial pallidum
Trillet (1990)	Hematoma Case 1	F/54	uk/uk	Amimia	Pedalling movements when standing, sucking, psychic akinesia	Verbal fluency		R head caudate nucleus, L lentiform head caudate, ant part putamen, PET frontal bilateral hypoperfusion
	Infarct Case 2	F/56	uk/uk	Parkinsonism	Counting, scratching, psychic akinesia			R putamen
Maraganore (1991)	Infarct	M/17	No/uk	Motor initiation	Complex ritual of hand clapping, wild flailing arms, stereotyped verbal rituals before speaking	Attention	Few without improvement	R putamen
Penisson-Besnier (1992)	Degenerative	F/54	No/uk	Normal	Counting, sniffing, scraping	Verbal visual retention		Caudate atrophy
Hebebrand (1993)	Infarct	M/16	uk/uk	Normal	Checking, cleaning, washing rituals, anorexia nervosa			R caudal putamen
Kotrla (1994)	Mineralization	M/36	No/uk		Hand washing, fears of contamination, somatic complaints	Intelligence, visual construction		Basal ganglia calcification SPECT: hyperperfusion of anterior cingulate and mesial frontal
Smadja (1995)	Infections	F/34	uk/uk	Left hemiparesis	Compulsive stereotyped – apathia movements	Verbal fluency		R lentiform, L globus pallidus
Daniele (1997)	Infarct	F/63	Parkinsonian/one day		Obsessive thoughts, compulsive verbal iterations, coprolalia	Attention, verbal fluency WCST, learning		L putamen/SPECT L frontal, basal ganglia, L thalamic hypoperfusion

Notes:

uk = unknown; CO = carbon monoxide poisoning.

Table 11.3. Obsessive–compulsive disorder with frontal lobe lesions

First author/ year	Etiologies	Sex/age (years)	Last history/ onset delay	Neurological examination	Obsessive–compulsive symptoms	Neuropsychological deficits	Medication	Lesional sites
Paunovic (1984)	Infarct	M/45	10 months	Right hemiparesis, affecting primarily upper limb and face	Thoughts to kill his grandson	Visual memory	Diazepam AVC→OCD	Left anterior frontal
Eslinger (1985)	Tumor (meningioma)	M/35	No/uk	Normal	Shaving, hair washing, deciding, particulars clung to outdated	Comportemental		Orbital cortex (R>L) Mesial damage (R>L) cortex dorsolateral R/SPECT frontal hypoperfusion
Cambier (1988)	Tumor (glioblastoma)	F/67	No/uk	Grasping, apragmatism	Graphomania, ordering, arranging, verification, rituals	Fluency, attention, aphasia dynamic		R frontal int, R cingulate, corpus callosum, L frontal
Laplane (1988b)	Head trauma	F/59	No/uk	Apragmatism	Counting	Attention, efficiency, intelligence, memory		Frontal white matter (F2F3F1), anterior cingulate cortex, PET: frontal bilateral cortex hypoperfusion
Seibyl (1988)	Tumor (meningioma)	F/54	No/uk	Normal	Compulsions to repeat words, need to obsessively verify	Memory, attention, vigilance calculation	MAOI+ lithium	L dural based in the ant R frontal
Ward (1988)	Glioblastoma	F/59	No	Hemiparesis	Urge to walk to the left few seconds (EEG)			R frontal parietal
	Glioblastoma	M/43	uk	Right hemiparesis	Strong urge to shake his R arm, urge to shout			L frontal
Max (1995)	Head trauma	F/12	No/uk		Compulsive hand washing, ordering, arranging, counting rituals	Nonverbal intelligence, spatial memory visual motor speed, disinhibition	Cranioplasty after 8 months	R: premotor, dorsolateral, prefrontal, orbital; temporal; anterior cingulate cortex L: dorsolateral, prefrontal, orbital, temporal cortex
Swoboda (1995)	Infarct	M/70	No/uk		Verification, collected old newspapers	Mild constructional abnormal motor function L hand, learning difficulties	Clonazepam	Post R frontal region/SPECT: post frontal underlying white matter hypoperfusion

Notes:

AVC = cerebral infarct; MAOI = monoamine oxidase inhibitor;

uk = unknown; M = male; F = female.

Neuropsychological testing was performed in seven cases. Neuropsychological disorders were somewhat variable from one patient to another:

intellectual function remained within normal limits;

linguistic and gestural specific activities, calculation, and drawing were intact;

orientation in space and time was preserved;

mental control and recall were good;

cognitive slowing varied between patients;

reduced digit span revealed attention disorders;

verbal fluency was poor;

some patients had problems extracting a figure from a complex figure: the reproduction of the Rey's Figure from memory indicated that attention was directed toward the large rectangle or toward the details;

learning could be disturbed;

the elaboration of a new strategy, the shifting of attitude in order to adapt to a changing situation, and the sequential programming of activity were also disturbed.

Associated with the cognitive impairment, some patients exhibited unusual behavioral abnormalities (Tables 11.2 and 11.3). Some authors reported marked subjective slowness and delay in the execution of daily-living tasks that appeared to derive principally from difficulties in initiating goal-directed action, from difficulties in suppressing perseverative behaviors during the course of such action (Hymas et al., 1991), or from an inadequate early inhibition of competing internal cues (Galderisi et al., 1995). In some cases, symptoms were more important, and summarized as a 'loss of drive.' They included a marked decrease in spontaneous activity, a loss of affect, and a notable reduction of spontaneous thought content. These patients' inertia was apparently reversible by external stimulation. First to describe these symptoms under the term of pure psychic akinesia, Laplane et al. (1982) associated them with bilateral lesions of the basal ganglia. Since then, other single cases reports have been published (Ali-Chérif et al., 1984; Trillet et al., 1990).

The premorbid personality of patients who develop OCD after a cerebral lesion is rarely considered as pathological. In most cases, authors reported no past psychiatric history (Tables 11.2 and 11.3, 20/31 cases). An anterior psychopathy (Laplane et al., 1988a) was described in one case, but for the other patients the past history is unknown (14/31 cases).

Etiologies

Acquired obsessive–compulsive disorder has been described after various neurologic diseases affecting principally the basal ganglia and frontal lobes.

A-OCD with basal ganglia pathology (Table 11.2)

Infarcts

Infarcts were very frequently described and affected different structures. Focal lesions of striatum affecting the putamen have been related with unilateral infarct (Maraganore, Lees and Marsden, 1991; Hebebrand et al., 1993; Daniele et al., 1997).

Combined lesions of caudate and putamen nuclei have been described: Williams, Owen and Heath (1988) reported an infarct in caudate nuclei and the right putamen; Weilburg et al. (1989) described a young man with left caudate and putamen lesions after neonatal infarct. Similarly, Croisile et al. (1989) and Trillet et al. (Case 2, 1990) reported infarcts of the bilateral head of caudate nuclei and anterior part of putamen. Case 1 of Trillet et al. (1990) had associated lesions of the head of the right caudate nucleus and the left lentiform nucleus. Desi et al. (1990) published the report of a case of bilateral medial pallidum lesions after infarct.

Anoxia

Carbon monoxide intoxication was a frequent etiology affecting globus pallidus. Laplane et al. (1982, 1984, 1988a) and Ali-Chérif et al. (1984) have reported several such cases.

The lentiform nucleus could also be concerned. Anoxia (Durand, Vercken and Goulon, 1989; Laplane et al., 1989, Cases 5 and 6) affected bilateral lentiform nucleus. After encephalopathy, lesions are more diffuse with right head caudate lesion and bilateral globus pallidus and putamen damage (Laplane et al., 1981).

Degenerative disease

OCD symptoms related to caudate lesions have been described in degenerative cases. Bilateral caudate atrophy was associated with OCD (Tonkonogy and Barreira, 1989; Wyszynski et al., 1989; Penisson-Besnier, Le Gall and Dubas, 1992).

OCD symptoms without focal lesion but in association with neurodegenerative disease affecting basal ganglia have been related. Disorders affecting the caudate nuclei, such as Parkinson's disease (Tomer, Levin and Weiner, 1993; Müller et al., 1997), Sydenham's choreas (Swedo et al., 1989), and Huntington's disease (Cummings and Cunningham, 1992), could be associated with OCD symptoms. In supranuclear paralysis, Destee et al. (1990) described compulsive symptoms. In the same way, in postencephalitis parkinsonism (Schilder, 1938; Jellife, 1932, in McGuire, 1995) or manganese intoxication (Mena et al., 1967), obsessions and compulsions could be observed.

Various etiologies

Smadja et al. (1995) described a case of a seropositive woman with right lentiform and left pallidum lesions caused by toxoplasmic abscesses. A left basal ganglia lesion associated with a right cerebellar peduncle has also been described (Ward, 1988). All the nuclei could be affected with bilateral striopallidodentate calcifications (Kotrla et al., 1994).

A-OCD after frontal lesions (Table 11.3)

Tumors

Tumors are the most frequent etiology. Bilateral mesial and orbital damage with right dorsolateral cortex lesion is described by Eslinger and Damasio (1985) after surgical intervention for a bilateral meningioma. Cambier et al. (1988) reported glioblastoma affecting right frontal internal, left frontal lesion and right anterior cingulum damage with graphomania. A dural-based lesion in the anterior right frontal lobe is described with a meningioma in the case of Seibyl et al. (1988). Sometimes, the lesion can be unilateral. Ward (1988) described two cases with frontal right (Case 1) and left (Case 2) lesion with transient OCD symptoms related to epileptic status.

Infarcts

Infarcts have been described by Paunovic (1984) with left anterior frontal hypoperfusion, and by Swoboda and Jenike (1995) with a right frontal lesion and right posterior frontal underlying white matter hypoperfusion.

Head injury

Head trauma induced frontal white matter and anterior cingulum lesions (Laplane et al., 1988b) or diffuse anterior lesions (Max et al., 1995). Kant, Smith-Seemiller and Duffy (1996) reported (in their Case 3) a young man who suffered a closed head injury with a small right frontal depressed fracture (computerized tomography, CT scan).

Degeneration

In degenerative cases with bilateral frontotemporal atrophy, obsessive behaviors are known but reports of OCD are rare. Ames et al. (1994) have described OCD in frontal degeneration with hypoperfusion in the caudate nuclei (single-photon emission computerized tomography, SPECT).

Diffuse encephalitic pathologies

A-OCD has also been described in some diffuse encephalitic pathologies such as head injury, with meningitis (Khanna et al., 1985), without evident lesions

(McKeon et al., 1984; Kant et al., 1996), normal pressure hydrocephalus (Abbruzzese, Scarone and Colombo, 1994), multiple sclerosis (George, Kellner and Fossey, 1989), hypoglycemia (Rippere, 1984), chronic epidemic encephalitis (Wohlfart, Ingvar and Hellberg, 1961), Creutzfeldt-Jakob disease (Lopez et al., 1997), diabetes insipidus (Barton, 1965), cerebellar brain tumor (Moriarty, Trimble and Hayward 1993; Paradis et al., 1992), and epilepsy (Kettl and Marks, 1986; Cascino and Sutula, 1989; Levin and Duchowny, 1991; Kroll and Drummond, 1993).

The etiologies are various, and it is therefore difficult to confirm whether OCD symptoms are induced by a particular disease, because the association could be coincidental.

Physiopathology

Implication of frontal lobes and basal ganglia in the regulation of action

The role of the frontal system in programming, regulating, and verifying ongoing activities is well known. According to Luria (1973), the mental representation of specific movements prior to their execution is a frontal lobe function. The frontal lobes are connected intimately with the limbic, sensory, and motor areas. They are responsible for the control and modulation of goal-directed behavior and the adaptation of such behavior to the changing demands of the external environment (Luria, 1966; Stuss and Benson, 1984). Frontal lobes have a role in 'policing' behavior, preventing impulsive actions, and selecting actions that are optimal for prevailing goals.

The basal ganglia are responsible for the synthesis of simple motor programs in complex motor programs (Marsden, 1982).

The frontal lobes, the basal ganglia, and their interconnections with limbic structures have a role in the modulation of goal-directed behaviors and the assignment of meaning to environmental stimuli. The frontal cortex, the basal ganglia, and the thalamus are units in circuits that mediate motor activity, eye movements, and behavior (Alexander, DeLong and Strick, 1986). The factor of all frontal subcortical circuits (Fig. 11.1) is their origin in the frontal lobes, with excitatory projections to striatal structures. Two pathways emanate from the striatum, a direct projection to the globus pallidus interna and substantia nigra, and an indirect projection from the striatum to the globus pallidus externa that in turn connects to the subthalamic nucleus, which projects back to the globus pallidus interna and substantia nigra. These structures also have connections to thalamic nuclei which complete these circuits by projecting back to the frontal lobes. The direct and indirect pathways through the circuit exert opposing influences. The direct pathway, with two consecutive inhibitory gamma-aminobutyric acid (GABA)-ergic neurons, tends to disinhibit the thalamus. The indirect pathway, with excitatory glutamatergic neurons

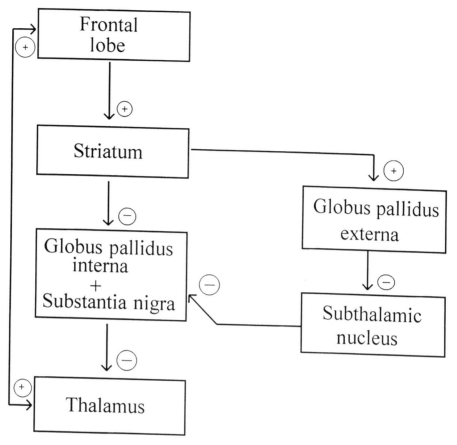

Fig. 11.1   Structure of frontal subcortical circuits.

as well as two inhibitory GABA-ergic neurons, exerts an inhibitory influence on the thalamus, balancing the disinhibiting (excitatory) effects of the direct pathway (Alexander, Crutcher and DeLong, 1990). Three circuits originating in the prefrontal cortex (the dorsolateral, the orbitofrontal, and the anterior cingulate) subserve, respectively, executive functions, personality, and motivation. The dorsolateral prefrontal subcortical circuit mediates the organization of information to facilitate a response. The lateral orbitofrontal subcortical circuit allows the integration of limbic and emotional information into contextually appropriate behavioral responses. The anterior cingulate subcortical circuit is required for motivated behavior.

Specific structural lesions may induce obsessive–compulsive behavior

To date, the majority of these lesions have involved frontal regions or the basal ganglia, leading to speculation about the neuronal circuitry underlying such complex behavioral repertoires (Alexander et al., 1986; Modell et al., 1989).

A defect in control of the action by the frontal lobes

The dorsolateral frontal zones have been hypothesized to be involved in the monitoring of ongoing activity in relation to environmental changes. Disruption of this system may result in difficulty terminating behavioral acts or emotional arousal. As a result, information about ongoing motor programs may not reach the limbic system, and overarousal and persistence in the response may occur. Compulsions are an example of perseverative behavior in which the frontal lobe may be unable to inhibit the motor or cognitive programs of the basal ganglia, with the recurrent execution of motor plans or programs. Sandson and Albert (1987) explained perseverative behavior with the functional absence of the Supervisory Attentional System of Shallice and Burgess (1991). Action schemas are triggered directly by environmental stimuli or by current activity leading to response perseveration and difficulty in shifting mental set. The inability to inhibit inappropriate responses should diminish the ability of the subject to dismiss obsessions and compulsions (Martinot et al., 1990). A functional disconnection between sensory systems and response output or emotional systems could also explain persistent arousal and compulsive and perseverative behavior (Otto, 1992).

The disorganization in activity that can follow frontal lobe damage is characterized by fragmented sequences of action, relevant parts being omitted and irrelevant parts being introduced (Duncan, 1986).

Dysfunction of basal ganglia circuits

Neurological diseases with obsessive–compulsive symptoms, neurosurgical procedures to treat OCD, and functional brain imaging with single-photon emission tomography (SPECT) and positron emission tomography (PET) have been the primary bases for current hypotheses about abnormalities in cortical striatal thalamic–cortical loop circuits in OCD (Rapoport and Wise, 1988; Modell et al., 1989; Insel, 1992a; Cummings, 1993)

Overaccess of sensory or interoceptive stimuli to emotional or response systems has also been suggested by Baxter et al. (in Otto, 1992) and Modell et al. (1989). The basal ganglia and the ventral caudate are thought to be a 'gating station' for sensory information. Dysfunction of this gating station or afferent input beyond the gating properties of the caudate were hypothesized to leave afferent information from the frontal lobes improperly regulated, resulting in inappropriate behavioral or cognitive responses, particularly perseverative responses.

Modell et al. (1989) identified the orbitofrontal cortex as one source of afferent input that exceeds the gating properties of the caudate. Baxter et al. (1996) reported that neural efferents from the orbital prefrontal cortex preferentially activated the direct basal ganglia pathway. However, elevated activity in the orbitofrontal regions is thought to reflect an attempt to compensate for these ungated sensations and thoughts, or chronic anxiety (Martinot et al., 1990). This would lead to disinhibition of the thalamocortical limb and increased orbitofrontal and caudate activity. Disinhibition might allow information that would normally be inhibited in the thalamus to flow freely through the mediodorsal nucleus of the thalamus, leading to the release of information to the orbitofrontal cortex (Baxter, 1990). Symptoms might be divided into a compulsive (behavioral drive) component and an inhibitory (loss of control) component. Orbitothalamic overactivity is proposed to give rise to the compulsive component of symptoms, whereas the basal ganglia may be central to the inhibitory component. Obsessive–compulsive symptoms would thus be expected to appear or increase when striatopallidothalamic activity is abnormally decreased (disinhibition), or when reciprocal orbitothalamic activity is abnormally increased (Modell et al., 1989). The apparent paradox of the occurrence of OCD in conjunction with both hypermetabolism of the caudate in I-OCD and hypometabolism of the caudate in certain cases studies reported earlier or in Huntington's disease (Cummings and Cunningham, 1992) is unexplained. Weilburg et al. (1989) described OCD symptoms after a lesion in the left caudate nucleus and discussed the fact that, whereas Baxter et al. (1987) found caudate hypermetabolism, their case was associated with hypoactivity. They suggested that the lesion in the left caudate nucleus could induce a state of relative hyperactivity in the right caudate nucleus. A finding of differential involvement of cell populations with excitatory or inhibitory neurotransmitters could solve the conundrum (Ames et al., 1994).

Dysfunction of the frontal subcortical circuits can be seen with involvement of several structures (Mega and Cummings, 1994)

These findings are consistent with reports of OCD acquired after basal ganglia lesions and with animal studies. Lesions of the caudate nucleus are associated with overresponsivity to certain sensory stimuli, such that immediate and sustained responses to stimuli occur despite the absence of appropriate environmental feedback (Otto, 1992). In the literature, most basal ganglia lesions are bilateral. However, a few cases have been described with unilateral damage. The case of Daniele et al. (1997) is doubtful because the patient was parkinsonian and could have a bilateral subcortical dysfunction. Nevertheless, Maraganore et al. (1991) and Hebebrand et al. (1993) reported unilateral lesions, and Weilburg et al. (1989) described two left-sided lesions. The case described by Croisile et al. (1989) is interesting because after a unilateral infarct of the head of caudate nucleus, the disturbances were transient, but persistent obsessive behavior occurred only when infarction of the caudate nucleus was bilateral. This is consistent with studies in animals in which the disturbances are persistent only with bilateral lesions (Iversen, 1979).

Unilateral frontal lesion could be able to provoke obsessive or compulsive symptoms. In the two cases of Ward (1988), the malignant tumor could have bilateral results because of edema. In animal experiments performed with monkeys, electrical stimulations and ablations in orbitomedial prefrontal cortex elicited alterations in anxious displays and reproduced emotional and cognitive symptoms present in OCD (Iversen and Mishkin, 1970; Raleigh and Steklis, 1979).

In degenerative cases, Ames et al. (1994) described OCD symptoms in patients with frontal degenerations with the common co-occurrence of basal ganglia pathology and frontal degenerative changes.

Biochemical alterations as well as direct lesion effects may play a role in the pathophysiological alterations mediating the aberrant behavior. The two principal fast-acting transmitters of the frontal subcortical circuits are GABA and glutamate. GABA is the most ubiquitous inhibitory transmitter in the nervous system, and glutamate is the most abundant excitatory transmitter. Dopamine, serotonin, and acetylcholine have modulatory roles in the frontal subcortical circuits (Cummings, 1995). Goodman, Price and Delgado (1990) suggested that in some forms of I-OCD, the pathology may involve not only serotonergic dysfunction, but also perturbation of dopaminergic systems. Dopamine excess in the hyperkinetic disorders produces cortical excitation by reducing inhibition of the thalamo-cortical projections by the globus pallidus (DeLong, 1990). A direct lesion of the globus pallidus has the same neurophysiological effect (Cummings and Cunningham, 1992). Treatment with levodopa may precipitate compulsions in parkinsonian patients (Hardie, Lees and Stern, 1984).

A better understanding of physiopathology is important to explain some therapeutic attempts.

Therapeutic aspects

Some authors think that neurobehavioral disorders associated with a precise lesion are treatment resistant. For Seibyl et al. (1988), the presence of neurological disease does not obviate the utility of pharmacotherapy. The circuits involve a number of transmitters, receptor subtypes, and second messengers that can be manipulated pharmacologically (Mega and Cummings, 1994).

Serotonin receptors are differentially distributed in the frontal subcortical circuits. The serotonin 5HT1 receptor is the most abundant serotonin receptor in the basal ganglia. The ventral striatum, the principal striatal structure of the anterior cingulate subcortical circuit, is the exception in that the 5HT3 receptor predominates there.

Depletion of serotonin in experimental animals leads to increased expression of normally suppressed behaviors, whereas treatment of obsessive compulsions with serotonergic antidepressants seems to reduce metabolic overactivity in fronto-cingulate and striatal regions, suggesting a serotonergic effect on activity at these sites (McGuire, 1995). Mann et al. (1966) reported a method for evaluating in-vivo serotonin responsivity in the human prefrontal cortex, the role of serotonergic dysfunction in a variety of psychiatric disorders, as well as the effects of treatment.

It is important to consider studies with I-OCD. In one double-blind study, clomipramine but not nortriptyline (a weak inhibitor of serotonin receptors) was significantly better than placebo in reducing the severity of obsessive–compulsive symptoms. In double blind crossover trials, clomipramine was found to be more effective than the relatively selective norepinephrine receptor inhibitor desipramine. The serotonin receptor properties of an antidepressant drug may be crucial to its efficacy as an antiobsessive–compulsive agent (Goodman, McDougle and Price, 1992; Insel, 1992b).

Piccinelli et al. (1995), in a meta-analysis, showed that antidepressant drugs are effective in the short-term treatment of patients suffering from OCD (clomipramine, fluoxetine, fluvoxamine, sertraline). Direct comparison between clomipramine and selective serotonin reuptake inhibitors showed that they had similar efficacy in the treatment of obsessive–compulsive symptoms. On Y-BOCS, the increase in improvement rate over placebo was between 61.3% and 21.6%. Clomipramine and fluvoxamine had greater therapeutic efficacy than antidepressant drugs with no selective serotonergic properties. Others (e.g. Marks et al., 1988) found that clomipramine had a limited, brief effect.

The therapeutic strategy could be a combined treatment. A trial with monoamine oxidase inhibitor may be an option in OCD patients with comorbid panic disorder.

The rationale for the majority of combination strategies has been to add agents to ongoing serotonin reuptake inhibitor therapy that may modify serotonergic function, such as fenfluramine, lithium, buspirone, neuroleptic. Lithium could be used when there are prominent depressive symptoms. Goodman et al.'s (1992) clinical impression is that buspirone addition may be most helpful in OCD patients with comorbid generalized anxiety disorder.

Neuroleptics alone do not appear effective in OCD, but there is emerging evidence that serotonin reuptake inhibitor with neuroleptic treatment may be beneficial in some cases in particular patients with a comorbid chronic tic disorder (Goodman et al. 1992).

Electroconvulsive therapy may have a role in the severely depressed patient with OCD who has been refractory to pharmacologic and behavioral approaches. This indication is for I-OCD and has never been utilized in A-OCD.

Surgical ablation of the orbitofrontal cortex or the medial thalamic nuclei has been very effective in ameliorating the symptoms of OCD (Modell et al., 1989). The effects of psychosurgery are explained because destruction of the anterior cingulate cortex, its thalamic input, its efferent pathways to the caudate nucleus, or the caudate itself would eliminate the excitatory drive to the internal motivation detector (Jenike et al., 1991). Nevertheless, neurosurgery is a controversial treatment (Sachdev and Hay, 1996), with a gradual decline in the number of operations performed (Poynton, Bridges and Bartlett, 1988). Stereotactic surgical methods are not utilized for A-OCD.

Examination of the published case studies shows that few patients have had treatment, and evolution is rarely reported (see Tables 11.1 and 11.2). Seibyl et al. (1988) used monoamine oxidase inhibitor with lithium, with notable improvement, while others have used benzodiazepine (diazepam for Paunovic, 1984; clonazepam for Swoboda and Jenike, 1995), or medications with anticholinergic effects (diphenydramine, Wyszinski et al., 1989). Antidepressant drugs with serotoninergic properties, such as clomipramine (Laplane et al., 1981) or trazodone (Ames et al., 1994), are also prescribed. Laplane et al. (1988a) used clembuterol with some improvement.

Conclusion

Obsessive–compulsive disorder after focal cerebral lesion is one of the best examples of a psychopathological organic disorder which may mimic a classical psychiatric syndrome. Scales and neurological examination are not always sufficient to distinguish idiopathic from acquired behavior. Nevertheless, age at onset, clinical history with sudden onset of the symptoms, and the pathological context (stroke, head injury, extrapyramidal diseases) may largely orient the diagnosis. The physiopathology of the disorder is still obscure, with some unexplained paradoxes. A-OCD is the result of a defect in the control of action with frontal or subcortical dysfunction, and described after focal brain lesions affecting frontal lobes and basal ganglia. Nevertheless, the relative rarity of these symptoms is surprising.

Are the symptoms of obsession and compulsion neglected in the clinical examination? Patients do not readily relate abnormal behavior, and symptoms could appear secondarily after onset of the disease. It would be interesting to perform a prospective investigation using Y-BOCS on a series of patients with focal frontal and basal ganglia lesions, patients with degeneration of the frontal lobes, or parkinsonian patients after stereotaxic surgery (no case of OCD has been reported to date, nor any significant deterioration, Soukup et al., 1997). Such a study could be justified by the relative rarity of A-OCD and by the difficulties inherent in the anatomoclinical correlations (Goldman-Rakic, 1987; Laplane et al., 1989).

It would appear premature to attempt an explanation of OCD based on a single physiopathological hypothesis (Turner, Beidel and Nathan, 1985). An association of different factors to explain the occurrence of OCD is suspected. It is possible that premorbid obsessional personality, genetic predisposition, neuroanatomical involvement, and biochemical abnormalities may contribute to the pathogenesis of OCD, each in varying degrees.

REFERENCES

Abbruzzese, M., Ferri, S. and Scarone, S. (1995). Wisconsin Card Sorting Test performance in obsessive–compulsive disorder: no evidence for involvement of dorsolateral prefrontal cortex. *Psychiatry Res* 58: 37–43.

Abbruzzese, M., Scarone, S. and Colombo, C. (1994). Obsessive–compulsive symptomatology in normal pressure hydrocephalus: a case report. *J Psychiatry Neurosci* 19(5): 378–80.

Alexander, G.E., Crutcher, M.D. and DeLong, M.R. (1990). Basal ganglia thalamo-cortical circuits: parallel substrates for motor, oculomotor, prefrontal and limbic functions. In *Progress in Brain Research*, Vol. 85, ed. H.B.M. Uylings, C.G. Van Eden, J.P.C. DeBruin, M.A. Corner and M.G.P. Feenstra, pp. 119–46. New-York: Elsevier Science Publishers.

Alexander, G.E., DeLong, M.R. and Strick, P.L. (1986). Parallel organization of functionally segregated circuits linking basal ganglia and cortex. *Annu Rev Neurosci* 9: 357–81.

Ali-Chérif, A., Royere, M.L., Gosset, A. et al. (1984). Troubles du comportement et de l'activité mentale après intoxication oxycarbonée. *Rev Neurol* 140(6–7): 401–5.

American Psychiatric Association (1994). *Diagnostic and Statistical Manual of Mental Disorders* (DSM IV), 4th edn. Washington, DC: American Psychiatric Association.

Ames, D., Cummings, J.L., Wirshing, W.C., Quinn, B. and Mahler, M. (1994). Repetitive and compulsive behavior in frontal lobe degenerations. *J Neuropsychiatry Clin Neurosci* 6(2): 100–13.

Barton, R. (1965). Diabetes insipidus and obsessional neurosis. A syndrome. *Lancet* 16: 133–5.

Baxter, L.R. (1990). Brain imaging as a tool in establishing a theory of brain pathology in obsessive compulsive disorder. *J Clin Psychiatry* 51(8): 32–5

Baxter, L.R. (1992). Neuroimaging studies of obsessive compulsive disorder. *Psychiatr Clin North Am* 15: 871–84.

Baxter, L.R., Phelps, M.E., Mazziotta, J.C. et al. (1987). Local cerebral glucose metabolic rates in obsessive compulsive disorder. *Arch Gen Psychiatry* 44: 211–18.

Baxter, L.R., Saxena, S., Brody, A.L. et al. (1996). Brain mediation of obsessive compulsive disorder symptoms: evidence from functional brain imaging studies in the human and nonhuman primate. *Semin Clin Neuropsychiatry* 1(1): 32–47.

Baxter, L.R., Schwartz, J.M., Guze, B.H., Bergman, K. and Szuba, M.P. (1990). PET imaging in obsessive compulsive disorder with and without depression. *J Clin Psychiatry* 51 (4 Suppl.): 61–9.

Berthier, M.L., Kulisevsky, J., Gironell, A. and Heras, J.A. (1996). Obsessive–compulsive disorder associated with brain lesions: clinical phenomenology, cognitive function, and anatomic correlates. *Neurology* 47: 353–61.

Cambier, J., Masson, C., Benammou, S. and Robine, B. (1988). La graphomanie, activité graphique compulsive. Manifestation d'un gliome fronto-calleux. *Rev Neurol* 144(3): 158–64.

Cascino, G.D. and Sutula, T.P. (1989). Thirst and compulsive water drinking in medial basal limbic epilepsy: an electroclinical and neuropathological correlation. *J Neurol Neurosurg Psychiatry* 52: 680–1.

Croisile, B., Tourniaire, D., Confavreux, C., Trillet, M. and Aimard, G. (1989). Bilateral damage to the head of the caudate nuclei. *Ann Neurol* 25(3): 313–4.

Cummings, J.L. (1993). Frontal–subcortical circuits and human behavior. *Arch Neurol* 50: 873–80.

Cummings, J.L. (1995). Anatomic and behavioral aspects of frontal subcortical circuits. *Ann N Y Acad Sci* 769: 1–13.

Cummings, J.L. and Cunningham, K. (1992). Obsessive–compulsive disorder in Huntington's disease. *Biol Psychiatry* 31: 263–70.

Daniele, A., Bartolomeo, P., Cassetta, E. et al. (1997). Obsessive–compulsive behaviour and cognitive impairment in a parkinsonian patient after left putaminal lesion. *J Neurol Neurosurg Psychiatry* 62: 288–302.

DeLong, M.R. (1990). Primate models of movement disorders of basal ganglia origin. *Trends Neurosci* 13: 281–5.

Desi, M., Klein, J., Parman, Y., Seibel, N. and Segobia, R. (1990). Adynamia and repetitive behaviour in a case of bilateral subcortical lesions. *J Neurol* 237 (Suppl. 1): 28.

Destee, A., Gray, F., Parent, M. et al. (1990). Comportement compulsif d'allure obsessionnelle et paralysie supranucléaire progressive. *Rev Neurol* 146(1): 12–18.

Duncan, J. (1986). Disorganisation of behaviour after frontal damage. *Cogn Neuropsychol* 3(3): 271–90.

Durand, M.C., Vercken, J.B. and Goulon, M. (1989). Syndrome extra-pyramidal après incompétence cardio-circulatoire. *Rev Neurol* 145(5): 398–400.

Eslinger, P.J. and Damasio, A.R. (1985). Severe disturbance of higher cognition after bilateral frontal lobe ablation: patient EVR. *Neurology* 35: 1731–41.

Galderisi, S., Mucci, A., Catapano, F., Colucci D'Amato, A. and MAJ, M. (1995). Neuropsychological slowness in obsessive–compulsive patients. Is it confined to tests involving the fronto-subcortical systems? *Br J Psychiatry* 167: 394–8.

George, M.S., Kellner, C.H. and Fossey, M.D. (1989). Obsessive–compulsive symptoms in a patient with multiple sclerosis. *J Nerv Ment Dis* 177(5): 304–5.

Goldman-Rakic, P.S. (1987). Circuitry of primate prefrontal cortex and regulation of behavior by representational memory. In *Secondary Circuitry of Primate Prefrontal Cortex and Regulation of Behavior by Representational Memory*, ed. V.B. Mountcastle, F. Plum and S.R. Geirger, pp. 373–417. Bethesda, MD: American Physiological Society.

Goodman, W.K., McDougle, C.J. and Price, L.H. (1992). Pharmacotherapy of obsessive compulsive disorder. *J Clin Psychiatry* 53 (4 Suppl.): 29–37.

Goodman, W.K., Price, L.H. and Delgado, P.L. (1990). Specificity of serotonin reuptake inhibitors in the treatment of obsessive–compulsive disorder: comparison of fluvoxamine and desipramine. *Arch Gen Psychiatry* 47: 577–85.

Goodman, W.K., Price, L.H., Rasmussen, S.A. et al. (1989). The Yale–Brown Obsessive Compulsive Scale. I. Development, use, and reliability. *Arch Gen Psychiatry* 46: 1006–11.

Hardie, R.J., Lees, A.J. and Stern, G.M. (1984). On–off fluctuations in Parkinson's disease. A clinical and neuropharmacological study. *Brain* 107: 487–506.

Hebebrand, J., Siemon, P., Lutcke, A., Marib, G. and Remschmidt, H. (1993). A putaminal lesion in an adolescent with obsessive–compulsive disorder and atypical anorexia nervosa. *J Nerv Ment Dis* 181: 520–1.

Hymas, N., Lees, A., Bolton, D., Epps, K. and Head, D. (1991). The neurology of obsessional slowness. *Brain* 114: 2203–33.

Insel, T.R. (1992a). Toward a neuroanatomy of obsessive–compulsive disorder. *Arch Gen Psychiatry* 49: 739–44.

Insel, T.R. (1992b). Neurobiology of obsessive compulsive disorder: a review. *Int Clin Psychopharmacol* 7 (Suppl. 1): 31–3.

Inversen, S.D. (1979). Behavior after neostriatal lesions in animals. In *The Neostriatum*, ed. I. Divac and R.G.E. Oberg, pp. 195–319. New York: Pergamon Press.

Iversen, S.D. and Mishkin, M. (1970). Perseverative interference in monkeys following selective lesions of the inferior prefrontal convexity. *Exp Brain Res* 11: 376–86.

Janet, P. (1903). *Les Obsessions et la Psychasthénie*. Paris: Alcan.

Jellife, S.E. (1929). Psychologic components in postencephalitic oculogyric crises. *Arch Neurol Psychiatry* 21: 491–532.

Jenike, M.A., Baer, L., Ballantine, H.T. et al. (1991). Cingulotomy for refractory obsessive–compulsive disorder. *Arch Gen Psychiatry* 48: 548–55.

Kant, R., Smith-Seemiller, L. and Duffy, J.D. (1996). Obsessive–compulsive disorder after closed head injury: review of literature and report of four cases. *Brain Inj* 10(1): 55–63.

Kettl, P.A. and Marks, I.M. (1986). Neurological factors in obsessive compulsive disorder. Two case reports and a review of the literature. *Br J Psychiatry* 149: 315–19.

Khanna, S., Narayanan, H.S., Sharma, S.D. and Mukundan, C.R. (1985). Post traumatic obsessive compulsive disorder, a case report. *Indian J Psychiatry* 27(4): 337–9.

Kotrla,K.J., Ardaman, M.F., Meyers, C.A., Novac, I.S. and Hayman, L.A. (1994). Unsuspected obsessive compulsive disorder in a patient with bilateral striopallidodentate mineralizations. *Neuropsychiatry Neuropsychol Behav Neurol* 7(2): 130–5.

Kroll, L. and Drummond, L.M. (1993). Temporal lobe epilepsy and obsessive–compulsive symptoms. *J Nerv Ment Dis* 181: 457–8.

Laplane, D., Baulac, M., Pillon, B. and Panayotopoulou-Achimastos I. (1982). Perte de l'autoactivation psychique. Activité compulsive d'allure obsessionnelle. Lésion lenticulaire bilatérale. *Rev Neurol* 138(2): 137–41.

Laplane, D., Baulac, M., Widlöcher, D. and Dubois, B. (1984). Pure psychic akinesia with bilateral lesions of basal ganglia. *J Neurol Neurosurg Psychiatry* 47: 377–85.

Laplane, D., Boulliat, J., Baron, J.C., Pillon, B. and Baulac, M. (1988a). Comportement compulsif d'allure obsessionnelle par lésion bilatérale des noyaux lenticulaires. Un nouveau cas. *L'encéphale* 14: 27–32.

Laplane, D., Dubois, B., Pillon, B. and Baulac, M. (1988b). Perte d'autoactivation psychique et activité mentale stéréotypée par lésion frontale. Rapports avec le trouble obsessivo–compulsif. *Rev Neurol* 144(10): 564–70.

Laplane, D., Levasseur, M., Pillon, B. et al. (1989). Obsessive–compulsive and other behavioural changes with bilateral basal ganglia lesions. *Brain* 112: 699–725.

Laplane, D., Widlöcher, D., Pillon, B., Baulac, M. and Binoux, F. (1981). Comportement compulsif d'allure obsessionnelle par nécrose circonscrite bilatérale pallidostriatale. Encéphalopathie par piqûre de guêfe. *Rev Neurol* 137(4): 269–76.

Leckman, J.F., Grice, D.E., Boardman, J. et al. (1997). Symptoms of obsessive–compulsive disorder. *Am J Psychiatry* 154(7): 911–17.

Levin, B. and Duchowny, M. (1991). Childhood obsessive–compulsive disorder and cingulate epilepsy. *Biol Psychiatry* 30: 1049–55.

Lopez, O.L., Berthier, M.L., Backer, J.T. and Boller, F. (1997). Creutzfeldt–Jakob disease with features of obsessive–compulsive disorder and anorexia nervosa: the role of cortical–subcortical systems. *Neuropsychiatry Neuropsychol Behav Neurol* 10(2): 120–4.

Luria, A.R. (1966). *Higher Cortical Functions in Man.* New York: Basic Books.

Luria, A.R. (1973). *The Working Brain. An Introduction to Neuropsychology.* New York: Basic Books.

Mann, J.J., Malone, K.M., Diehl, D.J. et al. (1996). Positron emission tomographic imaging of serotonin activation effects on prefrontal cortex in healthy volunteers. *J Cereb Blood Flow Metab* 16: 418–26.

Maraganore, D.M., Lees, A.J. and Marsden, C.D. (1991). Complex stereotypies after right putaminal infarction: a case report. *Mov Disord* 6(4): 358–61.

Marks, I.M., Lelliott, P., Basoglu, M. et al. (1988). Clomipramine, self-exposure and therapist-aided exposure for obsessive–compulsive rituals. *Br J Psychiatry* 152: 522–34.

Marsden, C.D. (1982). The mysterious motor function of the basal ganglia: the Robert Wartenberg Lecture. *Neurology* 32: 514–39.

Martinot, J.L., Allilaire, J.F., Mazoyer, B.M. et al. (1990). Obsessive–compulsive disorder: a clinical, neuropsychological and positron emission tomography study. *Acta Psychiatr Scand* 82: 233–42.

Max, J.E., Smith, W.L., Lindgren, S.D. et al. (1995). Case study: obsessive–compulsive disorder after severe traumatic brain injury in an adolescent. *J Am Acad Child Adolesc Psychiatry* 34(1): 45–9.

McGuire, P.K. (1995). The brain in obsessive–compulsive disorder. *J Neurol Neurosurg Psychiatry* 59: 457–9.

McKeon, J., McGuffin, P. and Robinson, P. (1984). Obsessive–compulsive neurosis following head injury. A report of four cases. *Br J Psychiatry* 144: 190–2.

Mega, M.S. and Cummings, J.L. (1994). Frontal–subcortical circuits and neuropsychiatric disorders. *J Neuropsychiatry Clin Neurosci* 6: 358–70.

Mena, I., Marin, O., Fuenzalida, S. and Cotzias, G.C. (1967). Chronic manganese poisoning. Clinical picture and manganese turnover. *Neurology* 17: 128–36.

Modell, J.G., Mountz, J.M., Curtis, G.C. and Greden, J.F. (1989). Neurophysiologic dysfunction in basal ganglia/limbic striatal and thalamocortical circuits as a pathogenetic mechanism of obsessive–compulsive disorder. *J Neuropsychiatry* 1: 27–36.

Moriarty, J., Trimble, M. and Hayward, R. (1993). Obsessive–compulsive disorder onset after removal of a brain tumor. *J Nerv Ment Dis* 181(5): 331.

Müller, N., Putz, A., Kathmann, N. et al. (1997). Characteristics of obsessive–compulsive symptoms in Tourette's syndrome, obsessive–compulsive disorder, and Parkinson's disease. *Psychiatry Res* 70: 105–14.

Otto, M.W. (1992). Normal and abnormal information processing. *Psychiatr Clin North Am* 15(4): 825–48.

Paradis, C.M., Friedman, S., Hatch, M. and Lazar, R.M. (1992). Obsessive–compulsive disorder onset after removal of a brain tumor. *J Nerv Ment Dis* 180: 535–6.

Paunovic, V.R. (1984). Syndrome obsessionnel au décours d'une atteinte cérébrale organique. *Ann Méd Psychol* 142(3): 379–82.

Penisson-Besnier, I., Le Gall, D. and Dubas, F. (1992). Comportement compulsif d'allure obsessionnelle (arithmomanie). Atrophie des noyaux caudés. *Rev Neurol* 148(4): 262–7.

Piccinelli, M., Pini, S., Bellantuono, C. and Wilkinson, G. (1995). Efficacy of drug treatment in obsessive–compulsive disorder. A meta-analytic review. *Br J Psychiatry* 166: 424–43.

Poynton, A., Bridges, P.K. and Bartlett, J.R. (1988). Psychosurgery in Britain now. *Br J Neurosurg* 2: 297–306.

Raleigh, M.J. and Steklis, H.D. (1979). The effects of orbitofrontal lesions in the aggressive behavior of vervet monkeys. *Exp Neurol* 66: 158–68.

Rapoport, J.L. and Wise, S.P. (1988). Obsessive–compulsive disorder: evidence for basal ganglia dysfunction. *Psychopharmacol Bull* 24(3): 380–4.

Rippere, V. (1984). Can hypoglycaemia cause obsessions and ruminations? *Med Hypotheses* 15: 3–13.

Sachdev, P. and Hay, P. (1996). Site and size of lesion and psychosurgical outcome in obsessive–compulsive disorder: a magnetic resonance imaging study. *Biol Psychiatry* 39: 739–42.

Sandson, J. and Albert, M.L. (1987). Perseveration in behavioral neurology. *Neurology* 37: 1736–41.

Schilder, P. (1938). The organic background of obsessions and compulsions. *Am J Psychiatry* 94: 1397–416.

Seibyl, J.P., Krystal, J.H., Goodman, W.K. and Price, L.H. (1988). Obsessive–compulsive symptoms in a patient with a right frontal lobe lesion. *Neuropsychiatry Neuropsychol Behav Neurol* 1(4): 295–9.

Shallice, T. and Burgess, P.W. (1991). Higher order cognitive impairments and frontal lobe lesions in man. In *Frontal Lobe Function and Dysfunction*, ed. H.S. Levin, H.M. Eisenberg and A.L. Benton, pp. 125–38. Oxford: Oxford University Press.

Smadja, D., Cabre, P., Prat, C. and Vernant, J.C. (1995). Perte d'auto-activation psychique. Comportements compulsifs d'allure obsessionnelle. Abcès toxoplasmiques des noyaux gris centraux. *Rev Neurol* 151(4): 271–3.

Soukup, V.M., Ingram, F., Schiess, M.C. et al. (1997). Cognitive sequelae of unilateral posteroventral pallidotomy. *Arch Neurol* 54: 947–50.

Stuss, D.T. and Benson, D.F. (1984). Neuropsychological studies of the frontal lobes. *Psychol Bull* 95: 3–28.

Swedo, S.E., Rapoport, J.L., Cheslow, D.L. et al. (1989). High prevalence of obsessive–compulsive symptoms in patients with Sydenham's chorea. *Am J Psychiatry* 146: 246–9.

Swoboda, K.J. and Jenike, M.A. (1995). Frontal abnormalities in a patient with obsessive–compulsive disorder: the role of structural lesions in obsessive–compulsive behavior. *Neurology* 45: 2130–4.

Tallis, F. (1997). The neuropsychology of obsessive–compulsive disorder: a review and consideration of clinical implications. *Br J Clin Psychol* 36: 3–20.

Tomer, R., Levin, B.E. and Weiner, W.J. (1993). Obsessive–compulsive symptoms and motor asymmetries in Parkinson's disease. *Neuropsychiatry Neuropsychol Behav Neurol* 6(1): 26–30.

Tonkonogy, J. and Barreira, P. (1989). Obsessive–compulsive disorder and caudate–frontal lesion. *Neuropsychiatry Neuropsychol Behav Neurol* 2(3): 203–9.

Trillet, M., Croisile, B., Tourniaire, D. and Schott, B. (1990). Perturbations de l'activité motrice volontaire et lésions des noyaux caudés. *Rev Neurol* 146(5): 338–44.

Turner, S.M., Beidel, D.C. and Nathan, R.S. (1985). Biological factors in obsessive–compulsive disorders. *Psychol Bull* 97(3): 430–50.

Veale, D.M., Sahakian, B.J., Owen, A.M. and Marks, I.M. (1996). Specific cognitive deficits in tests sensitive to frontal lobe dysfunction in obsessive–compulsive disorder. *Psychol Med* 26: 1261–9.

Von Economo, C. (1931). *Encephalitis Lethargica: its Sequelae and Treatment*. Oxford: Oxford University Press. Translated by K.O. Newman.

Ward, C.D. (1988). Transient feelings of compulsion caused by hemispheric lesions: three cases. *J Neurol Neurosurg Psychiatry* 51: 266–8.

Weilburg, J.B., Mesulam, M.M., Weintraub, S. et al. (1989). Focal striatal abnormalities in a patient with obsessive–compulsive disorder. *Arch Neurol* 46: 233–5.

Williams, A.C., Owen, C. and Heath, D.A. (1988). A compulsive movement disorder with cavitation of caudate nucleus. *J Neurol Neurosurg Psychiatry* 51: 447–8.

Wohlfart, G., Ingvar, D.H. and Hellberg, A.M. (1961). Compulsory shouting (Benedek's 'Klazomania') associated with oculogyric spasms in chronic epidemic encephalitis. *Acta Psychiatr Scand* 36: 369–77.

Wyszynski, B., Merriam, A., Medalia, A. and Lawrence, C. (1989). Choreoacanthocytosis. Report of a case with psychiatric features. *Neuropsychiatry Neuropsychol Behav Neurol* 2: 137–44.

12

Emotional dysprosody and similar dysfunctions

Diana Van Lancker and Caterina Breitenstein

Introduction

The importance of intonation meanings is generally well understood. However, until recently, relatively little attention has been paid to prosodic deficits following focal brain damage. In the nineteenth century, Hughlings Jackson (1874, 1915) described preserved singing and emotional speech in aphasia, thought to be 'duplicated' in the right hemisphere. The American neurologist Mill (1912) spoke of the 'zone of emotion and emotional expression as especially developed in the right cerebral hemisphere,' referencing facial and behavioral but not vocal examples (p. 167). Critchley (1964) noted expletives and other emotive expressions as residual aphasic speech. The first focused investigation was Monrad-Krohn's (1947) now famous description of a selective 'melody of speech' disorder, but the deficit was linguistic (see Moen, 1991) and did not involve 'emotional prosody' (Monrad-Krohn, 1963). Except for these few important efforts, more interest over the past century has been devoted to the related topics of facial emotional expression and the experience of emotion, until the inception in 1975 of emotional prosody studies in patients with brain lesions.

Despite the obvious correspondences between facial and vocal emotional expression, and some findings of impairments in common (Cancelliere and Kertesz, 1990), the extent to which they share processors in the adult brain is unclear (Starkstein et al., 1994; Hornak, Rolls, and Wade, 1996; Stone et al., 1996). Bowers et al. (1996) as well as Breitenstein, Daum, and Ackermann (1998), recently reported a double dissociation between the identification of facial and vocal emotional expressions, suggesting independence of these functions. In the child, the ability to judge the emotional meaning in facial expression develops significantly earlier than the ability to correctly identify vocal emotions (Brosgole and Weisman, 1995). This chapter does not attempt to resolve the relationship between emotional expression in the two modalities (with gesture as a third), but instead focuses on the effects of brain lesions on vocal emotional processing in adults.

Emotions research can be broadly cast into three components: emotional behavior (e.g., autonomic responses, overt behavior), emotional feelings/experiences (subjective reports), and the communication of emotion through tone of voice (prosody), facial expressions, and gestures (Heilman, 1997). Benson (1984) uses the term 'mood' to refer to a 'subjective feeling tone,' with the term 'affect' referring to 'the observable physical manifestations of emotion,' adding the notions 'drive' and 'motivation' to 'characterize the energy of emotions' (Benson, 1996, p. 91). The following review aims to explore the neural basis of vocal communication of emotions. By the term 'emotional prosody' (or 'affective prosody') we refer to nonverbal or 'suprasegmental' (not pertaining to phonemes) aspects of speech which carry information about the speaker's feelings and attitudes (Johnson et al., 1986). Although words communicate emotional content, it has been estimated that more than 90% of a message's affect is conveyed by nonverbal information (Mehrabian, 1972).

One aspect of related topics on emotion that might pertain is the 'valence hypothesis,' which proposes a differential involvement of the two cerebral hemispheres in negative (right-sided) and positive (left-sided) emotional expressions (Sackeim and Gur, 1978; Sackeim et al., 1982; Silberman and Weingartner, 1986; Gainotti, 1989). In a related view, Gainotti, Caltagirone, and Zoccolotti (1993) claim that the right (frontal) hemisphere has a stronger involvement in autonomic emotional reactions whereas the left (frontal) hemisphere mediates intentional emotional responses (laughing, crying). In addition, both animal and human studies provide evidence of an emotion-specific involvement of the amygdalar complex in the perception of fear and to a lesser degree anger (Adolphs et al., 1994; Clark, 1995; LeDoux, 1995; Calder et al., 1996; Scott et al., 1997; but see also Hamann et al., 1996). A selective impairment of disgust recognition was also described in (presymptomatic) Huntington's disease carriers (Gray et al., 1997). Whereas hemispheric differences and specific neural structures underlying emotional behaviors have been observed in some neurological conditions, clinical studies of emotional–prosodic (speech) perception and expression in brain-damaged patients do not support the valence theory, in that deficits are usually observed across both positive and negative emotional categories (Borod, 1992, 1993; Heilman, Bowers, and Valenstein, 1993).

Definitions

Prosodic information is 'backgrounded' in speech, in that people are more 'aware' and more educable in the classical linguistic elements, such as phonology, grammar, and lexicon, than they are in the 'paralinguistic' elements which make up prosody. Secondly, prosodic parameters entail other difficult-to-define domains, such as emotions and attitudes. Acoustically, measurable attributes include fundamental frequency (pitch), intensity (loudness), aspects of timing, and voice quality. Fundamental frequency is measured in terms of mean, variation, direction, and range. The control of intensity requires special care in data acquisition because its unit of measurement, the decibel, is relative, and it is particularly sensitive to differences in auditory acuity. The third attribute, timing, applies to units such as sounds, words phrases, and to relations such as pausing, rate, and rhythm. The fourth attribute, voice quality, is difficult to submit to quantification or reliable perceptual judgments (Kent, 1996; Kreiman, 1996; Kreiman and Garrett, 1996), and has been least studied in the context of emotional prosody. Timing and fundamental frequency are the most frequently utilized in prosody studies. The acoustic measures are more or less straightforward; knowing the significance of these acoustic parameters with respect to prosodic meanings remains the greatest challenge for future studies.

Although the details are complex, it is agreed that prosody signals various types of meanings through these acoustic cues. Linguistic meanings include those that, in English, indicate statement and question, and noun or verb (e.g., *im*port versus im*port*). Emotional prosody includes attitudes and emotions, with the experimental focus on emotional meanings, including happiness, anger, sadness, and fear.

Theoretical perspective

An early proposal about prosody and brain, the 'functional lateralization' hypothesis, stated that acoustic/motoric features of prosody that are utilized functionally as linguistic (those at the level of phoneme, syllable, word, or clause) are lateralized to the left hemisphere, while those involved in attitudinal/emotional and personal voice quality recognition will be lateralized to the right hemisphere (Van Lancker, 1980). Some limited support for parts of this 'functional lateralization' hypothesis has appeared using linguistic tonal stimuli (e.g., Van Lancker and Fromkin, 1973; Ryalls and Reinvang, 1986; Gandour et al., 1993b), word-level of phrase-level linguistic contrasts (Blumstein and Cooper, 1974; Ouellette and Baum, 1993), and emotional prosody in a tonal language (Gandour et al., 1995) and in English (Ross, 1981; Bryden and Ley, 1983). In their recent review of the neural bases of prosody for receptive and expressive prosody, Baum and Pell (1999) concluded that the left hemisphere may be particularly involved in the processing of phonemic and lexical tone contrasts (segmental and word-level prosody), whereas 'the effects of the functional load of prosodic cues' become less clear at the sentential level. However, several studies have reported linguistic–prosodic deficits following right hemisphere damage (Weintraub, Mesulam, and Kramer, 1981; Behrens, 1989; Baum, 1992), whereas others found no differences between left hemisphere damaged (LHD) and right hemisphere damaged (RHD) groups using linguistic

(Cooper et al., 1984; Baum and Pell, 1997) or emotional stimuli (e.g., Schlanger, Schlanger, and Gerstman, 1976; Van Lancker and Sidtis, 1992; Baum and Pell, 1997; Breitenstein et al., 1998). In a study of 42 patients with acute middle cerebral artery infarctions (26 RHD, 16 LHD), only four (three RHD, one LHD) had emotional–prosodic comprehension deficits (Darby, 1993). In two studies, patients with transcortical aphasia following LHD, who retained a repetition ability, were not able to repeat emotional–prosodic sentences accurately; they were not able to utilize intact right hemisphere function to accomplish this task (Speedie, Coslett, and Heilman, 1984; Bertier-Marcelo et al., 1996). Another example of contrary findings is the report of a double dissociation for linguistic and emotional–prosodic tasks in two patients with comparable bilateral lesions of the rostral superior temporal cortex (Peretz et al., 1994). It is likely that other factors besides the cognitive–functional one, which may indeed play a small part, account for the varied findings in the processing of both linguistic and emotional–prosodic cues.

Similarly, the proposal of a unitary emotional–prosodic competence lateralized to the right cortical hemisphere, varying by processing mode (production, repetition, comprehension) with the anterior–posterior hemispheric axis (Ross, 1981), has been only weakly supported or not supported at all. We will see that only about 50% of studies report performance differences between LHD and RHD groups, and almost none supports the intrahemispheric proposal. Findings in brain-damaged patients suggest the neuroanatomic independence of the two processing modes, perception and production (Borod et al., 1990, 1996; Borod, 1992). Further, studies point to a selective ability of the right hemisphere to perceive and produce pitch variations, indicating a role of complex motor and auditory function. In addition, the notion of preferential processing of emotional experiencing in the right hemisphere, including verbal labelling of these experiences, has come to light (Borod, 1993; Bowers, Bauer, and Heilman, 1993; Rapcsak, Comer, and Rubens, 1993). Finally, a predominant basal ganglia role in neurobehavioral syndromes which include dysprosody as a feature has emerged. Patients with lesions of the caudate nucleus, globus pallidus, or putamen and concomitant mood or motivational disturbance have been observed to have deficits in emotional–prosodic production (Bhatia and Marsden, 1994; Van Lancker et al., 1996). Some patients with basal ganglia damage associated with progressive neurological disorders (Parkinson's and Huntington's disease), known to have prosodic production deficits, have been observed also to be deficient in emotional–prosodic comprehension (Blonder, Gur, and Gur, 1989; Speedie et al., 1990; Breitenstein et al., 1998).

A basic question in emotional–prosodic research is whether there is a distinct, 'modular' competence or ability (Blonder, Bowers, and Heilman, 1991) to process emotional information in speech, or whether a combination of motor, perceptual, and neurobehavioral operations is coopted in orchestrating emotional–prosodic behaviors. The question is an important one, because focal lesions can be expected to affect a 'unitary' behavior differently from a constellation of disparate functions. This chapter presents evidence that emotional–prosodic behaviors are effected by a constellation of perceptual, motor, motivational, emotional, and cognitive–functional factors, which can be differentially dysfunctional following focal brain damage. Thus, a variety of 'causes' can lead to a clinical presentation of emotional dysprosody, or to inferior performance on emotional prosody tests.

As will be seen from the review below, the majority of neuropsychological studies cast emotional experience into categories, such as 'sad,' 'happy,' etc. Another approach is to describe emotions along dimensions, measuring valence or arousal ratings of emotional stimuli (Peper and Irle, 1997a, 1997b). Thus, it remains a basic question – not to be resolved here – whether to investigate emotional behaviors using a categorial or a dimensional concept of emotion (Young et al., 1997). It may be that a different paradigm for investigating prosodic deficits, such as described by Scherer (1986) and others in emotional psychology (e.g., Davidson, 1993a, 1993b), may help unravel some of the current discrepancies.

Methodological considerations: perception and production

Following the first studies of the effects of brain lesions on prosody in the middle 1970s, there has been an outpouring of literature on the topic. In a listing of publications catalogued in Psychological Abstracts accessed by the search term 'Prosody and Brain' of the (later) period from 1984 to 1999, 414 separate titles appear. It is obviously not possible to mention them all here. Instead, several methodological considerations pertaining to emotional–prosodic studies are reviewed, to aid the evaluation of these papers, followed by a critical review of representative studies.

Standard study design

Generally, the effects of focal brain damage on emotional prosody are studied through analyzing patients' performance in comprehension, repetition, and spontaneous production modes. If the investigator is interested in tapping 'real' abilities to produce and understand emotional information in speech, all of the formal techniques described here have limitations and failings of some type or other. In comprehension, study stimuli may be presented live by the experimenter (which lacks standardization but is more 'natural') or tape-recorded (which benefits from being controlled). Tasks involve discrimination (same/different judgments, which eliminate emotional meaning categories, for better or worse) or recognition/perception (choosing verbal labels or facial expressions, or both, in a multiple-choice format, which requires more cognitive processing). Stimuli are real (meaningful or nonsense) or acoustically treated speech (low pass filtered or altered in timing or pitch) of word, phrase, or sentence length. Responses in comprehension tests can be quantified in terms of accuracy or dimensional ratings and, in the case of production data, by listeners' evaluations and acoustic measures.

Various task demands

Task designs have proliferated to probe different questions about prosodic performance. In some studies, for example, sentences containing prosodic and semantic information are either congruent or incongruent. In the incongruent condition, a sentence such as 'The man held his dying son' is spoken on a happy intonation, and subjects make comprehension judgments about the prosodic meaning while ignoring the semantic content of the utterance. Although certainly justifiable as a study design and part of a widely used prosody testing protocol (Bowers, Blonder, and Heilman, 1991), the relation to normal prosodic function is indeterminate. In this and other task variants, the role of working memory or of 'metaprosodic' ability (thinking about the task rather than the content of the task) may be affecting performance results, as observed in several studies (Bowers et al., 1987; Blonder et al., 1991; Lalande et al., 1992; Breitenstein et al., 1998). Similarly, incongruent contexts for emotional prosody (using paragraphs) resulted in poorer performance of RHD patients in one study (Tompkins, 1991) and of LHD patients in another (Tompkins and Flowers, 1987). The number of responses, whether two or four choices, significantly determined performance in LHD patients in the study by Tompkins and Flowers (1985). Schmitt, Hartje, and Willmes (1997) compared 'unimodal' and 'multimodal' recognition tasks via videotaped scenes presented to LHD, RHD, and normal-control subjects, who judged the video sequences in terms of facial expression, emotional prosody, and the emotional meaning of the sentence spoken in the scene. They reported a right hemisphere superiority for the unimodal task. During the increased task demands of the multimodal condition, patients with LHD scored overall lower than the healthy control group (RHD and LHD patients did not differ from one another).

A study of children revealed a significant role of 'metaprosodic ability' – applying emotional–prosodic categories in a listening task. In a study using stimuli of a similar format to that of Heilman, Scholes, and Watson (1975), normal children under seven years were *unable* to match tape-recorded utterances ('Johnny is walking his dog') spoken with emotional–prosody (happy, angry, sad, surprised), to facial line-drawings presented with a verbal label (Van Lancker, Kreiman, and Cornelius, 1989). This result is troubling because there is ample evidence that children in the first year of life respond to nonverbal prosodic cues (Crystal, 1970; Mandel, Jusczyk, and Nelson, 1994; Mehler and Christophe, 1994; Vihman and De Boysson-Bardies, 1994). Similarly, other studies have also demonstrated that brain-damaged patients perform worse on tasks of cross-modal matching of prosodic sentences and facial expressions than on either task separately (Blonder et al., 1991; Breitenstein et al., 1996, 1998).

Posed versus spontaneous expression

This parameter pertains either to presentation of stimuli, or to the type of response, and is most viable in the study of facial expression. Facial expression performance for 'posed' versus 'spontaneous' emotional–facial expressions has been much compared. As Davidson (1993a) and others (e.g., Borod, 1992) pointed out, the underlying brain mechanisms for posed and spontaneous expression of emotion may be very different and results may not be directly comparable. For prosody, the weak analog for spontaneous expression is 'elicited' (e.g., 'Say this sentence with a sad meaning') versus repeated/imitated speech. It is unconvincing to claim that these conditions approximate natural ones, and yet there are few alternatives. One technique is to 'induce' emotional states by getting subjects to produce emotional prosody after reading mood-laden paragraphs. Shapiro and Danly (1985) presented paragraphs containing an emotional target sentence (happy or sad) to be read aloud by experimental subjects, as did House, Rowe, and Standen (1987), whose instructions to subjects were to read three passages (sad, neutral, or excited) 'imparting as much emotion in the reading as possible' (p. 911). In Gandour et al.'s (1995) study, Thai patients read target sentences aloud with simulated emotional meaning; the sentences were embedded in emotional paragraphs.

Design feature discrepancies

The variety of task designs has led to difficulty comparing findings from one study to another. Some published papers have used tasks and methods either frankly lacking in adequate design features or describing variant results dependent on an esoteric detail of the experimental design, e.g., using emotional 'sounds' (Hornak et al., 1996) or 'vowels' (Denes et al., 1984) instead of emotional–prosodic sentences. Hummed sentences did not produce differences between left and right brain-damaged patients in another study (Lalande et al., 1992). Generalizability of results is also very limited if only two emotional categories are included (e.g., Schmitt et al., 1997). A neutral category is included in some but not all test batteries. Although neutral is not an emotional choice (and thus does not 'fit' the emotion array), it might be argued that adding neutral provides a contrast category that allows subjects to express uncertainty with the emotional choices.

In a study of the 'sensory speech' abilities in Parkinson's disease, categories used to study the 'affective functions of prosody' (Scott, Caird, and Williams, 1984, p. 841) were one tape-recorded stimulus each expressing 'sarcasm,' 'caring advice,' 'officious and abrupt greeting,' and 'pleasant greeting.' Patients 'commented on the emotional features presented' (p. 481). The subtest included performance on four 'grammatical' functions, which were summed with the attitudinal data. Although the stimuli here are too few and the response categories too vague to obtain a valid result, this is one of the few studies the authors are aware of that utilized attitudinal rather than emotional categories (see also Tompkins and Mateer, 1985). However, Caekebeke et al. (1991), studying 21 patients with Parkinson's disease, were unable to replicate the Scott et al. (1984) finding for perceptual prosodic deficits.

Earlier studies (e.g., Ross, 1981; Ross, Anderson, and Morgan-Fisher, 1989) used a small number of 'live' trials with questionable reliability for the comprehension testing; and for the production material, patients were subjectively evaluated by the experimenter. As has been seen, 'trained phoneticians' argue about the acoustic parameters alleged to be present in speech samples, we are confident that subjective judgments by the examiner are not sufficient to draw conclusions about impaired performance. Listeners' ratings should be used to provide a measure of the 'goodness' of the prosodic utterances. Although the meaning of acoustic measurements in normal speakers overall remains controversial (Scherer, 1986), acoustic cues measured in patients' performance can be compared with premorbid speech, with patients' speech in different modes (e.g., elicited versus repeated, or affective compared to propositional modes), or, when focused on certain categories, with speech from the normal-control group.

In order to resolve some of the uncertainties deriving from multifarious study designs, Pell and Baum (1997a) incorporated different task levels into a single experimental design. They compared nine RHD (without neglect), ten aphasic LHD (nine nonfluent) stroke patients, and ten age-matched controls in discrimination and identification of linguistic and emotional–prosodic stimuli which contained different degrees of linguistic structure (speech-filtered/phonetic, nonsense/syntactic, semantically well-informed/semantic). Neither patient group was impaired compared to controls in discriminating or recognizing emotional prosody on either task level, but patients with LHD showed deficits in tasks requiring semantics. The authors conclude that the results of previous studies reporting significant emotional–prosodic deficits following RHD may have been confounded by the coexistence of lasting visual neglect.

Testing of groups

In the early clinical studies of prosody, most testing was performed on people with right hemisphere damage, with normal-control subjects usually used as the comparison group. LHD patients were not included because aphasic symptoms were thought to complicate the test procedure. This was an unfortunate enterprise, as low versus high 'speech melody' (Goodglass and Kaplan, 1972) and impaired intonation (Luria, 1966) had classicallly been associated with LHD. One of the early published measures of dysprosody in LHD erroneously presented two single cases as anomalies (Ross, Anderson, and Morgan-Fisher, 1989). Some studies failed to include a normal-control group or selected a LHD group with relatively mild deficits (Heilman, Scholes, and Watson, 1975). Others failed to match the control group for variables such as age, sex, and general intellectual performance, which have been associated with performance in the recognition of emotional prosody (Alvarez et al. 1989; Weddell, 1994; Breitenstein et al., 1996). In a recent report of right hemisphere emotional–prosodic dominance (Ross, Thompson, and Yenkosky, 1997), patients with RHD were on average 17 years older than those in either the LHD or the control group. Some deficits may be due to age-related changes in hearing (Harford and Dodds, 1982), neuropsychological functioning (especially working memory), laryngeal structures (Hagen, Lyons, and Nuss, 1996), or specific emotional perception (McDowell, Harrison, and Demaree, 1994).

Patient selection

Patient selection criteria may also present an important factor with regard to the divergence of findings between research groups. As mentioned above, it is a difficult decision whether to exclude or include neurological patients with aphasia or hemi-neglect. If patients with these symptoms are included, the effects on emotional processing must be controlled for (e.g., using covariate analysis). There is always a danger that differences in emotional–prosodic performance are related in part to overall reduced attentional capabilities in a RHD group or linguistic deficits in a LHD group. Lesion size may obviously have a crucial effect on extent of impairment (Silberman and Weingartner, 1986), but few studies consider this variable. In the study by Blonder et al. (1991), for example, more than 50% of subjects presented with lesions extending over three lobes. Similarly, intrahemispheric site of lesion has been carefully considered in only a few studies (e.g., Cancelliere and Kertesz, 1990; Darby, 1993; Peper and Irle, 1997a), although presence or absence of temporoparietal damage as crucial to prosodic performance has been a topic of controversy (Heilman, 1993). There is also evidence that the etiology of brain lesion affects the severity of deficits (Borod, 1993; Breitenstein et al., 1998), with stroke patients being more impaired in emotional recognition tasks than patients with brain tumors or head trauma. Bradvik et al. (1990) reported no emotional–prosodic perception deficits in a RHD group which included 14 infarct and seven transient ischemic attack patients, but a later study involving 20 patients with right-sided infarcts did report deficits, in both emotional and linguistic prosodic perception (Bradvik et al., 1991).

In most group studies, individuals with RHD are included in comparison studies without regard to whether or not they have clinical prosodic deficits. It may be that clearer results will emerge when brain-damaged people who have demonstrated dysprosody are evaluated, as has long been the tradition for studying people with aphasia following left brain damage.

Time post onset

In one study, patients in the test group varied from one month to nearly 15 years post onset of injury (Blonder et al., 1991). This is not unusual for group studies of emotional prosody. While the impact of wide ranges of post-onset time is difficult to evaluate, some have claimed that time post onset is a crucial variable in emotional–prosodic function, with important findings present only in the acute phase. It has previously been reported that RHD patients with a time interval since lesion of shorter than 100 days presented with a narrower F0 range than RHD patients who were tested after a longer time interval post onset (Ryalls, Joanette, and Feldman, 1987), which points to the possibility of spontaneous remission of symptoms even after 100 days. Darby's (1993) results on prosodic comprehension deficits in four patients with acute RHD reported resolution of the symptoms after a few weeks. However, deficits noted acutely may not accurately reflect intrinsic structure–function correlations of interest to behavior studies, but may reflect transitory processes, of which a prime example is brain swelling with related pressure changes.

Studies in normal subjects

As experimental paradigm, dichotic listening has been the most prominently used in normal subjects. A range of auditory patterns has been applied. For emotional tones of voice, a left ear/right hemisphere dominance has been reported (Bryden, 1982; Ley and Bryden, 1982; Shipley-Brown et al., 1988). Blumstein and Cooper (1974) utilized the dichotic listening procedure in a test of grammatical use of intonation, and found a right ear advantage. These results support the notion of a functional laterality hypothesis. However, several studies support the notion that in nonlinguistic contexts, the right hemisphere preferentially processes pitch patterns. This has been demonstrated in uses of the *Complex Pitch Perception Test* (Sidtis, 1980, 1982). Here, a right hemisphere dominance for pitch processing in both normal and brain-damaged populations has been consistently seen (Sidtis and Volpe, 1988; Sidtis and Feldmann, 1990).

Recently, a few EEG studies of emotional prosody have been performed on normal subjects. Pihan, Altenmueller, and Ackermann (1997) reported significant differences in right hemispheric slow-wave potentials in association with fundamental frequency changes in the stimulus sentences. Evoked responses in patients with hemispheric damage revealed abnormal endogenous evoked response potential (ERP) components on pitch functions in RHD subjects, compared to abnormal responses in the LDH patients on the semantic task (Twist et al., 1991). Another study of auditory evoked responses to happy and angry utterances (as well as phonological and grammatical stimuli) in native and non-native speakers of English (native Japanese) reported the largest P300 amplitudes to the emotional stimuli, similar in both language groups. In contrast, only the English speakers discriminated between 'rip' and 'lip,' indicating a cultural constraint on discriminating a linguistic contrast, while suggesting a universality of brain responses to emotional–prosodic stimuli (Buchwald et al., 1994).

A few neuroimaging studies are using positron emission topography (PET) procedures to investigate prosody. A study of linguistic–prosodic stimuli using labelled (radioactive) oxygen (O^{15}) (in water) PET scanning replicated the earlier dichotic listening but no speakers of English were found to process tone-words in Thai in the left hemisphere. A study of emotional prosody reported a selective activation of the right prefrontal cortex (George et al., 1996). However, the finding may be attributable, at least in part, to working memory functions found in other studies to be associated with frontal lobe activity. Zatorre et al. (1992) attributed a right prefrontal activation during a pitch discrimination task to the working memory load of the task. It may be premature to base firm conclusions regarding brain function for prosody from PET results, as many questions remain about the interpretation of activation in PET studies using O^{15} to measure blood flow changes (Friston et al., 1996; Sidtis et al., 1996; Jennings et al., 1997).

Subjects with neurological disorders other than focal lesions

More recently, progressive neurological disorders associated with subcortical disease, such as Parkinson's and Huntington's disease, have been studied. These findings are important to the broader picture of emotional–prosodic function, and will be mentioned in that regard but not described in detail here. Deficits in emotional–prosodic production are known to accompany the motor speech disorders seen in these diseases (Darley, Aronson, and Brown, 1975; Duffy, 1995), but in addition, deficient emotional–prosodic comprehension is also reported (Blonder, Gur, and Gur, 1989 Speedie et al., 1990; Breitenstein et al., 1996, in press; Pell, 1996). Using attitudinal and grammatical prosody tasks, Scott et al. (1984) reported a 'sensory speech disorder' in parkinsonian patients (see above).

A study of speech prosody using the WADA test recorded deficient ability to repeat emotionally intoned sentences following right-sided injection of barbiturate (Ross et al., 1988). Several methodological flaws obviate the value of this finding, in particular the failure to compare performance on nonemotional speech and to evaluate speech melody during left-sided WADA. It is likely that the barbiturate is the immediate cause of a transient dysarthria, which included pitch and voice quality changes. Two related studies are by LaFramboise, Snyder, and Cogen (1997), claiming hemispheric differences in perception of formant transitions (acoustic cues for consonants), a finding not easy to place in any context; and Lee et al. (1990), who found statistically significantly greater laughter associated with right hemisphere injection and crying with left hemisphere injection.

Critical overview of focal lesion studies of emotional dysprosody

Studies on emotional–prosodic comprehension

The inception of the current era of lesion studies of emotional prosody must be credited to Heilman et al. (1975), who reported on six LHD and six RHD patients, all with temporoparietal or parietal damage (seven due to stroke), listening to 'bidemensional' sentences – those with neutral semantic content as well as emotional–prosodic meanings, in a task that required matching to line drawings of facial emotions. LHD subjects (one anomic and five with conduction aphasia) performed as well as RHD patients (all with neglect) on matching semantic meaning (e.g., 'The man is showing the girls the bird seed') to drawings. In fact, *all* patients performed at ceiling on the semantic task. In contrast, the LHD group performed significantly better than the RHD group in matching the emotional–prosodic meaning.

Soon the notion that the normal, intact right hemisphere subserves emotional prosody caught hold, despite the finding shortly thereafter by Schlanger et al. (1976) of no differences between patients with RHD and LHD (all aphasic) in the perception of emotionally toned, 'nonsense' sentences (spoken happy, angry, sad) with line drawings/verbal labels as response sheets. Interestingly, low-verbal aphasics presented with significantly lower scores than high-verbal aphasics, suggesting that the severity of aphasic symptoms may have affected performance (compared with the mild comprehension deficits of the LHD group in the study by Heilman et al., 1975). As for the Schlanger et al. (1976) study, critics noted that only three of 20 RHD patients had suffered damage to temporoparietal areas, the putative site of emotional–prosody processing.

In subsequent studies, the prosody test format was expanded to include discrimination (same/different judgments of 32 pairs), with RHD patients performing worse than LHD subjects on both discrimination (32 pairs) and identification (16 sentences) (Tucker, Watson, and Heilman, 1977). Using only vowels as stimuli, Denes et al. (1984) reported that right posterior and, to a lesser degree, right anterior damaged patients were impaired in the discrimination of emotional–prosodic vowels compared to patients with LHD and the control group. Analysis of confusion errors suggested nonutilization of an acoustic criterion in patients with right posterior lesions. A later study analyzed confusions of LHD and RHD subjects, who had not differed from one another in an emotional–prosodic comprehension task, and found that LHD patients erred more on pairs that were distinguished predominantly by temporal cues, while the RHD subjects made more errors related to pitch cues (Van Lancker and Sidtis, 1992). A similar analysis performed on their data by Pell and Baum (1997b) did not replicate these results. A number of studies suggest that temporal versus pitch processing in certain auditory tasks may correspond to left and right hemisphere processing respectively (e.g., Robinson and Solomon, 1974; Sidtis, 1980; Klouda et al., 1988; Robin, Tranel, and Damasio, 1990; Baum, 1998), but contradictory reports exist. Harrington, Haaland, and Knight (1998) reported sensory timing deficits in RHD patients; Griffiths et al. (1997) described a temporal locus as a perceptual deficit in music perception (amusia) in a RHD patient; Hird and Kirsner (1993) reported shorter durations for linguistic–prosodic productions in RHD patients than in three other groups tested. Another model of prosody places the 'tempo' of speech in limbic structures, the frontal lobe, and the substantia nigra (Merewether and Alpert, 1990). Some resolution might come with the careful study of the features called 'temporal' in these and related studies.

Later investigations involved adjusting task design to probe different dimensions of performance. Heilman et al. (1984) tested LHD and RHD patients using low-pass filtered sentences. The tasks were to identify the emotional (happy, sad, angry) and linguistic (statement, questions, imperative) prosodic meanings. Both RHD and LHD patients performed significantly worse than the control group in both the emotional and linguistic tasks, but the RHD patients were more impaired than the LHD patients in the emotional–prosodic test. The possibility exists that the patients were more distracted than normal subjects by the artificiality of the filtered stimulus material. This is supported by studies using incongruent (semantic versus prosodic meanings) sentences (Bowers et al., 1987; Blonder et al., 1991; Lalande et al., 1992; Breitenstein et al., 1998), in which RHD patients (and to a lesser degree LHD patients) performed significantly worse for prosodic sentences with a conflicting content.

Several studies have revealed a significant role of basal ganglia structures in emotional–prosodic function, for both comprehension and production (production is reviewed below). In the Cancelliere and Kertesz (1990) study, 46 stroke patients were tested two weeks to three months post onset using a battery for emotional perception and expression modelled psychometrically on the Western Aphasia Battery (Kertesz, 1982). No effect of hemispheric group membership on any of the emotional–prosodic subtests was found, but coordinating lesion areas of patients with deficits across tasks revealed a common basis of basal ganglia damage. Later, a single case study reported a young woman who had suffered a stroke to the right basal ganglia (putamen and body of the caudate nucleus), who performed poorly on a perceptual test of emotional prosody (Cohen, Riccio, and Flannery, 1994). Similarly, Starkstein et al. (1994) found the greatest deficit in RHD patients with lesions involving the temporoparietal cortex or basal ganglia. Weddell's (1994) study of the role of lesions of the third ventricle (affecting hypothalamic function), compared with cortical and basal ganglia damage, included (among other emotional protocols) tests of perception of verbally expressed emotion. A main finding was an association of basal ganglia damage with impaired 'perception of verbally expressed emotion' (p. 171), without regard to hemispheric side. Similar findings in progressive neurological disorders involving basal ganglia structures have been reported. Speedie et al. (1990) reported deficient comprehension and discrimination of emotional and linguistic prosody in nondemented patients with Huntington's disease, while Blonder et al. (1989), Pell (1996) and Breitenstein et al. (1998) found deficient emotional–prosodic comprehension in Parkinson's disease patients, with no differences between those with left-sided versus right-sided symtoms.

Studies on emotional–prosodic expression

The elicitation and evaluation of expression data present several challenges. Strategies vary for obtaining speech samples. Evaluative methods used are examiner judgments, listeners' ratings, classifications, and acoustic analyses. Tucker et al. (1977) used accuracy ratings by three judges to evaluate affective–prosodic utterances elicited from RHD subjects, while Ross and Mesulam (1979) and Gorelick and Ross (1987) relied on their clinical observations, risking the inherent bias. In a study by Van Lancker et al. (1996), a group of listeners judged whether emotional–prosodic utterances were good exemplars of the intended category, and then they identified the category of randomized utterances. This provided two independent measures of the performance of emotional–prosodic productions.

A group of raters was also used by House et al. (1987). RHD and LHD patients, depressed patients, and control subjects were instructed to read passages with different tones of voice (sad, neutral, excited). Raters judged the prosody of patients with RHD, LHD, and depression as very similar, in that all patient groups scored lower than the control group in all three emotional categories.

A number of production studies have performed acoustic analyses on the speech of patients with LHD or RHD, yielding diverse results. A higher pitch has been reported for Broca's aphasia (Danly and Shapiro, 1982; Ryalls, 1982; Cooper et al., 1984; Van Lancker et al., 1988). Abnormal intonational characteristics have been found in fluent and nonfluent aphasic patients (Danly, Cooper, and Shapiro, 1983; Ryalls and Behrens, 1988). De Bleser and Poeck (1985) studied the prosody in the spontaneous speech of nine patients with global aphasia. Their results contradicted the clinical impression of preserved prosodic function: intonation contours were stereotyped and constricted. Klouda et al. (1988) acoustically measured emotional–prosodic speech over the course of a year in a female patient who suffered a hemorrhage from a left pericallosal aneurysm. Four weeks following callosal disconnection, the patient presented with lowered pitch mean and variability during the production of emotional sentences. No acoustic changes in neutral speech following right brain damage were found by Ryalls et al. (1987). Thai RHD patients' happy, sad, or neutral utterances, which were poorly identified by listeners, differed acoustically from normal productions in duration and loudness variability, but not in pitch measures (Gandour et al., 1995).

Shapiro and Danly (1985), who obtained linguistic and emotional–prosodic utterances from RHD patients who read aloud sentences embedded in paragraphs, reported reduced fundamental frequency mean and variability in association with anterior damage, while posterior damage was associated with elevated values. In a single case study by Blonder et al. (1995), analysis of discourse in a 77-year-old woman before and after a stroke involving the right-sided fronto-temporo-parietal area and the basal ganglia revealed a slight overall diminution in pitch contour and range. In contrast, Colsher, Cooper, and Graff-Radford (1987) reported an overall increase in mean fundamental frequency in two RHD subjects reading three types of emotional–prosodic sentences (happy, sad, angry). Acoustic analysis of a single case of bilateral subcortical stroke reported by Van Lancker et al. (1996) revealed reduced pitch mean and variability, worse in spontaneous (as compared with elicited) utterances.

In a few studies, durational characteristics have emerged, although usually not for emotional–prosodic utterances. An exception lies in durational abnormalities measured in RHD Thai patients' emotional utterances (Gandour et al., 1995). In a study of nonfluent aphasic speech with impaired 'melody,' Danly and Shapiro (1982) found the source of the dysprosody lay more in timing features than in pitch. Similarly, abnormal timing was observed for words (Gandour et al., 1993a) and for sentences (Gandour et al., 1994) in LHD Thai patients. In a study by Hird and Kirsner (1993), wherein only duration was tested, RHD patients produced significantly shorter noun phrases than the control group, but no group differences emerged for the linguistic and emotional–prosodic productions. The Blonder et al. (1995) single RHD case study reported an increased speech rate postmorbidly. Two of seven Broca's aphasics, those judged as having 'labored' speech, displayed longer durations than the five nonfluent patients not judged as having labored speech (Williams and Seaver, 1986). In Behrens' (1988) study of linguistic stress in RHD subjects, patients used duration more than pitch cues in sentence emphasis, whereas most normal-control subjects used pitch to cue the emphasis. In a single case study of a right-sided basal ganglia stroke, the 'impression' of faster postmorbid speech was revealed by acoustic analysis not to be due to an actual difference in rate, but to significantly shorter breath groups (Van Lancker et al., 1996).

Similarly to the perception studies mentioned above, also for emotional prosodic production, recent findings in the scientific literature on emotional processing point to a role of the basal ganglia. Several papers describing aspects of the basal ganglia pertinent to emotional–prosodic deficits have appeared in the past five years. Although the behavioral descriptions have not always included detailed references to speech, defective prosody is sometimes described, and other comments imply an involvement. Tranel (1992, p. 82) associates 'defects in articulation and prosody' with lesions of the putamen. In clinical characterizations of behaviors associated with basal ganglia disease, terms such as 'emotional limitations' (Saint-Cyr, Taylor, and Nicholson, 1995, p. 14) are used. In three patients with bilateral basal ganglia lesions, affect is described as 'disturbed' in the sense of an 'indifferent attitude' (p. 377), 'impaired' in the sense of 'inactive,' and dramatically 'passive' (p. 379) (Laplane et al., 1984). In two patients who suffered bilateral globus pallidus lesions following carbon monoxide intoxication, an 'apparent affective indifference connected with a lack of spontaneous expression of the affects' was described (Ali-Chérif et al., 1984, p. 401). These authors state that the patients are able to 'témoigner de leurs sentiments et de leurs émotions, mais toujours de façon froide et purement verbale' (p. 404). These comments may well be referring to a lack of 'feeling' in the voice. These clinical descriptions often do not specify whether facial, vocal, and/or gestural behaviors are the basis of the observation (as noted by Weddell, 1994). The authors speculate that it is unlikely that one mode of expression is consistently, uniquely spared in these cases. Saint-Cyr et al. (1995) speak of 'reduced drive or motivation' (p. 14), seen in frontal lobe damage, Parkinson's disease, and focal basal ganglia lesions, and attribute to the basal ganglia, among other things, 'the establishment and selection of emotional responses' (p. 20). Poncet and Habib (1994), describing 'motivational' (p. 588) disorders in association with damage to (bilateral) globus pallidus and adjacent structures, observe that 'l'expression spontanée des sentiments and des émotions est absente ou très pauvre;' they further state that 'le contenu des réponses et la qualité de la prosodie avec laquelle elles sont énoncées pourraient faire penser que l'évaluation émotionnelle elle-même est altérée' (p. 591). Yet these patients can say whether or not they are enjoying situations. Caplan et al. (1990), in discussing behavioral changes in motivational capacity, or abulia, following caudate damage, refer to 'decreased speech' (p. 135). Caplan et al. (1990, p. 139) explicitly follow Fisher (1983) in characterizing abulia as 'lacking in spontaneity of action and speech . . . Verbal responses are late, terse, incomplete, and emotionally flat, but the intellectual content is normal.' These authors state that their abulic patients 'conformed in every detail' with the descriptions provided by Fisher (1983). Partially taking these literal comments, and partially utilizing inference, the authors believe that it is likely that one of the indicators of 'abulia' and motivational disorders lies in 'flat speech,' but that this symptom has not been specifically mentioned in many cases. For example, in a study of behavioral changes following subcortical damage, Mendez, Adams, and Lewandowski (1989) described a group of patients with lesions in the caudate nucleus as being in an 'apathetic state,' with verbalization consisting of a few words. We might safely infer that speech in these cases would be dysprosodic – low in pitch and intensity mean, range, and variability, without articulatory disturbances. The term 'abulia' doubtless flows at least in part from the presentation of the speech pattern.

In the most comprehensive of these recent studies, Bhatia and Marsden (1994) concluded from the analysis of disturbances in 240 patients with focal basal ganglia lesions (the majority presenting with a vascular lesion etiology) that the most common behavioral symptom (seen in 28% of the unilateral damage to the caudate nucleus) is a loss of spontaneous emotional and cognitive responses, or 'abulia.' Bilateral lesions of the globus pallidus are also associated with abulia (p. 868), for which a defining feature is the 'loss of emotional affective expression' (p. 860). 'Dysarthria with dysprosody' (p. 863) was associated with small unilateral putamenal lesion, while 'hypophonia' was seen in a patient with unilateral caudate and lentiform lesions. Whereas some authors conclude that the observed parkinsonian prosodic deficits are limited to the expressive mode and therefore of motor origin (Ackermann, Hertrich, and Ziegler, 1993), several recent studies (as reviewed above) suggest a general supramodal impairment with both perceptive and expressive emotional–prosodic deficits in Parkinson's disease patients in more advanced stages of the disease (Breitenstein, 1996; Breitenstein et al., 1998).

The role of fronto-subcortical circuits in identifiable neurobehavioral syndromes has become generally known (e.g., Cummings, 1993). As an example, Weddell (1994) concluded from his data obtained in a large sample of (mostly) brain tumor patients that social–emotional skills may be controlled by at least two similar parallel neural networks, as 'fronto-striatal damage impaired emotional recognition and expression, right medial temporal lobe damage impaired recognition but not expression' (p. 187).

Conclusions and perspectives for future research

As adumbrated in our introduction, an overview of the laterality results of emotional–prosodic studies (Tables 12.1 and 12.2) reveals that, whether assessing comprehension or production, only about half of the compiled studies report greater performance deficit associated with RHD (than with comparison groups). Further, a strict functional differentiation between the linguistic and emotional

Table 12.1. Studies of emotional–prosodic perception in patients with focal cerebral lesions

Study	Objective	Subjects	Methods	Results
Heilman et al. (1975)	Recognition of emotional prosody	6 RHD, 6 LHD (most conduction aphasia, all temporoparietal lesions)	Tasks: 16 emotional sentences (happy, angry, sad, indifferent) and 16 content of sentences Response: picture-matching	No group differences for recognition of content Emotional prosody: RHD<LHD
Schlanger et al. (1976)	Recognition of emotional prosody	20 RHD (85% CVA), 40 aphasic LHD	60 emotionally toned sentences (10 meaningful and 10 meaningless) recorded in angry, happy, sad prosody Response: picture-matching	Low-verbal aphasic LHD<high-verbal aphasics No difference between RHD and LHD groups
Tucker et al. (1977)	Discrimination and recognition of emotional prosody	11 RHD (all with neglect), 7 LHD (all with conduction aphasia)	Four different sentences read with angry, happy, sad, or indifferent tone of voice Recognition: 16 sentences Discrimination: 32 pairs	Recognition and discrimination: RHD<LHD RHD subjects scored at chance
Denes et al (1984)	Discrimination and recognition of emotional prosody in CVA	15 RHD (9 anterior, 6 posterior), 15 asphasic LHD (6 anterior, 9 posterior), 6 HC	Discrimination and recognition of vocal emotions expressed in vowels (happy, frightened, angry, sad, disgust)	Posterior RHD<anterior RHD< anterior/posterior LHD, HC
Heilman et al. (1984)	Recognition of linguistic and emotional prosody	8 RHD and 9 LHD (all CVA), 15 HC	Recognition of linguistic (declarative, interrogative, imperative) and emotional prosody (happy, sad, angry) using speech filtered stimuli	Linguistic task: RHD, LHD<HC Emotional task: RHD<LHD<HC
Tompkins and Flowers (1985)	Influence of task difficulty on recognition of emotional prosody	11 RHD and 11 LHD (all CVA), 11 HC	Paragraphs with neutral content read happy, angry, frightened, neutral tones three different task levels: (a) easiest (discrimination) (b) intermediate (two-choice) (c) demanding (four-choice)	RHD<HC (all three task levels) LHD<HC ('demanding' level) Significant correlation of emotional prosody performance and age

Study	Aim	Participants	Task	Results
Bowers et al. (1987)	Influence of task demands on recognition of emotional prosody	9 RHD and 8 LHD (all CVA), 8 HC	(a) Distraction task: 32 sentences spoken with happy, sad, angry, or indifferent tone (semantic content was either congruent or incongruent with prosody) (b) Processing task: 16 sentences spoken with happy, sad, angry, or indifferent tone (neutral semantic content), filtered (content unintelligible) and unfiltered	Distraction task: RHD<LHD, HC in both congruent and incongruent conditions; Processing task: RHD<LHD, HC for filtered and unfiltered conditions; Conclusion: both distraction and processing defects are present in RHD
Cancelliere and Kertesz (1990)	Recognition and production of emotional expression using adaptation of aphasia instrument	28 RHD and 18 LHD (all acute CVA), 20 HC	Identification of emotional prosody (19 sentences with happy, angry, sad, or neutral tone of voice); Score less than 2 SD below the mean of the HC considered impaired	75% of RHD and 78% of LHD classified as 'aprosodic'; Lesion mapping: patients with damage to basal ganglia and anterior temporal pole most severely impaired
Borod et al. (1990)	Perception and recognition of facial and vocal emotion	19 RHD (CVA), 21 HC	Happy, sad, angry, and indifferent tones of voice (16 trials for recognition, 32 pairs for discrimination)	No group differences for discrimination; Recognition: RHD<HC
Blonder, et al. (1991)	Processing of ideational versus prosodic aspects of emotional meaning	10 RHD and 10 LHD (all CVA, in most cases lesion involved both anterior and posterior regions), 10 HC	Tasks: Part 2, Florida Affect Battery – Revised (discrimination and recognition of happy, sad, angry, frightened, and neutral); 'Nonverbal' condition: Descriptions (e.g., 'She smiled'); 'Verbal' condition: sentences containing emotion words; Response: Labelling	Emotional prosody: RHD<LHD, HC; 'Nonverbal' condition: RHD<LHD, HC; 'Verbal' emotional meaning: no group differences

Table 12.1. (*cont.*)

Study	Objective	Subjects	Methods	Results
Lalande et al. (1992)	Compare prosodic vs semantic categorizations	12 RHD and 10 LHD (all CVA), 16 HC	(a) Verbal task: 36 sentences in emotional setting (neutral tone) (b) Prosody task: 36 sentences hummed (joy, anger, fear, disgust, surprise, sadness) (c) Emotional concordance task: 36 sentences on congruent or incongruent prosody (same–different judgments)	Prosody task: RHD<HC RHD = LHD RHD: lower score in emotional concordance task
Van Lancker and Sidtis (1992)	Use of acoustic cues by RHD and LHD patients in perception of emotional prosody	13 RHD and 24 aphasic LHD (all CVA), 37 HC	16 sentences with neutral content spoken with sad, angry, happy, surprised tones Acoustic analysis (duration) F0, amplitude) Discriminant analyses: (a) Acoustic cues that best differentiate the four emotions (b) Predicting patients' misclassifications	RHD = LHD<HC in perception of emotional prosody F0 variability was major cue in emotion differentiation Error analysis: RHD relied on duration cues, LHD on F0 information
Peretz et al. (1994)	Two case studies with bilateral damage compared to 5 HC	Case CN: female (35 years) superior temporal gyrus Case GL: male (61 years) with LH temporal and inferior frontal and RH superior temporal insula and inferior frontal	Task: recognition of emotional tones of voice in meaningless syllables (joy, sadness, fear, anger, neutral) Response: multiple choice	Only patient GL had marked impairments compared to control subjects
Starkstein et al. (1994)	Neuroradiologic correlates of emotional prosody perception	59 acute stroke patients (<1 week post stroke!), 17 HC	Emotional prosody tasks: (a) neutral content, happy/sad/angry prosody	Patients with aprosody (especially with right temporoparietal or basal ganglia lesion)<patients with no-aprosody in incongruent stimuli

Study	Aim	Subjects	Method	Results
Hornak, et al. (1996)	Patients with frontal (ventral) and nonventral brain damage	12 patients with uni/bilateral damage to orbital or ventrolateral cortex, 11 with other damage (nonventral group), 18 HC	(b) semantically congruent or incongruent content (sad, happy) Classification into aprosody and no-aprosody groups based on performance; correlation with neuropsychological performance and lesion location. Identification of emotional sounds (sad, angry, frightened, disgusted, puzzled, contented, neutral) in a multiple-choice design	Patients with aprosody larger frontal horn contralateral to brain damage and larger third ventricle. Ventral group<nonventral group <HC
Pell and Baum (1997a)	Compare linguistic (phonetic, syntactic, semantic) and emotional prosody	9 RHD (without neglect) and 10 aphasic LHD (all CVA), 10 HC	Emotional prosodic (angry, sad, happy) and linguistic prosodic utterances (declarative, interrogative, imperative) Discrimination and recognition tasks: (a) speech-filtered (b) nonsensical (c) semantically well formed	No group differences in discrimination or recognition emotional prosody. Pooled across the linguistic and emotional prosodic tasks: (a) Filtered and nonsense sentences: RHD = LHD<HC (b) Semantically well-formed sentences: LHD<HC
Pell and Baum (1997b)	Acoustic analysis; errors by of LHD and RHD patients in linguistic and emotional prosodic tasks	9 RHD (without neglect) and 10 aphasic LHD (all CVA), 10 HC	Nonsensical utterances (taken from Pell and Baum, 1997a) presented in linguistic and emotional (angry, sad, happy) prosodic task conditions. Acoustic analyses of stimuli: extraction of F0, syllable duration, amplitude (mean and variation)	Mean F0 and F0 variability best differentiated angry/happy from sad prosody (76% of variance); followed by syllable duration (11% of variance). LHD and RHD patients' responses not biased by acoustic parameters (contradicts Van Lancker and Sidtis,

Table 12.1. (*cont.*)

Study	Objective	Subjects	Methods	Results
Peper and Irle (1997a)	Comparison of categorical and dimensional decoding of emotional prosody	19 RHD (12 anterior, 7 posterior lesions), 21 LHD (12 anterior, 9 posterior lesions), and 12 HC (non-neurological patients) All neurological patients had recent brain tumor extirpations	Semantically meaningless utterances spoken with emotional tones (joy, fear, sadness, anger), each stimulus presented twice. Four different rating conditions: (a) Categorical (multiple-choice or cross-modally to one or two facial expressions) (b) Dimensional (cross-modally matching the prosody to one of two facial expressions with respect to valence or arousal)	All patient groups overall impaired to HC. Cross-modal categorical labelling: RHD<HC Dimensional decoding: (a) Valence: LHD (especially with ventral frontal lesions)<HC (b) Arousal: RHD (especially with temporoparietal lesions)<HC
Ross, et al. (1997)	Explore effects of aphasia on emotional prosody (all CVA) (only 5 LHD, 10 RHD used in analysis)	12 RHD, 10 LHD, 16 HC (RHD 17 years older on average) Testing 5–6 weeks poststroke	Perception of affective prosody with words, monosyllables, asyllabic. Stimuli spoken with neutral, happy, sad, surprised, angry, disinterested prosody. Tasks: discrimination of 24 pairs: low-pass stimuli	RHD, LHD<HC (but LHD improved in mono- and asyllabic condition) No correlation with aphasia: greater deficits in RHD cortical/subcortical/basal ganglia lesions; LHD lesions by corpus callosum
Schmitt, Hartje and Willmes (1997)	Comparison of unimodal and simultaneous multimodal perception of emotional attitude	27 RHD and 25 LHD (all CVA), 26 HC	Unimodal task: emotional prosodic nonsense sentences/facial expressions/propositional content presented separately. Multimodal task: video- and audio-recordings by actor with happy, frightened, and neutral attitudes; video scenes were either incongruent or	Unimodal task: RHD<LHD, HC (facial expressions, emotional prosody). Multimodal task: RHD<HC (overall, facial expressions, emotional prosody), LHD<HC (overall, propositional content), RHD<LHD (facial expressions)

Study	Aim/Design	Subjects	Tasks	Results
			congruent Response: name the valence for (a) facial expression, (b) emotional prosody, (c) propositional content	
Scott et al. (1997)	Single case study	Patient DR presenting with selective bilateral damage to the amygdala 12 HC	Auditory perception tasks (e.g., identification of environmental sounds, understanding verbal emotional meanings, perception of happy, angry, sad, frightened, and disgusted vocal expressions, recognition of linguistic prosody)	Deficits in linguistic and emotional prosody Impairment most pronounced for perception of angry or frightened (spoken words and non-verbal sound patterns)
Breitenstein, et al. in press	Contribution of the frontostriatal circuitry to perception of emotional prosody	16 RHD (8 anterior, 8 posterior), 16 LHD (8 anterior, 8 posterior), 14 patients with Parkinson's disease, 10 HC	Standardized tests of emotional prosody (discrimination, recognition)	Patients with anterior lesions (RHD, LHD), patients in more advanced stages of Parkinson's disease<HC

Notes:

RHD = patients with right hemisphere damage; LHD = patients with left hemisphere damage; HC = healthy control subjects; CVA = cerebral vascular accident; MPO = months post onset; F0 = fundamental frequency (auditory equivalent is 'pitch').

Table 12.2. Studies of emotional prosodic expression in patients with focal cerebral lesions

Study	Objective	Subjects	Methods	Results
Tucker, et al. (1977)	Compare RHD with HC on emotionally intoned sentences	8 RHD (all with neglect), 8 HC (non-neurological, medical conditions)	Subjects repeated sentences (presented with neutral tone) with happy, sad, angry, or indifferent prosody Accuracy ratings by three judges	RHD<HC
Ross and Mesulam (1979)	Spontaneous expression of emotional prosody	2 RHD (CVA) with both anterior and posterior lesions (frontoparietal)	Clinical observation	Patients presented with paucity of nonverbal emotional expression
Danly and Shapiro (1982)	Acoustic measures of aphasic prosody	5 LHD patients with Broca's aphasia, 5 HC	Task: patients read aloud sentences of various lengths with varying sentence accents. Measures: final F0 fall, F0 declination, and timing measures	F0 fall present at the end of sentences; declination absent in longer sentences; prepausal lengthing was absent 'Speech melody' partly intact, partly impaired
Shapiro and Danly (1985)	Linguistic and affective prosody production	11 RHD and 5 LHD (94% CVA), 5 HC	Task: reading of a paragraph with happy or sad prosody Acoustic analysis: extraction of F0 peaks and valleys (F0 variation)	RHD with anterior/central lesions: less F0 variation than LHD RHD with posterior lesions: higher F0 variation than HC All LHD patients posterior lesions, no intragroup comparisons possible
Gorelick and Ross (1987)	Posed and spontaneous expression of emotional prosody	14 RHD (CVA), mean MPO<1	Repetition and spontaneous production of emotional prosody Two examiners judged performance	RHD impaired

Study	Aim	Subjects	Task/Measures	Results/Conclusion
House et al. (1987)	Emotional prosody in stroke patients without mood disorder	10 RHD, 10 LHD, depressed and physically ill control subjects	Task: reading of three passages with 'as much emotion as possible' (content of passages: sad, neutral, or excited) Measures: 12 judges rated intensity (seven-point scale with end-points sad–excited)	Intensity ratings: RHD, LHD <physically ill controls No differences between RHD, LHD, and depressed subjects
Colsher, et al. (1987)	Acoustic analysis of RHD: evaluate mean F0 level	2 RHD (CVA), 3 HC	Task: subjects read four semantically neutral sentences, with three emotions (happy, sad, angry) Measure: acoustic analysis: extraction of lowest and highest F0 (and their SDs)	RHD presented with higher mean F0 peaks and valleys, in all utterance types Conclusion: mean F0 has to be taken into account in discussions of F0 variability
Klouda et al. (1988)	Single case study: role of callosal connections in	Female (39 years): damage to anterior corpus callosum	Assessments: 4 weeks, 4 months, and 1 year post surgery Task: reading of four sentences (neutral content) in happy, sad, angry or neutral tones Acoustic analyses: durational measures, F0 Six judges rated accuracy	Mean peak F0 and F0 variability lower at first assessment than 4 months/1 year post surgery; sentence duration was longest 4 weeks post; listeners' accuracy increased with time
Ross et al. (1988)	Acoustic analysis of emotional prosody during right-sided WADA	5 patients with partial complex seizures, evaluated for epilepsy surgery	Task: model examiner's tone (neutral, sad, happy, surprised, bored, angry) Assessments: pre-, during-right-sided WADA, post-WADA Acoustic analysis: extraction of 12 parameters (based on F0, duration, amplitude), values pooled across emotional types	Flattening of emotional prosody during WADA involved different aspects of F0 and overall lengthening Problem: no sample of RH nonemotional speech or of speech during LH WADA

Table 12.2. (cont.)

Study	Objective	Subjects	Methods	Results
Cancelliere and Kertesz (1990)	Recognition and production of emotional expression using adaptation of asphasia instrument	28 RHD and 18 LHD (all acute CVA), 20 HC	Task: 'elicitation:' listen to emotionally neutral sentence and produce one with happy, sad, angry, or neutral tone. Repetition: repeat an emotionally intoned sentence. Three judges rated accuracy/minimum and maximum F0	Both reading and repetition tasks: RHD=LHD<HC. Lesion mapping: patients with damage to basal ganglia, anterior temporal pole, insula most severely impaired
Borod et al. (1990)	Examining components of emotional processing (facial/vocal, expression/recognition)	19 RHD (CVA), 21 HC	Task: subjects posed each emotional expression (happy, pleasant surprise, interest, sad, angry, fear, disgust) to oral command, transforming one of two neutral sentences. Measures: four judges rated accuracy and intensity	Accuracy: RHD<HC. Intensity: RHD<HC
Hird and Kirsner (1993)	Acoustic bases of prosodic production in RHD subjects	10 RHD (CVA), 10 HC	Task: subjects read 10 sentences with happy, sad, angry, neutral tones. Acoustic analyses: mean F0, intensity, duration; only duration was analyzed	No significant group differences for production of emotional prosody
Cohen, et al. (1994)	Single case study	Female (16 years); stroke to right basal ganglia (putamen, body of caudate nucleus)	Testing: acutely and at 4 months. Tasks: emotional prosodic recognition (happy, sad, mad tones of voice), repetition and spontaneous expression of emotional prosody (two judges rated accuracy)	First assessment: marked prosodic production deficit, perception of emotional prosody depressed. Second assessment: normal performance in perception task, but no improvement in prosodic expression

| Van Lancker et al. (1996) | Postmorbid dysprosody in two single cases with selective basal ganglia damage | Patient 1: 36-year-old black female, bilateral damage to globus pallidus and medial putamen

Patient 2: 48-year-old white male, damage to right putamen and globus pallidus | Recognition of emotional prosody (sentences with neutral content)

Tasks: elicited and repeated emotional prosody (listeners' ratings, acoustic analyses)

Comparison of premorbid with current speech samples (Patient 2) | Patient 1: emotional prosodic recognition preserved, elicited expression worse than repetition; F0 variability higher during repetition than elicited

Patient 2: no receptive or expressive emotional prosodic deficits, but prestroke higher mean F0, F0 variability, and longer breath groups |
| Ross, et al. (1997) | Explore the effect of aphasic syndromes on emotional prosodic production in LHD (CVA) | 12 RHD and 10 LHD, 16 HC (RHD 17 years older on average)

Testing 5–6 weeks poststroke

Only 7 LHD, 5 RHD included in analysis | Tasks:

(a) Repetition of words, monosyllables, or asyllabic speech: neutral, happy, sad, surprised, angry, disinterested prosody (initial and final stress)

(b) Spontaneous production: description of personally relevant life events (10 s samples)

(c) Extraction of mean F0 variation coefficient

(d) Three judges rated accuracy and intensity | (a) Repetition: RHD, LHD<HC on all task levels but LHD improved with reduced verbal load

Correlations between F0 variations and judges' ratings; no correlation between F0 and aphasic symptoms (fluency)

(b) Spontaneous speech: RHD, LHD<HC

(c) Conclusion: deficits in RHD cortex/basal ganglia; LHD near corpus callosum |

Notes:

RHD = patients with right hemisphere damage; LHD = patients with left hemisphere damage; HC = healthy control subjects; CVA = cerebral vascular accident; MPO = months post onset; F0 = fundamental frequency (or 'pitch').

functions of prosodic cues associated with left and right hemispheric performance respectively has not been borne out. Thus, the hypothesis proposing a right hemisphere specialization for emotional–prosodic competence is not supported because half the studies are contradictory; the functional hypothesis describing separate lateralization of emotional and linguistic prosody, while suggested, is not strongly supported because damage to either hemisphere may affect both kinds of processing; the notion that emotional–prosodic performance is a unitary cortical function is not tenable, or at least must be considered with extreme caution, because brain damage at various sites affects prosodic performance.

In the earlier studies, little attempt was made to distinguish responses due to 'impaired planning' from those merely 'poorly produced' (Ryalls and Behrens, 1988). The important notion of neurological 'levels,' from peripheral to central, as underlying the deficits must be carefully considered before an understanding of prosodic deficits is possible. What has been called a central deficit in emotional–prosodic prosody may be dysphonia, a basic phonation problem, referencing the important difference between impairment of 'planning of an intonation contour and its execution' (Ryalls and Behrens, 1988). Comparisons with musical–melodic functions are important in understanding the nature of the deficit (Sidtis, 1984), as the role of motor and perceptual function may be key in the performance of some patients. In particular, aspects of prosodic function may depend crucially and selectively on the ability to control and perceive pitch, temporal information, and voice quality in the paralinguistic signal.

Findings in normal subjects may help us to understand better the discrepant results from lesion studies. In normal subjects, complex pitch or timbre (Sidtis, 1980, 1984), chords (Gordon, 1970), melodies (Zatorre, 1979), and personal voice information (Van Lancker and Canter, 1982) are relatively better processed by the right hemisphere. These are all complex auditory 'patterns,' containing complex pitch information as the salient perceptual cue. It is likely that the right hemisphere is specialized for processing steady-state harmonic information, contributing to its apparent advantage for some musical functions, and probably in part to its contribution to the prosody of fluent speech (Sidtis, 1984). In the comprehension mode, emotional–prosodic stimuli have in common with these other auditory patterns a key reliance on pitch information. On the other hand, temporal cues are found in some studies to be better processed by the left hemisphere. As emotional–prosodic information contains at least these two kinds of acoustic cues as important information, it is likely that both hemispheres are engaged to some extent in handling prosodic material, and that at the perceptual level, damage on either side can affect the performance of emotional–prosodic comprehension, especially regarding stimuli longer than words. Although structures in the basal ganglia were formerly thought to perform primarily motor functions, recent studies indicate an association of damage to subcortical areas with defective emotional–prosodic comprehension, possibly related to the role of these structures in the regulation of mood and motivation. It is likely, as suggested by Ryalls (1988), that prosody is 'more distributed throughout the brain and less lateralized' than proposed by the earlier models (p. 337).

In production, dysprosodic speech is seen clinically and described in acoustic studies in patients with LHD (Danly et al., 1983; De Bleser and Poeck, 1985; Ryalls and Behrens, 1988). Yet subjective clinical observations of retained prosodic function in some people with aphasia originally supported notions of intonational abilities of the right hemisphere. These ideas led to the development of Melodic Intonation Therapy (MIT), theoretically utilizing preserved intonational output in nonfluent patients (Helm-Estabrooks and Albert, 1991). However, MIT has proven a therapy of highly selected patient applicability and limited success. It is unclear why this practice does not have better results. Here, again, questions arise about: (1) the extent to which both hemispheres contribute to prosodic output, and (2) how significant a role is played by the basal ganglia, which may often be damaged in patients with severe nonfluent aphasia. Pitch control for familiar songs has been clearly identified with right hemisphere function in clinical subjects (Smith, 1966; Gordon and Bogen, 1981). It is likely that some patients believed to have selective emotional–prosodic production deficits (or, as previously designated, 'motor aprosodia') are equally unable to produce modulated speech in linguistic–prosodic functions or singing (e.g., Sudia, Bolon, and Van Lancker, 1998). A subcortical involvement is associated with dysprosodic production, most notably in patients with Parkinson's and Huntington's disease, but, as described above, also in patients with focal damage to subcortical structures (e.g., Bhatia and Marsden, 1994), with accompanying neurobehavioral alterations, including changes in mood.

Depression and other affective disturbances (Mayeux, 1983; Mendez et al., 1989; Cummings, 1993) have been described in basal ganglia disorders. At least some of the Parkinson's disease patients (30–60%) may have a mood disorder which is independent of the motor disability, and which is not viewed as reactive to the disability (Santamaria and Tolosa, 1992). The observed dysprosody in Parkinson's disease may best be considered a feature of this fronto-subcortical syndrome, which includes motor/movement initiation, mood, and speech deficits. Interestingly, in his original article, Monrad-Krohn described the prosodic deficit in Parkinson's disease as a 'simple loss of the melody of language' and suggested that it be termed 'aprosodia' (p. 414). For prosodic production, it is long known that clinically depressed subjects show alteration in specific acoustic parameters, one being an increase in mean pitch and a reduction in pitch variation (Ellgring and Scherer, 1996). Poststroke dysprosody following a right-sided caudate lesion was associated with a mood change toward 'irritability' in a recent single case study (Van Lancker et al., 1996).

Due to the known effects of lesions on mood following cortical lesions (which may or may not include subcortical damage: Robinson et al., 1984), it is essential to take into account the effect of mood changes in studies on emotional–prosodic expression. Indeed, in an emotional–prosodic reading task, House et al. (1987) reported that listeners evaluated stroke (in both hemispheric groups and without clinical mood disturbance) and depressed patients as significantly more 'depressed' than hospital control subjects. Although depression scores have in some cases not correlated with performance in emotional–prosodic comprehension in patients with cortical lesions (e.g., Starkstein et al., 1994), in some patient groups emotional–prosodic disturbance may be related to mood or motivational state as part of a neurobehavioral syndrome.

Early on, from a literature review and visual–acoustic records of single cases, Kent and Rosenbek (1982) presented a model of speech production that has proven to be a workable scheme for expressive prosodic disturbances, presenting multiple cerebral sites. They correctly observed 'many similarities between the speech pattern of patients with right-cerebral lesion and patients with Parkinson's disease' (p. 260) and they included dysprosody associated with left hemisphere, as well as cerebellar, damage. A similar overview of production is given by Ackermann et al. (1993), reviewing dysprosodic output deficits in LHD, RHD, Huntington's and Parkinson's disease patients. These authors also consider the respective roles of 'planning' or higher control versus peripheral (articulatory and phonatory) functions as variously underlying the clinical presentation of dysprosody.

There is another source of explanation for the discrepant findings of emotional–prosodic studies. Despite the bilateral neuroanatomical basis of structures known to be involved in emotional functions (Papez, 1937), by the 1980s there was evidence that emotional experiencing has greater representation in the right hemisphere, manifest in findings for lexical, facial, and gestural processing (Wechsler, 1973; Cicone, Wapner, and Gardner, 1980; Bear, 1983; TenHouten et al., 1986; Borod, 1992, 1993; Hornak et al., 1996). The term 'nonverbal affect lexicon' has been coined to describe the specialized abilities of the right hemisphere (Bowers, Bauer, and Heilman, 1993). Borod et al. (1996) recorded RHD and LHD subjects during the description of personally relevant emotional (seven emotions) and nonemotional (characteristics of people) experiences in an attempt to elicit spontaneous emotional expression. From two raters' judgments of 'emotionality' on a six-point scale, RHD patients produced less emotional content than the control group, but did not differ from the LHD group. Related are observations that emotional disorders are often associated with RHD (Heilman, Watson, and Bowers, 1983; Robinson et al., 1984; Cummings, 1985; Cutting, 1990). Interestingly, this is not really a new idea; as stated by Mill (1912, p. 167): 'It is not a new idea that the right hemicerebrum plays a larger part in the realization, control and excitation of emotions than the left.'

While some understanding of the complex role of emotional–prosodic information in speech has emerged from these scientific studies, many more questions, and a great variety of other kinds of research, are imaginable. First, there is a need for the application of available research in prosodic function in normal speech (e.g., Crystal, 1969; Bolinger, 1986; Banse and Scherer, 1996; Ladd, 1996) to lesion and other neurological studies. In this spirit, Lance (1994) applied Crystal's framework in a phonological analysis of ataxic speech. For further lesion studies, to determine the role of neurological deficits in prosodic disturbance more responsibly, single case studies will be useful, evaluating brain-damaged people who have demonstrated dysprosody in careful association with their neurobehavioral symptoms and related musical and linguistic abilities. How frontal and prefrontal lobe functions specifically involve prosodic abilities remains to be carefully studied (Zatorre et al., 1992; Dykstra, Gandour, and Stark, 1995). The lateral orbital circuit, which receives input from auditory and visual association areas of the temporal lobe (Alexander, Crutcher, and DeLong, 1990), is involved in emotion-related learning and social behavior (Rolls, 1990; Hornak et al., 1996; Peper and Irle, 1997a, 1997b; Masterman and Cummings, 1997). This could explain why patients with right frontal or temporal cortical lesions (e.g., Kolb and Taylor, 1981; Shapiro and Danly, 1985; Starkstein et al., 1994; Breitenstein et al., 1998), as well as patients with basal ganglia functions (e.g., Cancelliere and Kertesz, 1990; Starkstein et al., 1994; Scott et al., 1997), overall show the strongest deficit in processing emotional stimulus material.

A focus on prosodic deficits following basal ganglia lesions, especially when accompanied by normal articulation, is a high priority. We have not spoken here of the anterior cingulate gyrus, and yet there is a great deal of animal and human evidence for an important role of this structure in mediating emotion (Devinsky, Morrell, and Vogt, 1995). Although vocal emotional involvement in humans has not been presented, it is not impossible that structures in the limbic system may be found to have a role in emotional prosody. Others invoke a role of the thalamus in speech deficits seen in subcortical disease, including dysprosody (Critchley, 1981). The notion of prosody as forming part of a separate signaling system in humans, deriving from phylogenetically earlier structures but only distantly related to a cortical language system, remains to be explored in patients with cerebral lesions (e.g., Robinson, 1976; Ploog, 1979). As for experimental paradigms, dimensional rather than categorial performance data may reveal still another perspective. Investigation of attitudinal information, surely the most common in everyday speech interaction, has yet to be undertaken in lesion studies. Here, the role of voice quality will be salient. A more detailed questioning of the role of acoustic parameters in perception has just begun: studies can utilize speech synthesis procedures, with systematic variation of acoustic parameters, to directly demonstrate failure or appropriate use of a specific acoustic parameter, such as timing, intensity, or pitch in association with neurological condition.

These diverse studies on perceptual and motor control, as well as studies of processing of emotional–linguistic and emotional–experiential cognition, will best serve to explicate prosodic functioning in human speech. As for cerebral correlates, in summary, the authors agree with Baum (1998) that there is some support for the representation of linguistic–prosodic contrasts in the left hemisphere. This is consistent with the broader domain of left hemisphere specialization for sequential and discrete sets of entities, like phonemes, syntactic elements, numbers, and Morse code elements (Papçun et al., 1974). Thus, the specialization is best not viewed as one for 'prosody' but for elements organized in a sequentially and hierarchically structured system (Bogen, 1969). Findings for emotional–prosodic deficits in RHD are probably attributable to problems in processing the emotional content of the stimuli, auditory patterns, especially those involving pitch, and mood, social–behavioral, and motivational changes following frontal and/or subcortical damage. Overall, the picture derived from the author's review of studies since 1975 mirrors something closer to that drawn by Monrad-Krohn (1947) for prosodic production: 'Co-operation of the whole brain is probably needed' (p. 415). This perspective is also fitting for prosodic comprehension.

REFERENCES

Ackermann, H., Hertrich, I. and Ziegler, W. (1993). Prosodische Störungen bei neurologischen Erkrankungen – eine Literaturübersicht [Prosodic disorders in neurological diseases – a review of the literature]. *Fortschr Neurol Psychiatr* 61: 241–53.

Adolphs, R., Tranel, D., Damasio, H. and Damasio, A. (1994). Impaired recognition of emotion in facial expressions following bilateral damage to the human amygdala. *Nature* 372 669–72.

Alexander, G.E., Crutcher, M.D. and DeLong, M.R. (1990). Basal ganglia-thalamocortical circuits: parallel substrates for motor, oculomotor, 'prefrontal', and 'limbic' functions. *Prog Brain Res* 85: 119–46.

Ali-Chérif, A., Royere, M.L., Gosset, A. et al. (1984). Troubles du comportement et de l'activité mentale après intoxication oxycarbonée: lesions pallidales bilaterales. *Rev Neurol* 140: 401–5.

Alvarez, G., Araya, F., Verdugo, R. and Quinteros, O. (1989). Prosody, socioeconomic level, and the right hemisphere. *Arch Neurol* 46: 480.

Banse, R. and Scherer, K.R. (1996). Acoustic profiles in vocal emotion expression. *J Pers Soc Psychol* 70: 614–36.

Baum, S.R. (1992). The influence of word length on syllable duration in aphasia: acoustic analyses. *Aphasiology* 6: 501–13.

Baum, S.R. (1998). The role of fundamental frequency and duration in the perception of linguistic stress by individuals with brain damage. *J Speech Lang Hear Res* 41: 31–40.

Baum, S.R. and Pell, M. (1997). Production of affective and linguistic prosody by brain-damaged patients. *Aphasiology* 11: 177–98.

Baum, S.R. and Pell, M.D. (1999). The neural bases of prosody: insights from lesion studies and neuroimaging. *Aphasiology* 13(8): 581–608.

Bear, D.M. (1983). Hemispheric specialization and the neurology of emotion. *Arch Neurol* 40: 195–202.

Behrens, S.J. (1988). The role of the right hemisphere in the production of linguistic stress. *Brain and Language* 33: 104–127.

Behrens, S.J. (1989). Characterizing sentence intonation in a right-hemisphere-damaged population. *Brain Lang* 37: 181–200.

Benson, D.F. (1984). The neurology of human emotion. *Bull Clin Neurosci* 49: 4923–42.

Benson, D.F. (1996). *The Neurology of Thinking*. Oxford: Oxford University Press.

Bertier-Marcelo, L., Fernandez, A.-M., Celdran, E.M. and Kulisevsky, J. (1996). Perceptual and acoustic correlates of affective prosody repetition in transcortical aphasias. *Aphasiology* 10: 711–12.

Bhatia, K.P. and Marsden, C.D. (1994). The behavioral and motor consequences of focal lesions of the basal ganglia in man. *Brain* 117: 859–76.

Blonder, L.X., Bowers, D. and Heilman, K.M. (1991). The role of the right hemisphere in emotional communication. *Brain* 114: 1115–27. [Published erratum (1992) *Brain* 115: 654.]

Blonder, L.X., Gur, R. and Gur, R. (1989). The effects of right and left hemiparkinsonism on prosody. *Brain Lang* 36: 193–207.

Blonder, L.X., Pickering, J.E., Heath, R.L., Smith, C.D. and Butler, S.M. (1995). Prosodic characteristics of speech pre- and post-right hemisphere stroke. *Brain Lang* 51: 318–35.

Blumstein, S. and Cooper, W. (1974). Hemispheric processing of intonation contours. *Cortex* 10: 146–58.

Bogen, J.E. (1969). The other side of the brain: an appositional mind. *Bull LA Neurol Soc* 34: 135–62.

Bolinger, D. (1986). *Intonation and its Parts*. Stanford: Stanford University Press.

Borod, J.C. (1992). Interhemispheric and intrahemispheric control of emotion: a focus on unilateral brain damage. *J Consult Clin Psychol* 60: 339–48.

Borod, J.C. (1993). Cerebral mechanisms underlying facial, prosodic, and lexical emotional expression: a review of neuropsychological studies and methodological issues. *Neuropsychology* 7: 445–63.

Borod, J.C., Rorie, K.D., Haywood, C.S. et al. (1996). Hemispheric specialization for discourse reports of emotional experiences: relationships to demographic, neurological, and perceptual variables. *Neuropsychologia* 34: 351–9.

Borod, J.C., Welkowitz, J., Alpert, M. et al. (1990). Parameters of emotional processing in neuropsychiatric disorders: conceptual issues and a battery of tests. *J Commun Disord* 23: 247–71.

Bowers, D., Bauer, R.M. and Heilman, K.M. (1993). The nonverbal affect lexicon: theoretical perspectives from neurological studies of affect perception. *Neuropsychology* 7: 433–44.

Bowers, D., Blonder, L.X. and Heilman, K.M. (1991). The Florida Affect Battery – Manual. Unpublished manuscript at the Center for Neuropsychological Studies, University of Florida, Gainesville, FL.

Bowers, D., Blonder, L.X., Slomine, B. and Heilman, K.M. (1996). Nonverbal affect signals: patterns of impairment following hemispheric strokes using the Florida Affect Battery. Poster presented at the Annual Meeting of the American Psychological Society, San Francisco, CA, USA.

Bowers, D., Coslettt, H.B., Bauer, R.M., Speedie, L.J. and Heilman, K.M. (1987). Comprehension of emotional prosody following unilateral hemisphere lesions: processing defect versus distraction defect. *Neuropsychologia* 25: 317–28.

Bradvik, B., Dravins, C., Holtas, S. et al. (1990). Do single right hemisphere infarcts or transient ischaemic attacks result in aprosody? *Acta Neurol Scand* 81: 61–70.

Bradvik, B., Dravins, C., Holtas, S. et al. (1991). Disturbances of speech prosody following right hemisphere infarcts. *Acta Neurol Scand* 84: 114–26.

Breitenstein, C. (1996). Affektverarbeitung nach kortikaler und subkortikaler Hirnschaedigung [Affective processing following cortical and subcortical brain damage]. Doctoral dissertation, University of Tübingen, Germany.

Breitenstein, C., Daum, I. and Ackermann, H. (1997). Affective prosody in patients with Parkinson's disease. In *Clinical Phonetics and Linguistics*, ed. W. Ziegler and K. Deger, pp. 382–6. London: Whurr Publishers.

Breitenstein, C., Daum, I. and Ackermann, H. (1998). Affective processing following cortical and subcortical brain damage: contribution of the fronto-striatal circuitry. *Behav Neurol* 11: 29–42.

Breitenstein, C., Daum, I., Ackermann, H., Luetgehetmann, R. and Mueller, E. (1996). Erfassung der Emotionswahrnehmung bei zentralnerven Lesionen und Erkrankungen: Psychometrische Gütekriterien der 'Tübinger Affekt Batterie' [Assessment of deficits in emotional perception following cortical and subcortical brain damage: psychometric properties of the 'Tübingen Affect Battery']. *Neurol Rehab* 2: 93–101.

Brosgole, L. and Weisman, J. (1995). Mood recognition across the ages. *Int J Neurosci* 82: 169–89.

Bryden, M.P. (1982). *Laterality: Functional Asymmetry in the Intact Brain.* New York: Academic Press.

Bryden, M. and Ley, R. (1983). Right-hemisphere involvement in the perception and expression of emotion in normal humans. In *Neuropsychology of Human Emotion*, ed. K. Heilman and P. Satz, pp. 6–44. New York: The Guilford Press.

Buchwald, J.S., Van Lancker, D., Erwin, R.J., Guthrie, D. and Schwafel, J. (1994). Influence of language structure on brain–behavior development. *Brain Lang* 46: 607–19.

Caekebeke, J.F.V., Jennekens-Schinkel, A., van der Linden, M.E., Buruma, O.J.S. and Roos, R.A.C. (1991). The interpretation of dysprosody in patients with Parkinson's disease. *J Neurol Neurosurg Psychiatry* 54: 145–8.

Calder, A.J., Young, A.W., Rowland, D. et al. (1996). Facial emotion recognition after bilateral amygdala damage: differentially severe impairment of fear. *Cogn Neuropsychol* 13: 699–745.

Cancelliere, A. and Kertesz, A. (1990). Lesion localization in acquired deficits of emotional expression and comprehension. *Brain Cogn* 13: 133–47.

Caplan, L.R., Schmahmann, J.D., Kase, C.S. et al. (1990). Caudate infarcts. *Arch Neurol* 47: 133–43.

Cicone, M., Wapner, W. and Gardner, H. (1980). Sensitivity to emotional expressions and situations in organic patients. *Cortex* 16: 145–58.

Clark, R.G. (1995). Fear and loathing in the amygdala. *Curr Biol* 5: 246–8.

Cohen, M.J., Riccio, C.A. and Flannery, A.M. (1994). Expressive aprosodia following stroke to the right basal ganglia: a case report. *Neuroposychology* 8: 242–5.

Colsher, P.L., Cooper, W.E. and Graff-Radford, N. (1987). Intonational variability in the speech of right-hemisphere damaged patients. *Brain Lang* 32: 379–83.

Cooper, W., Soares, C., Nicol, J., Michelow, D. and Goloskie, S. (1984). Clausal intonation after unilateral brain damage. *Lang Speech* 27: 17–24.

Critchley, E.M.R. (1981). Speech disorders of Parkinsonism: a review. *J Neurol Neurosurg Psychiatry* 44: 751–8.

Critchley, M. (1964). The neurology of psychotic speech. *Br J Psychiatry* 110: 353–64.

Crystal, D. (1969). *Prosodic Systems and Intonation in English*. Cambridge, UK: Cambridge University Press.

Crystal, D. (1970). Prosodic systems and language acquisition. In *Prosodic Feature Analysis*, ed. P. Leon, G. Faure and A. Rigault, pp. 77–90. Montreal: Librairie Didier.

Cummings, J.L. (1985). *Clinical Neuropsychiatry*. Orlando, FL: Grune & Stratton.

Cummings, J.L. (1993). Frontal–subcortical circuits and human behavior. *Arch Neurol* 50: 873–80.

Cutting, J. (1990). *The Right Cerebral Hemisphere and Psychiatric Disorders*. Oxford: Oxford University Press.

Danly, M., Cooper, W. and Shapiro, B. (1983). Fundamental frequency, language processing, and linguistic structure in Wernicke's aphasia. *Brain Lang* 19: 1–24.

Danly, M. and Shapiro, B. (1982). Speech prosody in Broca's aphasia. *Brain Lang* 16: 171–90.

Darby, D.G. (1993). Sensory aprosodia: a clinical clue to lesions of the inferior division of the right middle cerebral artery? *Neurology* 43: 567–72.

Darley, F.L., Aronson, A.E. and Brown, J.R. (1975). *Motor Speech Disorders*. Philadelphia: W.B. Saunders.

Davidson, R.J. (1993a). Cerebral asymmetry and emotion: conceptual and methodological conundrums. *Cogn Emotion* 7: 115–38.

Davidson, R.J. (1993b). Parsing affective space: perspectives from neuropsychology and psychophysiology. *Neuropsychology* 7: 464–75.

De Bleser, R. and Poeck, K. (1985). Analysis of prosody in the spontaneous speech of patients with CV-recurring utterances. *Cortex* 21: 405–15.

Denes, G., Caldognetto, E.M., Semenza, C., Vagges, K. and Zettin, M. (1984). Discrimination and identification of emotions in human voice by brain-damaged subjects. *Acta Neurol Scand* 69: 154–62.

Devinsky, O., Morrell, M.J. and Vogt, B.A. (1995). Contributions of anterior cingulate cortex to behavior. *Brain* 118: 279–306.

Duffy, J.R. (1995). *Motor Speech Disorders*. St Louis, MI: Mosby.

Dykstra, K., Gandour, J. and Stark, R. (1995). Disruption of prosody after frontal lobe seizures in the nondominant hemisphere. *Aphasiology* 9: 453–76.

Ellgring, H. and Scherer, K.R. (1996). Vocal indicators of mood change in depression. *J Nonverb Behav* 20: 83–110.

Fisher, C.M. (1983). Abulia minor versus agitated behavior. *Clin Neurosurg* 31: 9–31.

Friston, K.J., Price, C.J., Fletcher, P. et al. (1996). The trouble with cognitive subtraction. *Neuroimage* 4: 97–104.

Gainotti, G. (1989). The meaning of emotional disturbances resulting from unilateral brain injury. In *Emotions and the Dual Brain*, ed. G. Gainotti and C. Caltagirone, pp. 173–202. Heidelberg: Springer Verlag.

Gainotti, G., Caltagirone, C. and Zoccolotti, P. (1993). Left/right and cortical/subcortical dichotomies in the neuropsychological study of human emotion. *Cogn Emotion* 7: 71–93.

Gandour, J., Dechongkit, S., Ponglorpisit, S. and Khunadorn, F. (1994). Speech timing at the sentence level in Thai after unilateral brain damage. *Brain Lang* 46: 419–38.

Gandour, J., Dechongit, S., Ponglorpisit, S., Khunadorn, F. and Poongird, P. (1993a). Intraword timing relations in Thai after unilateral brain damage. *Brain Lang* 45: 160–79.

Gandour, J., Larsen, J., Dechongkit, S., Ponglorpisit, S. and Khunadorn, F. (1995). Speech prosody in affective contexts in Thai patients with right hemisphere lesions. *Brain Lang* 51: 422–43.

Gandour, J., Ponglorpisit, S., Dechongkit, S. et al. (1993b). Anticipatory tonal coarticulation in Thai noun compounds after unilateral brain damage. *Brain Lang* 45: 1–20.

Gandour, J., Wong, D., Hsieh, L., Weinzapfel, B., Van Lancker, D. and Hutchins, G. (2000). A crosslinguistic PET study of tone perception. *Cogn Neurosci* 12(1): 207–22.

George, M.S., Parekh, P.I., Rosinsky, N. et al. (1996). Understanding emotional prosody activates right hemisphere regions. *Arch Neurol* 53: 665–70.

Goodglass, H. and Kaplan, E. (1972). *Assessment of Aphasia and Related Disorders*. Philadelphia: Lea and Febiger.

Gordon, H. (1970). Hemispheric asymmetries for the perception of musical chords. *Cortex* 6: 387–98.

Gordon, H. and Bogen, J.E. (1981). Hemispheric lateralization of singing after intracarotid sodium amylobartitone. *J Neurol Neurosurg Psychiatry* 37: 727–38.

Gorelick, P.B. and Ross, E.D. (1987). The aprosodias: further functional–anatomical evidence for the organization of affective language in the right hemisphere. *J Neurol Neurosurg Psychiatry* 50: 553–60.

Gray, J.M., Young, A.W., Barker, W.A., Curtis, A. and Gibson, D. (1997). Impaired recognition of disgust in Huntington's disease gene carriers. *Brain* 120: 2029–38.

Griffiths, T.D., Rees, A., Witton, C. et al. (1997). Spatial and temporal auditory processing deficits following right hemisphere infarction. *Brain* 120: 785–94.

Hagen, P., Lyons, G.D. and Nuss, W. (1996). Dysphonia in the elderly: diagnosis and management of age-related voice changes. *South Med J* 89: 204–7.

Hamann, S.B., Stefanacci, L., Squire, L.R. et al. (1996). Recognizing facial emotion. *Nature* 379: 497.

Harford, E.R. and Dodds, E. (1982). Hearing status of ambulatory senior citizens. *Ear Hear* 3: 105–9.

Harrington, D.L., Haaland, K.Y. and Knight, R.T. (1998). Cortical networks underlying mechanisms of time perception. iJ Neurosci 18: 1085–95.

Heilman, K.M. (1993). A response to Van Lancker and Sidtis (1992). *J Speech Hear Res* 36: 1191.

Heilman, K.M. (1997). The neurobiology of emotional experience. *J Neuropsychiatry Clin Neurosci* 9: 439–48.

Heilman, K.M., Bowers, D., Speedie, L. and Coslett, H.B. (1984). Comprehension of affective and nonaffective prosody. *Neurology* 34: 917–21.

Heilman, K.M., Bowers, D. and Valenstein, E. (1993). Emotional disorders associated with neurological diseases. In *Clinical Neuropsychology*, 3rd edn, ed. K.M. Heilman and E. Valenstein, pp. 461–97. New York: Oxford University Press.

Heilman, K.M., Scholes, R. and Watson, R.T. (1975). Auditory affective agnosia. *J Neurol Neurosurg Psychiatry* 38: 69–72.

Heilman, K.M., Watson, R.T. and Bowers, D. (1983). Affective disorders associated with hemispheric disease. In *Neuropsychology of Human Emotion*, ed. K.M. Heilman and P. Satz, pp. 45–64. New York: The Guilford Press.

Helm-Estabrooks, N. and Albert, M.L. (1991). *Manual of Aphasia Therapy*. Austin, TX: Pro-Ed.

Hird, K. and Kirsner, K. (1993). Dysprosody following acquired neurogenic impairment. *Brain Lang* 45: 46–60.

Hornak, J., Rolls, E.T. and Wade, D. (1996). Face and voice expression identification in patients with emotional and behavioral changes following ventral frontal lobe damage. *Neuropsychologia* 34: 247–61.

House, A., Rowe, D. and Standen, P.J. (1987). Affective prosody in the reading voice of stroke patients. *J Neurol Neurosurg Psychiatry* 50: 910–12.

Hughlings Jackson, J. (1874). On the nature of the duality of the brain. Reprinted in J. Taylor (ed.) (1932). *Selected Writings of John Hughlings Jackson*, Vol. 2, pp. 129–45. London: Hodder & Stoughton.

Hughlings Jackson, J. (1915). On affections of speech from diseases of the brain. *Brain* 38: 101–86.

Jennings, J.M., McIntosh, A.R., Kapur, S., Tulving, E. and Houle, S. (1997). Cognitive subtractions may not add up: the interaction between semantic processing and response mode. *Neuroimage* 5: 229–39.

Johnson, W.F., Emde, R.N., Scherer, K.R. and Klinnert, M.D. (1986). Recognition of emotion from vocal cues. *Arch Gen Psychiatry* 43: 280–3.

Kent, R.D. (1996). Hearing and believing: some limits to the auditory–perceptual assessment of speech and voice disorders. *Am J Speech–Lang Pathol* 5: 7–24.

Kent, R.D. and Rosenbek, J. (1982). Prosodic disturbance and neurologic lesion. *Brain Lang* 15: 259–91.

Kertesz, A. (1982). *The Western Aphasia Battery*. New York: Grune and Stratton.

Klouda, G.V., Robin, D.A., Graff-Radford, N.R. and Cooper, W.E. (1988). The role of callosal connections in speech prosody. *Brain Lang* 35: 154–71.

Kolb, B. and Taylor, L. (1981). Affective behavior in patients with localized cortical excisions: role of lesion site and side. *Science* 214: 89–91.

Kreiman, J. (1996). Listening to voices: theory and practice in voice perception. In *Talker Variability in Speech Processing*, ed. K. Johnson and J.W. Mullenis, pp. 85–108. New York: Academic Press.

Kreiman, J. and Garrett, B. (1996). The perceptual structure of pathological voice quality. *J Acoust Soc Am* 100: 1787–95.

Ladd, D.R. (1996). *Intonational Phonology*. Cambridge, UK: Cambridge University Press.

LaFramboise, M., Synder, P. and Cohen, H. (1997). Cerebral hemispheric control of speech during the intracarotid sodium amytal procedure: an acoustic exploration. *Brain Lang* 60: 243–54.

Lalande, S., Braun, C.M., Charlebois, N. and Whitaker, H.A. (1992). Effects of right and left hemisphere cerebrovascular lesions on discrimination of prosodic and semantic aspects of affect in sentences. *Brain Lang* 42: 165–86.

Lance, J.E. (1994). Prosodic deviation in dysarthria: a case study. *Eur J Disord Commun* 29: 61–76.

Laplane, D., Baulac, M., Widlöcher, D. and DuBois, B. (1984). Pure psychic akinesia with bilateral lesions of basal ganglia. *J Neurol Neurosurg Psychiatry* 47: 377–85.

LeDoux, J. (1995). Emotion: clues from the brain. *Ann Rev Psychol* 46: 209–35.

Lee, G.P., Loring, D.W., Meador, K.J. and Brooks, B.B. (1990). Hemispheric specialization for emotional expression. A reexamination of results from intracarotic administration of sodium amobartital. *Brain Cogn* 12: 267–80.

Ley, R. and Bryden, M. (1982). A dissociation of right and left hemisphere effects for recognizing emotional tone and verbal content. *Brain Cogn* 1: 3–9.

Luria, A.R. (1966). *Higher Cortical Functions in Man*. New York: Basic Books.

Mandel, d., Jusczyk, P.W. and Nelson, D.G. (1994). Does sentential prosody help infants organize and remember speech information? *Cognition* 53: 155–80.

Masterman, D.L. and Cummings, J.L. (1997). Frontal–subcortical circuits: the anatomic basis of executive, social, and motivated behaviors. *J Psychopharmacol* 11: 107–14.

Mayeux, R. (1983). Emotional changes associated with basal ganglia disorders. In *Neuropsychology of Human Emotion*, ed. K. Heilman and P. Satz, pp. 141–64. New York: The Guilford Press.

McDowell, C.L., Harrison, D.W. and Demaree, H.A. (1994). Is right hemisphere decline in the perception of emotion a function of aging? *Int J Neurosci* 79: 1–11.

Mehler, J. and Christophe, A. (1994). Language in the infant's mind. *Philos Trans R Soc Lond* 346: 13–20.

Mehrabian, A. (1972). *Nonverbal Communication*. Chicago: Aldine Atherton.

Mendez, M., Adams, N.L. and Lewandowski, K.S. (1989). Neurobehavioral changes associated with caudate lesions. *Neurology* 39: 349–54.

Merewether, F.C. and Alpert, M. (1990). The components and neuroanatomic bases of prosody. *J Commun Disord* 23: 325–36.

Mills, C.K. (1912). The cerebral mechanism of emotional expression. *Trans Coll Phys Philadelphia* 34: 381–90.

Moen, I. (1991). Functional lateralization of pitch accents and intonation in Norwegian: Monrad-Krohn's study of an aphasic patient with altered 'melody of speech'. *Brain Lang* 41: 538–54.

Monrad-Krohn, G.H. (1947). Dysprosody or altered 'melody of speech.' *Brain* 70: 405–15.

Monrad-Krohn, G.H. (1963). The third element of speech prosody and its disorders. In *Problems of Dynamic Neurology*, ed. L. Halpern, pp. 101–18. Jerusalem: Hebrew University.

Ouellette, G.P. and Baum, S.R. (1993). Acoustic analysis of prosodic cues in left- and right-hemisphere-damaged patients. *Aphasiology* 8: 257–83.

Papçun, G., Krashen, S., Terbeek, D., Remington, R. and Harshman, R. (1974). Is the left hemisphere specialized for speech, language and/or something else? *J Acoust Soc Am* 55: 319–27.

Papez, J.W. (1937). A proposed mechanism of emotion. *Arch Neurol Psychiatry* 38: 725–43.

Pell, M.D. (1996). On the receptive prosodic loss in Parkinson's disease. *Cortex* 32: 693–704.

Pell, M.D. and Baum, S.R. (1997a). The ability to perceive and comprehend intonation in linguistic and affective contexts by brain-damaged adults. *Brain Lang* 57: 80–99.

Pell, M.D. and Baum, S.R. (1997b). Unilateral brain damage, prosodic comprehension deficits, and the acoustic cues to prosody. *Brain Lang* 57: 195–214.

Peper, M. and Irle, E. (1997a). Categorical and dimensional coding of emotional intonations in patients with focal brain lesions. *Brain Lang* 58: 233–64.

Peper, M. and Irle, E. (1997b). The decoding of emotional concepts in patients with focal cerebral lesions. *Brain Cogn* 34: 360–87.

Peretz, I., Kolinsky, R., Tramo, M. et al. (1994). Functional dissociations following bilateral lesions of auditory cortex. *Brain* 117: 1283–301.

Pihan, H., Altenmueller, E. and Ackermann, H. (1997). The cortical processing of perceived emotion: a DC-potential study on affective speech prosody. *NeuroReport* 8: 623–7.

Ploog, D. (1979). Phonation, emotion, cognition, with reference to the brain mechanisms involved. In *Brain and Mind. Ciba Foundation Symposium* 69, pp. 79–98. Amsterdam: Excerpta Medica.

Poncet, M. and Habib, M. (1994). Atteinte isolée des comportements motivés et lésions des noyaux gris centraux. *Rev Neurol* 150: 588–93.

Rapcsak, S.Z., Comer, J.F. and Rubens, A.B. (1993). Anomia for facial expressions: neuropsychological mechanisms and anatomical correlates. *Brain Lang* 45: 233–52.

Robin, D.A., Tranel, D. and Damasio, H. (1990). Auditory perception of temporal and spectral events in patients with focal left and right cerebral lesions. *Brain Lang* 39: 539–55.

Robinson, B.W. (1976). Limbic influences on human speech. *Ann N Y Acad Sci* 280: 761–71.

Robinson, G.M. and Solomon, D.J. (1974). Rhythm is processed by the speech hemisphere. *J Exp Psychol* 102: 508–11.

Robinson, R., Kubos, K., Starr, L., Rao, K. and Price, T. (1984). Mood disorders in stroke patients: importance of location of lesion. *Brain* 197: 81–93.

Rolls, E.T. (1990). A theory of emotion, and its application to understanding the neural basis of emotion. *Cogn Emotion* 4: 161–90.

Ross, E.D. (1981). The aprosodias: functional–anatomical organization of the affective components of language in the right hemisphere. *Arch Neurol* 38: 561–9.

Ross, E.D., Anderson, B. and Morgan-Fisher, A. (1989). Crossed aprosodia in strongly dextral patients. *Arch Neurol* 46: 206–9.

Ross, E.D., Edmondson, J.A., Seibert, G.B. and Homan, R.W. (1988). Acoustic analysis of affective prosody during right-sided Wada Test: a within-subjects verification of the right hemisphere's role in language. *Brain Lang* 33: 128–45.

Ross, E.D. and Mesulam, M.-M. (1979). Dominant language functions of the right hemisphere? Prosody and emotional gesturing. *Arch Neurol* 36: 144–8.

Ross, E.D., Thompson, R.D. and Yenkosky, J. (1997). Lateralization of affective prosody in brain and the collosal integration of hemispheric language functions. *Brain Lang* 56: 27–54.

Ryalls, J. (1982). Intonation in Broca's aphasia. *Neuropsychologia* 20: 355–60.

Ryalls, J. (1988). Concerning right-hemisphere dominance for affective language. *Arch Neurol* 45: 337–8.

Ryalls, J. and Behrens, S.J. (1988). An overview of changes in fundamental frequency associated with cortical insult. *Aphasiology* 2: 107–15.

Ryalls, J., Joanette, Y. and Feldman, L. (1987). An acoustic comparison of normal and right-hemisphere-damaged speech prosody. *Cortex* 23: 685–94.

Ryalls, J. and Reinvang, I. (1986). Functional lateralization of linguistic tones: acoustic evidence from Norwegian. *Lang Speech* 29: 389–98.

Sackeim, H.A., Greenberg, M.S., Weiman, M.A. et al. (1982). Hemispheric asymmetry in the expression of positive and negative emotions. *Arch Neurol* 39: 210–18.

Sackeim, H.A. and Gur, R.C. (1978). Lateral asymmetry in intensity of emotional expression. *Neuropsychologia* 16: 473–81.

Saint-Cyr, J.A., Taylor, A.E. and Nicholson, K. (1995). Behavior and the basal ganglia. In *Behavioral Neurology of Movement Disorders. Advances in Neurology*, Vol. 65, ed. W.J. Weiner and A.E. Lang, pp. 1–28. New York: Raven Press.

Santamaria, J. and Tolosa, E. (1992). Clinical subtypes of Parkinson's disease and depression. In *Parkinson's Disease: Neurobehavioral Aspects*, ed. S.J. Huber and J.L. Cummings, pp. 217–28. New York: Oxford University Press.

Scherer, K.R. (1986). Vocal affect expression: a review and a model for future research. *Psychol Bull* 99: 145–65.

Schlanger, B.B., Schlanger, P. and Gerstman, L.J. (1976). The perception of emotionally toned sentences by right hemisphere-damaged and aphasic subjects. *Brain Lang* 3: 396–403.

Schmitt, J.J., Hartje, W. and Willmes, K. (1997). Hemispheric asymmetry in the recognition of emotional attitude conveyed by facial expression, prosody, and propositional speech. *Cortex* 33: 65–81.

Scott, S., Caird, F. and Williams, B. (1984). Evidence for an apparent sensory speech disorder in Parkinson's disease. *J Neurol Neurosurg Psychiatry* 47: 840–3.

Scott, S.K., Young, A.W., Calder, A.J. et al. (1997). Impaired auditory recognition of fear and anger following bilateral amygdala lesions. *Nature* 385: 254–7.

Shapiro, B.E. and Danly, M. (1985). The role of the right hemisphere in the control of speech prosody in propositional and affective contexts. *Brain Lang* 25: 19–36.

Shipley-Brown, F., Dingwall, W.O., Berlin, C.I., Yeni-Komshian, G. and Gordon-Salant, S.

(1988). Hemispheric processing of affective and linguistic information contours in normal subjects. *Brain Lang* 33: 16–26.

Sidtis, J.J. (1980). On the nature of the cortical function underlying right hemisphere auditory perception. *Neuropsychologia* 18: 321–30.

Sidtis, J.J. (1982). Predicting brain organization from dichotic listening performance: cortical and subcortical functional asymmetries contribute to perceptual asymmetries. *Brain Lang* 17: 287–300.

Sidtis, J.J. (1984). Music, pitch perception, and the mechanisms of cortical hearing. In *Handbook of Cognitive Neuroscience*, ed. M.S. Gazzaniga, pp. 91–114. New York: Plenum Press.

Sidtis, J., Anderson, J.R., Rehm, K. et al. (1996). Are brain functions really additive? *Neuroimage* 3: S93.

Sidtis, J.J. and Feldmann, E. (1990). Transient ischemic attacks presenting with a loss of pitch perception. *Cortex* 26: 469–71.

Sidtis, J.J. and Volpe, T.B. (1988). Selective loss of complex-pitch or speech discrimination after unilateral cerebral lesion. *Brain Lang* 34: 235–45.

Silberman, E. and Weingartner, H. (1986). Hemispheric lateralization of functions related to emotions. *Brain Cogn* 5: 322–53.

Smith, A. (1966). Speech and other functions after left (dominant) hemispherectomy. *J Neurol Neurosurg Psychiatry* 29: 467–71.

Speedie, L.J., Brake, N., Folstein, S., Bowers, D. and Heilman, K. (1990). Comprehension of prosody in Huntington's disease. *J Neurol Neurosurg Psychiatry* 53: 607–10.

Speedie, L.J., Coslett, H.B. and Heilman, K.M. (1984). Repetition of affective prosody in mixed transcortical aphasia. *Arch Neurol* 41: 268–70.

Starkstein, S., Federoff, J., Price, T., Leigarda, R. and Robinson, R. (1994). Neuropsychological and neuroradiologic correlates of emotional prosody comprehension. *Neurology* 44: 515–22.

Stone, V.E., Nisenson, L., Eliassen, J.C. and Gazzaniga, M.S. (1996). Left hemisphere representations of emotional facial expressions. *Neuropsychologia* 34: 23–9.

Sudia, S., Bolon, D. and Van Lancker, D. (1998). Linguistic–prosodic performance in dysprosodic apraxia following left versus right hemisphere damage: two 'matched' case studies. Poster presented at the Annual Meeting of the International Neuropsychological Society, Honululu, Hawaii.

TenHouten, W.D., Hoppe, K.D., Bogen, J.E. and Walter, D.O. (1986). Alexithymia: an experimental study of cerebral commissurotomy patients and normal control subjects. *Am J Psychiatry* 143: 312–16.

Tompkins, C.A. (1991). Automatic and effortful processing of emotional intonation after right or left hemisphere brain damage. *J Speech Hear Res* 34: 820–30.

Tompkins, C.A. and Flowers, C.R. (1985). Perception of emotional intonation by brain-damaged adults: the influence of task processing levels. *J Speech Hear Res* 28: 527–38.

Tompkins, C.A. and Flowers, C.R. (1987). Contextual mood priming following left and right hemisphere damage. Brain Cogn 6: 361–76.

Tompkins, C.A. and Mateer, C.A. (1985). Right hemisphere appreciation of prosodic and linguistic indications of implicit attitude. *Brain Lang* 25: 185–203.

Tranel, D. (1992). Neuropsychological correlates of cortical and subcortical damage. In *Textbook of Neuropsychiatry*, Vol. II, ed. S.C. Yudofsky and R.E. Hales, pp. 57–88. Washington, DC: American Psychiatric Press.

Tucker, D., Watson, R.T. and Heilman, K.M. (1977). Discrimination and evocation of affectively intoned speech in patients with right parietal disease. *Neurology* 27: 947–50.

Twist, D., Squires, N., Spielholz, N. and Silverglide, R. (1991). Event-related potentials in disorders of prosodic and semantic linguistic processing. *Neuropsychiatry Neuropsychol Behav Neurol* 4: 281–304.

Van Lancker, D. (1980). Cerebral lateralization of pitch cues in the linguistic signal. *Int J Hum Commun* 13: 201–27.

Van Lancker, D. and Canter, G.J. (1982). Impairment of voice and face recognition in patients with hemispheric damage. *Brain Cogn* 1: 185–95.

Van Lancker, D. and Fromkin, V. (1973). Hemispheric specialization for pitch and 'tone': evidence from Thai. *J Phonetics* 1: 101–9.

Van Lancker, D., Hanson, W., Jackson, C. et al. (1988). Prosodic changes in speech following brain damage. Acoustic and neuroradiographic measures. *J Acoust Soc Am* 84 Abstract.

Van Lancker, D., Kreiman, J. and Cornelius, C. (1989). Recognition of emotional prosodic cues in normal, autistic, and schizophrenic children. *Dev Neuropsychol* 5: 207–26.

Van Lancker, D., Pachana, N.A., Cummings, J.L., Sidtis, J.J. and Erickson, C. (1996). Dysprosodic speech following basal ganglia stroke: role of fronto-subcortical circuits. *J Int Neuropsychol Soc* 2: S5.

Van Lancker, D. and Sidtis, J.J. (1992). The identification of affective–prosodic stimuli by left- and right-hemisphere-damaged subjects: all errors are not created equal. *J Speech Hear Res* 35: 963–70.

Vihman, M.M. and De Boysson-Bardies, B. (1994). The nature and origins of ambient language influence on infant vocal production and early words. *Phonetica* 51: 159–69.

Wechsler, A. (1973). The effect of organic brain disease on recall of emotionally charged vs. neutral narrative texts. *Neurology* 23: 130–5.

Weddell, R.A. (1994). Effects of subcortical lesion site on human emotional behavior. *Brain Cogn* 25: 161–93.

Weintraub, S., Mesulam, M.-M. and Kramer, L. (1981). Disturbances in prosody: a right-hemisphere contribution to language. *Arch Neurol* 38: 742–4.

Williams, S. and Seaver, E. (1986). A comparison of speech sound durations in three syndromes of aphasia. *Brain Lang* 29: 171–82.

Young, A.W., Rowland, D., Calder, A.J. et al. (1997). Facial expression megamix: tests of dimensional and category accounts of emotion recognition. *Cognition* 63: 271–313.

Zatorre, R.J. (1979). Recognition of dichotic melodies by musicians and nonmusicians. *Neuropsychologia* 17: 607–17.

Zatorre, R.J., Evans, A., Meyer, E. and Gjedde, A. (1992). Lateralization of phonetic and pitch discrimination in speech processing. *Science* 256: 846–9.

13

Temporal lobe behavioral syndromes

Serge Bakchine

Introduction

Although the importance of the temporal lobes in behavior and mood has long been recognized by clinicians, the role of these structures is yet to be understood. The literature of the middle third of the twentieth century offers both rich anatomo-clinical studies and the first attempts to conceptualize models of behavioral control, with the description by Papez in 1937 of the limbic system (Papez, 1937). Subsequently, experimental studies in animals, especially primates, allowed descriptions of behavioral disturbances directly related to temporolimbic structures. Some of these syndromes, such as the Klüver–Bucy syndrome, were observed, almost unchanged, in humans. During recent years, knowledge about behavioral syndromes related to temporal lobes has progressed very little compared with the important advances accomplished in the study of cognitive processes. A series of facts may explain this slow rate of progress.

1 The theoretical framework of human emotions is still controversial, and there are several rival models attempting to explain emotional control (Feyereisen, 1989; Heilman and Watson, 1989; Rolls, 1995; LeDoux, 1996; Heilman, 1997).

2 Although the cerebral structures integrating human emotions are better delineated, it has been suggested that they may constitute a complex, 'parallel distributed processing' network widely distributed within the brain (Mega and Cummings, 1994; Halgren and Marinkovic, 1995; LeDoux, 1995, 1996). Many authors have also insisted on the functional importance of cortico-subcortical circuits (Cummings, 1993a). This type of organization lessens the anatomoclinical value of temporal syndromes.

3 Apart from their role in emotional functions, the temporal lobes participate in several important congitive capacities, such as memory, language, and access to semantic knowledge, which are frequently impaired when the temporal lobes are damaged. Although these functions are not usually considered to be directly involved in emotional behavior, their impairment results in cognitive deficits, for example aphasia, that make more complex the exploration of behavioral

disturbances. Cognitive impairment can be viewed as part of the mechanism of behavioral disturbances. For instance, language allows anticipation of actions and could participate in conscious processes (Rolls, 1995). Language impairment could mediate important aspects of behavioral dysfunctioning. It is interesting to note that some recent theories have put forward the idea that schizophrenia could be considered, 'as a failure of hemispheric dominance for language' (Crow, 1997).

4 Studies of behavior and mood disturbances in brain-damaged patients are hampered by methodological weaknesses. Precise localization of the damaged or dysfunctioning areas is not always possible (see discussion for epileptic foci in Strauss, 1989). Tools (criteria, scales, inventories, questionnaires etc.) used to assess behavior and mood in this peculiar population are far less developed compared to those for cognitive assessment (for further discussion, see Chapter 2). Researchers often use tools directly derived from psychiatric practice. Yet, in many situations, brain-damaged patients may develop psychoaffective disturbances that do not present as the typical 'psychiatric' syndromes and therefore would not fit with the usual diagnostic criteria or be assessed reliably by psychiatric scales. Moreover, the expression of behavioral disturbances may vary considerably with the type of interaction in which the patient is involved, and with the patient's environment (Fayada and Bakchine, 1998). Thus, the validity and reliability of several tools used by investigators in brain-damaged patients are far from being demonstrated (Bakchine, 1991, 1998a).

The aim of this chapter is threefold. First, it briefly describes the main contributions of temporal structures to networks integrating human emotions and behaviors. Then it presents the most frequent pathologies associated with focal temporal lesions. Finally, it reviews behaviors and mood disturbances associated with temporal lesions.

The contribution of temporal structures to networks integrating human emotions

As stated by Mega et al. (1997), the limbic system is the border zone where psychiatry meets neurology. Since the original description of the Papez's loop, the concept of a temporolimbic system has evolved and this is now considered as a widely distributed circuit, a 'parallel distributed processing network,' including several cortical and subcortical structures and pathways. The present vision of the temporolimbic system comports two main subdivisions: the medial limbic circuits and the lateral limbic circuits (Byrum et al., 1997; Trimble, Mendez, and Cummings, 1997).

The medial circuit (an archicortical division) includes hypothalamus, anterior thalamic nuclei, cingulate gyrus, hippocampus, and related tracts. It is connected with the brainstem reticular formation. It mediates important aspects of learning, memory, and attentional control, as well as information related to internal states.

The lateral (or basolateral) circuit (a paleocortical division) consists of the amygdala, dorsomedial thalamic nuclei, and the orbitofrontal, insular, and temporal polar cortices. It has extensive connections with dorsolateral prefrontal cortex and posterior parietal association cortex. It processes information concerning the external world, the implicit integration of affect, drives, and social–personal interactions.

These two circuits function together to integrate thought, feeling, and action.

Recently, Alheid and Heimer (1996) proposed the concept of 'extended amygdala,' which they defined as a complex pathway extending from the central and medial amygdaloid nuclei through subpallidal gray matter to the nucleus accumbens. It exchanges rich connections with temporal and frontal cortices, with ventral striatum, with ventral tegmental area, the substantia nigra, the periaqueductal gray region, and nuclei in the reticular formation. Thus, extended amygdala influences areas thought to be related to emotional motor behaviors, or to the coordination of autonomic and somatomotor behavior.

Focal pathologies of the temporal lobes

There is a large and heterogeneous corpus of literature concerning the study of behavior disturbances associated with focal lesions of the temporal lobes in humans. A very important part of this corpus comes from studies of temporal lobe epilepsy (TLE), in which frequent and various behavioral disturbances have been extensively investigated. These important data are considered below.

Another major component comes from the studies of focal brain lesions such as strokes and tumors. During the middle third of the twentieth century, several studies conducted with large series of patients (Keschner, Bender and Strauss, 1936; Bingley, 1958) demonstrated that temporal lobe sites produce perhaps the highest incidence of affective and behavioral disturbances, just behind those of the frontal lobe (Lishman, 1989). These disturbances may appear during the evolution of a diagnosed tumor, but may also reveal the illness. This semiology may be particularly misleading, when right temporal tumors are revealed by anxiety symptoms or panic attacks, or left temporal tumors by depressive symptoms (Malamud, 1975; Druback and Kelly, 1989). For correlation study purposes, however, investigators avoid brain tumors because of the many factors that weaken the localization value (mass effect, diffuse extension, etc.). Recently, most studies have concentrated on stroke, because this pathology offers a higher localization reliability after the acute period. Studies with stroke patients have allowed major advances in the comprehension of behavioral and mood disturbances (see Chapters 5 and 7). In stroke, in contrast to tumors, diagnosis is rarely masked by the behavioral disturbances. Misleading situations are rare, and mainly observed for posterior cerebral artery strokes, especially right sided, that may be associated with delusional states or psychotic symptoms (Lishman, 1968; Ghika-Schmid and Bogousslavsky, 1997).

Traumatic head injury frequently produces psychoaffective disturbances, because this pathology frequently damages at least one of the two brain areas that are critical to behavior: the frontal lobes, especially in their orbital part, or the temporal lobes, in their anterior and basomedial parts. Many behavioral or mood disturbances have been observed in head-injured patients, but none is specific, and when both temporal and frontal lobes are involved, it is difficult to discriminate between the consequences of each lesion site (Lishman, 1968, 1989; Shukla et al., 1987; Jorge et al., 1993a; Roberts et al., 1995). However, head injury is the most common cause of the rare postlesional manic syndromes (Starkstein, Boston and Robinson, 1988a; Jorge et al., 1993b).

The encephalitis due to herpes simplex virus forms the last important etiopathological group (Trimble et al., 1997). The HSV encephalitis has a specific tropism toward the temporal lobes, especially in basal and medial parts. Behavioral or pseudopsychiatric disturbances may be the sole manifestations during the initial period. Therefore, unfortunately, patients may be mistakenly treated for psychiatric illness, thus delaying antiviral treatment, with dramatic consequences on the outcome. Among the many possible behavioral sequelae, the Klüver–Bucy syndrome is the most typical of this etiology.

Temporal lobe behavior and mood syndromes

Behavioral syndromes in temporal lobe epilepsy

Although most epileptic patients present no behavioral problems, TLE has frequently been associated with emotional disturbances manifesting as ictal phenomena, directly related to the seizure discharge, or interictal behavior, occurring between overt seizures. A controversy still exists regarding the nature of the relationship between emotional disturbances and TLE (for a detailed review see Strauss, 1989). Advances in this domain have been hindered by methodological weaknesses (insufficient definition and diagnosis of TLE, lack of appropriate control groups) (Strauss, 1989). Moreover, epileptics, as a group, are more prone to reactional psychological problems than people without epilepsy (Hermann and Whitman, 1984). Nevertheless, studies of such emotional manifestations provide important data which may be helpful to understanding the neural mechanisms that underlie emotions, because they allow for direct correlation between specific aspects of affective behavior and localized dysfunction (Geschwind, 1979).

Ictal disturbances

The literature describes a wide variety of emotional responses to ictal discharge or electrical stimulation (Struass, 1989; Spiers et al., 1992). Most of the cases involve limbic structures of the temporal lobes. The most frequent ictal emotions are fear or anxious feelings, with depression with flat mood feelings being less frequent. Other emotional ictal states are rare or exceptional: euphoria or pleasure, laughter, crying, aggressive behavior, or sexual sensations.

Fear and anxiety

Ictal fear is often considered as a typical symptom of temporal lobe seizures (Cherlow and Serafetinides, 1977; Gloor et al., 1982; LeDoux, 1995). It occurs in about 20% of patients (Gloor et al., 1982). Ictal fear arises suddenly, out of context, and is not specifically directed. It is the 'fear which comes by itself – the symptom of fear' as described by Hughlings Jackson (1931). Fear rarely occurs as an isolated syndrome, but is usually associated with other (visceral) symptoms. The duration and intensity of ictal fear seem quite variable (Spiers et al., 1992). It seems to have no lateralizing value. However, prolonged attacks of fear seem more frequent with seizures originating from the right temporal lobe (McLachlan and Blume, 1980).

Data converge to indicate that amygdala could be the critical structure in the induction of the fear response (Gloor et al., 1982; LeDoux, 1995, 1996). Penfield (Penfield and Jasper, 1954) has already noted that the most effective sites for producing fear were located in the medial areas of the temporal lobe. Studies of chronic limbic stimulation have shown that fear was a frequent symptom, but that it was related to the subject's personality (Gloor et al., 1982; Halgren and Marinkovic, 1995). In some TLE patients, attacks of fear could be stopped after temporal lobectomy, which included removal of portions of the amygdala (McLachlan and Blume, 1980).

Depression

'Ictal depression' is a rare symptom, reported in less than 10% of patients with TLE (Perini, 1986; Strauss, 1989; Altshuler et al., 1990; Hermann et al., 1991; Spiers et al., 1992). It may occur as an aura of the seizure, during the seizure, or as a sequel to the seizure. It is more often reported as a feeling of sadness that appears unmotivated to the patient, rather than as a true depression. The feelings may sometimes last for several minutes, but more frequently persist for days or weeks after the attack (Strauss, 1989). Many studies report feelings of emotional distress in the form of depression or other unpleasant emotional states during stimulation of the temporal–limbic regions (Penfield and Jasper, 1954; Perini, 1986; Altshuler et al., 1990; Spiers et al., 1992).

Laughter and crying (gelastic and dacrystic seizures)
Gelastic epilepsy refers to seizures in which laughter is a prominent ictal event (Daly and Mulder, 1957). Ictal laughter is rare, reported in less than 0.2% of epileptic patients, the majority of the cases having TLE (Sethi and Rao, 1976). The laughter does not necessarily occur during a pleasant experience, and may be experienced as an unpleasant, incongruous happening. The duration is usually brief, up to one or two minutes. The laughter may or may not be accompanied by mood changes (Yamada and Yoshida, 1977). Gelastic seizures originating from temporal lobes are more frequent than those from frontal cortex or diencephalic regions, and could be associated with more affective components.

Crying is a very uncommon ictal manifestation, termed 'dacrystic epilepsy' or 'quiritarian epilepsy' (Sethi and Rao, 1976). Although no specific area could be associated with ictal crying, it seems more frequent with right-sided lesions (Spiers et al., 1992). There is no report of dacrystic seizure obtained during focal stimulation. Contrary to crying, laughter is rarely elicited by electrical stimulation of the temporal lobe (Gloor et al., 1982; Halgren and Marinkovic, 1995).

Euphoria and pleasure
Feelings of gladness or euphoria seem to be quite rare in epilepsy, occurring almost exclusively in temporal lobe epilepsy. As already observed for other ictal feelings, these pleasurable experiences may be inappropriate with regard to circumstances. Reports based on electrical stimulation are quite confusing (Strauss, 1989): most authors failed to produce feelings of joy or pleasure (Gloor et al., 1982; Spiers et al., 1992; Halgren and Marinkovic, 1995). Positive responses have been reported for medial stimulation of the amygdala (Strauss, 1989).

Ictal anger or aggressive behavior
For a long time, an increase in aggressive behavior has been accepted as directly related to epilepsy, especially in temporal lobe epilepsy. This issue was even considered for legal purposes, because epilepsy was used as a defence in the courts (Pincus, 1981; Trieman, 1986). More recently, the validity of the concept of ictal aggression, whether associated with temporal lobe discharge or electrical stimulation, has been the subject of intense study and debate (Strauss, 1989). It is now admitted that true ictal aggression is an extremely rare phenomenon, mostly observed in patients suspected of having a temporal lobe focus, particularly the hippocampus and amygdala (Mark and Sweet, 1974; Kiloh and Smith, 1978; Ramani and Gumnit, 1981; Devinsky and Bear, 1984; Devinsky and Vaquez, 1993).

In many cases, aggression appears not as an ictal phenomenon, but rather as the result of postictal confusion (Rodin, 1973; Devinsky and Bear, 1984). Most of the recorded cases have shown aggression while being restrained at the end of a seizure, rather than directed and planned aggression (Delgado-Escueta et al., 1981). Truly ictal aggressive acts are usually simple, stereotyped and unplanned (Delgado-Escueta et al., 1981; Trieman, 1986). Among cases of violence allegedly due to an epileptic attack, very few present sufficient evidence to established the ictal nature of the violent episode (Mark and Sweet, 1974; Trieman, 1986). Finally, many studies have shown that temporolimbic stimulation rarely evokes anger or aggression (Gloor et al., 1982).

Erotic or sexual sensations

Although regarded as typical symptoms of temporal lobe epilepsy, erotic manifestations are rarely reported during spontaneous or electrically provoked seizures, and when reported they are more often by women than by men (Gloor et al., 1982; Strauss, 1989). The nature of ictal sexual symptoms seems to discriminate between temporal lobe epilepsy, in which sexual experiences occur (erotic feelings, with or without genital feelings or sensations of orgasm), and frontal foci, in which sexual behavior seems characterized by automatism as exhibitionism or masturbatory activity (Taylor, 1969b; Bancaud et al., 1971; Blumer, 1971; Shukla, Srivastava and Katiyar, 1979a; Remillard et al., 1983). Lateralization of the epileptogenic foci is predominantly, though not invariably, right sided (Bancaud et al., 1971; Heath, 1972; Remillard et al., 1983; Daniele et al., 1997).

Interictal manifestations

Although many authors reported a high prevalence of interictal behavioral disturbances in temporal lobe epilepsy patients, there is still a controversy about the proposal that this population is at special risk. A high proportion of these patients appear to suffer from, or to be hospitalized because of, psychological disturbances. In a recent study by Devinsky and Vaquez (1993) these proportions were respectively 51% and 21% in a population of temporal lobe epilepsy patients, as compared with 29% and 7% in a general population of epileptic patients. The factors determining the development of the interictal behaviors are not precisely known. A dysfunction of the limbic system could be critical in altering emotional control. However, interictal behavioral disturbances present large interindividual and within-individual variations. These disturbances could depend on an interaction with many other factors, such as an individual's past experience and psychosocial situation (Waxman and Geschwind, 1975; Bear and Fedio, 1977; Dodrill and Batzel, 1986; Strauss, 1989; Devinsky et al., 1994). Strauss (1989) reviewed four types of manifestations: disorders of personality, aggressiveness, emotional disturbances (anxiety, fear, depression), and disorders of sexuality.

Disorders of personality and the Gastaut–Geschwind syndrome

A wide variety of interictal personality traits has been associated with epilepsy, especially in temporal lobe epilepsy (Spiers et al., 1992).

Some authors, such as Gastaut (1956), Pincus and Tucker (1974) Geschwind (1979; Waxman and Geschwind, 1975), and Bear (1997; Bear and Fedio, 1977), stressed a series of interictal traits that seemed specific to temporal lobe epilepsy. The Gastaut–Geschwind syndrome, which includes these traits, is characterized by three main clusters of symptoms.

The first cluster comprises a tendency to develop intense metaphysical pre-occupation with hyperreligiosity, and exaggerated philosophic or moral concerns. These patients are often reported as serious, humourless, with a tendency to emotional behavior (depression, paranoia, irritability).

The second group of traits relates to a behavioral 'viscosity,' with overinclusiveness in verbal (circumstantiality), motor (stickiness), and writing (hypergraphia) behaviors. 'Viscosity' is considered as the most important characteristic of the Gastaut–Geschwind syndrome (Benson, 1991; Bear, 1997). It refers to various behaviors: 'stickiness' of thought processes, adherence to ideas, interpersonal adhesiveness, increased social adhesion (Rao et al., 1992). Patients exhibit altered interpersonal behavior, with a tendency to prolong exaggeratedly interpersonal encounters, with obsessive preoccupation with detail, and circumstantiality of speech. They tend to provide excessively detailed background information or to write copiously about their thoughts and feelings, with often a moral or religious content (Hermann, Whitman and Arntson, 1983; Naito and Matsui, 1988). In some patients, hypergraphia is associated with excessive drawing or painting.

The third cluster relates to alterations of physiological drives, such as sexuality (typically hyposexuality), aggression, and fear (Benson, 1991).

As the Minnesota Multiphasic Personality Inventory (MMPI) proved insensitive to most of the specific traits attributed to temporal lobe epilepsy, Bear and Fedio (1977) designed two questionnaires (a self-report form, the Personal Inventory, and an informant form, the Personal Behavior Survey) specifically to detect 18 personality features. These authors found a higher prevalence of 'TLE syndrome' among temporal lobe epilepsy patients as compared with normal subjects. They also observed an effect of the involved side: right temporal lobe epilepsy patients were more likely to exhibit emotional tendencies and denial, whereas patients with left temporal lobe epilepsy showed ideational disturbances and exaggerated concerns (Bear and Fedio, 1977; Bear, 1997). Similar personality traits have also been described after temporal lobectomy, with a more frequent impairment after right lobectomy (Robinson and Saykin, 1992). Bear (Bear, Schenk and Benson, 1981; Bear, 1997) suggested that this syndrome may stem from a 'sensory–limbic hyper-connection,' an increased functional connectivity between temporal neocortex and limbic structures, that could produce deepened associations to overtly neutral events.

However, since these authors have used no control group with other types of seizures, the specificity of these changes has been challenged by subsequent controlled studies using the same tools, or the MMPI, or other specific tools. Except for some other uncontrolled studies (Perini, 1986; Persinger, 1991), most attempts (mainly controlled studies) to replicate Bear and Fedio's findings have failed to define a personality profile specific to TLE epileptic patients, or to show any difference in trait scores between patients with right or left temporal lobe foci (Mungas, 1982; Rodin and Schmaltz, 1984; Hermann and Whitman, 1992). However, a large proportion of the variance in the trait scores seems attributable to the presence or absence of associated psychiatric illness, and, thus, temporal lobe epilepsy could make no discernible contribution of its own (Mungas, 1982).

Several cardinal signs of the syndrome, such as hyperreligiosity or hypergraphia, appear nonspecific (Mungas, 1982; Hermann et al., 1983; Tucker, Novelly and Walker, 1987; Saver and Rabin, 1997). However, Rao et al. (1992) showed that the 'sticky' interpersonal style is common in temporal lobe epilepsy patients with a left-sided temporal lobe seizure focus, and could arise from subtle interictal language disturbances, although other mechanisms are possible.

Strauss stated that no strong conclusion can be derived from the literature (Strauss, 1989). Although patients with temporal lobe epilepsy demonstrate significantly more behavioral difficulties than normal controls, it is uncertain whether they show more disturbances than people with other chronic illnesses or other types of seizure. Methodological issues seem important, since results depend heavily upon the evaluation tools employed. If there is a characteristic constellation of traits of temporal lobe epilepsy, it appears to be difficult to demonstrate with current procedures. Finally, some risk factors have been identified, such as an early age of seizure onset, the presence of multiple seizure types, seizures with an aura of fear, and mediobasal temporal foci (Hermann and Whitman, 1984; Spiers et al., 1992).

Delusions, psychosis

Early authors reported 'schizophreniform' traits observed as a chronic interictal disturbance in patients with temporal lobe epilepsy (see review in Strauss, 1989). Delusions, mostly of the paranoid type, appear frequently in these patients (Trimble, 1991; Spiers et al., 1992; Mendez et al., 1993). Some studies reported that about 11% of temporal lobe epilepsy patients exhibited an overt schizophrenia-like psychosis (Pritchard, Lombroso and McIntyre, 1980; Trimble, 1991), a frequency which represented a higher incidence than in a control group of patients with generalized seizures (Shukla et al., 1979b). Patients with psychosis or delusions were reported to have more frequent left-sided foci (Prithchard et al., 1980; Jibiki et al., 1993). However, other studies presented contradictory results, and most have failed to show a higher than expected incidence of psychosis in temporal lobe epilepsy (Davison and Bagley, 1969; Taylor, 1975; Hermann et al., 1981; Roberts, Done and Crow, 1990; Schomer, 1997). Factors other than the type of seizures and the location of foci may be important, such as a history of poorly controlled seizures with frequent secondary generalization. An antagonism between delusions and the control of the ictal activity has been reported: when some patients get worse with the increase in seizure frequency, some others may paradoxicially have more delusion when epilepsy is controlled. Finally, surgical treatment may fail to prevent the prolongation, or the secondary development, of psychosis and delusions (Bladin, 1992).

Emotional disturbances

Patients with temporal lobe epilepsy have a high prevalence of interictal emotional problems, mostly anxiety and depression (Perini, 1986; Altshculer et al., 1990).

Depression occurs frequently in epileptic patients (7.5% to 25%) and does not seem related to a psychological reaction to having a chronic illness (Mendez, Cummings and Benson, 1986). Depression seems more frequent in patients with left-sided foci, and could be more specifically related to a limbic dysfunction (Mendez et al., 1986; Altshuler et al., 1990; Hermann et al., 1991). The intactness of the frontal lobe may be of some importance (Hermann et al., 1991). Many studies reported an increased risk of suicide in epileptics (up to three-fold or five-fold compared with the nonepileptic population; Barraclough, 1987), although these findings have been recently challenged (Diehl, 1997; Harris and Barraclough, 1997). However, temporal lobe epilepsy patients appear at particular risk for suicide (Barraclough, 1987), and that risk seems to be related more with psychotic behaviors and psychic auras than with major depression or the psychosocial burden of being epileptic (Mendez et al., 1986; Mendez and Doss, 1992). Temporal surgery may lower the incidence of depression, but does not clearly modify the risk of suicide (Bladin, 1992; Guldvog et al., 1994).

Interictal anxiety or panic attacks are also relatively common in temporal lobe epilepsy. Anxiety may be particularly related to right-sided foci (Druback and Kelly, 1989; Ross, 1997); however, this point is not clearly established (Altshuler et al., 1990; Hermann et al., 1991). Roth has reported a strong association between temporal lobe epilepsy and phobic anxiety, which he described as a 'phobic–anxiety–depersonalization' syndrome (Roth and Argyle, 1988). Recently, Toni et al. (1996) suggested that panic disorder–agoraphobia (the current equivalent of 'phobic–anxiety–depersonalization') could have a greater than chance association with seizures, maybe because of a common neurophysiological substrate.

Aggression

Like ictal aggressiveness, interictal aggressiveness has raised many medicolegal controversies. During the past half-century, it was often reported that a high proportion of temporal lobe epilepsy patients present with interictal aggressiveness (Strauss, 1989). Several surveys of aggressive criminals have found a significant incidence of temporal lobe epilepsy. However, several factor variables were associated with an increased risk of aggressive behavior: male sex, left-sided epileptic focus, early onset of seizures, low IQ, and poor early environment (Taylor, 1969a; Hermann and Whitman, 1984). Thus, the high prevalence of aggressiveness in temporal lobe epilepsy may be due to some confounding variables (Hermann and Whitman, 1984). When patients with psychiatric disorders or subnormal intelligence are excluded, there is no increased evidence of violence. The frequency of violent crimes is similar among prisoners with temporal lobe epilepsy and those with other epilepsies (Hermann and Whitman, 1984; Trieman, 1986).

Recently, Devinsky et al. (1994) have suggested that lateralization of the seizure focus in patients with temporal lobe epilepsy may alter the expression of aggressive behavior. They compared the profile on the Buss–Durkee Hostility Inventory (BDHI), a standardized questionnaire of aggressive tendencies, of adult patients with left, right, or bilateral temporal lobe epilepsy, or with absence epilepsy, and normal controls. Patients with left temporal lobe seizure foci scored higher on the suspicion scale than did other patients or controls. The groups differed in their pattern on three factor scores provided by a factor analysis (hostile feelings, covert aggression, and overt aggression). Patients with left temporal lobe epilepsy scored higher than other groups on hostile feelings; bitemporal patients scored higher on overt aggression. Patients with absence seizures did not differ from controls: both groups scored higher on covert aggression. Thus, the impression of a higher aggressiveness in patients with temporal lobe epilepsy may simply stem from a more overt expression of hostile feelings.

Sexual behavior

Various studies have described an unusually common incidence of sexual and reproductive dysfunction in patients affected by temporal lobe epilepsy (Shukla et al., 1979a; Daniele et al., 1997). The rare studies that have contrasted TLE patients and individuals with other seizures (Shukla et al., 1979a; Strauss, 1989) found constantly that TLE patients showed more sexual dysfunction.

Hyposexuality (reduced libido or impotence) is the more common disorder in TLE, ranging from 40% to 70% of patients (Taylor, 1969b). Sexual disorders seem more frequent for mediobasal temporal foci as compared to temporal lobe convexity (Cogen, Antunes and Correll, 1979), and more frequent for right-sided sites as compared to left (Daniele et al., 1997). The close physiological relationship of medial temporal areas with the hypothalamus could explain a functional alteration of the hypothalamic–pituitary control of gonadotropin secretion (Pritchard et al., 1982; Herzog et al., 1986; Gallagher, 1987). In some patients, temporal lobectomy may restore normal sexual function (Blumer and Walker, 1967; Taylor, 1969b; Cogen et al., 1979); however, temporal lobectomy may itself induce sexual disturbances (Blumer and Walker, 1967; Cherlow and Serafetinides, 1977; Shukla et al., 1979a; Christianson et al., 1995). Sexual deviations or hypersexuality seem exceedingly rare (Shukla et al., 1979a). At the present time, no firm conclusions can be drawn about the relationship between sexual disturbance and TLE, because a number of other factors may also influence sexual behavior. Factors such as anxiety, depression, availability of social relationships, and side-effects of anticonvulsant therapies may also play an important role.

Critical analysis

Although literature devoted to disturbances of emotional behavior in epilepsy constitute the largest available corpus of data regarding the role of temporal lobes in behavior, these data must be used very carefully. Strauss (1989) has highlighted three main methodological issues that may hinder the accurate assessment of behavior disturbance in temporal lobe epilepsy. The first point is related to a rather imprecise definition of temporal lobe epilepsy. Many variations have been observed in the nomenclature, in the diagnostic criteria, and in the adequacy of the EEG techniques. The second point is that the majority of studies have used patients with generalized epilepsy as control subjects, when a more appropriate comparison would have been patients with partial epilepsy originating from other cerebral regions. The third and major issue is that TLE does not represent a well-defined homogeneous entity. Thus, behavioral trends that are observed may represent a mean of the characteristics of various subtypes and not the profile of precise temporal foci. The most robust correlation could, however, be established with medial temporal regions. Recent studies have demonstrated that approximately 60% to 80% of patients who have complex partial seizures have pathological evidence of medial temporal sclerosis (Tien et al., 1993). Magnetic resonance imaging (MRI) could provide a reliable technique of exploration as it has demonstrated an 80% accuracy in determining this sclerosis in vivo by an increased signal in T2-weighted images of FLAIR sequences (Byrum et al., 1997).

Klüver–Bucy syndrome

The Klüver–Bucy syndrome is considered as the most typical temporolimbic syndrome because of its specificity for bilateral anterior temporal lesions (Trimble et al., 1997). As the Klüver–Bucy syndrome is detailed elsewhere in this volume, only the most salient features are presented here.

The original description is due to Klüver and Bucy (1937, 1939), who reported a characteristic pattern of behavioral changes occurring in rhesus monkeys after bilateral resection of major portions of the temporal lobes. In adult rhesus monkeys, the complete syndrome includes the following (Trimble et al., 1997): tameness, with loss of fear and anxiety, or diminished aggression; dietary changes, with bulimia and loss of alimentary selectivity (animals may eat previously rejected foods); aberrant sexual behavior, with increased autoerotic, homosexual, or heterosexual activities, or inappropriate sexual object choice; hypermetamorphosis, defined as an excessive visual exploration of the environment; hyperorality, with a tendency to examine all objects by mouth; 'psychic blindness' corresponding to a visual agnosia.

After the original report in monkeys, similar syndromes have repeatedly been reported in various human pathologies. The first case was described after a bilateral temporal lobectomy for intractable seizures (Terzian and Dalle Ore, 1955), but the most frequent cause is herpes simplex encephalitis (Pilleri, 1966; Marlowe, Mancall and Thomas, 1975; Lilly et al., 1983; Bakchine, Chain and Lhermitte, 1986; Goscinski et al., 1997; Trimble et al., 1997). The Klüver–Bucy syndrome is excessively rare in humans, especially in its complete form. The diagnosis requires the presence of at least three of the six symptoms listed above. The human syndrome usually presents with some differences compared with the syndrome observed in monkeys. The most common symptoms are placidity, bulimia, hyperorality, and indiscriminate dietary behavior (Bakchine and Derouesne, 1989), whereas loss of sexual interest is much more common than hypersexuality (Bakchine et al., 1986). In these authors' experience, hypersexuality is excessively rare, with the exception of transitory compulsive masturbation that may be observed during the early stages. During chronic stages, hyposexuality associated with a tendency to make silly and childish sexual proposals directed indifferently to either sex was observed more often than true hypersexuality. Bulimia, if not strictly controlled, may lead to major gain in weight (ranging from 25 to 48 kg after six months in a personal series: Bakchine and Derouesne, 1989). The hyperorality behavior may lead to life-threatening situations (Mendez and Foti, 1997): one patient underwent three gastroscopies and one bronchoscopy in one year to remove nonalimentary material. He finally died three years after disease onset from pharmacological intoxication after swallowing the entire contents of the family medicine chest, unfortunately left unlocked by his wife. Another characteristic feature of the Klüver–Bucy syndrome in humans is the high frequency of severe accompanying cognitive deficits, mainly amnesia, loss of semantic knowledge, aphasia, and visual or multimodal agnosia (Gerstenbrand et al., 1983; Damasio et al., 1985; Bakchine et al., 1986; Goscinski et al., 1997; Trimble et al., 1997).

Abundant data have demonstrated that amygdalae are the most important lesional sites within the temporal lobes to produce the Klüver–Bucy syndrome (LeDoux, 1992, 1996; Aggleton, 1993; Fukuda and Ono, 1993; King et al., 1993; Gallagher and Chiba, 1996; Mega et al., 1997; Pitkänen, Savander and LeDoux, 1997). In animals, the amygdala seems to have an important role in giving motivational and emotional meaning to sensory stimuli by learning to associate stimuli, mainly visual, with primary reinforcement, including both punishments and rewards (Aggleton, 1993; Rolls, 1995). Other studies in animals have shown that the amygdala contains neurons that respond selectively to the emotional and social significance of faces (Rolls, 1995; LeDoux, 1996). Both face identity and facial expression provide important information regarding social and emotional responses to other primates, which must be based on the identity of who is seen, as well as on the facial expression or gesture being made. In humans, both clinical and functional imaging studies – with positron emission tomography (PET) or functional MRI (fMRI) – have demonstrated that the amygdala may process emotional facial expressions, and could mediate pleasant or unpleasant emotions (Adolphs et al., 1994, 1996; George et al., 1995; Lane et al., 1997; Weniger et al, 1997; Morris et al., 1998). In line with these observations, many symptoms of the Klüver–Bucy syndrome may be considered as revealing a 'visual–limbic disconnection' (Aggleton, 1993; Rolls, 1995). Tameness of the Klüver–Bucy syndrome, and the inability of amygdalectomized monkeys to interact normally in a social group may be the consequences of damage to this system, which is specialized for processing faces.

Sexual behavior

Sexuality changes are frequently reported in temporal lesions. As described above, hyposexuality is more common than hypersexuality in TLE, and it is one of the main characteristics of the Gastaut–Geschwind syndrome. In other pathologies, as in TLE, hyposexuality seems to be more frequent after damage to medial temporal areas, with a higher incidence for right-sided lesions (Mandal et al., 1996; Cummings, 1997; Daniele et al., 1997). Biological studies suggest the possibility of a subclinical hypogonadotropic hypogonadism secondary to functional or anatomic damage to pathways connecting the medial temporal lobe with the hypothalamus (Herzog et al., 1986; Gallagher, 1987). However, other causes of hyposexuality, such as depression, anxiety, or side-effects of treatments (antiepileptics, hypotensive drugs), must be systematically checked in brain-damaged patients.

Depression, mania, and bipolar syndromes

Besides its high frequency in epilepsy (see above), depression is certainly a very common complication of brain focal lesions. Patients with strokes, brain tumors, or focal contusions in the left hemisphere have a high prevalence of depression

(Flor-Henry, 1979; Gainotti, 1989; Cummings, 1993b; Jorge et al., 1993a; Ghika-Schmid and Bogousslavsky, 1997; Robinson, 1997). Large series of clinical studies have shown that clinical correlates of postlesional depression include less severe aspects of physical and cognitive impairment than brain localization issues (Tucker and Liotti, 1989; Jorge et al., 1993a). Although the most frequent sites are the frontal lobe and the striatum (caudate nucleus), depression following anterior temporal lobe damage has also been reported (Starkstein, Robinson and Price, 1987b; Starkstein et al., 1988a; Gainotti, 1989; Joseph, 1992; Jorge et al., 1993a; LeDoux, 1996).

Mania is a far less frequent complication of brain lesions compared to depression, but also seems to be related to temporal lesions (Evans, Byerly and Greer, 1995; Ghika-Schmid and Bogousslavsky, 1997). Among various causal pathologies, such as stroke, tumors, and closed-head injury, the last-mentioned is the most frequent, with a nine times higher prevalence compared to strokes (Cummings and Mendez, 1984; Shukla et al., 1987; Starkstein et al., 1987a, 1990; Jorge et al., 1993b; Evans et al., 1995). Recent reports have emphasized the importance of lesion site. Almost all secondary manias are observed in right-hemisphere-damaged patients and seem to be associated with lesions resulting in direct or indirect (orbitofrontal cortex, thalamus) dysfunction of the basotemporal cortex in the right hemisphere (Bogousslavsky et al., 1988; Starkstein et al., 1988b, 1990; Bakchine et al., 1989; Jorge et al., 1993b). After brain damage, patients may also develop a bipolar affective disorder, the cycling succession of mania and depression. A study compared patients presenting with bipolar or pure mania and found differences with regard to the pattern of lesions: when all bipolar patients had subcortical lesions, those with pure mania showed a significantly higher frequency of cortical involvement as well as larger lesions (Starkstein et al., 1991).

The mechanism of secondary mania appears rather complex and is not clearly understood. Starkstein stated that the rare occurrence of secondary mania could be explained by the necessary confluence of several specific factors: anterior subcortical atrophy and a focal lesion of a limbic or limbic-connected region of the right hemisphere, or genetic loading and a limbic-connected right hemisphere lesion (Starkstein et al., 1987a). Recently, Starkstein and Robinson (1997) proposed that basotemporal and orbitofrontal regions could be critical structures for the emergence of postlesional disinhibited behaviors. Considering that both structures constitute the main cortical output to paralimbic areas, they hypothesized that any damage to those structures or to connecting pathways could result in emotional disinhibition.

Functional neuroimaging with PET, single positron emission tomography (SPECT), or fMRI may provide important insights into the neural substrate of mood and emotional behavior by showing how mood changes correlate with disturbances in a complex network involving mainly the temporolimbic structures (amygdala), the frontal lobes, the striatum (caudate), and the thalamus (Drevets and Raichle, 1995). Patients with depression showed asymmetric modifications of blood flow with an increase in the left thalamus, frontal, and temporolimbic regions (Drevets and Raichle, 1995; Gyulai et al., 1997). When the depression resolves, symmetry is restored. Studies of provoked emotions provide similar results (George et al., 1995; Lane et al., 1997).

Postlesional depression or mania may have a serious impact on social functioning, on rehabilitation efforts, and on long-term recovery after brain damage. It is highly recommended to treat these disturbances (Gustafson et al., 1995; Bakchine, 1998b).

Although antidepressant medication has been shown to be effective in treating postlesional depression, there are very few controlled trials that may help in the choice of a specific drug (Gustafson et al., 1995). Tricyclic antidepressants cannot be recommended because of the high frequency of contraindications and adverse effects. Various drugs have been proposed, such as imipramine or desipramine (Lauritzen et al., 1994), selective serotonin reuptake inhibitors (Andersen, 1995), psychostimulants (Masand, Murray and Pickett, 1991). Electroconvulsive therapy has been considered effective in severe forms (Gustafson et al., 1995). Since recent studies suggested that daily left prefrontal repetitive transcranial magnetic stimulation has antidepressant activity, this technique should be evaluated in the treatment of postlesional depression (Bakchine, 1998b).

The treatment of postlesional mania is not significantly different from the treatment of idiopathic manic troubles. Neuroleptics should be reserved for the acute phase treatment of intense manic troubles. Likewise, carbamazepine and lithium carbonate appear efficient (Cummings and Mendez, 1984; Bakchine et al., 1989; Zwil et al., 1993; Evans et al., 1995).

The reader will find a more detailed description and discussion of postlesional depression and mania elsewhere in this volume (see Chapters 5 and 7).

Anxiety and fear

Although less frequent than depression, anxiety is also observed with focal brain lesions, usually involving the temporolimbic lobe (Gainotti, 1989; Tucker and Liotti, 1989; Cummings, 1997). In animals, the amygdala is a key structure in fear conditioning (Gray, 1995; LeDoux, 1995; Rogan, Staubli and LeDoux, 1997). In humans, direct electrical stimulation of any limbic sector may evoke a visceral sensation or an emotion, usually fear or anxiety (Joseph, 1992; Halgren and Marinkovic, 1995). As described above, anxiety is a common interictal change and does not seem related to a specific side of the foci (Perini, 1986; Altshuler et al., 1990). Several studies reported that lesions could involve mainly right temporolimbic areas (Druback and Kelly, 1989; Hermann et al., 1991; Ross, 1997). Studies with stroke or closed-head injuries showed that anxiety may co-occur with depression and that anxious depression was also associated with right hemisphere lesions (Robinson and Starkstein, 1990; Jorge et al., 1993a).

Studies with PET scan showed contrasting results regarding temporolimbic involvement in anxiety: the right amygdala flow increased during induced anxiety, but no changes have been observed in the amygdala in panic disorder (Drevets and Raichle, 1995).

Aggressive and violent behaviors

Aggressive and violent behaviors have particular importance as patients exhibiting these behaviors may be involved in legal problems. There is also a recent shift in criminal defence strategies to present in court a 'neurologic defence' attempting to explain a defendant's criminal behaviors based upon the presence of brain disease (Miller et al., 1997). Therefore, investigators have tried to document an association between aggressive or criminal behaviors and brain illnesses, with two main strategies: first, assess these behaviors in patients with known brain pathologies; second, look for brain pathologies in violent subjects or in criminals. However, few studies have reached conclusive results.

The relationship between damage to temporal lobes and aggressive or violent behaviors has been noticed for many years (Blumer and Benson, 1975). The largest corpus of data comes from studies in patients with TLE (see above) that have documented the presence of interictal violence and aggression among other behavioral abnormalities. 'Episodic dyscontrol' is a much more controversial concept, which is characterized by intermittent explosive behavior, and sometimes temporal EEG abnormalities (Rickler, 1982). In other pathologies, the issue of whether patients with temporal (especially medial) injuries have a higher than expected frequency of violent behavior is controversial, although a majority of reports seem to confirm such a relationship (Mark and Sweet, 1974; Miller et al., 1997; Trieman, 1986; Suzuki et al., 1992; Raine, 1993). In animals, bilateral destruction of the amygdala usually results in reduced aggressiveness (Vochteloo and Koolhaas, 1987; LeDoux, 1995, 1996). In humans, bilateral amygdala surgical destruction has been reported to reduce violent behaviors (Kiloh et al., 1974; Kiloh and Smith, 1978).

Many studies have reported brain abnormalities in violent subjects of criminals (Mark and Ervin, 1970; Lewis et al., 1986, 1988; Raine, 1993). Unfortunately, the location of the abnormalities was often not well defined. When mentioned, the localization is often temporal or frontal (Lewis et al., 1986, 1988; Blake, Pincus and Buckner, 1995). An exemplary case has been reported by Sweet, Ervin and Mark (1969), who described the case of CV, a man who suddenly started to shoot indiscriminately at people from a tower at the University of Texas, killing 14 people and wounding 38. The autopsy revealed a tumor compressing the left amygdala.

Some metabolic studies provided data confirming the results of clinical studies. A recent study (Seidenwurm et al., 1997) showed a decrease in temporal lobe metabolism, especially in the medial part, in a selected population of violent subjects, results that confirmed similar data obtained in aggressive psychiatric patients (Volkow and Tancredi, 1987; Volkow et al., 1995) and in criminals (Raine, 1993). However, no specific pattern emerged from these studies. In some subjects, the major metabolic decrease was found within the temporal lobes, in others within the frontal regions. Similar variations were observed with regard to right/left asymmetries. Moreover, it is far from demonstrated that all subjects with hypometabolism in similar areas ever exhibit criminal or even aggressive behavior (Miller et al., 1995).

Finally, these results still appear to be somewhat uncertain, as a constellation of mitigating factors often observed in violent subjects (perinatal neglect, childhood physical or sexual abuse, sexual disturbance, low intellect) may hamper any definite conclusion (Mark and Sweet, 1974; Hermann and Whitman, 1984). Thus, further study is warranted to determine the role of structural or functional abnormalities in the brain in aggression and violent behaviors.

The reader will find a section specifically devoted to aggression in brain injury elsewhere in this volume (see Chapter 14).

Delusion, psychotic symptoms, and schizophrenia

Delusions and psychotic symptoms have been frequently described in various temporal lobe pathologies, such as tumors or strokes (Davison and Bagley, 1969; Malamud, 1975; Lishman, 1989; Heilman, Bowers and Valenstein, 1993), but have been especially studied in TLE patients (see above). Capgras syndrome is a variety of delusion in which patients regard people whom they know well, such as their spouses or parents, as being replaced by an impostor. Several neuroimaging studies showed the involvement of medial temporal regions, more frequently right than left, in various associations, often with right or bilateral frontal areas (Ellis, 1994; Forstl et al., 1994; Signer, 1994; Mentis et al., 1995; Sellal et al., 1996). These results may suggest that the mechanism of Capgras delusion lies in damage to neuroanatomical pathways responsible for appropriate emotional reactions to familiar visual stimuli (Young et al., 1993).

At the end of the twentieth century, schizophrenia offers a fascinating domain of controversy regarding the role of temporal lobes in behavior. Many recent contemporary findings appear consistent with models involving an aberrant development of temporal lobe structures in schizophrenia (Gray, 1995; Arnold, 1997; Bogerts, 1997; Crow, 1997). It is interesting to point out that, from his early description of the 'dementia praecox,' Kraepelin (1919) suggested that hallucinations and thought disorder may be related to an irritative damage to the temporal lobes. Later, many reports have highlighted the clinical similarities between schizophrenia and 'schizophrenia-like' syndromes observed after pathologies involving the temporal lobes. The idea of a link between temporal lobes and schizophrenia has received the support of converging evidence from the modern techniques of neurosciences (see the review in Arnold, 1997). Neuropsychological studies have shown that schizophrenic patients had, among other cognitive impairments, a more severe memory deficit (Saykin et al., 1994), especially in verbal learning, verbal, and visual memory. All these deficits may be related to temporomedial impairment, with a trend for a greater left-sided involvement, as verbal performances are often more altered (Saykin et al., 1994; Bogerts, 1997). Several authors report deficits of working memory (Schroder et al., 1996; Gold et al., 1997) which, together with deficits in frontal executive functions, may suggest that frontal regions may also make an important contribution to the pathophysiology of schizophrenia (Evans et al., 1997; Weinberger and Gallhofer, 1997). Recent results from transverse or longitudinal studies (Chua and Murray, 1996; Censits et al., 1997; Mockler, Riordan and Sharma, 1997) support a neurodevelopmental model of schizophrenia, by showing that patients demonstrated cognitive deficits from the first episode and did not show decline at follow-up or with age. Postmorten studies provide growing evidence for the hypothesis of an early acquired dysplasia and against a neurodegenerative disorder. Three main categories of anatomic findings support this hypothesis: (1) the demonstration of cytoarchitectural abnormalities in the temporal, limbic, and frontal areas; (2) the lack of gliosis in the affected regions; and (3) the absence of progressivity in tissue loss. Finally, convergent data from structural and functional neuroimaging studies demonstrate abnormalities in both the temporolimbic (mainly left) and the prefrontal (mainly right) structures (Crow, 1995; Schroder et al., 1995; Turetsky et al., 1995; Arnold, 1997; Kindermann et al., 1997). Many aspects remain unclear, such as the genetic, molecular, and cellular nature of these abnormalities. The physiopathological link between these structural abnormalities and the many clinical features of schizophrenia remain controversial (for a detailed discussion see Bogerts, 1997, and Gray, 1995). The role of medial temporal lobe is also under investigation for autism (Bachevalier, 1996).

Conclusion

Studies of patients with focal lesions to temporolimbic structures provide an extensive range of symptoms concerning emotion, personality, and social functioning. A large network including hippocampus, amygdala, and multiple cortical and subcortical circuits appears to modulate affect and emotional behavior. The connections with frontal orbital and prefrontal regions appear especially important. Although some syndromes appear to be specific to temporal lobe lesions, such as the Klüver–Bucy and the Gastaut–Geschwind syndromes, most symptoms are difficult to localize specifically to the temporal lobes, or to the left or right sides. This may be explained in terms of the extended temporolimbic system working as a parallel distributed processing network. Further research is warranted to further clarify the very complex neural network of emotion. Methodological issues are important, mainly the development of specific tools seems mandatory. Data that will come from anatomic and functional imaging studies may be particularly useful in developing neuropsychological theories on emotion. Research in this field may also provide valuable advances, allowing for a better comprehension of some of the most devastating illnesses for the mind – schizophrenia and autism.

Acknowledgment

Many thanks to Liliane Manning for revising the manuscript and helpful comments.

REFERENCES

Adolphs, R., Damasio, H., Tranel, D. and Damasio, A.R. (1996). Cortical systems for the recognition of emotion in facial expressions. *J Neurosci* 16: 7678–87.

Adolphs, R., Tranel, D., Damasio, H. and Damasio, A. (1994). Impaired recognition of emotion in facial expressions following bilateral damage to the human amygdala. *Nature* 372: 669–72.

Aggleton, J.P. (1993). The contribution of the amygdala to normal and abnormal emotional states. *Trends Neurosci* 16: 328–33.

Alheid, G.F. and Heimer, L. (1996). Theories of basal forebrain organisation and the 'emotional motor system'. In *The Emotional Motor System*, ed. G. Holstege, R. Bandler and C. Saper, pp. 461–84. Amsterdam: Elsevier.

Altshuler, L.L., Devinsky, O., Post, R.M. and Theodore, W. (1990). Depression, anxiety, and temporal lobe epilepsy. Laterality of focus and symptoms. *Arch Neurol* 47: 284–8.

Andersen, G. (1995). Treatment of uncontrolled crying after stroke. *Drugs Aging* 6: 105–11.

Arnold, S.E. (1997). The medial temporal lobe in schizophrenia. *J Neuropsychiatry Clin Neurosci* 9: 460–70.

Bachevalier, J. (1996). Brief report: medial temporal lobe and autism: a putative animal model in primates. *J Autism Dev Disord* 26: 217–20.

Bakchine, S. (1991). Problèmes méthodologiques rencontrés dans l'évaluation des perturbations comportementales dans les démences d'Alzheimer. *Rev Geriatr* 16: 59–64.

Bakchine, S. (1998a). Déficits non-cognitifs de la MA: une illustration des difficultés méthodologiques rencontrées dans l'abord de la psychopathologie lors des démences organiques. In *Troubles des Affects et de la Motivation en Neurologie. Rapport au Congrès de Psychiatrie et de Neurologie de Langue Française, 96e session*, ed. M. Habib and S. Bakchine. Paris: Masson.

Bakchine, S. (1998b). Dépressions et manies post-lésionnelles. In *Troubles des Affects et de la Motivation en Neurologie. Rapport au Congrès de Psychiatrie et de Neurologie de Langue Française, 96e session*, ed. M. Habib and S. Bakchine. Paris: Masson.

Bakchine, S., Chain, F. and Lhermitte, F. (1986). Syndrome de Kluver–Bucy humain complet après une encéphalite à herpes simplex type 2. *Rev Neurol (Paris)* 142: 126–32.

Bakchine, S. and Derouesne, C. (1989). Le syndrome de Kluver–Bucy chez l'homme: étude des troubles du comportement alimentaire. *Rev Prat* 39: 399–401.

Bakchine, S., Lacomblez, L., Benoit, N. et al. (1989). Manic-like state after bilateral orbitofrontal and right temporoparietal injury: efficacy of clonidine. *Neurology* 39: 777–81.

Bancaud, J., Favel, P., Bonis, A. et al. (1971). Paroxysmal sexual manifestations and temporal epilepsy. *Electroencephalogr Clin Neurophysiol* 30: 371.

Barraclough, B.M. (1987). The suicide rate of epilepsy. *Acta Psychiatr Scand* 76: 339–45.

Bear, D.M. (1997). Interictal behavior in temporal lobe epilepsy. In *Behavioral Neurology and the Legacy of Norman Geschwind*, ed. S.C. Schacter and O. Devinsky, pp. 213–22. Philadelphia: Lippincott-Raven.

Bear, D.M. and Fedio, P. (1977). Quantitative analysis of interictal behavior in temporal lobe epilepsy. *Arch Neurol* 34: 454–67.

Bear, D., Schenk, L. and Benson, H. (1981). Increased autonomic responses to neutral and emotional stimuli in patients with temporal lobe epilepsy. *Am J Psychiatry* 138: 843–5.

Benson, D.F. (1991). The Geschwind syndrome. *Adv Neurol* 55: 411–21.

Bingley, T. (1958). Mental symptoms in temporal lobe epilepsy and temporal lobe gliomas. *Acta Psychiatr Neurol Scand* 33: 136–51.

Bladin, P.F. (1992). Psychosocial difficulties and outcome after temporal lobectomy. *Epilepsia* 33: 898–907.

Blake, P.Y., Pincus, J.H. and Buckner, C. (1995). Neurological abnormalities in murderers. *Neurology* 45: 1641–7.

Blumer, D. (1971). The sexual behavior of patients with temporal lobe epilepsy before and after surgical treatment. Observations on the part played by the limbic system in the regulation of sexual activity. *J Neurovisc Relat* 20 Suppl.: 10: 469–76.

Blumer, D. and Benson, D.F. (1975). Personality changes with frontal and temporal lobe lesions. In *Psychiatric Aspects of Neurological Disease*, ed. D.F. Benson and D. Blumer, pp. 151–70. New York: Grune and Stratton.

Blumer, D. and Walker, A.E. (1967). Sexual behavior in temporal lobe epilepsy. A study of the effects of temporal lobectomy on sexual behavior. *Arch Neurol* 16: 37–43.

Bogerts, B. (1997). The temporolimbic system theory of positive schizophrenic symptoms. *Schizophr Bull* 23: 423–35.

Bogousslavsky, J., Ferrazini, M., Regli, F. et al. (1988). Manic delirium and frontal-like syndrome with paramedian infarction of the right thalamus. *J Neurol Neurosurg Psychiatry* 51: 116–19.

Byrum, C.E., Thompson, J.E., Heinz, E.R., Krishnan, K.R. and Tien, R.D. (1997). Limbic circuits and neuropsychiatric disorders: functional anatomy and neuroimaging findings. *Neuroimaging Clin N Am* 7: 79–99.

Censits, D.M., Ragland, J.D., Gur, R.C. and Gur, R.E. (1997). Neuropsychological evidence supporting a neurodevelopmental model of schizophrenia: a longitudinal study. *Schizophr Res* 24: 289–98.

Cherlow, D.G. and Serafetinides, E.A. (1977). The measurement of emotional concepts in patients with temporal lobe epilepsy. *Dis Nerv Syst* 38: 613–16.

Christianson, S.A., Silfvenius, H., Saisa, J. and Nilsson, M. (1995). Life satisfaction and sexuality in patients operated for epilepsy. *Acta Neurol Scand* 92: 1–6.

Chua, S.E. and Murray, R.M. (1996). The neurodevelopmental theory of schizophrenia: evidence concerning structure and neuropsychology. *Ann Med* 28: 547–55.

Cogen, P.H., Antunes, J.L. and Correll, J.W. (1979). Reproductive function in temporal lobe epilepsy: the effect of temporal lobectomy. *Surg Neurol* 12: 243–6.

Crow, T.J. (1995). Brain changes and negative symptoms in schizophrenia. *Psychopathology* 28: 18–21.

Crow, T.J. (1997). Schizophrenia as failure of hemispheric dominance for language. *TINS* 20: 339–43.

Cummings, J.L. (1993a). Frontal–subcortical circuits and human behavior. *Arch Neurol* 50: 873–80.

Cummings, J.L. (1993b). The neuroanatomy of depression. *J Clin Psychiatry* 54 Suppl.: 14–20.

Cummings, J.L. (1997). Neuropsychiatric manifestations of right hemisphere lesions. *Brain Lang* 57: 22–37.

Cummings, J.L. and Mendez, M.F. (1984). Secondary mania with focal cerebrovascular lesions. *Am J Psychiatry* 141: 1084–7.

Daly, D.D. and Mulder, D.W. (1957). Gelastic epilepsy. *Neurology* 7: 189–92.

Damasio, A.R., Eslinger, P.J., Damasio, H., Van Hoesen, G.W. and Cornell, S. (1985). Multimodal amnesic syndrome following bilateral temporal and basal forebrain damage. *Arch Neurol* 42: 252–9.

Daniele, A., Azzoni, A., Bizzi, A. et al. (1997). Sexual behavior and hemispheric laterality of the focus in patients with temporal lobe epilepsy. *Biol Psychiatry* 42: 617–24.

Davison, K. and Bagley, C.R. (1969). Schizophrenia-like psychoses associated with organic disorders of the central nervous system: a review of the literature. In *Current Problems in Neuropsychiatry*, ed. R.N. Herrington, pp. 113–84. Ashford: Royal Medico-psychological Association, Headley Brothers, Ltd.

Delgado-Escueta, A.V., Mattson, R.H., King, L. et al. (1981). Special report. The nature of aggression during epileptic seizures. *N Engl J Med* 305: 711–16.

Devinsky, O. and Bear, D. (1984). Varieties of aggressive behavior in temporal lobe epilepsy. *Am J Psychiatry* 141: 651–6.

Devinsky, O., Ronsaville, D., Cox, C. et al. (1994). Interictal aggression in epilepsy: the Buss–Durkee Hostility Inventory. *Epilepsia* 35: 585–90.

Devinsky, O. and Vaquez, B. (1993). Behavioral changes associated with epilepsy. *Neurol Clinics* 11: 127–49.

Diehl, L.W. (1997). Epilepsy and suicide – a new evaluation. Prevalence and classification of methods. *Versicherungsmedizin* 49: 203–8.

Dodrill, C.B. and Batzel, L.W. (1986). Interictal behavioral features of patients with epilepsy. *Epilepsia* 27 Suppl. 2: S64–76.

Drevets, W.C. and Raichle, M.E. (1995). Positron emission tomographic imaging studies of human emotional disorders. In *The Cognitive Neurosciences*, ed. M.S. Gazzaniga, pp. 1153–64. Cambridge, MA: The MIT Press.

Druback, D.A. and Kelly, M.P. (1989). Panic disorder associated with a right paralimbic lesion. *Neuropsychiatry Neuropsychol Behav Neurol* 2: 282–9.

Ellis, H. (1994). The role of the right hemisphere in the Capgras delusion. *Psychopathology* 27: 177–85.

Evans, D.L., Byerly, M.J. and Greer, R.A. (1995). Secondary mania: diagnosis and treatment. *J Clin Psychiatry* 56 Suppl. 3: 31–7.

Evans, J.J., Chua, S.E., McKenna, P.J. and Wilson, B.A. (1997). Assessment of the dysexecutive syndrome in schizophrenia. *Psychol Med* 27: 635–46.

Fayada, C. and Bakchine, S. (1998). Entre cognition et émotion: réflexions à propos de l'expérience d'une consultation de troubles du comportement. In *Troubles des Affects et de la Motivation en Neurologie. Rapport au Congrès de Psychiatrie et de Neurologie de Langue Française, 96e session*, ed. M. Habib and S. Bakchine. Paris: Masson.

Feyereisen, P. (1989). Theories of emotions and neuropsychological research. In *Handbook of Neuropsychology*, 1st edn, ed. F. Boller and J. Grafman, Vol. 3, *Section 6: Emotional Behavior and its Disorders*, ed. L. Squire and G. Gainotti, pp. 271–82. Amsterdam: Elsevier.

Flor-Henry, P. (1979). On certain aspects of the localization of the cerebral systems regulating and determining emotion. *Biol Psychiatry* 14: 677–98.

Forstl, H., Besthorn, C., Burns, A. et al. (1994). Delusional misidentification in Alzheimer's disease: a summary of clinical and biological aspects. *Psychopathology* 27: 194–9.

Fukuda, M. and Ono, T. (1993). Amygdala–hypothalamic control of feeding behavior in monkeys: single cell responses before and after reversible blockade of temporal cortex or amygdala projections. *Behav Brain Res* 55: 233–41.

Gainotti, G. (1989). Disorders of emotions and affect in patients with unilateral brain damage. In *Handbook of Neuropsychology*, 1st edn, ed. F. Boller and J. Grafman, Vol. 3, *Section 6: Emotional Behavior and its Disorders*, ed. L. Squire and G. Gainotti, pp. 345–62. Amsterdam: Elsevier.

Gallagher, B.B. (1987). Endocrine abnormalities in human temporal lobe epilepsy. *Yale J Biol Med* 60: 93–7.

Gallagher, M. and Chiba, A.A. (1996). The amygdala and emotion. *Curr Opin Neurobiol* 6: 221–7.

Gastaut, H.(1956). Etude électroclinique des épisodes psychotiques survenant en dehors des crises cliniques chez les épileptiques. *Rev Neurol* 94: 587–94.

George, M., Ketter, T., Parekh, P. et al. (1995). Brain activity during transient sadness and happiness in healthy women. *Am J Psychiatry* 152: 341–51.

Gerstenbrand, F., Poewe, W., Aichner, F. and Saltuari, L. (1983). Kluver–Bucy syndrome in man: experiences with posttraumatic cases. *Neurosci Biobehav Rev* 7: 413–17.

Geschwind, N. (1979). Behavioral changes in temporal lobe epilepsy. *Psychol Med* 9: 217–19.

Ghika-Schmid, F. and Bogousslavsky, J. (1997). Affective disorders following stroke. *Eur Neurol* 38: 75–81.

Gloor, P., Olivier, A., Quesney, L.F., Andermann, F. and Horowitz, S. (1982). The role of the limbic system in experiential phenomena of temporal lobe epilepsy. *Ann Neurol* 12: 129–44.

Gold, J.M., Carpenter, C., Randolph, C., Goldberg, T.E. and Weinberger, D.R. (1997). Auditory working memory and Wisconsin Card Sorting Test performance in schizophrenia. *Arch Gen Psychiatry* 54: 159–65.

Goscinski, I., Kwiatkowski, S., Polak, J., Orlowiejska, M. and Partyk, A. (1997). The Kluver–Bucy syndrome. *J Neurosurg Sci* 41: 269–72.

Gray, J.A. (1995). A model of the limbic system and basal ganglia: application to anxiety and schizophrenia. In *The Cognitive Neurosciences*, ed. M.S. Gazzaniga, pp. 1165–76. Cambridge, MA: The MIT Press.

Guldvog, B., Loyning, Y., Hauglie-Hanssen, E., Flood, S. and Bjornaes, H. (1994). Surgical treatment for partial epilepsy among Norwegian adults. *Epilepsia* 35: 540–53.

Gustafson, Y., Nilsson, I., Mattson, M., Astrom, M. and Bucht, G. (1995). Epidemiology and treatment of post-stroke depression. *Drugs Aging* 7: 298–309.

Gyulai, L., Alavi, A., Broich, K. et al. (1997). A I-123 iofetamine single-photon computed emission tomography in rapid cycling bipolar disorder: a clinical study. *Biol Psychiatry* 41: 152–61.

Halgren, E. and Marinkovic, K. (1995). Neurophysiological networks integrating human emotions. In *The Cognitive Neurosciences*, ed. M.S. Gazzaniga, pp. 1137–52. Cambridge, MA: The MIT Press.

Harris, E.C. and Barraclough, B. (1997). Suicide as an outcome for mental disorders. A meta-analysis. *Br J Psychiatry* 170: 205–28.

Heath, R.G. (1972). Pleasure and brain activity in man. Deep and surface electroencephalograms during orgasm. *J Nerv Ment Dis* 154: 3–18.

Heilman, K.M. (1997). The neurobiology of emotional experience. *J Neuropsychiatry Clin Neurosci* 9: 439–48.

Heilman, K.M., Bowers, D. and Valenstein, E. (1993). Emotional disorders associated with neurological diseases. In *Clinical Neuropsychology*, ed. K.M. Heilman and E. Valenstein, 3rd edn, pp. 461–96. Oxford: Oxford University Press.

Heilman, K.M. and Watson, R.T. (1989). Arousal and emotions. In *Handbook of Neuropsychology*, 1st edn, ed. F. Boller and J. Grafman, Vol. 3, *Section 6: Emotional Behavior and its Disorders*, ed. L. Squire and G. Gainotti, pp. 403–18. Amsterdam: Elsevier.

Hermann, B.P., Schwartz, M.S., Whitman, S. and Karnes, W.E. (1981). Psychosis and epilepsy: seizure-type comparisons and high-risk variables. *J Clin Psychol* 37: 714–21.

Hermann, B.P., Seidenberg, M., Haltiner, A. and Wyler, A.R. (1991). Mood state in unilateral temporal lobe epilepsy. *Biol Psychiatry* 30: 1205–18.

Hermann, B.P. and Whitman, S. (1984). Behavioral and personality correlates of epilepsy: a review, methodological critique, and conceptual model. *Psychol Bull* 95: 451–97.

Hermann, B. and Whitman, S. (1992). Psychopathology in epilepsy. The role of psychology in altering paradigms of research, treatment, and prevention. *Am Psychol* 47: 1134–8.

Hermann, B.P., Whitman, S. and Arntson, P. (1983). Hypergraphia in epilepsy: is there a specificity to temporal lobe epilepsy? *J Neurol Neurosurg Psychiatry* 46: 848–53.

Herzog, A.G., Seibel, M.M., Schomer, D.L., Vaitukaitis, J.L. and Geschwind, N. (1986). Reproductive endocrine disorders in men with partial seizures of temporal lobe origin. *Arch Neurol* 43: 347–50.

Jackson, J.H. (1931). Lectures on the diagnosis of epilepsy. In *On Epilepsy and Epileptiform*

Convulsions, Selected Writings of John Huglings Jackson, Vol. 1, ed. J. Taylor, pp. 276–307. London: Hodder and Stoughton.

Jibiki, I., Maeda, T., Kubota, T. et al. (1993). 123I-IMP SPECT brain imaging in epileptic psychosis: a study of two cases of temporal lobe epilepsy with schizoprenia-like syndrome. *Neuropsychobiology* 28: 207–11.

Jorge, R.E., Robinson, R.G., Starkstein, S.E. and Arndt, S.V. (1993a). Depression and anxiety following traumatic brain injury. *J Neuropsychiatry Clin Neurosci* 5: 369–74.

Jorge, R.E., Robinson, R.G., Starkstein, S.E. et al. (1993b). Secondary mania following traumatic brain injury. *Am J Psychiatry* 150: 916–21.

Joseph, R. (1992). The limbic system: emotion, laterality, and unconscious mind. *Psychoanal Rev* 79: 405–56.

Keschner, M., Bender, M. and Strauss, I. (1936). Mental symptoms in cases of tumors of the temporal lobe. *Arch Neurol Psychiatry* 35: 572–96.

Kiloh, L.G., Gye, R.S., Rushworth, R.G., Bell, D.S. and White, R.T. (1974). Stereotactic amygdaloidotomy for aggressive behavior. *J Neurol Neurosurg Psychiatry* 37: 437–44.

Kiloh, L.G. and Smith, J.S. (1978). The neural basis of aggression and its treatment by psychosurgery. *Aust N Z J Psychiatry* 12: 21–8.

Kindermann, S.S., Karimi, A., Symonds, L., Brown, G.G. and Jeste, D.V. (1997). Review of functional magnetic resonance imaging in schizophrenia. *Schizophr Res* 27: 143–56.

King, B.M., Kass, J.M., Cadieux, N.L. et al. (1993). Hyperphagia and obesity in female rats with temporal lobe lesions. *Physiol Behav* 54: 759–65.

Klüver, H. and Bucy, P.C. (1937). 'Psychic blindness' and other symptoms following bilateral temporal lobectomy in rhesus monkeys. *Am J Physiol* 119: 352–3.

Klüver, H. and Bucy, P. (1939). Preliminary analysis of functions of the temporal lobes in monkeys. *Arch Neurol Psychiatry* 42: 979–1000.

Kraepelin, E. (1919). *Dementia Praecox and Paraphrenia*. Edinburgh: Livingstone.

Lane, R.D., Reiman, E.M., Bradley, M.M. et al. (1997). Neuroanatomical correlates of pleasant and unpleasant emotion. *Neuropsychologia* 35: 1437–44.

Lauritzen, L., Bendsen, B.B., Vilmar, T. et al. (1994). Post-stroke depression: combined treatment with imipramine or desipramine and mianserin. A controlled clinical study. *Psychopharmacology* 114: 119–22.

LeDoux, J.E. (1992). Brain mechanisms of emotion and emotional learning. *Curr Opin Neurobiol* 2: 191–7.

LeDoux, J.E. (1995). In search of an emotional system in the brain: leaping from fear to emotion and consciousness. In *The Cognitive Neurosciences*, ed. M.S. Gazzaniga, pp. 1049–62. Cambridge, MA: The MIT Press.

LeDoux, J.E. (1996). *The Emotional Brain*. New York: Simon & Schuster.

Lewis, D.O., Pincus, J.H., Bard, B. et al. (1988). Neuropsychiatric, psychoeducational, and family characteristics of 14 juveniles condemned to death in the United States. *Am J Psychiatry* 145: 584–9.

Lewis, D.O., Pincus, J.H., Feldman, M., Jackson, L. and Bard, B. (1986). Psychiatric, neurological, and psychoeducational characteristics of 15 death row inmates in the United States. *Am J Psychiatry* 143: 838–45.

Lilly, R., Cummings, J.L., Benson, D.F. and Frankel, M. (1983). The human Klüver–Bucy syndrome. *Neurology* 33: 1141–5.

Lishman, W.A. (1968). Brain damage in relation to psychiatric disability after brain injury. *Br J Psychiatry* 114: 373–410.

Lishman, W.A. (1989). *Organic Psychiatry: the Psychological Consequences of Cerebral Disorder.* Boston: Blackwell Scientific Publications.

Malamud, N. (1975). Organic brain disease mistaken for psychiatric disorders. In *Psychiatric Aspects of Neurologic Diseases*, ed. D.F. Benson and D. Blumer. New York: Grune and Stratton.

Mandal, M.K., Mohanty, A., Pandey, R. and Mohanty, S. (1996). Emotion-specific processing deficit in focal brain-damaged patients. *Int J Neurosci* 84: 87–95.

Mark, V.H. and Ervin, F.R. (1970). *Violence and the Brain.* New York: Harper and Row.

Mark, V.H. and Sweet, W.H. (1974). The role of limbic brain dysfunction in aggression. *Res Publ Assoc Res Nerv Ment Dis* 52: 186–200.

Marlowe, W.B., Mancall, E.L. and Thomas, J.J. (1975). Complete Kluver–Bucy syndrome in man. *Cortex* 11: 53–9.

Masand, P., Murray, G.B. and Pickett, P. (1991). Psychostimulants in post-stroke depression. *J Neuropsychiatry Clin Neurosci* 3: 23–7.

McLachlan, R.S. and Blume, W.T. (1980). Isolated fear in complex partial status epilepticus. *Ann Neurol* 8: 639–41.

Mega, M.S. and Cummings, J.L. (1994). Frontal–subcortical circuits and neuropsychiatric disorders. *J Neuropsychiatry Clin Neurosci* 6: 358–70.

Mega, M.S., Cummings, J.L., Salloway, S. and Malloy, P. (1997). The limbic system: an anatomic, phylogenetic, and clinical perspective. *J Neuropsychiatry Clin Neurosci* 9: 315–30.

Mendez, M.F., Cummings, J.L. and Benson, D.F. (1986). Depression in epilepsy. Significance and phenomenology. *Arch Neurol* 43: 766–70.

Mendez, M.F. and Doss, R.C. (1992). Ictal and psychiatric aspects of suicide in epileptic patients. *Int J Psychiatry Med* 22: 231–7.

Mendez, M.F. and Foti, D.J. (1997). Lethal hyperoral behaviour from the Kluver–Bucy syndrome. *J Neurol Neurosurg Psychiatry* 62: 293–4.

Mendez, M.F., Grau, R., Doss, R.C. et al. (1993). Schizophrenia in epilepsy: seizure and psychosis variables. *Neurology* 43: 1073–7.

Mentis, M.J., Weinstein, E.A., Horwitz, B. et al. (1995). Abnormal brain glucose metabolism in the delusional misidentification syndromes: a positron emission tomography study in Alzheimer disease. *Biol Psychiatry* 38: 438–49.

Miller, B., Mena, I., Cummings, J.L. et al. (1995). Neuroimaging in clinical practice. In *Comprehensive Textbook of Psychiatry*, ed. H.I. Kaplan and B.J. Sadock, Vol. VI. Baltimore: Williams and Wilkins.

Miller, B.L., Darby, A., Benson, D.F., Cummings, J.L. and Miller, M.H. (1997). Aggressive, socially disruptive and antisocial behavior associated with fronto-temporal dementia. *Br J Psychiatry* 170: 150–4.

Mocker, D., Riordan, J. and Sharma, T. (1997). Memory and intellectual deficits do not decline with age in schizophrenia. *Schizophr Res* 26: 1–7.

Morris, J.S., Friston, K.J., Büchel, C. et al. (1998). A neuromodulatory role for the human amygdala in processing emotional facial expressions. *Brain* 121: 47–57.

Mungas, D. (1982). Interictal behavior abnormality in temporal lobe epilepsy. A specific syndrome or nonspecific psychopathology? *Arch Gen Psychiatry* 39: 108–11.

Naito, H. and Matsui, N. (1988). Temporal lobe epilepsy with ictal ecstatic state and interictal behavior of hypergraphia. *J Nerv Ment Dis* 176: 123–4.

Papez, J.W. (1937). A proposed mechanism of emotion. *Arch Neurol Psychiatry* 38: 725–43.

Penfield, W. and Jasper, H. (1954). *Epilepsy and the Functional Anatomy of the Human Brain.* Boston: Little Brown.

Perini, G.I. (1986). Emotions and personality in complex partial seizures. *Psychother Psychosom* 45: 141–8.

Persinger, M.A. (1991). Canonical correlation of a temporal lobe signs scale with schizoid and hypomania scales in a normal population: men and women are similar but for different reasons. *Percept Mot Skills* 73: 615–18.

Pilleri, G. (1966). The Kluver–Bucy syndrome in man. A clinico-anatomical contribution to the function of the medial temporal lobe structures. *Psychiatr Neurol (Basel)* 152: 65–103.

Pincus, J.H. (1981). Violence and epilepsy [editorial]. *N Engl J Med* 305: 696–8.

Pincus, J.H. and Tucker, G.J. (1974). *Behavioral Neurology.* New York: Oxford University Press.

Pitkänen, A., Savander, V. and LeDoux, J.E. (1997). Organization of intra-amygdaloid circuitries in the rat: an emerging framework for understanding functions of the amygdala. *TINS* 20: 517–23.

Pritchard, P.B., Lombroso, C.T. and McIntyre, M. (1980). Psychological complications of temporal lobe epilepsy. *Neurology* 30: 227–32.

Pritchard, P.B., Wannamaker, B.B., Sagel, J. and Devillier, C. (1982). Endocrine dysfunction in temporal lobe epilepsy [letter]. *Arch Neurol* 39: 786–7.

Raine, A. (1993). *The Psychopathology of Crime: Criminal Behavior as a Clinical Disorder.* San Diego: Academic Press.

Ramani, V. and Gumnit, R.J. (1981). Intensive monitoring of epileptic patients with a history of episodic aggression. *Arch Neurol* 38: 570–1.

Rao, S.M., Devinsky, O., Grafman, J. et al. (1992). Viscosity and social cohesion in temporal lobe epilepsy. *J Neurol Neurosurg Psychiatry* 55: 149–52.

Remillard, G.M., Andermann, F., Testa, G.F. et al. (1983). Sexual ictal manifestations predominate in women with temporal lobe epilepsy: a finding suggesting sexual dimorphism in the human brain. *Neurology* 33: 323–30.

Rickler, K.C. (1982). Episodic dyscontrol. In *Psychiatric Aspects of Neurological Disease*, ed. D.F. Benson and D. Blumer. New York: Grune and Stratton.

Roberts, M.A., Manshadi, F.F., Bushnell, D.L. and Hines, M.E. (1995). Neurobehavioral dysfunction following mild traumatic brain injury in childhood: a case report with positive findings on positron emission tomography (PET). *Brain Inj* 9: 427–36.

Roberts, O.W., Done, D.J. and Crow, T.J. (1990). A 'mock up' of schizophrenia: temporal-lobe epilepsy and schizophrenia-like psychosis. *Biol Psychiatry* 28: 127–43.

Robinson, L. and Saykin, A.J. (1992). Psychological and psychosocial outcome of anterior temporal lobectomy. In *The Neuropsychology of Epilepsy*, ed. T.L. Bennet, pp. 181–97. New York: Plenum Press.

Robinson, R.G. and Starkstein, S.E. (1990). Current research in affective disorders following stroke. *J Neuropsychiatry Clin Neurosci* 2: 1–14.

Rodin, E.A. (1973). Psychomotor epilepsy and aggressive behavior. *Arch Gen Psychiatry* 28: 210–13.

Rodin, E. and Schmaltz, S. (1984). The Bear–Fedio personality inventory and temporal lobe epilepsy. *Neurology* 34: 591–6.

Rogan, M.T., Staubli, U.V. and LeDoux, J.E. (1997). Fear conditioning induces associative long-term potentiation in the amygdala [see comments]. *Nature* 390: 604–7.

Rolls, E.T. (1995). A theory of emotion and consciousness, and its application to understanding the neural basis of emotion. In *The Cognitive Neurosciences*, ed. M.S. Gazzaniga, pp. 1091–106. Cambridge, MA: The MIT Press.

Ross, E.D. (1997). Right hemisphere syndromes and the neurology of emotion. In *Behavioral Neurology and the Legacy of Norman Geschwind*, ed. S.C. Schacter and O. Devinsky, pp. 183–91. Philadelphia: Lippincott-Raven.

Roth, M. and Argyle, N. (1988). Anxiety, panic and phobic disorders: an overview. *J Psychiatr Res* 22 Suppl. 1: 33–54.

Saver, J.L. and Rabin, J. (1997). The neural substrates of religious experience. *J Neuropsychiatry Clin Neurosci* 9: 498–510.

Saykin, A.J., Shtasel, D.L., Gur, R.E. et al. (1994). Neuropsychology deficits in neuroleptic naive patients with first-episode schizophrenia. *Arch Gen Psychiatry* 51: 124–31.

Schomer, D.L. (1997). Behavioral aspects of temporal lobe epilepsy. In *Behavioral Neurology and the Legacy of Norman Geschwind*, ed. S.C. Schacter and O. Devinsky, pp. 195–206. Philadelphia: Lippincott-Raven.

Schroder, J., Buchsbaum, M.S., Siegel, B.V., Geider, F.J. and Neithammer, R. (1995). Structural and functional correlates of subsyndromes in chronic schizophrenia. *Psychopathology* 28: 38–45.

Schroder, J., Tittel, A., Stockert, A. and Karr, M. (1996). Memory deficits in subsyndromes of chronic schizophrenia. *Schizophr Res* 21: 19–26.

Seidenwurm, D., Pounds, T.R., Globus, A. and Valk, P.E. (1997). Abnormal temporal lobe metabolism in violent subjects: correlation of imaging and neuropsychiatric findings. *Am J Neuroradiol* 18: 625–31.

Sellal, F., Fontaine, S.F., van der Linden, M. Rainville, C. and Labrecque, R. (1996). To be or not to be at home? A neuropsychological approach to delusion for place. *J Clin Exp Neuropsychol* 18: 234–48.

Sethi, P.K. and Rao, T.S. (1976). Gelastic, quiritarian, and cursive elipsepy, A clinicopathological appraisal. *J Neurol Neurosurg Psychiatry* 39: 823–8.

Shukla, G.D., Srivastava, O.N. and Katiyar, B.C. (1979a). Sexual disturbances in temporal lobe epilepsy: a controlled study. *Br J Psychiatry* 134: 288–92.

Shukla, G.D., Srivastava, O.N., Katiyar, B.C., Joshi, V. and Mohan, P.K. (1979b). Psychiatric manifestations in temporal lobe epilepsy: a controlled study. *Br J Psychiatry* 134: 411–17.

Shukla, S., Cook, B., Mukherjee, S., Godwin, C. and Miller, M. (1987). Mania following head trauma. *Am J Psychiatry* 144: 93–6.

Signer, S.F. (1994). Localization and lateralisation in the delusion of substitution: Capgras syndrome and its variants. *Psychopathology* 27: 168–76.

Spiers, P.A., Schomer, D.L., Blume, H.W. and Hochanadel, G.S. (1992). Behavioral alterations in temporo-limbic epilepsy. In *The Neuropsychology of Epilepsy*, ed. T.L. Bennet, pp. 97–137. New York: Plenum Press.

Starkstein, S.E., Boston, J.D. and Robinson, R.G. (1988a). Mechanisms of mania after brain injury. 12 case reports and review of the literature. *J Nerv Ment Dis* 176: 87–100.

Starkstein, S.E., Fedoroff, P., Berthier, M.L. and Robinson, R.G. (1991). Manic–depressive and pure manic states after brain lesions. *Biol Psychiatry* 29: 149–58.

Starkstein, S.E., Mayberg, H.S., Berthier, M.L. et al. (1990). Mania after brain injury: neuroradiological and metabolic findings. *Ann Neurol* 27: 652–9.

Starkstein, S.E., Pearlson, G.D., Boston, J. and Robinson, R.G. (1987a). Mania after brain injury. A controlled study of causative factors. *Arch Neurol* 44: 1069–73.

Starkstein, S.E. and Robinson, R.G. (1997). Mechanism of disinhibition after brain lesions. *J Nerv Ment Dis* 185: 108–14.

Starkstein, S.E., Robinson, R.G., Berthier, M.L., Parikh, R.M. and Price, T.R. (1988b). Differential mood changes following basal ganglia vs thalamic lesions. *Arch Neurol* 45: 725–30.

Starkstein, S.E., Robinson, R.G. and Price, T.R. (1987b). Comparison of cortical and subcortical lesions in the production of poststroke mood disorders. *Brain* 110: 1045–59.

Strauss, E. (1989). Ictal and interictal manifestations of emotions in epilepsy. In *Handbook of Neuropsychology*, 1st edn, ed. F. Boller and J. Grafman, Vol. 3, *Section 6: Emotional Behavior and its Disorders*, ed. L. Squire and G. Gainotti, pp. 315–44. Amsterdam: Elsevier.

Suzuki, T., Iwakuma, A., Tanaka, Y. et al. (1992). Changes in personality and emotion following bilateral infarction of the posterior cerebral arteries. *Jpn J Psychiatry Neurol* 46: 897–903.

Sweet, W.H., Ervin, F. and Mark, V.H. (1969). The relationship of violent behavior in nonhuman primates. In *Aggressive Behavior*, ed. M. Reite and T. Fields. New York: John Wiley & Sons.

Taylor, D.C. (1969a). Aggression and epilepsy. *J Psychosom Res* 13: 229–36.

Taylor, D.C. (1969b). Sexual behavior and temporal lobe epilepsy. *Arch Neurol* 21: 510–16.

Taylor, D.C. (1975). Factors influencing the occurrence of schizophrenia-like psychosis in patients with TLE. *Psychol Med* 5: 249–54.

Terzian, H. and Dalle Ore, G. (1955). Syndrome of Klüver–Bucy reproduced in man after bilateral removal of temporal lobes. *Neurology* 5: 373–80.

Tien, R.D., Felsberg, G.J., Castro, C.C. et al. (1993). Complex partial seizures and mesial temporal sclerosis: evaluation with fast spin-echo MR imaging. *Radiology* 189: 835–42.

Toni, C., Cassano, G.B., Perugi, G. et al. (1996). Psychosensorial and related phenomena in panic disorder and in temporal lobe epilepsy. *Compr Psychiatry* 37: 125–33.

Trieman, D. (1986). Epilepsy and violence: medical and legal issues. *Epilepsia* 27 Suppl. 2: S77–S104.

Trimble, M.R. (1991). *The Psychosis of Epilepsy*. New York: Raven Press.

Trimble, M.R., Mendez, M.F. and Cummings, J.L. (1997). Neuropsychiatric symptoms from the temporolimbic lobes. *J Neuropsychiatry Clin Neurosci* 9: 429–38.

Tucker, D.M. and Liotti, M. (1989). Neuropsychological mechanisms of anxiety and depression. In *Handbook of Neuropsychology*, 1st edn, ed. F. Boller and J. Grafman, Vol. 3, *Section 6: Emotional Behavior and its Disorders*, ed. L. Squire and G. Gainotti, pp. 443–76. Amsterdam: Elsevier.

Tucker, D.M., Novelly, R.A. and Walker, P.J. (1987). Hyperreligiosity in temporal lobe epilepsy: redefining the relationship. *J Nerv Ment Dis* 175: 181–4.

Turetsky, B., Cowell, P.E., Gur, R.C. et al. (1995). Frontal and temporal lobe brain volumes in schizophrenia. Relationship to symptoms and clinical subtype. *Arch Gen Psychiatry* 52: 1061–70.

Vochteloo, J.D. and Koolhaas, J.M. (1987). Medial amygdala lesions in male rats reduce aggressive behavior. *Physiol Behav* 41: 99–102.

Volkow, N.D. and Tancredi, L. (1987). Neural substrates of violent behavior. A preliminary study with positron emission tomography. *Br J Psychiatry* 151: 668–73.

Volkow, N.D., Tancredi, L.R., Grant, C. et al. (1995). Brain glucose metabolism in violent psychiatric patients: a preliminary study. *Psychiatry Res* 61: 243–53.

Waxman, S.G. and Geschwind, N. (1975). The interictal behavior syndrome of temporal lobe epilepsy. *Arch Gen Psychiatry* 32: 1580–6.

Weinberger, D.R. and Gallhofer, B. (1997). Cognitive function in schizophrenia. *Int Clin Psychopharmacol* 12 Suppl. 4: S29–36.

Weniger, G., Irle, E., Exner, C. and Rüther, E. (1997). Defective conceptualization of emotional facial expressions during T2 signal enhancement of the right amygdala. *Neurocase* 3: 259–66.

Yamada, H. and Yoshida, H. (1977). Laughing attack: a review and report of nine cases. *Folia Psychiatr Neurol Jpn* 31: 129–37.

Young, A., Reid, I., Wright, S. and Hellawell, D. (1993). Face-processing impairments and the Capgras delusion. *Br J Psychiatry* 162: 695–8.

Zwil, A.S., McAllister, T.W., Cohen, I. and Halpern, L.R. (1993). Ultra-rapid cycling bipolar affective disorder following a closed-head injury. *Brain Inj* 7: 147–52.

14

Neural correlates of violent behavior

Daniel Tranel

Introduction

The neurologist Richard Restak has written that 'there is not evidence . . . that damage in any area of the brain leads inevitably to a specific violent act.' This statement is, in this author's view, entirely correct, and it has abundant scientific support. Nonetheless, cases abound in which violent behavior has been attributed largely or entirely to some kind of brain malfunction. Such attributions have become more common than ever in recent years. There are numerous examples in the popular press of mass murderers and other violent criminals who were eventually discovered to have a brain lesion (e.g., tumor); in several cases, this discovery was made after the person had been put to death for a crime. Such examples have attracted considerable sympathy for the notion that some brain-damaged people may not be capable of controlling their violent behavior, and perhaps should even be exonerated for their acts of violent (Cohen, 1998). The issue is not simple, and compelling arguments can be proffered on both sides.

Violent and aggressive behavior[1] has been associated with a number of neurological and neuropsychiatric conditions, especially head injury, seizure disorder, and brain tumors, and, to a lesser extent, stroke, Alzheimer's disease and other degenerative conditions, movement disorders (e.g., Huntington's disease), mental retardation, and psychosis (Silver and Yudofsky, 1997). However, the fact remains that in all of these conditions, the vast majority of affected people do *not* commit violent acts. Moreover, in cases in which violence does occur, acute situational factors (particularly drug and alcohol intoxication) and constitutional and psychosocial characteristics (e.g., a lifelong history of antisocial personality) nearly always figure in the equation (Goldstein, 1974; Herzberg and Fenwick, 1988). Cases in which a sober, placid, well-adjusted person suddenly goes berserk are extremely uncommon. Also, understanding of the nature of cause-and-effect relationship between brain maladies and violent behavior has been hindered by the fact that a large majority of cases are dominated by thorny legal considerations, and in the course of sorting out the forensic issues, scientific integrity is often stretched well beyond reasonable limits. As Wortis (1990) has put it, 'interest in the biological determinants of violent behavior should not serve as a means of getting away with murder.'

Ideally, the principal focus of this chapter from a strict neuroscience perspective would be on violent and aggressive behavior that develops in connection with focal brain injury, following the onset of a neurological condition, in individuals whose personality development was previously normal. Such a focus is necessary if we are to gain some idea of direct cause-and-effect relationships between neural factors and acts of violence. That being said, though, it turns out that nearly all of the literature on human violence and the brain has involved psychiatric patients, and it is impossible to provide a decent review of the field without looking at studies of this type. But the fact remains that in these patients, many of whom have extensive psychiatric histories, long-term institutionalization, chronic medication, and so on, it is very difficult to determine to what extent neural factors alone may be contributing to the picture. Thus, it is necessary to review some literature which has focused on psychiatric patients, with the caution that brain–behavior relationships in these patients can be rather murky.

The discussion also includes a brief review from the other side of the coin: specifically, an analysis of neural structure and function in people who are known to have committed violent acts (Raine, 1993). These different lines of inquiry have provided some convergent evidence on the neural correlates of violent and aggressive behavior. Finally, a brief sketch of a neurobiological model of social conduct and emotion is presented, so as to provide a framework for interpreting the results of extant studies, and of posing questions for future research.

Before reviewing the current literature, though, a case that was studied in considerable detail a few years ago is presented (Relkin et al., 1996). The case is remarkable for a number of features, especially as an illustration of how a brain injury (in this case, a growing arachnoid cyst) can lead to a shocking act of brutal violence in an individual who had absolutely no premorbid history of aggressive behavior, and who committed the act in perfectly 'cold blood,' with no influence from drugs or alcohol, or, from what we can tell, even from heated emotion. A combination of orbital frontal and left temporal lobe dysfunction appeared to be the direct cause of the violent eruption. Following Norman Relkin's lead, the patient is referred to here as Spyder Cystkopf.[2]

A case report: Spyder Cystkopf

Description and history

The patient is a 65-year-old, fully right-handed man who suddenly strangled his wife in the course of a domestic argument, and then attempted to disguise her death as a suicide. His behavior was totally out of character, as he had for his entire life been a law-abiding, non-violent, socially conforming individual. In an attempt to explore potential explanations for this dramatic latelife eruption of violence, the man was subjected to a variety of detailed neurological, neuropsychological, psychophysiological, psychiatric, and other specialized evaluations (see Paradis et al., 1994; Relkin et al., 1996).

Cystkopf was the product of a normal upbringing, and was raised in an intact, nonviolent family. He was entirely well until age 22, when he developed two months of left-sided headaches, and then the acute onset of left-sided ptosis, hyperreflexia, and word-finding difficulties. No cause for these symptoms was uncovered at the time, and the problems resolved spontaneously. He was discharged from medical care after seven weeks, and suffered no residual symptoms. Cystkopf went on to lead a highly successful, productive life. He obtained a masters degree in business, and then achieved considerable economic success as an advertizing executive. He had been married to his first wife for 25 years when she died of cancer. He remarried, and was ten years into his second marriage at the time of the homicidal incident. The second marriage was described as 'idyllic,' and friends and family concurred that Cystkopf and his second wife seemed completely happy together. Neither spouse had any history of violent behavior. Cystkopf had never received psychiatric treatment, and he had no history of alcohol or drug abuse. He was, by all accounts, well adjusted and highly socialized, a fully productive and conforming member of society.

On a winter morning in 1991, Cystkopf and his wife became involved in an argument over family matters. The verbal exchange intensified, but Cystkopf remained calm and controlled. His wife, apparently angered by his lack of emotion, suddenly began scratching his face. He abruptly, and reportedly without any great sense of emotion, strangled her. Some minutes later, realizing she was dead, he threw her body out of the window of their 12th floor apartment, in an attempt to disguise her death as a suicide. Even then, he remained calm and unemotional; he retrieved his briefcase and left the apartment to go to his office. However, his neighbors identified him to police, and he was arrested when it was found that he had fresh scratch marks on his face and that there was blood on the carpet in his apartment. Cystkopf initially denied any knowledge of his wife's death. Later, he admitted to having caused her demise, but he could not explain what had prompted his behavior, and he remained adamant that he had never felt angry, frustrated, or emotionally upset. He reported the facts of the incident accurately and fluently, but entirely devoid of emotion, or any hint of the distress that might be expected under such grisly circumstances. In fact, in the months that followed, he continued living in the same apartment (to the dismay of neighbors who knew of his role in his wife's death). While still under indictment for his wife's murder, he began dating and eventually remarried.

Neuropsychological examination

A neuropsychological evaluation conducted about two months after this event yielded some early clues about possible cortical dysfunction (Paradis et al., 1994). For example, while most of his cognitive abilities were intact, Cystkopf produced an average score on the digit span subtest of the WAIS-R, significantly below his superior scores on all other verbal subtests. He had a 40-point split on the Wechsler Memory Scale – Revised, with a far higher score on visual memory (99th percentile) compared to verbal memory (45th percentile). Also, fine motor speed was relatively deficient in the dominant right hand. These findings hinted at possible left cerebral dysfunction, and prompted referral for neurological evaluation.

Supplemental neuropsychological testing was completed several months later (in the Benton Neuropsychology Laboratory at the University of Iowa Hospitals; see Tranel, 1996), and the findings were remarkable in several respects. (1) There was a mild impairment in *prospective* memory, which refers to the capacity of remembering to remember. This type of memory has been associated with the ventromedial prefrontal cortices. (2) Sequential digit learning was mildly defective; however, sequential learning of nonverbal spans was normal. (3) He demonstrated a mild impairment on the Category Test, which requires abstract problem-solving, rule formation, and cognitive flexibility. These findings, consistent with those obtained earlier, again pointed to dysfunction of the ventromedial prefrontal and left temporal regions.

An extensive personality evaluation was also conducted, using a variety of interview techniques and personality inventories (e.g., Minnesota Multiphasic Personality Inventory, California Personality Inventory, Eysenck Personality Questionnaire). The results painted the picture of an individual who experiences very little anxiety and fear, and who has cultivated an overcontrolled, highly rational approach to the world. However, the assessment was not diagnostic of a sociopathic personality, but, instead, revealed a person who relies on rationalization and verbal agility to deal with psychological dissonance and emotional stress. These findings were consistent with the patient's history, which was remarkable for the use of verbal mechanisms, rather than physical aggression, for dealing with stress and conflict.

Neurological, electroencephalographic, and neuroimaging evaluations

General neurological evaluation was entirely normal, as were all basic laboratory studies. An EEG, however, showed mild intermittent amplitude attentuation over the left hemisphere, interpreted as indicative of mild left-sided cerebral dysfunction. A magnetic resonance imaging (MRI) study revealed a region of abnormal signal in the left hemisphere, extending from the posterior portion of the sylvian fissure to the orbital frontal region. The findings were interpreted as consistent with a congenital arachnoid cyst. A follow-up MRI study was conducted, and the resultant data were quantified and interpreted using a special analysis program (Damasio and Frank, 1992). This study revealed that there was upward displacement by the cyst of the ventral surface of the left frontal lobe, by as much as 2 cm; also, there was comparable displacement of the left temporal lobe in a caudal and ventral direction (Fig. 14.1). Mesial temporal structures, including the amygdala, were extant, but displaced. The findings suggested that the cyst had enlarged during Cystkopf's adult life, between the time of his undiagnosed illness at the age of 22 and the occasion of his homicide.

Positron emission tomography

Cerebral glucose metabolism was measured with a resting FDG PET, using standard methodology (see Relkin et al., 1996). The study showed decreased glucose metabolism in

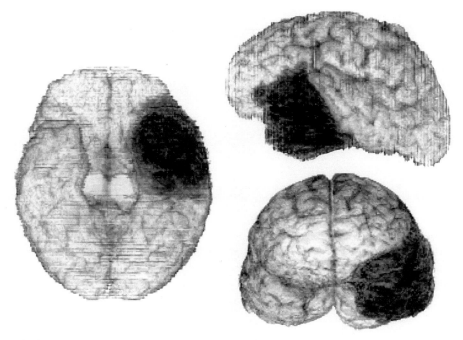

Fig. 14.1   A high-resolution, thin slice MRI was performed in Spyder Cystkopf, and analyzed with
Brainvox. The three-dimensional reconstruction revealed the presence of an arachnoid
cyst occupying most of the left middle fossa. The cyst displaces left temporal cortices
upward and backward, and also displaces the left orbital frontal region upward.

several left hemisphere structures, including lateral and mesial temporal regions, the frontal
operculum, and medial and lateral prefrontal regions.

Psychophysiological studies

Cystkopf was evaluated with a series of procedures that have been developed to investigate
autonomic responses to socially charged stimuli (Damasio, Tranel and Damasio, 1990;
Tranel, 1994). Briefly, this involved recording skin conductance responses (SCRs) from the
left and right hands, while the subject viewed slides with neutral (e.g., farm scenes) or
socially charged (e.g., nudes, mutilations) content. Normal subjects produce large-ampli-
tude SCRs to the socially charged pictures. Such responses were entirely absent in Cystkopf,
as he failed to show any difference in his SCRs to the neutral stimuli versus the socially
charged ones (Fig. 14.2). This happened in spite of the fact that Cystkopf had normal skin
conductance during passive resting, and was capable of producing normal responses to
basic orienting stimuli, such as a loud noise. Thus, his autonomic response impairment was
specific to socially charged stimuli. The experiment was repeated on consecutive days, and
the findings proved highly reliable. In fact, the nature of Cystkopf's performance in this task
was virtually identical, qualitatively and quantitatively, to the pattern observed in neurological patients with bilateral ventromedial prefrontal damage and acquired disturbances of

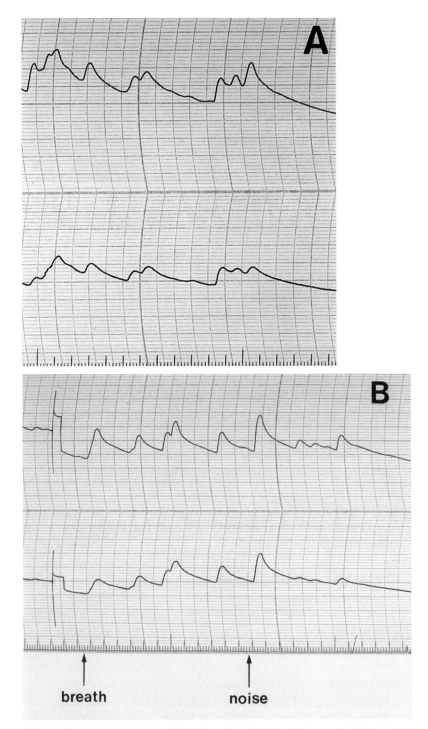

Fig. 14.2   Skin conductance responses (SCRs) from the right hand (upper tracing) and left hand (lower tracing) of Spyder Cystkopf. A. Skin conductance during passive resting. There are several nonspecific SCRs, and these and other aspects of the record are entirely normal.

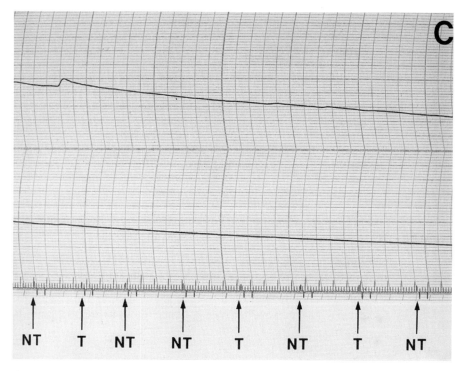

Fig. 14.2 (*cont.*)

B. Skin conductance during presentation of two basic orienting stimuli (deep breath, loud noise), marked by the arrows. The orienting SCRs, depicted by the rise in skin conductance about one to two seconds following stimulus onset, are normal. C. Skin conductance during presentation of target (T) and nontarget (NT) pictures. The absence of SCRs to the target stimuli is severely abnormal.

social conduct (Damasio et al., 1990; Tranel, 1994). This suggested that the ventromedial dysfunction in Cystkopf was probably bilateral.

In summary, the weight of the evidence in this case ended up supporting quite convincingly the conclusion that the sudden eruption of violent behavior in Cystkopf was the direct consequence of brain dysfunction. In the first place, and perhaps most impressively, his act of homicide was a radical departure from past behavior, which was devoid of any hint of unusual aggression. Neuropsychological testing, EEG findings, and the PET results pointed consistently to left frontotemporal dysfunction. Finally, the striking pattern of abnormal autonomic responses to socially charged stimuli was highly reminiscent of the profile from patients with bilateral ventromedial prefrontal damage, suggesting a similar pattern of neural abnormality in Cystkopf. In short, this case depicts an example of unchecked violent behavior related to focal brain dysfunction, in the setting of normal personality development, no acute catalysts such as drugs and alcohol, and a relatively trivial eliciting stimulus (the scratching). The neural correlates appear to be the ventromedial prefrontal region, and the left anterior and mesial temporal regions. As will be seen below, this is consistent with the general picture that can be gleaned from available human and animal studies.

Some neural correlates of violent behavior

Discussions of the neural correlates of violent and aggressive behavior have focused on structures in the so-called *limbic system* (Fig. 14.3), including the amygdala, hypothalamus, cingulate gyrus, septal nucleus, anterior thalamus, and anterior temporal lobe (Moyer, 1976; Volavka, 1995). Another brain region that has received considerable attention in connection with violent and aggressive behavior is the frontal lobes, especially the orbital and lower mesial portions. Some of the more consistent findings are reviewed below.

Hypothalamus

Earlier reviews of the nonhuman animal literature documented extensively the relationship between damage to the ventromedial hypothalamic region and the development of aggressive, rage-like behavior (Moyer, 1976; Valzelli, 1981). A similar relationship has been hinted at in humans (Weiger and Bear, 1988). According to Malamud (1967), most destructive lesions in the hypothalamic region associated with aggressive behavior and rage reactions are neoplastic in nature, and most are bilateral.

Amygdala and anterior temporal lobe

The importance of the amygdala and nearby anterior temporal lobe structures in the modulation of aggressive behavior has been emphasized in a number of studies, in humans and other animals. Dysfunction of these structures has been associated with violent and aggressive behavior in psychiatric patients and patients with a history of epilepsy (Volkow and Tancredi, 1987; Garyfallos, Manos and Adamopoulou, 1988; Tonkonogy, 1991). Convergent evidence comes from studies which have shown that electrical stimulation of the amygdala sometimes produces rage outbursts and other aggressive behavioral manifestations (Mark and Ervin, 1970; Egger and Flynn, 1981; see Kling, 1986, for review). Less specifically, the anterior temporal lobes in general have been associated with violent behavior. Volkow and Tancredi (1987) found that in four patients with repetitive acts of violence, there were blood flow and metabolic abnormalities in the left temporal lobe (as shown by PET scanning). Two of the patients also had abnormalities in the frontal cortex. Unilateral or bilateral amygdalotomy has been used to control aggressive behavior, often with favorable outcomes (for reviews, see Goldstein, 1974; Lee et al., 1988). Lee and his colleagues have published details of two patients with bilateral amygdalotomy, both of whom showed significant improvement of uncontrollable aggressive behavior following their surgeries (Lee et al., 1988, 1995).

In a number of well-studied neurological cases with bilateral amygdala lesions, the patients have actually been shown to have *less* aggression than normal (Tranel

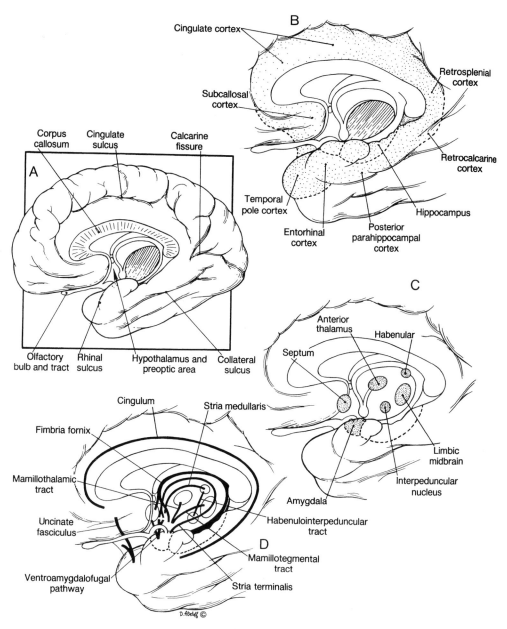

Fig. 14.3   Schematic depiction of the major neuroanatomical components of the 'limbic system,'
shown in mesial views of the cerebral hemisphere. A. Limbic system landmarks and
boundaries. B. The so-called limbic lobe, which includes major cortical components of the
limbic system. C. Subcortical components of the limbic system. D. Major pathways and
interconnections of limbic system components. (From Damasio, A.R., Van Hoesen, G.W.
and Tranel D. (1998). In *Surgery of the Third Ventricle*, 2nd edn., ed. M.L.J. Apuzzo.
Baltimore: Williams & Wilkins. Used with permission.)

and Hyman, 1990; Adolphs al., 1994, 1995, 1998). The author and his colleagues have studied three patients with extensive bilateral mesial temporal lobe lesions (which include the amgydala), all of whom have a remarkable preference for positive affect, and an equally impressive proclivity to avoid negative affect. The patient known as Boswell, who has complete bilateral damage to the entire mesial temporal region, provides a striking illustration (Tranel, Adolphs and Damasio, 1997). For example, when asked to explain what is happening in a picture showing people leaping off a burning ship into the ocean, Boswell said that the people are 'swimming, going for a dip.' Shown a film clip in which military people are gunning down a fleeing crowd of civilians, Boswell said that the people are 'jogging, exercising.' Boswell's behavior in other situations is similar; for example, he is very uncomfortable when placed in situations of social conflict (e.g., when asked to decide which of two experimenters is 'nicer').

The findings reviewed here emphasize the fact that it is not possible to draw simple conclusions about cause-and-effect relationships between amygdala dysfunction and violent behavior (cf. Treiman, 1991; Garza-Trevino, 1994). Nonetheless, the weight of the evidence points to a close relationship between amygdala function and modulation of emotion, including regulation of at least some aspects of aggressive behavior. It is interesting to note in this context that the amygdala's role in emotional processing appears to be heavily weighted to negatively valenced emotions, especially fear and anger (Adolphs et al., 1998). For example, recent studies have demonstrated a robust relationship between amygdala function and the recognition of fear (and possibly anger) in facial expressions (Adolphs et al., 1994, 1995; Breiter et al., 1996; Calder et al., 1996; Morris et al., 1996) and in tone of voice (Scott et al., 1997; for review, see Tranel, 1997). These findings are quite consistent with the idea that the amygdala is a critical part of neural systems on which the modulation of aggressive behavior, especially in response to aversive or threatening stimuli, depend.

The frontal lobes

A number of lines of evidence have supported the idea that the frontal lobes are related to violent and aggressive behavior, although, as with the case for the amygdala, the relationship is far from simple.

A critical review of the literature was published by Kandel and Freed (1989), who concluded that 'the evidence for the association between specifically violent criminal behavior and frontal-lobe dysfunction is weak at best.' Nevertheless, the authors note that in *all* studies which have explored brain–behavior relationships in regard to violent and psychopathic behavior, it has been concluded that the anterior regions of the brain, including the frontal lobes and anterior temporal lobes, are the most likely neuroanatomical correlates. The fact that there are no exceptions

Table 14.1. Characteristic features of organic aggressive syndrome

Reactive	Triggered by modest or trivial stimuli
Nonreflective	Usually does not involve premeditation or planning
Nonpurposeful	Aggression serves no obvious long-term aims or goals
Explosive	Build-up is *not* gradual
Periodic	Brief outbursts of rage and aggression, punctuated by long periods of relative calm
Ego-dystonic	After outbursts, patients are upset, concerned, and/or embarrassed, as opposed to blaming others or justifying behavior

Source: Reprinted with permission from Yudofsky et al. (1990).

to this pattern supports the conclusion that there is probably at least some credibility to the idea that dysfunction of anterior brain regions (frontal/temporal) could be related to the development of violent and aggressive behavior, provided the needed catalysts are in place.

Another clue comes from studies of patients who sustained frontal lobe injuries early in life, and then went on to have severe impairments in comportment (Grattan and Eslinger, 1991). For example, two cases of this type published by Price et al. (1990) both exhibited significant aggressive and violent behavior. However, it is important to keep in mind that the principal focus of abnormality in these cases, and in virtually all similar cases published to date, is in the realm of *social conduct*: the patients make very poor decisions regarding friends, sexual encounters, and occupational pursuits (see review in Tranel, Anderson and Benton, 1994). As Price et al. note, the behavioral features of these developmental cases seem to be qualitatively similar to, but quantitatively more severe than, those exhibited by patients who acquire bilateral prefrontal lesions in adulthood. Specifically, social misconduct is a central feature, but blatant violence and aggression are not necessarily the predominant manifestations.

Another line of evidence comes from studies of patients who have sustained head injuries. These injuries often result in damage to orbital prefrontal cortices, and they have been associated with a very high incidence of aggressive behavior (see Silver and Yudofsky, 1994, for review). In fact, such behavior is frequently the most challenging aspect for rehabilitation and management. Silver and Yudofsky (1994) have presented a compelling argument for classifying this condition as a special form of psychiatric disorder, namely, *organic aggressive syndrome*, rather than as a 'personality change' as currently designated in the DSM-IV nosology (see Table 14.1).

With regard to the frontal lobes, as was the case for the amygdala, there is a sort of paradox. The ventromedial prefrontal region is clearly important for the regulation of behavior, social conduct in particular, and for decision-making, and there is little question that dysfunction of this region can lead to maladaptive behavior. However, the vast majority of patients with focal damage to this region do *not* engage in violent or aggressive behavior. Many, in fact, became rather placid and affectively flat. But this does not explain why so many patients with head injury have aggressive and violent behavior. Perhaps the critical feature is a *combination* of orbital prefrontal injury and anterior temporal lobe injury; this conclusion appears quite consistent with the case report of Relkin et al. (1996) summarized above. In any event, I would wholeheartedly agree with the conclusion by Heinrichs (1989) that 'there is little evidence to indicate that frontal lesions cause aggression per se.'

Brain abnormalities in mass murderers

Adrian Raine has taken a different approach to understanding the neural correlates of violence and aggression. He and his colleagues have studied subjects who have a well-documented history of violent behavior – namely, murderers – and have applied modern imaging techniques to investigate the neural architecture of these individuals (Raine, 1993; Raine et al., 1994, 1997, 1998).

Raine et al. (1994) studied a group of 22 subjects who had been charged with murder, and 22 controls matched for gender, age, and psychiatric status. An FDG PET imaging procedure was applied while the subjects were performing a continuous performance test. The results showed that the murderers had significant reductions of glucose metabolism in the anterior medial prefrontal region, and in a region the authors describe as the 'higher supraventricular superior frontal cortex.' In general, relatively widespread prefrontal dysfunction was noted in the murderers, compared to controls. Moreover, the metabolic abnormalities were specific to the prefrontal region, as there were no significant reductions in other brain regions, including the posterior frontal, temporal, and parietal sectors. These PET findings are consistent with the idea that functional prefrontal abnormalities may be related to violent and aggressive behavior, a conclusion very much in line with the findings reviewed above in connection with lesion studies.

Raine et al. (1997) have replicated and extended these findings in a larger sample of murderers ($n=41$). A PET approach was used again, while subjects performed the continuous performance test. The findings showed a significant reduction of glucose metabolism in the prefrontal cortex; also, abnormal 'asymmetries of activity' were detected in the amygdala, thalamus, and medial temporal lobe, and there were reductions of metabolism in several other brain regions. The authors interpreted their findings as showing 'a network of abnormal cortical and subcortical brain processes that may predispose to violence in murderers . . .' Actually, the widespread nature of metabolic abnormalities detected in this study, and the odd 'asymmetries' in several regions, are rather puzzling and somewhat difficult to interpret. Nonetheless, the findings are at least consistent with regard to the prefrontal cortices.

The somatic marker hypothesis

It is interesting to consider the findings summarized above in the context of the *somatic marker hypothesis*, which was developed to account for the striking changes in social conduct, planning, and decision-making which characterize patients with ventromedial prefrontal damage (Damasio et al., 1990; Damasio, 1994, 1995). The hypothesis is centered on the notion that the ventromedial prefrontal region is a crucial neural substrate for the capacity to use emotions and feelings to help guide behavior. In particular, this region provides access to somatic guideposts that normally mark various behavioral alternatives as positive or negative, which in turn facilitates advantageous decision-making. Structures in ventromedial prefrontal cortex provide the neural substrate for learning associations between complex situations, on the one hand, and the types of bioregulatory states (including emotional states) usually associated with such situations in prior experience, on the other. The ventromedial prefrontal region holds linkages between the facts that make up a given situation, and the predominant emotion previously paired with that situation in an indivudal's experience. It is important to note that these linkages are *dispositional*. They do not hold explicitly representations of the situation or of the emotional state, but rather, the potential to reactivate an emotion by evoking activity in pertinent cortical and subcortical structures. The ventromedial prefrontal region helps establish a linkage between the disposition for a certain aspect of a situation, and the disposition for the type of emotion that has been associated with the situation.

People are confronted at various times with situations which call for decisions and courses of action regarding social behavior, and, in some cases, the situations will require a decision about whether or not aggressive behavior is called for or is appropriate. In these situations, according to our somatic marker formulation, dispositions are activated in higher-order association cortices, leading to the recall of pertinent facts and other related knowledge. Pertinent ventromedial prefrontal linkages are activated concurrently. This leads to activation of the emotional disposition apparatus (e.g., various limbic structures, such as the amygdala, cingulate, and insular cortex), and the net result is a reconstruction of a previously learned factual–emotional set. The reactivation of the emotional disposition network can occur via two routes: (1) *a body loop*, in which somatic units (e.g., musculoskeletal, visceral, and other internal milieu components of the soma) actually change, with the changes being relayed to somatosensory cortices; and (2) an *'as if' body loop*, in which the reactivation signals bypass the body and get relayed to the somatosensory cortices directly, with the latter adopting the appropriate pattern without bodily input. Also, the instantiation of a somatosensory pattern can occur either overtly or covertly. The somatosensory pattern evoked by a particular situation is then displayed concurrently with factual knowledge pertinent to the situation.

As far as decision-making is concerned, a key function of the somatosensory pattern is to constrain the process of reasoning over multiple options and multiple future outcomes. For example, when the somatosensory image which defines a particular emotional response is codisplayed with the images which describe a particular future scenario, the somatosensory pattern marks the scenario as good or bad (or inbetween). Hence, the images of the scenario are judged and marked by the juxtaposed images of the somatic state. When utilized in complex decision-making situations, this process greatly facilitates the operation of logical reasoning. Somatic markers allow certain option–outcome pairs to be rapidly endorsed or rejected, making the decision-making space manageable for a logic-based cost–benefit analysis. In situations in which there is a lot of uncertainty regarding which course of action is optimal, the constraints imposed by somatic markers would allow the individual to decide efficiently within reasonable time intervals, and to decide in a manner that is consistent with applicable social norms and with the best interests of the principal parties to the situation. This decision-making process would apply in particular in situations involving possible aggressive or even violent behavior.

Without somatic markers, response options and outcomes become more or less equalized. The processes of decision-making and response selection would then depend entirely on logic operations over many potential alternatives, a strategy that can be inordinately time consuming, and that may fail to take into account previous experience. Decision-making and response selection would not be timely, accurate, or propitious, and may become random or impulsive. The somatic marker hypothesis goes against the notion that reasoning and decision-making are optimal when a person is cool, calm, and calculating, and helps explain why too little emotion might be just as bad for decision-making as too much emotion. This could account for the seemingly inexplicable behavior of patients such as Spyder Cystkopf, and other patients who suffer damage to the ventromedial prefrontal region. Also, it is possible to conjecture that developmental abnormalities in this region, as might be the case in developmental forms of sociopathy, could contribute to social conduct disorders and, specifically, to inappropriate violent and aggressive behavior.

Treatment considerations

Unfortunately, it is very difficult to write sanguinely about the treatment of individuals who are prone to violent and aggressive behavior. The treatment of such individuals when they have no history of acquired brain injury is tenuous at best, and the prospects for success are reduced even further when brain damage is added to the equation. With regard to psychopathic individuals, who comprise the main segment of the population most at risk for violent and aggressive behavior, a traditional teaching is that the 'burn-out' principle is probably as hopeful as any – specifically, the idea that beyond the age of 40 or so, most psychopaths lose their energy, drive, and enthusiasm for committing violent acts, and hence gradually cease such behavior without any particular form of intervention. A good deal of research backs this up: interventions of all natures have proved to have little long-term effect on violent and aggressive behavior, when compared to the mere passage of time (e.g., Weiss, 1973; Cleckley, 1976; Hare, McPherson, and Forth, 1988; also see Sutker, 1994).

In dealing with brain-damaged individuals who manifest violent and aggressive behavior, it is often more productive to focus treatment efforts on the people around the patients, rather than on the patients themselves. For example, considerable positive influence can be imparted by dealing directly with family members, caretakers, and others who are in regular contact with the patient. Such people can be taught why patients behave the way they do, what situations and stimuli are likely to trigger such behavior, and how to intervene early to abort a cascade of catalytic events. Often, this tack is far more likely to produce positive results than an approach that is aimed directly at the brain-damaged individual. Patients are, in a sense, not in control of their actions, as the review of the literature earlier in this chapter made clear. Hence, it is fruitless to invest huge resources in treating the brain-damaged person directly; such treatment often proves to be completely unhelpful in altering the real-world, day-to-day behavior of the patient. Moreover, the patient may have learning and memory defects that interfere even further with the implementation of coping strategies taught in therapy.

One particular factor that warrants emphasis is the importance of prohibiting patients from consuming alcohol and other drugs. As noted above, alcohol and drug consumption are highly common catalysts in the execution of violent acts; this is true of normal individuals and even more true of psychopaths (e.g., Raine, 1993). Again, adding brain damage to the equation exacerbates the situation even further; psychopathic individuals are much more prone to the influence of alcohol and drugs than normal individuals, and often respond adversely to even low levels of intoxication. In short, it is imperative that brain-damaged patients be prevented from access to alcohol and drugs, if at all possible, and this alone can go a long way toward reducing the chances that such individuals will engage in violent and aggressive behavior.

Pharmacological management of violence and aggression, in both psychiatric populations and in patients with acquired brain injury, is common, although the efficacy of this approach is inconsistent at best (see Silver, Hales, and Yudofsky, 1997, for a review). The most commonly used medications include antipsychotics, sedatives and hypnotics, and anticonvulsants. Drug treatment is much more likely to be successful if careful consideration is given in each individual case to factors such as premorbid personality, the presumed etiology of the aggressive behavior, age, and comorbid conditions. There is some evidence that drugs that act primarily or specifically on serotonin (e.g., reuptake blockers) are particularly effective in the management of aggression, although, as Silver et al. (1997) point out, no drug has been specifically approved by the Food and Drug Administration in the USA for the treatment of aggression. Also, in all cases of drug treatment, the clinician must maintain constant vigilance regarding potential drug misuse and abuse, and medication side-effects.

Finally, it should be mentioned that neurosurgical intervention for the treatment of violence and aggression is, on occasion, a reasonable option. For example, as noted earlier, amygdalectomies have been used with some success to treat uncontrollable aggressive behavior (Goldstein, 1974; Lee et al., 1988). One major indication for this type of treatment approach is the presence of refractory seizures – in such cases, surgical intervention, usually in conjunction with follow-up medical management, may greatly reduce or even eliminate the seizures, and a significant concomitant reduction in violence and aggression becomes a reasonable expectation. Cingulotomies and prefrontal lobotomies and leukotomies have also been used to control violent and aggressive behavior; however, although these operations may, in fact, often reduce the unwanted behavior, they produce far too many 'side-effects' to make them reasonable courses of treatment in all but very rare cases (see Damasio, 1975).

Conclusion

The determinants of violent and aggressive behavior are obviously multiple and complex. Neural factors certainly play a role, but it is very difficult to find unequivocal cases that help pinpoint specific brain–behavior relationships. Structures for which there appears to be a fair degree of convergent evidence are the amygdala and ventromedial prefrontal cortex, but even here, the stories are far from simple. The introduction of functional imaging techniques, especially PET, may allow important new advances to be made in the understanding of the neural basis of violent and aggressive behavior. No less important is the development of testable theoretical formulations, which can help guide research in this domain and facilitate productive question asking. As the numbers of senseless acts of violence and aggression skyrocket the world over, and legal systems struggle with tricky questions about degrees of individual culpability, scientific advances in this domain are of obvious importance.

Notes

1   Some authors have emphasized a distinction between *violence*, which can be considered 'the forceful infliction of abuse or damage onto another individual or object,' and *aggression*, which can be considered 'an offensive action directed toward another individual or object with the intent to harm, threaten, or control' (Treiman, 1991; Gerard et al., 1998). This distinction may be especially important in studying the violent behavior of patients with seizure disorders. In the current chapter, however, violence and aggression are considered together, as more or less different parts of a common, more general construct. Actually, insofar as current understanding of the neural correlates of violent behavior are concerned, the distinction may not be all that crucial, although this could obviously change as more knowledge is accrued in this domain.

2   Norman Relkin invested an enormous amount of time and energy in studying the patient known as Spyder Cystkopf, and Relkin deserves credit for the careful original published description of the case (see Relkin et al., 1996). The description here follows the general outline provided by Relkin.

Acknowledgments

Supported by Program Project Grant NINDFS NS19632 and the Mathers Foundation. I thank my colleagues especially, Antonio Damasio, Hanna Damasio, and Norman Relkin, for their collaboration in much of the work reported here, and I thank Hanna Damasio for help with the figures.

REFERENCES

Adolphs, R., Tranel, D. and Damasio, A.R. (1998). The human amygdala in social judgments. *Nature* 393: 470–4.

Adolphs, R., Tranel, D., Damasio, H. and Damasio, A.R. (1995). Fear and the human amygdala. *J Neurosci* 15: 5879–91.

Adolphs, R., Tranel, D., Damasio, H. and Damasio, A.R. (1994). Impaired recognition of emotion in facial expressions following bilateral damage to the human amygdala. *Nature* 372: 669–72.

Breiter, H.C., Etcoff, N.L., Whalen, P.J. et al. (1996). Response and habituation of the human amygdala during visual processing of facial expression. *Neuron* 17: 875–87.

Calder, A.J., Young, A.W., Rowland, D. et al. (1996). Facial emotion recognition after bilateral amygdala damage: differentially severe impairment of fear. *Cogn Neuropsychol* 13: 699–745.

Cleckley, H. (1976). *The Mask of Sanity*, 5th edn. St Louis: Mosby.

Cohen, E. (1998). Broken brains. *Notre Dame Magazine* 26: 22–6.

Damasio, A.R. (1975). Egas Moniz, pioneer of angiography and leucotomy. *Mt Sinai J Med* 42: 502–13.

Damasio, A.R. (1994). *Descartes' Error: Emotion, Reason and the Human Brain*. New York: Grosset/Putnam.

Damasio, A.R. (1995). On some functions of the human prefrontal cortex. In *Structure and Functions of the Human Prefrontal Cortex*, eds. J. Grafman, K. Holyoak and F. Boller, pp. 241–51. New York: The New York Academy of Sciences.

Damasio, A.R., Tranel, D. and Damasio, H. (1990). Individuals with sociopathic behavior caused by frontal damage fail to respond autonomically to social stimuli. *Behav Brain Res* 41: 81–94.

Damasio, A.R., Van Hoesen, G.W. and Tranel, D. (1998). Pathological correlates of amnesia and the anatomical basis of memory. In *Surgery of the Third Ventricle*, 2nd edn, ed. M.L.J. Apuzzo, pp. 187–204. Baltimore: Williams & Wilkins.

Damasio, H. and Frank, R. (1992). Three-dimensional *in vivo* mapping of brain lesions in humans. *Arch Neurol* 49: 137–43.

Egger, M.D. and Flynn, J.P. (1981). Effects of electrical stimulation of the amygdala on hypothalamically elicited attack behavior in cats. *J Neurophysiol* 26: 705–20.

Garyfallos, G., Manos, N. and Adamopoulou, A. (1988). Psychopathology and personality characteristics of epileptic patients: epilepsy, psychopathology and personality. *Acta Psychiatr Scand* 78: 87–95.

Garza-Trevino, E.S. (1994). Neurobiological factors in aggressive behavior. *Hosp Commun Psychiatry* 45: 690–9.

Gerard, M.E., Spitz, M.C., Towbin, J.A. and Shantz, D. (1998). Subacute postictal aggression. *Neurology* 50: 384–8.

Goldstein, M. (1974). Brain research and violent behavior. *Arch Neurol* 30: 1–35.

Grattan, L.M. and Eslinger, P.J. (1991). Frontal lobe damage in children and adults: a comparative review. *Dev Neuropsychol* 7: 283–326.

Hare, R.D., McPherson, L.M. and Forth, A.E. (1988). Male psychopaths and their criminal careers. *J Consult Clin Psychol* 56: 710–14.

Heinrichs, R.W. (1989). Frontal cerebral lesions and violent incidents in chronic neuropsychiatric patients. *Biol Psychiatry* 25: 174–8.

Herzberg, J.L. and Fenwick, P.B.C. (1988). The aetiology of aggression in temporal-lobe epilepsy. *Br J Psychiatry* 153: 50–5.

Kandel, E. and Freed, D. (1989). Frontal-lobe dysfunction and antisocial behavior: a review. *J Clin Psychol* 45: 404–13.

Kling, A.S. (1986). The anatomy of aggression and affiliation. In *Emotion: Theory, Research, and Experience*, Vol. 3, ed. R. Plutchik and H. Kellerman, pp. 237–64. New York: Academic Press.

Lee, G.P., Arena, J.G., Meador, K.J. et al. (1988). Changes in autonomic responsiveness following bilateral amygdalotomy in humans. *Neuropsychiatry Neuropsychol Behav Neurol* 1: 119–29.

Lee, G.P., Reed, M.F., Meador, K.J., Smith, J.R. and Loring, D.W. (1995). Is the amygdala crucial for cross-modal association in humans? *Neuropsychology* 9: 236–45.

Malamud, N. (1967). Psychiatric disorder with intracranial tumors of limbic system. *Arch Neurol* 17: 113–23.

Mark, V.H. and Ervin, F.R. (1970). *Violence and the Brain*. New York: Harper & Row.

Morris, J.S., Frith, C.D., Perrett, D.I. et al. (1996). A differential neural response in the human amygdala to fearful and happy facial expressions. *Nature* 383: 812–15.

Moyer, K.E. (1976). *The Psychobiology of Aggression*. New York: Harper & Row.

Paradis, C.M., Horn, L., Lazar, R.M. and Schwartz, D.W. (1994). Brain dysfunction and violent behavior in a man with a congenital subarachnoid cyst. *Hosp Commun Psychiatry* 45: 714–16.

Price, B.H., Daffner, K.R., Stowe, R.M. and Mesulam, M.M. (1990). The comportmental learning disabilities of early frontal lobe damage. *Brain* 113: 1383–93.

Raine, A. (1993). *The Psychopathology of Crime*. New York: Academic Press.

Raine, A., Buchsbaum, M. and LaCasse, L. (1997). Brain abnormalities in murderers indicated by positron emission tomography. *Biol Psychiatry* 42: 495–508.

Raine, A., Buchsbaum, M.S., Stanley, J. et al. (1994). Selective reductions in prefrontal glucose metabolism in murderers. *Biol Psychiatry* 36: 365–73.

Raine, A., Stoddard, J., Bihrle, S. and Buchsbaum, M. (1998). Prefrontal glucose deficits in murderers lacking psychosocial deprivation. *Neuropsychiatry Neuropsychol Behav Neurol* 11: 1–7.

Relkin, N., Plum, F., Mattis, S., Eidelberg, D. and Tranel, D. (1996). Impulsive homicide associated with an arachnoid cyst and unilateral frontotemporal cerebral dysfunction. *Semin Clin Neuropsychiatry* 1: 172–83.

Scott, S.K., Young, A.W., Calder, A.J. et al. (1997). Impaired auditory recognition of fear and anger following bilateral amygdala lesions. *Nature* 385: 254–7.

Silver, J.M., Hales, R.E. and Yudofsky, S.C. (1997). Neuropsychiatric aspects of traumatic brain injury. In *Textbook of Neuropsychiatry*, 3rd edn, ed. S.C. Yudofsky and R.E. Hales, pp. 521–60. Washington DC: American Psychiatric Press.

Silver, J.M. and Yudofsky, S.C. (1994). Aggressive disorders. In *Neuropsychiatry of Traumatic Brain Injury*, ed. J.M. Silver, S.C. Yudofsky and R.E. Hales, pp. 313–53. Washington, DC: American Psychiatric Press.

Silver, J.M. and Yudofsky, S.C. (1997). Violence and the brain. In *Behavioral Neurology and Neuropsychology*, ed. T.E. Feinberg and M.J. Farah, pp. 711–17. New York: McGraw Hill.

Sutker, P.B. (1994). Psychopathy: traditional and clinical antisocial concepts. In *Progress in Experimental Personality and Psychopathology Research*, Vol. 17, ed. D.C. Fowles, P. Sutker, and S.H. Goodman, pp. 73–120. New York: Springer.

Tonkonogy, J.M. (1991). Violence and temporal lobe lesion: head CT and MRI data. *J Neuropsychiatry* 3: 189–96.

Tranel, D. (1994). 'Acquired sociopathy': the development of sociopathic behavior following focal brain damage. In *Progress in Experimental Personality and Psychopathology Research*, Vol. 17, ed. D.C. Fowles, P. Sutker and S.H. Goodman, pp. 285–311. New York: Springer.

Tranel, D. (1996). The Iowa–Benton school of neuropsychological assessment. In *Neuropsychological Assessment of Neuropsychiatric Disorders*, 2nd edn, ed. I. Grant and K.M. Adams, pp. 81–101. New York: Oxford University Press.

Tranel, D. (1997). Emotional processing and the human amygdala. *Trends Cogn Sci*: 46–7.

Tranel, D., Adolphs, R. and Damasio, A.R. (1997). Knowledge of emotions following extensive bilateral damage to limbic system in humans. *Soc Neurosci* 23: 570.

Tranel, D., Anderson, S.W. and Benton, A.L. (1994). Development of the concept of 'executive function' and its relationship to the frontal lobes. In *Handbook of Neuropsychology*, Vol. 9, ed. F. Boller and J. Grafman, pp. 125–48. Amsterdam: Elsevier.

Tranel, D. and Hyman, B.T. (1990). Neuropsychological correlates of bilateral amygdala damage. *Arch Neurol* 47: 349–55.

Treiman, D.M. (1991). Psychobiology of ictal aggression. *Adv Neurol* 55: 341–56.

Valzelli, L. (1981). *Psychobiology of Aggression and Violence*. New York: Raven Press.

Volavka, J. (1995). *Neurobiology of Violence*. Washington, DC: American Psychiatric Press.

Volkow, N.D. and Tancredi, L. (1987). Neural substrates of violent behavior: a preliminary study with positron emission tomography. *Br J Psychiatry* 151: 668–73.

Weiger, W.A. and Bear, D.M. (1988). An approach to the neurology of aggression. *J Psychiatr Res* 22: 85–98.

Weiss, J.M.A. (1973). The natural history of antisocial attitudes: what happens to psychopaths? *J Geriatr Psychiatry* 6: 236–42.

Wortis, J. (1990). Getting away with murder. *Biol Psychiatry* 28: 555.

Yudofsky, S.C., Silver, J.M. and Hales, R.E. (1990). Pharmacologic management of aggression in the elderly. *J Clin Psychiatry* 51 Suppl. 10: 22–8.

15

Focal lesions and psychosis

Terri Edwards-Lee and Jeffrey L. Cummings

Introduction

Focal lesions leading to psychosis are relatively rare. For example, of 1821 men with focal brain lesions due to trauma, only 21 showed psychotic symptoms (six with paranoid psychosis and 15 with schizophrenia-like psychosis) (Hillbom, 1951). Lesions in many areas have been implicated in the causation of psychosis; however, there are no areas that, when lesioned, reliably produce psychotic symptoms. This chapter reviews the location of lesions that have been associated with psychosis and factors that contribute to the expression of psychosis. Lesions associated with psychosis found in epilepsy, stroke, demyelinating syndromes, neoplasms, trauma, and focally degenerative diseases are described. Conditions associated with psychosis and the brain regions commonly involved are summarized in Table 15.1.

Definitions

Psychosis has many possible definitions; the definition employed in this chapter is 'the inability to distinguish reality from fantasy with impaired reality testing and the creation of a new reality' (Kaplan and Saddock, 1995) manifested by the presence of delusions or hallucinations. Other definitions of psychosis include impairment of personal and social functioning and thought disorder, but these qualities extend beyond the core syndrome and would include many patients with uncomplicated neurological disorders. Delusions will be defined as false beliefs based on incorrect inferences about external reality and firmly held in spite of evidence to the contrary (Cummings, 1995b). Hallucinations will be defined as sensory perceptions occurring without appropriate external stimulation of the relative sensory organ, and are only manifestations of psychosis if the perceiver believes them to be real. They will be included in this discussion only if the hallucinations are psychotic manifestations.

Table 15.1. Summary of focal abnormalities leading to psychosis

Type of lesion	Area(s) most commonly implicated
Epilepsy	Temporal lobe
	Primarily medial temporal lobe
	Left>right in association with Schneiderian first-rank symptoms
Stroke	Temporo-parietal/temporo-parietal-occipital (most common)
	Deep gray matter
	Right>left
White matter ischemic lesions	Frontal lobe
	Temporo-parieto-occipital area
Demyelinating syndromes	
Multiple sclerosis	Temporo-parietal area
	Frontal lobe
	Periventricular area
Metachromatic leukodystrophy	Frontal lobe
Adrenoleukodystrophy	Temporo-parietal area
Neoplasms	Temporal lobe and limbic structures (most common)
	Pituitary
	Suprasellar region
	Hippocampus
	Amygdala
	Cingulate gyrus
	Frontal lobe
	Diencephalon
Trauma	Temporal lobe
	Frontal lobe
	Laterality
	Left hemisphere involvement more common with schizophrenia-like psychosis
	Right hemisphere involvement more common with delusions and hallucinations not associated with a schizophrenia-like illness
Focal subcortical degeneration	
Huntington's disease	Caudate more specifically the medial aspect of the caudate head
Parkinson's disease	
Idiopathic calcification of the basal ganglia	
Wilson's disease	
Focal cortical degeneration	
Alzheimer's disease	Temporo-parietal area
Frontotemporal dementia	Temporal lobe

Epilepsy

Epilepsy is one of the more frequent neurologic disorders associated with psychosis and also one of the most controversial. Though a number of studies have failed to find a relationship between seizures and psychosis (Bartlett, 1957; Small, Milsstein and Stevens, 1962; Betts, 1974; Stevens, 1991), and some have reported a decrease in the incidence of epilepsy in patients with schizophrenia (Stevens, 1991), many others have found a predilection for psychosis when epilepsy is present (Gibbs, 1951; Slater, Beard and Glithero, 1963; Flor-Henry, 1969, Slater and Moran, 1969; Wing, Cooper and Sartorius, 1974; Perez et al., 1985; Roberts et al., 1990; Rabins, Starkstein and Robinson, 1991). Studies examining the relationship between lesions and psychosis indicate that lesions accompanied by seizures appear more likely to cause psychotic symptoms (Levine and Finklestein, 1982; Peroutka et al., 1982; Rabins et al., 1991; Starkstein, Robinson and Berthier, 1992).

The area of the brain more implicated in psychosis and epilepsy is the temporal lobe. In 1948, Gibbs, Gibbs and Furster reported a higher than expected prevalence of psychopathology among patients with temporal lobe epilepsy. Since that time, many other studies have found a similar relationship between temporal lobe epilepsy and psychopathology. Flor-Henry (1969) observed that in patients with epilepsy, the chance of developing psychosis was ten times greater in temporal lobe epilepsy than in centrencephalic epilepsy. He also found that significantly more patients with phychosis had left temporal lobe foci. Perez and colleagues (1985) also noted an increased frequency of schizophreniform psychosis in epileptics with left temporal lobe seizures. Some investigators have failed to confirm this laterality of delusion-inducing lesions (Kristensen and Sindrup, 1978b; Jensen and Larsen, 1979). Both Stevens (1991) and Perez et al. (1985) point out that the diagnosis of schizophreniform psychosis in the studies that have found lateralized abnormalities used Schneider's first-rank symptoms, which are based largely on verbal phenomena. These symptoms include thought intrusion, thought broadcast, thought commentary, thought withdrawal, voices talking about the patient, primary delusions, and delusions of control or of alien penetration.

Studies of temporal lobe epilepsy defining the exact structures associated with psychosis have found involvement primarily in the medial temporal lobe. Kristensen and Sindrup (1978b), using electroencephalography employing sphenoidal electrodes, found that patients with temporal lobe epilepsy and psychosis had a significant preponderance of temporal mediobasal spike foci when compared to those with temporal lobe epilepsy and no psychosis. Roberts et al. (1990) analyzed pathological and clinical data from temporal lobectomies to determine factors related to the development of schizophrenia-like psychosis. They found that the schizophrenia-like psychosis was significantly associated with lesions occurring in the fetal or perinatal period and affecting the medial temporal lobe, particularly the left temporal lobe. Gangliogliomas were disproportionately associated with risk of psychosis. Further support of the involvement of deep temporal structures in schizophrenia-like psychosis is provided by depth electrode studies (Stevens, 1991). Stimulation of these structures with depth electrodes or spontaneously occurring seizures recorded with depth electrodes have produced many of the subjective sensations observed in schizophrenia and schizophrenia-like psychosis.

It is paradoxical that there is a tendency for fewer seizures to occur in patients with psychosis and epilepsy than in those afflicted with epilepsy alone. Flor-Henry (1969) found a significantly lower frequency of seizures in the patients with temporal lobe epilepsy and psychosis than in those with temporal lobe epilepsy alone. He noted that this had previously been observed by a number of other earlier investigators (Flor-Henry, 1969). More recent investigators (Slater and Moran, 1969; Kristensen and Sindrup, 1978a; Wolf and Trimble, 1985; Pakalnis et al., 1987a) have also noted an apparent antagonism between the frequency of seizures or epileptic discharges by EEG and the occurrence of psychosis. Flor-Henry (1969) concluded that it is not the epilepsy itself that predisposes one to psychotic symptoms, but the underlying patterns of abnormal neuronal activity in the dominant temporal lobe.

In summary, temporal lobe epilepsy is a risk factor for the development of psychosis. The area of the temporal lobe most often implicated is the deep, medial temporal lobe. When the epileptic focus is lateralized to the left hemisphere, the patient is more likely to manifest Schneiderian first-rank symptoms. The presence of frequent seizures appears to exert a protective effect from psychosis in those who have temporal lobe epilepsy. Psychosis in patients with epilepsy may represent a phenomenon caused by the combination of hyperfunctioning and hypofunctioning of limbic structures.

Strokes

Focal lesions caused by strokes as well as diffuse cerebral white matter damage on a vascular basis have been reported to cause psychosis. Strokes involving the temporoparietal cortex are most frequently reported to produce delusional syndromes and visual hallucinations (Cummings, 1992; Starkstein et al., 1992), though deep gray matter lesions may also cause delusions. The literature supports a right-sided preponderance of lesions leading to psychosis, though left-sided lesions also are implicated, particularly in cases of Wernicke's aphasia. A predisposing condition for the development of psychosis, both singularly and in combination with other lesions, is the presence of white matter ischemic disease or cerebral atrophy.

Single strokes leading to psychosis are rare, but right hemisphere strokes are reported comparatively frequently as inciting events that lead to psychosis. The region of the right hemisphere that most commonly leads to psychosis when affected by a stroke is the right temporo-parieto-occipital junction (Robinson and Downhill, 1995; Cummings, 1997). Rabins and colleagues (1991) described five patients who developed schizophreniform psychosis following stroke. These represented the only patients who had been admitted to a psychiatric unit following stroke over a nine-year period. Interestingly, all five had right hemisphere strokes. Four of the five patients had cortical lesions involving the right temporo-parieto-occipital junction. Price and Mesulam (1985) reported the development of psychosis in five patients with right hemisphere lesions (presumed to represent stroke) identified by focal neurological findings, EEG, or computerized axial tomography (CAT). Of these five cases, four involved the parietal or temporal area by CAT scan of EEG (one of the four also had frontal involvement). Levine and Finklestein (1982) described the development of psychosis in seven patients following stroke (four ischemic, three following hemorrhage) involving the posterior right cerebrum. They noted that they had not observed similar psychoses in patients with lesions situated in homologous areas of the left hemisphere. The predominance of right hemisphere strokes leading to psychosis may be a reflection of the role of the right hemisphere in monitoring the external environment and integrating it into personally relevant information (Borod, 1992). A misperception created by defective environmental monitoring could lead to either delusions or hallucinations.

Anosognosia refers to denial of an acquired deficit in patients with stroke or other lesions, usually involving the right hemisphere (Cummings, 1997). This is a delusional syndrome in which the patient denies weakness or disability of the left limbs and may even deny ownership of the paretic limbs. The delusion concerns only the left side of the body and occurs with other signs of unilateral neglect. It is maintained by the patient despite evidence to the contrary.

Factors predisposing to psychosis in patients with focal strokes include cerebral atrophy and development of seizures. Levine and Finkelstein (1982) found seizures in seven of eight patients who developed psychosis following right hemisphere lesions. The seizures were often temporally related to the onset of psychosis. Rabins et al. (1991) compared patients with psychosis to controls with lesions of comparable size and location but without psychosis. They found that those who developed psychosis had a more severe subcortical atrophy.

White matter lesions are the most frequently identified cerebral abnormality in patients with late-onset psychosis (Miller et al., 1989; Breitner et al., 1990; Lesser et al., 1991, 1992). Delusions in vascular dementia are found more commonly in patients with multiple and bilateral lesions than in those with single infarctions (Cummings et al., 1987). The location of the affected white matter has included the frontal white matter, with involvement of the frontal–subcortical circuits (Merriam and Hegarty, 1989; Miller et al., 1989; Flint, Rifat and Eastwood, 1991) or the temporo-parieto-occipital area (Pakalnis, Drake and Kellum, 1987b; Breitner et al., 1990; Cummings, 1992, 1997) involving auditory or visual pathways and association areas.

Demyelinating syndromes

Demyelinating diseases, including multiple sclerosis, metachromatic leuko-dystrophy, and adrenoleukodystrophy, have frequently been associated with psychosis. All three of these diseases have been misdiagnosed in the early stages as a primary psychiatric illness, including schizophrenia. The localization of lesions leading to psychosis in these diseases is difficult to determine due to their wide-spread or multifocal demyelination.

Multiple sclerosis is commonly associated with psychiatric disturbances. Up to 50% of patients with multiple sclerosis show psychiatric symptoms including psychosis (Mahler, 1992; Nasrallah, 1994). Mania or symptoms of bipolar affective disorder (Joffe et al., 1987, 1988; Pine et al., 1995; Schifferdecker, Krahl and Krekel, 1995), depression (Mahler, 1992), and psychosis (Geocaris, 1957; Kohler, Heilmeyer and Volk, 1988; Feinstein, du Boulay and Ron, 1992; Filley and Gross, 1992; Pine et al., 1995; Schifferdecker et al., 1995) are reported frequently in multiple sclerosis patients. Not infrequently, psychosis has been diagnosed and multiple sclerosis discovered during further examination of the patient (Geocaris, 1957; Drake, 1984; Kohler et al., 1988; Carson and Searle-White, 1996).

Psychosis in patients with multiple sclerosis is most often found with involvement of the temporal–parietal area by the demyelinating process, but other areas have also been implicated. Ron and Logsdail (1989) studied 116 patients with multiple sclerosis and found the presence of delusions and thought disorder correlated with the degree of demyelination in the temporal–parietal region. Honer and colleagues (1987) had previously found a similar relationship. Others have found predominantly frontal involvement (Ramani, 1981), periventricular involvement (Ramani, 1981), or involvement of the basal ganglia, thalamus, hypothalamus, and hippocampus (Salguero, Itabashi and Gutierrez, 1969).

Two other demyelinating diseases that often cause prominent psychiatric disturbances are metachromatic leukodystrophy and adrenoleukodystrophy. Metachromatic leukodystrophy is an autosomal recessive disease that is caused by abnormal lipid storage and the subsequent accumulation of sulfatides in the central and peripheral nervous system. It may begin at any stage of life and is divided into three forms, the infantile, juvenile, and adult forms. With infantile or juvenile onset, white matter involvement is diffuse, but in the adult form multifocal lesions occur in the white matter with a propensity for the frontal lobes (Grossman and Yousem, 1994). The presence of psychiatric symptoms in this disease is well documented (Skomer, Stears and Austin, 1983; Finelli, 1985; Fisher, Cope and Lishman, 1987; Merriam, Hegarty and Miller, 1989; Merriam and Hegarty, 1989; Filley and Gross, 1992; Hyde, Ziegler and Weinberger, 1992; Shapiro et al., 1994). Hyde and colleagues reviewed 129 neuropathologically or biologically confirmed published cases. They noted that psychosis was present in the subjects with adolescent or early adult onset. Because of the presence of psychosis and the initial absence of neurological findings, this subset of patients was often misdiagnosed as having schizophrenia. Involvement of the frontal lobe and subsequent involvement of the mesolimbic dopaminergic system are hypothesized to lead to the psychiatric manifestations (Merriam et al., 1989; Merriam and Hegarty, 1989), though others have hypothesized that the psychiatric manifestations arise from periventricular (Hyde et al., 1992) or temporolimbic involvement (Filley and Gross, 1992).

Adrenoleukodystrophy is an X-linked disorder caused by impairment in the β-oxidation of very long chain fatty acids by peroxisomes, resulting in the accumulation of very long chain fatty acids in the cerebral white matter, adrenal cortex, and body fluids. The accumulation of fatty acids leads to demyelination that is most pronounced in the parieto-occipital regions (Schochet, 1993). Change in behavior followed by intellectual deterioration are the disease's initial manifestations. The disease then causes blindness, quadriparesis, and eventually death due to debilitation (Cummings and Benson, 1992). The psychosis in this disorder arises from temporoparietal involvement (Cummings, 1992).

Neoplasms

Psychosis has been associated with tumors in a variety of locations, e.g. the pituitary (Davison and Bagley, 1969; Galasko, Kwo-on-yuen and Thal, 1988; Stevens, 1991), temporal lobes (Malamud, 1967; Davison and Bagley, 1969; Galasko et al., 1988; Roberts et al., 1990; Stevens, 1991), suprasellar region (Davison and Bagley, 1969; Galasko et al., 1988; Stevens, 1991), hippocampus, amygdala, cingulate gyrus, and frontal lobe (Malamud, 1967; Stevens, 1991), third ventricle (Malamud, 1967; Davison and Bagley, 1969), and diencephalon (Davison and Bagley, 1969; Galasko et al., 1988). Davison and Bagley (1969) found that schizophrenia was significantly associated with pituitary adenomas and that hallucinations were associated with temporal lobe and suprasellar tumors. In a series of 245 brain tumors, Malamud (1967) found schizophrenia-like psychosis associated with tumors in the hippocampus, amygdala, and cingulate gyrus. Twenty percent of tumors affecting the temporal lobes were associated with schizophrenia-like psychosis in a series by Mulder and Daly (1952; Galasko et al., 1988). Overall, psychosis is most common with tumors affecting temporal lobe and limbic structures.

Tumors of developmental origin are disproportionately represented among patients with epilepsy and psychosis. Roberts et al. (1990) analyzed the data from 249 temporal lobectomies performed for intractable TLE. They found that lesions that originated in the fetus or perinatally and involved neurons in the medial temporal lobe were correlated to the eventual development of psychosis. Taylor (1975) found that, of the patients with alien tissue (consisting of small tumors, hamartomas, and focal dysplasia), 23% were psychotic, compared to only 5% of 41 patients with mesial temporal sclerosis. Roberts et al. (1990) found the presence of gangliogliomas (neuro-developmental tumors of the medial temporal lobes) was disproportionately associated with the later development of psychosis.

Trauma

The temporal lobe is the most common site of trauma linked to the development of psychosis. Hillbom (1951) reviewed 1821 cases of brain injury that occurred during the wars between Russian and Finland. Of these, 81 soldiers developed psychosis, 20 of whom had schizophrenia-like disorders. Seventeen of the 20 had temporal lobe trauma with or without other lesions. There was also a greater number of left-sided than right-sided injuries. Hillbom (1960) later analyzed a random sample of 415 patients from among 3552 men with brain injury in the Russian–Finnish War. He noted that left-sided injuries were more common in patients with psychosis as well as other psychiatric disturbances, temporal lobe lesions were more frequent in patients with psychosis, and frontal lesions were slightly underrepresented in association with psychosis. Davison and Bagley (1969; Flor-Henry, 1976) studied 40 cases of post-traumatic psychosis and found significant associations between frontal and temporal lesions, left-hemisphere damage, closed head injury, and unconsciousness of more than 24 hours. Achte and colleagues (Achte, Hillbom and Aalberg, 1969; Stevens, 1991) re-analyzed the data of the aforementioned 3552 cases from the Russian–Finnish War. They found an 8.9% frequency of postinjury psychosis. Temporal lobe lesions were only slightly more common in the psychotic patients when compared to a group of nonpsychotic brain-injured men. Buckley et al. (1993) identified the left temporal lobe as the key area of involvement in three patients with postinjury schizophrenia-like psychosis.

Delusions and paranoia have been related commonly to right hemisphere pathology (Benson, Gardner and Meadows, 1976; Alexander, Stuss and Benson, 1979; Staton, Brumback and Wilson, 1982; Montevecchi and Maniscalco, 1983; Cummings, 1985, 1992; Fuji and Ahmed, 1996), including the right temporal/temporoparietal area (Alexander et al., 1979; Staton et al., 1982; Cummings, 1985, 1992; Fuji and Ahmed, 1996), and right frontal area (Benson et al., 1976; Alexander et al., 1979; Montevecchi and Maniscalco, 1983). Visual hallucinations are also associated commonly with right hemisphere lesions (Cummings, 1997). Left-sided temporal lobe lesions appear more likely in schizophrenia-like psychosis, while right frontal and temporal lesions are more frequently associated with psychosis not associated with a schizophrenia-like illness.

Focal degenerative diseases

Focal degenerative diseases affecting the basal ganglia, including Huntington's disease, Parkinson's disease, idiopathic calcification of the basal ganglia, and Wilson's disease, are known to produce psychotic symptoms as well as extrapyramidal disorders. Among patients with subcortical disorders, psychosis is most common when the caudate nuclei, specifically the medial aspect of the caudate head, are involved (Cummings, 1992, 1995a). Of diseases affecting the basal ganglia, Huntington's disease and idiopathic calcification of the basal ganglia exhibit a higher frequency of delusions; this probably reflects their greater involvement of the medial aspect of the head of the caudate. Delusions associated with extrapyramidal disorders are more difficult to treat and are associated with a relatively spared intellect when compared to other dementias.

Psychosis is commonly seen in degenerative disorders affecting the cortex, including Alzheimer's disease and frontotemporal dementia. Alzheimer's disease pathology predominantly involves the temporal and parietal lobes and is frequently accompanied by psychosis. The prevalence over a year is approximately 35% (Levy et al., 1996) in patients with mild to moderate cognitive impairment. Psychosis is less prevalent in frontotemporal dementia than in Alzheimer's disease, though patients with the temporal lobe variant (predominant involvement of the temporal lobe with relative sparing of the frontal lobes) may show a higher incidence of psychosis. In a recent analysis of data from ten patients with the temporal variant of frontotemporal dementia, two of the patients with predominantly right degeneration were delusional, but none of those with left predominant degeneration had delusional symptoms (Edwards-Lee et al., 1997).

Specific syndromes

Misidentification and reduplicative delusions are more common following right hemisphere injury. Capgras syndrome, the most common misidentification syndrome, is the delusional belief that someone (usually the patient's spouse or other family member) has been replaced by an identical-appearing impostor. This syndrome has been associated most often with right hemisphere pathology (Cummings, 1997). Feinberg and Shapiro (1989) reviewed 26 published cases of Capgras syndrome; they found a trend toward right hemisphere versus left hemisphere abnormality. Structural pathology reported in patients with Capgras syndrome has included isolated right hemisphere damage, diffuse cerebral atrophy, bilateral occipitotemporal and frontal lesions, and bilateral frontal and temporal lesions (Alexander et al., 1979; Lewis, 1987; Forstl, Almeida and Iacoponi, 1991).

Reduplication delusions or reduplication syndromes occur in several different forms and are also most frequently associated with right hemisphere pathology. These syndromes occur when minor changes are noted in a familiar object, place, or person. Patients cannot reconcile or integrate these minor changes with their pre-existing conception of the item in question, and thus imagine that a reduplication has occurred. A striking example of this variety of delusion is the syndrome of reduplicative paramnesia, the belief that a familiar location has been duplicated, despite overwhelming evidence to the contrary. Benson et al. (1976) associated this syndrome with damage involving bilateral frontal lobes and the right hemisphere. A greater association of this syndrome to right-sided lesions was also identified in 96 cases reviewed by Feinberg and Shapiro (1989). It has been suggested that the right hemisphere is responsible for directing attention to and monitoring the external environment (Borod, 1992). This property may cause faulty interpretation of environmental cues when the right hemisphere is damaged, and thus lead to reduplicative delusions.

Schizophrenia

Schizophrenia is the prototypic psychotic illnesses. It is a common disease without a known cause, despite the many well-designed studies of pathologic and functional data in this condition. A number of pathological findings have been identified in patients with schizophrenia and will be briefly reviewed (see Nasrallah, 1994, and Stevens, 1991, for more thorough discussion). Gross findings show that schizophrenics generally have smaller brain mass and volume, reflected by the presence of ventriculomegaly affecting predominantly the lateral and third venticle, smaller midsagittal craniums and cerebrums on magnetic resonance imaging (MRI) scans, smaller brain weight, widened sulci, and cerebellar vermis atrophy. They may have abnormal or reversed cerebral asymmetries compared to controls. The temporal lobe has a number of abnormalities in schizophrenics, including reduced temporal lobe gray matter, abnormal left temporal lobe size, temporal horn enlargement, reduced limbic temporal volume, and focal cortical atrophy. Specific areas with decreased volume at autopsy include the parahippocampal gyrus, hippocampus, amygdala, and internal pallidal segment, and narrowing of the paraventricular nuclei of the thalamus and hypothalamus. The corpus callosum has been found to be thicker or to show other pathology in some patients with schizophrenia.

Microscopic findings have suggested a neurodevelopmental disruption, possibly in the second trimester. Changes have been found in the usual histoarchitecture of brain tissue and a failure of certain neuronal cells to migrate to their normal location. The above catalogued changes in the brains of schizophrenics are not uniformly present, and can vary widely among individuals.

Functional imaging studies have shown differences in schizophrenics compared to normal controls. The frontal lobes have shown decreased cerebral blood flow and decreased glucose metabolism, particularly during tasks known to activate the frontal lobes. The basal ganglia may be metabolically hyperactive in unmedicated schizophrenics. In summary, a number of structural and functional differences commonly occur in schizophrenics, though no abnormality is a uniform finding in all patients suffering from this illness. Abnormalities in the frontal and temporal lobes are encountered most commonly.

Comments

Psychosis is a phenomenon with a variety of differing etiologies found in many conditions. This is a reflection of complex neural mechanisms underlying perception and cognition and the distribution of perceptive and integrative circuits in many brain regions. The lesions associated with psychosis occur in association cortex limbic areas, and other brain regions with extensive communication with the limbic areas (such as the frontal lobe and basal ganglia). Involvement of the association cortex by a disruptive lesion may cause psychosis by leading to less accurate processing of sensory information (visual or auditory). The limbic system is a final step in the integration of this information and its relevance to the organism. Lesions in the limbic or limbic-related areas may produce defective integration of perceptual information and its relevance. Therefore, lesions in these areas cause defective sensory processing and/or the attribution of erroneous relevance to incoming sensory information.

The right hemisphere and right-sided limbic circuits are involved in interpreting, integrating, and assigning relevance to visuospatial, perceptual, and affective information from the environment. When the right hemisphere/right limbic circuits are damaged or dysfunctional, external cues are misinterpreted. This leads to psychotic phenomena such as the reduplicative syndromes, and visual or auditory hallucinations.

The left hemisphere is concerned with the perception and interpretation of verbal information from the environment. When this hemisphere or its limbic circuits are dysfunctional, verbal information is misinterpreted or assigned erroneous relevance. This may give rise to many of the psychotic features described by Schneiderian first-rank symptoms.

Lesions arising in the perinatal period have a greater chance of causing psychosis than those that occur later in life. This is supported by two observations in patients with epilepsy: (1) patients with an earlier onset of seizures have a greater chance of developing psychopathology, including psychosis; and (2) surgical data from temporal lobectomies for seizure control show that lesions arising in the perinatal period are more likely to cause psychosis. This is also supported by pathologic findings in schizophrenia, where microscopic pathology, including abnormal neuronal cytoarchitecture and migration failure, suggests a developmental aberration in the fetus. Lesions in the developing fetus or in the neonatal period appear to be associated disproportionately with the development of psychosis, though lesions in later life can also lead to psychotic phenomena.

The co-occurrence of two or more processes disrupting brain function appears to have a synergistic effect on the development of psychosis. Psychosis is more frequently seen in stroke patients with a coexisting disorder such as cerebral atrophy, diffuse ischemic white matter disease, or seizures.

Dopamine and its balance with other neurotransmitters are commonly linked to the presence of psychosis. The three principal dopamine systems in the brain are: (1) one originating in the substantia nigra and projecting to the striatum, (2) another originating in the hypothalamus and projecting to the infundibulum of the pituitary, and (3) a third originating in the ventral tegmental area and projecting via the medial forebrain bundle to the amygdala, frontal cortex, anterior cingulate cortex, and medial temporal regions (Cummings, 1986). Interruption of these circuits may result in mesolimbic dopamine receptor denervation hypersensitivity similar to that seen in idiopathic schizophrenia (Cummings, 1986). Similarly, the administration of dopaminergic substances to patients with Parkinson's disease may produce psychosis as a side-effect.

Focal lesions do not precisely define the neurotransmitters involved in psychosis, but areas containing dopaminergic or cholinergic circuits are frequently involved (Stevens, 1991; Cummings, 1992). Dopaminergic/cholinergic balance may also be crucial in the genesis of psychosis (Cummings, 1992), Psychosis is frequently encountered in Alzheimer's disease, which has a severe cholinergic deficit but preserved dopaminergic function.

Treatment of psychosis associated with focal neurological lesions

Treatment of psychosis associated with focal brain lesions usually requires the use of antipsychotic agents. In some cases, treatment of the underlying neurological disorder will ameliorate the psychosis, but more often use of an antipsychotic agent will be required. Ictal psychotic events in patients with limbic epilepsy may respond to treatment with anticonvulsants, but interictal psychosis is treated with antipsychotic drugs. Psychotic episodes in multiple sclerosis may emerge and remit in concert with inflammatory CNS activity; an antipsychotic drug will usually be necessary during the episode of psychosis. Post-stroke psychosis may wane with CNS recovery; acute and persistent psychotic symptoms necessitate treatment with antipsychotic medications.

Antipsychotic agents include conventional neuroleptic compounds such as phenothiazines and butyrophenones as well as novel or atypical antipsychotic agents including clozapine, risperidone, olanzapine, and quetiapine. These two classes of agents have approximately equal efficacy, but differ in their side-effect profiles and adverse event liabilities. Conventional antipsychotic drugs are more likely to induce acute and chronic extrapyramidal syndromes, including dystonia, akathisia, parkinsonism, and tardive dyskinesia. Clozapine has induced a few cases of fatal agranulocytosis, and biweekly monitoring of the leukocyte count is required for patients receiving this agent. Interruption of therapy is essential if the white blood cell count declines. Sedation is common with both conventional and atypical antipsychotic agents; it may resolve after the first few days of therapy. There have been relatively few double-blind, placebo-controlled trials of the use of antipsychotic agents in patients with neurological disorders and psychosis. Risperidone has been studied in a double-blind, placebo-controlled trial, and has been shown to be superior to placebo in the treatment of psychosis and agitation in patients with Alzheimer's disease and vascular dementia (Katz et al., 1999).

Many patients with focal neurological lesions and psychosis are elderly. In these patients, application of the principles of geriatric psychopharmacology must be assiduously followed, including introducing drugs at low doses (typically half the dosage used in younger patients), increasing the dose slowly, and carefully monitoring for potential side-effects. Dosages should be advanced until an acceptable benefit has been observed or the limits of tolerability have been reached. Changes in the absorption, distribution, binding, and receptor sensitivity of elderly patients frequently mean that lower end doses will be achieved than is typical for younger patients. Increased frequencies of comorbid conditions and the co-administration of pharmacologic agents for the management of these conditions increase the chance of drug interactions and require constant vigilance (Jenike, 1989; Salzman, 1998: pp. 21–47).

In summary, three factors contribute to the development of psychosis following a focal lesion: (1) lesion location, (2) stage of cerebral development, and (3) concomitant brain pathology (see Table 15.2). Lesions in some areas, such as association cortex, limbic areas, or areas with extensive limbic connections, are more likely to lead to psychosis than lesions in other locations. The presence of a lesion during the developmental period is more likely to lead to psychosis. Concomitant brain pathologies such as diffuse ischemic white matter disease, atrophy or seizures increase the frequency of psychosis in patients with focal lesions.

Table 15.2. Factors contributing to the development of psychosis with a focal lesion

Location of lesion
   Limbic areas or areas with extensive limbic connections
   Association areas
Stage of cerebral development
   Presence of a lesion during the developmental period
Concomitant brain pathology
   Diffuse ischemic white matter disease
   Cerebral atrophy
   Seizures

Acknowledgments

This project was supported by a National Institute on Aging Alzheimer's Disease Center Grant (AG10123), an NIA training award, and the Sidell-Kagan Foundation.

REFERENCES

Achte, K.A., Hillbom, E. and Aalberg, V. (1969). Psychoses following war brain injuries. *Acta Psychiatr Scand* 45: 1–18.

Alexander, M.P., Stuss, D.T. and Benson, D.F. (1979). Capgras syndrome: a reduplicative phenomenon. *Neurology* 29: 334–9.

Bartlett, J. (1957). Chronic psychosis following epilepsy. *Am J Psychiatry* 114: 338–43.

Benson, D.F., Gardner, H. and Meadows, J.C. (1976). Reduplicative paramnesia. *Neurology* 26: 147–51.

Betts, T. (1974). *A follow-up study of a cohort of patients with epilepsy admitted to psychiatric care in an English city*, ed. P. Harris and C. Maudsley. Edinburgh: Churchill Livingstone.

Borod, J.C. (1992). Interhemispheric and intrahemispheric control of emotion: a focus on unilateral brain damage. Special section: The emotional concomitants of brain damage. *J Consult Clin Psychol* 60: 339–48.

Breitner, J.C., Husain, M.M., Figiel, G.S. et al. (1990). Cerebral white matter disease in late-onset paranoid psychosis. *Biol Psychiatry* 28: 266–74.

Buckley, P., Stack, J.P., Madigan, C. et al. (1993). Magnetic resonance imaging of schizophrenia-like psychoses associated with cerebral trauma: clinicopathological correlates. *Am J Psychiatry* 150: 146–8.

Carson, H.J. and Searle-White, D.J. (1996). Occult multiple sclerosis presenting with psychosis. *Can J Psychiatry* 41: 486–7.

Cummings, J. (1986). Organic psychosis, delusional disorders and secondary mania. *Psychiatric Clin N Am* 9: 293–311.

Cummings, J.L. (1985). Organic delusions: phenomenology, anatomical correlations, and review. *Br J Psychiatry* 146: 184–97.

Cummings, J.L. (1992). Psychosis in neurologic disease: neurobiology and pathogenesis. *Neuropsychiatry Neuropsychol Behav Neurol* 5: 144–50.

Cummings, J.L. (1995a). Behavioral and psychiatric symptoms associated with Huntington's disease. In *Behavioral Neurology of Movement Disorders*, Vol. 65, ed. W.J. Weiner and A.E. Lange, pp. 179–86. New York: Raven Press.

Cummings, J.L. (1995b). Neuropsychiatry: clinical assessment and approach to diagnosis. In *Comprehensive Textbook of Psychiatry*, Vol. 1, ed. H.I. Kaplan and B.J. Saddock, pp. 167–86. Baltimore: Williams and Wilkins.

Cummings, J.L. (1997). Neuropsychiatric manifestations of right hemisphere lesions. *Brain Lang* 57: 22–37.

Cummings, J.L. and Benson, D.F. (1992). *Dementia, a Clinical Approach.* Stoneham, MA: Butterworth–Heinemann.

Cummings, J.L., Miller, B., Hill, M.A. and Neshkes, R. (1987). Neuropsychiatric aspects of multi-infarct dementia and dementia of the Alzheimer type. *Arch Neurol* 44: 389–93.

Davison, K. and Bagley, C.R. (1969). Schizophrenia-like psychosis associated with organic disorders of the central nervous system: review of the literature. In *British Journal of Psychiatry Special Publication*, Vol., ed. R.N. Herrington, pp. 113–84. Ashford, Kent: Headley Bros Ltd.

Drake, M.E. (1984). Acute paranoid psychosis in multiple sclerosis. *Psychosomatics* 25: 60–5.

Edwards-Lee, T., Miller, B.L., Benson, D.F. et al. (1997). The temporal variant of frontotemporal dementia. *Brain* 120: 1027–40.

Feinberg, T.E. and Shapiro, R.M. (1989). Misidentification–reduplication and the right hemisphere. *Neuropsychiatry Neuropsychol Behav Neurol* 2: 39–48.

Feinstein, A., du Boulay, G. and Ron, M.A. (1992). Psychotic illness in multiple sclerosis: a clinical and magnetic resonance imaging study. *Br J Psychiatry* 161: 680–5.

Filley, C.M. and Gross, K.F. (1992). Psychosis with cerebral white matter disease. *Neuropsychiatry Neuropsychol Behav Neurol* 5: 119–25.

Finelli, P.F. (1985). Metachromatic leukodystrophy manifesting as a schizophrenic disorder: computed tomographic correlation. *Ann Neurol* 18: 94–5.

Fisher, N.R., Cope, S.J. and Lishman, W.A. (1987). Metachromatic leukodystrophy: conduct disorder progressing to dementia. *J Neurol Neurosurg Psychiatry* 50: 488–9.

Flint, A., Rifat, S. and Eastwood, R. (1991). Brain lesions and cognitive function in late-life psychosis. *Br J Psychiatry* 158: 866.

Flor-Henry, P. (1969). Psychosis and temporal lobe epilepsy. *Epilepsia* 10: 363–95.

Flor-Henry, P. (1976). Lateralized temporal–limbic dysfunction and psychopathology. *Ann N Y Acad Sci* 280: 777–97.

Flor-Henry, P. (1983). Determinants of psychosis in epilepsy: laterality and forced normalization. *Biol Psychiatry* 18: 1045–57.

Forstl, H., Almeida, O.P. and Iacoponi, E. (1991). Capgras delusion in the elderly: the evidence for a possible organic origin. *Int J Geriatr Psychiatry* 6: 845–52.

Fuji, D.E.M. and Ahmed, I. (1996). Psychosis secondary to traumatic brain injury. *Neuropsychiatry Neuropsychol Behav Neurol* 9: 133–8.

Galasko, D.R., Kwo-on-yuen, P.F. and Thal, L.J. (1988). Intracranial mass lesions associated with late-onset psychosis and depression. *Psychiatr Clin N Am* 11: 151–66.

Geocaris, K. (1957). Psychotic episodes heralding the diagnosis of multiple sclerosis. *Bull Menninger Clin* 21: 107–16.

Gibbs, F.A. (1951). Ictal and non-ictal psychiatric disorders in temporal lobe epilepsy. *J Nerv Ment Dis* 113: 522–8.

Gibbs, F.A., Gibbs, E.L. and Furster, B. (1948). Psychomotor epilepsy. *Arch Neurol* 60: 331–9.

Grossman, R.I. and Yousem, D.M. (1994). *Neuroradiology, the Requisites*, ed. J. Thrall. St. Louis, MI: Mosby-Year Book, Inc.

Hillbom, E. (1951). Schizophrenia-like psychoses after brain trauma. *Acta Psychiatr Neurol* 60 (Suppl.): 36–47.

Hillbom, E. (1960). After-effects of brain-injuries: research on the symptoms causing invalidism of persons in Finland having sustained brain-injuries during the wars of 1939–1940 and 1941–1944. *Acta Psychiatr Neurol* 142: 1–195.

Honer, W.G., Hurwitz, T.A., Li, D.K. et al. (1987). Temporal lobe involvement in multiple sclerosis patients with psychiatric disorders. *Arch Neurol* 44: 187–90.

Hyde, T.M., Ziegler, J.C. and Weinberger, D.R. (1992). Psychiatric disturbances in metachromatic leukodystrophy: insights into the neurobiology of psychosis. *Arch Neurol* 49: 401–6.

Jenike, M.A. (1989). *Geriatric Psychiatry and Psychopharmacology: a Clinical Approach*. Chicago: Mosby-Year Book.

Jensen, I. and Larsen, J.K. (1979). Psychoses in drug resistant temporal lobe epilepsy. *J Neurol Neurosurg Psychiatry* 42: 948–54.

Joffe, R.T., Lippert, G.P., Gray, T.A. et al. (1987). Mood disorder and multiple sclerosis. *Arch Neurol* 44: 376–8.

Joffe, R.T., Lippert, G.P., Gray, T.A. et al. (1988). Multiple sclerosis and mood disorders. *Adv Neurol* 5: 34–7.

Kaplan, H.I. and Saddock, B.J. (1995). Typical signs and symptoms of psychiatric illness. In *Comprehensive Textbook of Psychiatry*, Vol. 1, ed. H.I. Kaplan and B.J. Saddock, pp. 535–44. Baltimore, MD: Williams and Wilkins.

Katz, I.R., Jeste, D.V., Mintzer, J.E. et al. (1999). Comparison of risperidone and placebo for psychosis and behavioral disturbances associated with dementia: a randomized, double-blind trial. *J Clin Psychiatry* 60: 107–15.

Kohler, J., Heilmeyer, H. and Volk, B. (1988). Multiple sclerosis presenting as chronic atypical psychosis. *J Neurol Neurosurg Psychiatry* 51: 281–4.

Kristensen, O. and Sindrup, E.H. (1978a). Psychomotor epilepsy and psychosis: I. Physical aspects. *Acta Neurol Scand* 57: 361–9.

Kristensen, O. and Sindrup, E.H. (1978b). Psychomotor epilepsy and psychosis: II. Electroencephalographic findings (sphenoidal electrode recordings). *Acta Neurol Scand* 57: 370–9.

Lesser, I.M., Jeste, D.V., Boone, K.B. et al. (1992). Late-onset psychotic disorder, not otherwise specified: clinical and neuroimaging findings. *Biol Psychiatry* 31: 419–23.

Lesser, I.M., Miller, B.L., Boone, K.B. et al. (1991). Brain injury and cognitive function in late-onset psychotic depression. *J Neuropsychiatry Clin Neurosci* 3: 33–40.

Levine, D.N. and Finklestein, S. (1982). Delayed psychosis after right temporoparietal stroke or trauma: relation to epilepsy. *Neurology* 32: 267–73.

Levy, M.L., Cummings, J.L., Fairbanks, L.A. et al. (1996). Longitudinal assessment of symptoms of depression, agitation, and psychosis in 181 patients with Alzheimer's disease. *Am J Psychiatry* 153: 1438–43.

Lewis, S.W. (1987). Brain imaging in a case of Capgras' syndrome. *Br J Psychiatry* 150: 117–21.

Mahler, M. (1992). Behavioral manifestations associated with multiple sclerosis. *Psychiatric Clin N Am* 15: 427–38.

Malamud, N. (1967). Psychiatric disorders with intracranial tumors of limbic system. *Arch Neurol* 17: 113–23.

Merriam, A.E. and Hegarty, A.M. (1989). Brain white-matter lesions and psychosis. *Br J Psychiatry* 155: 868–9.

Merriam, A.E., Hegarty, A. and Miller, A. (1989). A proposed etiology for psychotic symptoms in white matter dementia. *Neuropsychiatry Neuropsychol Behav Neurol* 2: 225–8.

Miller, B.L., Lesser, I.M., Boone, K. et al. (1989). Brain white-matter lesions and psychosis. *Br J Psychiatry* 155: 73–8.

Montevecchi, M.T. and Maniscalco, G. (1983). Un caso di psicosi schizofreniforme postraumatica. [A case of post-traumatic schizophrenic psychosis.] *Riv Speriment Freniatr Med Legale Alien Ment* 107: 548–58.

Mulder, D.W. and Daly, D. (1952). Psychiatric symptoms associated with lesions of temporal lobe. *JAMA* 150: 173–6.

Nasrallah, H.A. (1994). The neuropsychiatry of schizophrenia. In *Synopsis of Neuropsychiatry*, ed. R.E.H. Stuart and C. Yudofsky, pp. 483–96. Washington, DC: American Psychiatric Press.

Pakalnis, A., Drake, M.E., John, K. and Kellum, J.B. (1987a). Forced normalization: acute psychosis after seizure control in seven patients. *Arch Neurol* 44: 289–92.

Pakalnis, A., Drake, M.E. and Kellum, J.B. (1987b). Right parieto-occipital lacunar infarction with agitation, hallucinations, and delusions. *Psychosomatics* 28: 95–6.

Perez, M.M., Trimble, M.R., Murray, N.M. and Reider, I. (1985). Epileptic psychosis: an evaluation of PSE profiles. *Br J Psychiatry* 146: 155–63.

Peroutka, S.J., Sohmer, B.H., Kumar, A.J., Folstein, M. and Robinson, R.G. (1982). Hallucinations and delusions following a right temporoparietooccipital infarction. *Johns Hopkins Med J* 151: 181–5.

Pine, D.S., Douglas, C.J., Charles, E. et al. (1995). Patients with multiple sclerosis presenting to psychiatric hospitals. *J Clin Psychiatry* 56: 297–306.

Price, B.H. and Mesulam, M. (1985). Psychiatric manifestations of right hemisphere infarctions. *J Nerv Ment Dis* 173: 610–14.

Rabins, P.V., Starkstein, S.E. and Robinson, R.G. (1991). Risk factors for developing atypical (schizophreniform) psychosis following stroke. *J Neuropsychiatry Clin Neurosci* 3: 6–9.

Ramani, S.V. (1981). Psychosis associated with frontal lobe lesions in Schilder's cerebral sclerosis: a case report with CT scan evidence. *J Clin Psychiatry* 42: 250–2.

Roberts, G.W., Done, D.J., Bruton, C. and Crow, T.J. (1990). A 'mock-up' of schizophrenia: temporal lobe epilepsy and schizophrenia-like psychosis. *Biol Psychiatry* 28: 127–43.

Robinson, R.G. and Downhill, J.E. (1995). Lateralization of psychopathology in response to focal brain injury. In *Brain Asymmetry*, ed. K.H. Richard and J. Davidson, pp. 693–711. Cambridge, MA: MIT Press.

Ron, M.A. and Logsdail, S.J. (1989). Psychiatric morbidity in multiple sclerosis: a clinical and MRI study. *Psychol Med* 19: 887–95.

Salguero, L.F., Itabashi, H.H. and Gutierrez, N.B. (1969). Childhood multiple sclerosis with psychotic manifestations. *J Neurol Neurosurg Psychiatry* 32: 572–9.

Salzman, C., ed. (1998). *Clinical Geriatric Psychopharmacology*, 3rd edn. Baltimore: Williams & Wilkins.

Schifferdecker, M., Krahl, A. and Krekel, N.O. (1995). Psychosen bei multipler Sklerose – eine Neubewertung. (Psychoses in multiple sclerosis: a reassessment.) *Fortschr Neurol Psychiatr* 63: 310–19.

Schochet, S.S. (1993). Intoxication and metabolic diseases of the central nervous system. In *Principles and Practice of Neuropathology*, ed. J.S. Nelson, J.E. Parisi and S.S. Schochet, pp. 302–43. St Louis, MO: Mosby-Year Book.

Shapiro, E.G., Lockman, L.A., Knopman, D. and Krivit, W. (1994). Characteristics of the dementia in late-onset metachromatic leukodystrophy. *Neurology* 44: 662–5.

Skomer, C., Stears, J. and Austin, J. (1983). Metachromatic leukodystrophy (MLD). XV. Adult MLD with focal lesions by computed tomography. *Arch Neurol* 40: 354–5.

Slater, E., Beard, A.W. and Glithero, E. (1963). The schizophrenia-like psychoses of epilepsy. *Br J Psychiatry* 109: 95–150.

Slater, E. and Moran, P.A. (1969). The schizophrenia-like psychoses of epilepsy: relation between ages of onset. *Br J Psychiatry* 115: 599–600.

Small, J.S., Milsstein, V. and Stevens, J.R. (1962). Are psychomotor epileptics different? *Arch Neurol* 7: 330–8.

Starkstein, S., Robinson, R. and Berthier, M.L. (1992). Post-stroke hallucinatory delusional syndromes. *Neuropsychiatry Neuropsychol Behav Neurol* 5: 114–18.

Staton, R.D., Brumback, R.A. and Wilson, H. (1982). Reduplicative paramnesia: a disconnection syndrome of memory. *Cortex* 18: 23–35.

Stevens, J.R. (1991). *Psychosis and the Temporal Lobe*, Vol. 55, ed. D. Smith, D. Treiman and M. Trimble. New York: Raven Press.

Taylor, D.C. (1975). Factors influencing the occurrence of schizophrenia-like psychosis in patients with temporal lobe epilepsy. *Psychol Med* 5: 249–54.

Wing, J.K., Cooper, J.E. and Sartorius, N. (1974). *The Description and Classification of Psychiatric Symptoms*. Cambridge: Cambridge University Press.

Wolf, P. and Trimble, M.R. (1985). Biological antagonism and epileptic psychosis. *Br J Psychiatry* 146: 272–6.

16

Alterations in sexual behavior following focal brain injury

John M. Ringman and Jeffrey L. Cummings

Introduction

The brain is the source of the motivating impulse, processor of the preparatory stimuli, and organizer of the required motoric activity for sexual activity. The motivating impulse, or libido, is the source of the behaviors of courting and romance. The notions of beauty and sense of family also arise from the brain. Lesions of the nervous system can derange this set of behaviors in many ways.

A variety of alterations in sexual behavior in association with neurological disease have been observed and reported. An analysis of this literature is of interest, not only because of its obvious clinical importance, but also as a means of studying the neurological basis of such behavior. Sexual activity is the result of a complex interaction of diverse influences, namely psychosocial, developmental, hormonal, and neurological. It is therefore subject to perturbation in many ways. An understanding of this interplay has far-reaching implications not only for the individual but also for the human species at large. This chapter reviews the literature on focal neurological lesions affecting sexual behavior and draws inferences on the neuroanatomy subserving such behavior. Finally, it addresses therapies aimed at modifying sexual function in the neurologically impaired.

Background and definitions

Despite many case reports and exhaustive animal research there are still many unanswered questions about the neurological basis for the human sexual response. It has proven to be a very difficult topic to study for a number of reasons. First, patients are not always forthcoming with observations or complaints regarding their sexuality. This may be because of self-consciousness, denial, or a lack of confidence in their physician's ability to deal with such issues. Second, most physicians themselves do not specifically ask questions regarding patients' sexual behavior. This may be secondary to discomfort in discussing these issues or because physicians underestimate their importance. In comparison to, for example, the ability to ambulate, sexual impairment may seem a secondary concern, but sexual dysfunction can be a major cause of distress and can affect quality of life dramatically. It is sometimes unclear with whom the appropriate expertise lies, whether in the realm of the urologist, gynecologist, endocrinologist, neurologist, psychologist, or psychiatrist. Third, the multifactorial nature of sexuality makes it difficult to analyze. The influences of unmeasurable factors such as family and religious values, past experiences, and partner availability make controlled observations impossible. One must often rely on patients' subjective histories for data regarding sexual behavior, a source which may be of limited value. Memory and insight may be lost in the neurologically impaired or patients may be ashamed or have other interests preventing them from representing themselves objectively. These reservations must be kept in mind when reading the literature. Fourth, sexual phenomena are difficult to study in controlled laboratory conditions for obvious logistic and ethical reasons. Finally, the great chasm between animal models and humans limits the generalizability of animal research. There is great variability among primates in their sexual behavior, for example in their display behavior and associated social hierarchy (MacLean, 1973). The differences between humans and nonhuman primate models are unquestionably great. Despite these limitations, we will attempt to draw tentative conclusions from the available human and animal data.

One metholodological issue in studying human sexual behavior lies in its definition. For example, if a couple experiences a decline in frequency of sexual activity, it could be because of decreased libido or decreased ability. In order to delineate the neurological mechanisms of the various aspects of human sexual behavior it is therefore necessary to define its different components and in turn see how these are affected in a specific context. A potentially useful classification scheme is to divide sexual behavior into *motivational* (pertaining to libido, or desire to engage in sexual activity), *orientational* (concerning the object of sexual desire), and *mechanical* (pertaining to the ability to engage in actual sexual acts) aspects. Cases are analyzed with respect to these dimensions, with an emphasis on the first two.

Alterations in sexual behavior occur after many different types of insults to the central nervous system (CNS). Physical trauma, ischemia, adverse drug effects, inflammation, degeneration, and metabolic derangements have all been reported to influence the sexual response by means of an effect on the brain and spinal cord. The influence of hormones on the development and expression of sexual behavior through their effect on the CNS is a discipline unto itself. Brain lesions are discussed that may ultimately exert their effect on sexual behavior via endocrinological changes without specific discussion of the hormonal changes themselves. For a discussion of this topic, see Bauer (1958) or Van de Poll and Van Goozen (1992). In addition, neurodegenerative diseases can influence sexual function (Cummings and Duchen, 1981; Federoff et al., 1994), but this chapter addresses focal lesions and will not review the sexual behavior changes associated with degenerative disorders. The focus of this chapter is on the many ways relatively discrete neurological lesions, regardless of their etiology, can affect sexual behavior.

Focal lesions producing altered sexual behavior

To discuss changes in sexual behavior coherently it is necessary to simplify and categorize these alterations. Changes in sexual activity are divided into those concerning *hyposexuality* (a decrease in libido or ability), *hypersexuality* (an increase in libido or ability), and in changes of *orientation* (altered sexual preference or paraphilias).

Hyposexuality

A decrease in sexual ability, desire, or both is the most common sexual complaint in the context of neurological illness. Its overall frequency is unknown. There is a complex interaction between sexual ability, sexual desire, and medical conditions. For example, sexual dysfunction is common in the context of diabetes mellitus. Impotency or erectile dysfunction has been reported to be present in 1–47% of men with insulin-dependent diabetes mellitus, depending on the duration of illness (Klein et al., 1996). Besides neuropathy, diabetes mellitus predisposes patients to cerebral ischemia and potentially to ischemia involving the genitals via impairment of the pelvic circulation, and it may be unclear in any particular case which is the most important factor affecting sexual function. Only with elaborate histories, examinations, and laboratory tests can such influences be distinguished.

Cerebrovascular lesions

Decreased sexual desire and/or ability is the most common sexual complaint following cerebrovascular accidents, its frequency varying among reports. A survey of a population of 35 male and female patients (Bray, DeFrank and Wolfe, 1981) found no decrease in sexual desire but significant changes in sexual ability and other aspects of sexual function after cerebrovascular accident. Only 11 of 18 men who could obtain erections normally and seven of 21 men who could ejaculate normally prior to their stroke continued to do so afterwards. In the women, two of the five who were still menstruating at the time of their cerebrovascular accident had interruptions in their patterns and only one of five remained orgasmic. Unfortunately, there were no data given in this series regarding the location of the strokes so no anatomical correlations can be made.

The information regarding a possible cerebral lateralization of sexual function is contradictory. In one series of 105 (Kalliomaki, Markkanen and Mustonen, 1961) post-stroke patients, the authors divided the sample into those with left hemiparesis, right hemiparesis, no hemiparesis, and subarachnoid hemorrhage. They asked the patients about change in libido and in coital frequency subsequent to their strokes and found that 37.8% of those with right hemiparesis and 16.7% with left hemiparesis had experienced a decrease in sexual drive. This difference between these groups was thought to be significant and the authors speculated that the left hemisphere is more important for sexual arousal. There was no difference between the genders in libido alterations. Of the males in this study for whom adequate data were available, 68% of those with left hemiparesis and 47.8% of those with right hemiparesis had decreased coital frequency. These data seem to indicate a trend for decreased coital frequency after stroke in males regardless of the side of infarct. The small number in this subgroup as well as the lack of a specification of the exact reasons for decreased coital frequency limit the interpretability of the study, but the observations favor a greater left-hemispheric involvement in sexual arousal.

In another study (Coslett and Heilman, 1986) damage to the right hemisphere was found to cause sexual dysfunction more frequently than damage to the left hemisphere. In this study, 26 male patients with hemispheric strokes (14 left hemisphere and 12 right hemisphere) were interviewed regarding their libido and frequency of intercourse before and after their strokes. Sixty-seven percent of the patients with right hemisphere strokes and 21% of those with left hemisphere strokes reported a decrease in libido. Seventy-five percent of right-hemisphere-damaged patients and 29% of left-hemisphere-damaged patients reported a decrease in their coital frequency. Most patients (18/26) underwent computerized tomography (CT), but there was no obvious correlation between presence or type of sexual dysfunction and pattern of lobar involvement.

The discrepancies between the findings in these two studies are probably explained by the different populations studied. In the study of Kalliomaki et al., there was little clinical information presented (and the study was done in the pre-CT era) and the patients were merely classified according to the side of hemiparesis. Brainstem lesions and subcortical lacunes which might not be comparable to hemispheric strokes were probably included. On the other hand, in an attempt to reduce confounding variables, the study by Coslett and Heilman had several exclusionary criteria. They excluded patients with depression, which is often associated with loss of libido and is more frequently seen in left hemisphere strokes (Robinson et al., 1984). Excluding this population may have artificially reduced the number of left-hemisphere-damaged patients with sexual dysfunction. Coslett and Heilman interpreted the reduced sexual function they observed in right-hemisphere-damaged patients as an aspect of the known laterality of *emotional* perception and expression. It is likely that cortical functions represented in both hemispheres, namely perception, language, and praxis, contribute to sexual function.

There have been few studies regarding sexual function after subarachnoid hemorrhage. This is especially unfortunate considering the predisposition of berry aneurysms, the most common cause of spontaneous subarachnoid hemorrhage, to be located in the area of the anterior cerebral artery and its bifurcations. The neural tissue underlying this vasculature (the hypothalamus, septal area, and orbito-frontal lobes) comprises areas of critical importance in the motivation and expression of sexual behavior, and the assessment of sexual behavior in subarachnoid hemorrhage patients would be of considerable interest. Kalliomaki et al. include 13 patients with subarachnoid hemorrhage involving unspecified structures in their series. They found that five (39%) of these patients experienced decreased libido, and all of the eight patients for whom they had adequate information regarding coital frequency experienced a decrease.

Though limited in number, these studies indicate a high incidence of sexual dysfunction in stroke patients. However, findings differ markedly among reports. Whether motivational or mechanical difficulties are encountered most frequently and whether or not there is an asymmetry in neocortical representation of sexuality are still uncertain.

Epilepsy

Though not a static CNS lesion, epilepsy is a focal lesion that periodically gives rise to more generalized manifestations. A number of different factors may contribute to changes in sexual behavior occurring in epilepsy: the continuous presence of a cerebral lesion, interictal spikes, ictal spreading of seizure activity, postictal depression of cerebral activity, hormonal changes secondary to seizures, and anticonvulsant medications.

As with most neurological illnesses, hyposexuality is the most common sexual complaint in epileptic patients. Rates of its occurrence range from 12% to 68% in different studies. In one series, Shukla, Srivastava and Katiyar (1979) found that 63% of temporal lobe epilepsy patients were hyposexual in comparison to only 12% of patients with generalized epilepsy. Other investigators have confirmed this finding (Blumer and Walker, 1967). In the series of 15 men with temporal lobe lesions (trauma: 5 patients; glioma: 4 patients; temporal lobe epilepsy: 4 patients; and possible capillary angioma: 1 patient) described by Hierons and Saunders (1966), the dysfunction was one of impotence rather than of decreased libido. Some of these patients were untreated at the time impotence was noted and the impotence resolved after anticonvulsants were given. The mechanism of hyposexuality in temporal lobe epilepsy is unclear but might be related to an inhibitory function of the temporal lobes on sexual behavior which is increased by interictal spike discharges. Further evidence for this is that removal of the temporal lobes or depression of their function postictally can result in *hypersexuality* (discussed below).

Prolactin causes a decrease in libido and may contribute to hyposexuality in some epileptic patients. Prolactin is released in surges with seizure activity. In addition, several reports (Murialdo et al., 1995; Isojarvi et al., 1995) have shown that impotence and decreased libido were associated with a decreased testosterone/estradiol ratio in male epileptic patients. This alteration occurs presumably because of an effect of anticonvulsants on hepatic metabolism.

Trauma

The reported incidence of sexual dysfunction in patients who have undergone traumatic brain injury varies from 4% to 71%. This wide range is hardly surprising considering the variable types of lesions in the populations studied. Not only do these patients vary in the type of head trauma sustained (blunt versus penetrating, diffuse versus focal injury), but also in the severity of traumatic brain injury, presence of trauma to other areas (e.g., the spinal cord), age, and time since the injury. Despite the diffuse nature of many brain injuries, traumatic brain injury is of interest because of the predilection of the anterior temporal and orbitofrontal lobes (areas known to be involved in sexuality) to damage in blunt head trauma.

Most early studies focused on the effect of traumatic brain injury on erectile function in men; the incidence varies from 4% to 57% in different studies. In a series of 739 men with head injuries sustained in World War II (Walker and Jablon, 1959), the prevalence was 8%, being more common in the more severely injured. Information regarding associated deficits and confounding variables such as medication was not given.

Sandel and colleagues (1996) studied 52 patients who had sustained severe traumatic brain injury. Seventy-five percent of the patients were men and they had their injury an average 3.7 years prior to the interview. The nature of sexual dysfunction and its relationship to type and severity of brain damage and cognitive impairment were studied. Using a self-reported semistructured interview format, these investigators found that their patients were below the norm in their experiences of sexual desire and orgasm, but total sexual functioning was not significantly impaired. There was no relationship between total sexual functioning and severity of injury as quantified by the initial Glascow Coma Scale (GCS) rating or length of post-traumatic amnesia. There was an inverse relationship between time since injury and degree of sexual arousal: the more recent the head injury, the higher the level of sexual arousal. Forty-two patients could be classified as to whether or not they had frontal lobe damage and 25 patients as to whether the left or right hemisphere was more affected. None of these groups differed from each other in their total sexual functioning scores, but patients with frontal lobe damage tended to score higher on the 'cognitions/fantasies' subscale and to be in the 'higher sexual functioning' group. Patients with predominant right hemisphere damage reported higher sexual arousal and had more sexual experiences. The possible effects of depression with left hemisphere lesions could not be deduced from these data.

This study is modestly encouraging with regard to the high level of sexual functioning in most of these patients with fairly severe brain damage. Conclusions regarding structure–function relationships must be tempered by the diffuse injury present in most of these patients.

Neurosurgery

The relatively controlled brain trauma that occurs during neurosurgery can also cause a decrease in sexual functioning. Meyers (1961) reported one woman and three men who underwent bilateral homologous ansotomy (surgical interruption of the pallidofugal pathway) for the control of hyperkinetic movement disorders. All of the men experienced a decrease in their libido and erectile function and the woman lost her libido and became anorgasmic. A fifth man in whom the lesions were performed in slightly different areas on each side did not experience post-operative loss of libido or potency. The author concluded that it was severance of the pallidofugal fibers that was responsible for the hyposexuality, while acknowledging that the areas lesioned probably included the 'ventral thalamic peduncle, the perifornical region, and the dorsal medial hypothalamic nuclei' as well as the pallidum and pallidofugal fibers. Recently a patient with Parkinson's disease who underwent stereotactic unilateral pallidotomy at UCLA (unpublished observation) became more sexually active despite a decrease in dosage of dopaminergic medications. The role of the globus pallidus in sexual behavior should be explored with the increasing numbers of patients undergoing pallidotomy for Parkinson's disease and hyperkinetic movement disorders.

Multiple sclerosis

Changes in sexual activity are commonly reported in the context of multiple sclerosis. The spinal cord is susceptible to multiple sclerosis lesions producing sensory and erectile dysfunction and hyposexuality is the most common sexually related complaint.

A recent survey (Mattson et al., 1995) of 101 multiple sclerosis patients (65% female) in which detailed questions regarding sexual function and satisfaction were asked revealed that 86% were interested in lovemaking around the time of interview and that this interest had decreased since the diagnosis of multiple sclerosis in 35%. Seventy-eight percent of men and 45% of women complained of general sexual dysfunction, with this dysfunction fluctuating with disease activity, especially in men. Specifically, 38% of women complained of no orgasms, 26% of decreased vaginal lubrication, and 12% of painful intercourse. Twenty-nine percent of men complained of trouble maintaining erections, 26% of decreased penile sensation, and 23% of absent orgasms. There was an expected association of such factors as urinary dysfunction and depression with sexual dysfunction. In 24% of patients, sexual dysfunction was believed to be the cause of marital problems. Besides the association with urinary disturbances, there was no attempt at making clinico-anatomical correlations in this study.

Hypersexuality

Though occurring less frequently than hyposexuality in the context of neurological illness, hypersexuality, or increased sexual activity over one's baseline, is more obvious when it arises. Hypersexuality can occur with relatively focal neurological conditions.

One well-described set of symptoms accompanied by hypersexuality is the Klüver–Bucy syndrome. In 1939, Klüver and Bucy observed in monkeys that had undergone bilateral temporal lobectomies a consistent constellation of behavioral abnormalities consisting of 'psychic blindness' (agnosia), hyperorality, 'hypermetamorphosis' (a tendency to explore objects either manually or orally), emotional placidity, and increased sexual activity. In 1955, Terzian and Dalle Ore described the first human case, and subsequently many cases with either the full syndrome or parts of it were added to the literature. Anatomically, the commonly affected areas in all verified cases are the amygdaloid nuclei bilaterally. Cerebrovascular accident, viral encephalitis, Alzheimer's disease, Pick's disease, trauma, adrenoleukodystrophy, bilateral temporal lobectomy or amygdalotomy, paraneoplastic limbic encephalitis, anoxia, hypoglycemia, toxoplasmic encephalitis, and possibly heat stroke (Lilly et al., 1983; Pitt et al., 1995) have all been reported to cause Klüver–Bucy syndrome.

Mania is another behavioral syndrome that can accompany hypersexuality in the context of either idiopathic psychiatric illness or neurological disease. This condition consists of increased energy, decreased need for sleep, and flight of ideas. These ideas and actions often pertain to grandiose themes, for example extreme sexual power.

Cerebrovascular lesions

Kalliomaki et al. (1961) found that 8.3% of their patients with left-sided paralysis and 4.4% of those with right-sided paralysis had increased libido. One of the ten patients without hemiparesis and none of the 12 patients with subarachnoid hemorrhage had a similar increase. Only one patient (who had right-sided paralysis) in the 68 for which they had adequate data reported increased frequency of coitus. Hypersexuality was not mentioned in the series of 35 patients with strokes interviewed by Bray et al. (1981) for altered sexual behavior. In the series by Coslett and Heilman (1986), only one of 26 male patients, who had aphasia and a mild right hemiparesis, reported increased libido and frequency of intercourse after his stroke.

In 1986, Monga et al. reported three cases of patients who had experienced unilateral temporal lobe strokes and subsequently developed hypersexuality. A 53-year-old man developed increasing desire for sex and improving erectile function in the months after his stroke, which involved the right anteromedial basal portion of the temporal lobe as well as the frontal lobe and caudate nucleus. By about ten months after the stroke, his sexuality had alienated his wife, at which time he had his first seizure. The second case was a 55-year-old woman who had an intracranial hemorrhage of unspecified etiology with subsequent ventriculoperitoneal shunt placement. After the stroke she was left with a resultant aphasia and right hemiplegia and then developed a tendency to hug everyone, strip inappropriately, and masturbate publicly. Her affect became more labile and her appetite increased to the point that she stole other people's food. Initial CT showed a hemorrhage in the left temporal lobe and near the atrium and occipital horn of the left lateral ventricle. The final case was a 47-year-old woman who had a stroke involving the right anterior temporal lobe in the area of the amygdala as well as the frontal lobe, internal capsule, and lentiform nucleus. Over the months after the stroke, she began to masturbate excessively by inserting whatever object seemed handy into her vagina. She also was verbally inappropriate, speaking openly of sex, and became hyperphagic. She was noted to eat other patients' food as well as abnormal items such as plant leaves, face powder, and baby oil. These cases are instructive in that they all involved the temporal lobes and, in the last two cases, other elements of the Klüver–Bucy syndrome were present. All three cases had seizures, with the hypersexuality manifesting before the seizures in the first and third case. It is possible that the hypersexuality and hyperphagia seen in these cases was a partial Klüver–Bucy syndrome arising in the context of bilateral temporal lobe dysfunction from seizures. Complicating the interpretation of the second case is the insertion of the ventriculoperitoneal shunt (discussed below).

Increases in sexual activity as a complication of ruptured cerebral aneurysms have been described. Miller et al. (1986) described two patients who developed hypersexuality following subarachnoid hemorrhage. The first was a 39-year-old man who, after the acute onset of altered mental status, began masturbating and propositioning his wife and other females in front of his hospital room mates. Over the next 24 hours he became comatose, and died within two weeks. Autopsy showed a ruptured aneurysm of the anterior cerebral artery with hemorrhage in the basal frontal areas bilaterally and involvement of the septal region. Another case involved a 31-year-old woman who had a ruptured right superior cerebellar artery aneurysm that was surgically clipped. Five days postoperatively, she developed a stroke, giving her a left hemiparesis and hemianesthesia. At the same time she began to talk incessantly about sexual matters and openly propositioned her physicians. She had increased appetite, disturbed sleep, and her verbal output was said to approach flight of ideas. A radiolucency in the right thalamic and hypothalamic area was present on CT. Her behavior was thought to represent a manic state with mania-related hypersexuality. Common to these two cases is involvement of the basal forebrain in the area of the septum and hypothalamus.

Secondary mania has produced hypersexuality in other cases. Cummings and Mendez (1984) described a case of a 63-year-old man with no past psychiatric history who underwent coronary bypass surgery. Six days after discharge he began sleeping less, becoming excessively talkative and expansive, and feeling sexually aroused for the first time in a year. At discharge he had a rendezvous with a prostitute. This behavioral pattern was a marked change from usual. On examination in the hospital, he was found to have a new mild left hemiparesis and hemianesthesia with a normal CT scan. His behavior resolved over the next four weeks, with residual left hand and leg paresthesias. A small right subcortical infarct possibly involving the thalamus was postulated. Focal lesions involving the right hemisphere, especially subcortically, gave rise to manic symptomatology more often than similar left hemisphere lesions (Cummings and Mendez, 1984). Occasionally, this mania is accompanied by a hypersexual state.

Review of the literature on cerebrovascular accidents suggests that an increase in sexual desire and activity can arise from infarction in the basal forebrain or in either temporal lobe, and that with temporal lobe infarcts and hypersexuality there is often associated seizure activity.

Epilepsy

In temporal lobe seizure disorders, heightened sexual activity can occur either during seizures (ictally), after seizures (postictally), or with seizure control (medically or surgically).

There have been many reports of sexual sensations occurring concomitantly with seizure activity. Erickson (1945) reported a 43-year-old woman who began having periodic sensations of being penetrated *on the left side* of her vagina associated with feeling the need to have sex. She also began being generally more desirous of sex. Her sexuality ultimately alienated her husband and family. Later, she began having intermittent jerking of the left leg and left side of the abdomen, and she gradually developed increasing spastic left hemiplegia. Sixteen years after the first symptom she underwent a craniotomy, and a meningioma between the falx and the upper portion of the rolandic sulcus was removed.

A series of 12 patients, all women, with sexual ictal manifestations was reported by Remillard et al. (1983). In all these cases, the feelings had an affective component and the sensations began after pubescence. In eight, the feelings were the initial sensation in an ictal event, in three there were associated vaginal secretions, and in four the feelings culminated in orgasm. Electrographic epileptiform activity could be recorded from the temporal lobes in ten (the right in six, the left in two, and bilaterally in two) of the patients, and of the four in whom the etiology could be identified, there was temporal lobe gliosis in two, a temporal lobe arteriovenous malformation in one, and a right temporal astrocytoma in one. The authors noted the preponderance of females in their cases and concluded that there is a sexual dimorphism in mesial temporal lobe structures and their connections with the hypothalamus.

Orgasmic seizures were described in another case report (Calleja, Carpizo and Berciano, 1988) involving a 38-year-old woman who had the sensation of an electrical discharge in the neck which awoke her from sleep and spread to the right leg. She later developed accompanying paresthesias in the right lateral abdomen and pubic region, followed by a sensation of vaginal dilatation and orgasm. Interictal electroencephalogram (EEG) showed left central parietal paroxysmal activity which became briefly generalized in synchrony with the experience of orgasm. The authors speculated that the spread of seizure activity to subcortical structures such as the hypothalamus during generalization gave rise to the experience of orgasm.

The cases described above indicate that epileptic activity in the temporal lobes can give rise to sexual sensations and orgasm, probably through their connections with limbic structures such as the amygdala and hypothalamus. The epileptogenic medial parietal lobe lesions are of interest because they appear to originate from the portion of somatosensory cortex in which the genitals are represented. Irritative foci in this region give rise to both erotic and sexually neutral genital sensations (Penfield and Rasmussen, 1950). The erotic senations may be due to spread of activity from the somatosensory regions via corticofugal pathways or by direct irritation of the adjacent limbic cingulate gyrus. These cases of sexual sensation in the conscious patient should be distinguished from the undressing and masturbatory phenomena that often occur during complex partial seizures. The latter automatisms may represent 'release' of subcortical behaviors for which the patients are usually amnestic.

Excessive sexual behavior is also described postictally. It has been reported to occur in six of 50 patients with temporal lobe epilepsy (Blumer, 1970) in one series and in four of 47 patients in another (Walker, 1972). An illustrative case was described by Anson and Kuhlman (1993) in which a 24-year-old woman underwent a left temporal lobectomy during intractable status epilepticus. Five years later, she was brought to the hospital after a seizure and was noted to be lethargic and unresponsive. She was left unattended and found 30 minutes later performing fellatio on a patient in an adjacent room. An hour later she was alert and neurologically intact with no memory of the episode. Family members reported that recent seizures had been followed by sexual behavior including masturbating in public and soliciting intercourse from them as well as from neighbours. During these episodes, she was also noted to be apathetic, did not recognize family members, and ate voraciously. She returned to normal one to two hours after the event and recalled none of it. The patient's behavior was interpreted as transient Klüver-Bucy syndrome, possibly due to a postictal 'Todd's paralysis' of the remaining temporal lobe.

Though temporal lobe epileptics are often relatively hyposexual, they may become at least temporarily hypersexual after successful seizure control. Increased libido and sexual activity with improved medical control of seizures have been reported by many authors (Hierons and Sanders, 1966). In one series, three of 42 patients treated with temporal lobectomy (Blumer, 1970) had hypersexual episodes postoperatively. Episodes of hypersexuality after surgery were more common in patients with improved seizure control and in those with preserved interictal sexual behavior preoperatively.

Trauma

Lilly et al. (1983) presented 12 patients with Klüver–Bucy syndrome of varying etiologies. In two of their 12 patients the cause was trauma. One patient had been in a traffic accident and had undergone bilateral craniotomies for evacuation of hematomas. During surgery, the inferior aspects of both temporal lobes were noted to be severely macerated. In the month after discharge, he exhibited all the components of Klüver–Bucy syndrome, but was greatly improved by two months.

Neurosurgery

Neurosurgically induced behavioral changes can be the most informative regarding brain–behavior relationships because the lesions are relatively circumscribed and their location known. There are many reports of increased sexual behavior induced inadvertently during surgery.

Klüver–Bucy syndrome, including the first reported human case, may arise postoperatively. Terzian and Dalle Ore (1955) reported a 19-year-old man with complex partial seizures and rage attacks associated with foci in both temporal lobes. The patient underwent bilateral temporal lobectomies extending posteriorly to the vein of Labbe and subsequently developed the full Klüver–Bucy syndrome with the exception of hyperorality. Klüver–Bucy syndrome has also been sought intentionally through bilateral amygdalectomy in an effort to treat violence in schizophrenics (Sawa et al., 1954). The human syndrome in these cases is very similar to the animal model and confirms the necessity to remove the amygdalae to produce it. Increased or altered sexual behavior is a component of these surgically induced Klüver–Bucy syndrome cases.

Neurosurgical observations also indicate a role for the frontal lobes in the expression of sexual behavior. Miller et al. (1986) reported a 59-year-old man who had a subfrontal meningioma that was removed surgically. His interest in sex increased postoperatively such that his usual urge for intercourse increased from about once a week to one to four times per day. He engaged in prolonged intercourse and had difficulty attaining orgasms. This ultimately led to a breakup with his girlfriend. Over the next two years he developed a manic state with increasing sexuality, masturbating openly in the hospital, and propositioning both male and female patients. CT showed infarction of the basal frontal lobes bilaterally.

Levine and Albert (1950) reported on sexual behavior after prefrontal lobotomy in 40 patients. Their patient population had various psychiatric diagnoses and the specific psychosurgical technique and lesion locations were not indicated. Of 25 female patients, 13 had a decrease in sexual drive, five had an increase, three had no change, and six could not be evaluated. Among the 15 males, three had a decrease in sexual interest, six had an increase, five had no change, and one could not be evaluated. The authors felt that there was a decrease in 'inhibitory forces' such as guilt, modesty, embarrassment, and anxiety associated with sexual behavior, but that this did not necessarily lead to an increase in drive *per se.* Four patients, two men and two women, exhibited troublesome sexual behavior postoperatively. One man became promiscuous and sexually aggressive and the other exhibited disinhibited verbal outbursts of a sexual nature. The two women, both of whom exhibited sexual psychopathology prior to their operations, were described as 'flirtatious' and 'seductive' after the procedures. These observations indicate that disconnection of the frontal lobes can result in a disinhibited state that may include sexually provocative behavior.

The most discrete human lesion reported to result in hypersexuality is damage to the septal region occurring with the placement of ventriculoperitoneal shunts. Gorman and Cummings (1992) reported two men in whom markedly increased sexual behavior arose after placement of such shunts. CT showed that the catheter tips were in the area of the septal nuclei. These cases were complicated by coexistent neurological disease (previous herpetic encephalitis in one case and cerebrovascular accident of unspecified location in the other), but no overt seizure activity was observed and the hypersexuality was temporally related to the shunt placements. Animal and human studies suggest a role of the septal nuclei in sexual expression. Figure 16.1 shows the CT of a patient with hypersexuality following shunt-related septal injury.

There is a report (Uitti et al., 1989) of two male patients with Parkinson's disease who had a dramatic but transient increase in sexual desire and activity after bilateral thalamotomy for their movement disorders. In one patient, the increase was noted to occur after a right-sided operation (he had a previous left-sided thalamotomy). Both patients were described as being 'overactive sexually' prior to the onset

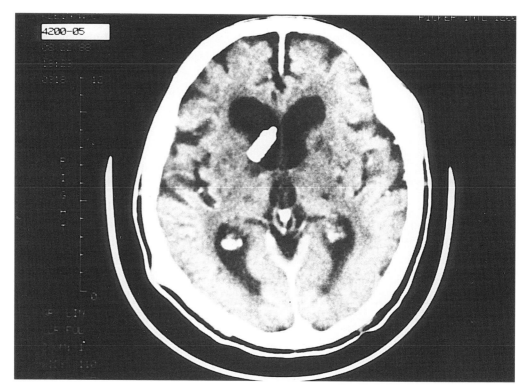

Fig. 16.1   Computerized tomogram of a patient with hypersexuality following shunt-related septal injury.

of Parkinson's disease. The operations may have allowed the patients to return to their usual baseline level of sexual activity, at least partly through improvement of their motor functioning. Alternatively, they may have had hypersexuality induced surgically or related to dopamimetic therapy.

The surgical cases contribute to our understanding of the neuroanatomical basis of sexual behavior, and they indicate roles for the temporal lobes, amygdalae, frontal lobes, septal area, hypothalamus, and possibly the thalamus in the regulation of sexual behavior.

Multiple sclerosis

In a series of 108 multiple sclerosis patients (Surridge, 1969) in which many neuro-psychiatric symptoms were assessed, four were found to be 'hypersexual,' but further details regarding how this was defined were not presented. This rate was not thought to be different from that in a control group of 39 patients with muscular dystrophy.

Encephalitis

Encephalitis can damage the nervous system directly via infection and subsequent infarction or hemorrhage as well as through secondary autoimmune mechanisms. This damage can cause permanent neurological disability and behavioral sequelae, including hypersexuality and other alterations of sexual behavior.

Of the 12 cases of Klüver–Bucy syndrome reported by Lilly et al. (1983), four were thought to be the result of herpes simplex encephalitis, reflecting the predisposition of this infection to damage the temporal lobes.

Poeck and Pilleri (1965) reported the case of a child who developed divergent strabismus, right hemiparesis, and clumsiness associated with an 'illness' at the age of two. At the age of 11 she became withdrawn, apathetic, and somnolent, and months later began having jerky, irregular, involuntary movements, which were worse in the right arm and leg. At the same time she also became aggressive and quarrelsome, stealing things and running away from her parents. When examined at the age of 15, she had partial paralysis of the right oculomotor nerve, a mild *left* hemiparesis with a gross tremor of the left side, and autonomic instability. She remained intermittently obstinate and uncooperative and had intermittent excessive sexual activity, flirting with her father's male friends over the phone, inviting passersby from the window to come and make love to her, and masturbating excessively. She died suddenly in the night at the age of 24 for unknown reasons. At autopsy, her brain showed cystic lesions in the ventral caudate nuclei bilaterally, greater on the left side than on the right. The substantia nigra was pale and there was a small lesion in the right basal thalamus near the subthalamic nucleus. There were also lesions in the hypothalamus, red nucleus, and in the area of the right oculomotor nucleus. There was no significant damage to the amygdalae or other parts of the temporal lobes. Encephalitis lethargica was the presumed etiology.

The caudate nuclei have been implicated in another patient in whom a change in sexual behavior accompanied by other behavioral changes occurred with bilateral lesions of uncertain etiology (Richfield, Twyman and Berent, 1987). A 25-year-old woman with no prior neurological or psychiatric history experienced headache, nausea, and vomiting for several weeks. She disappeared for three days and when found was noted to have profoundly altered affect, motivation, cognition, and self-care. CT showed abnormal enhancement of both caudate nuclei. She continued to have abnormal behaviors consisting of vulgarity, impulsiveness, easy frustration, violent outburst, hypersomnia, increased appetite, polydipsia, poor hygiene, and hypersexuality with exhibitionism. Repeat CT eight months later showed hypodense areas in the heads of the caudate nuclei without any other abnormality. EEG was normal and treatment with phenytoin and carbamazepine was without benefit. The etiology and exact pathology in this patient remain uncertain.

Among the various behaviors reported to occur in rabies encephalitis is heightened sexuality including nymphomania and satyriasis. Reportedly, one infected man attempted to have sexual intercourse 30 times in one day (Kaplan, Turner and Warrell, 1986), and indecent exposure and attempted rape have been reported. There is an initial proclivity for the virus to affect the diencephalon, hippocampus, and brainstem, potentially explaining the early sexual changes.

Changes in sexual orientation

Alterations in sexual orientation or paraphilias (sexual urges involving nonhuman objects, children or nonconsenting individuals, or suffering or humiliation of oneself or one's partner) occurring with neurological insults have been recorded in the literature.

Pedophilia and exhibitionism are the two types of paraphilic behavior most commonly reported in patients with neurological diseases. Of 239 individuals who had committed sexual offenses and were referred to a forensic mental health center (Henn, Herjanic and Vanderpearl, 1976), 'organic mental syndromes' (14.4%) and mental retardation (13.5%) were common.

Cerebrovascular lesions

Miller and Cummings (1991) described a 64-year-old man with an inoperable right frontal arteriovenous malformation. This lesion extended into the region of the septum, basal ganglia, and hypothalamus. Six months later, he was arrested for having sex with a 16-year-old boy. The patient had no history of pedophilia and the frontal lesion may have contributed to the behavior.

Pedophilia has followed global cerebral hypoxia in two reported cases (Regestein and Reich, 1978). Both were men with multiple cardiac risk factors in their thirties and forties who had myocardial infarctions and underwent cardioversion. The first had an antecedent history of car theft and extramarital affairs; after his cardiac event he sexually molested his two daughters. The other patient was said to have become more passive following his myocardial infarction, suffered sudden crying spells, and flew into childish rages. He became more sexually demanding from his wife, requesting unstated activities she described as 'disgusting.' He then made sexual advances toward his 16-year-old daughter.

Epilepsy

There are several reports of paraphilias occurring in association with temporal lobe epilepsy (Epstein, 1961; Hunter, Logue and McMenemy, 1963; Walinder, 1965; Kolarsky et al., 1967). An unusual case of a patient with complex partial seizures induced by the sight of a safety pin was reported by Mitchell, Falconer and Hill (1954). These authors describe a man whose typically heterosexual orientation was replaced by sexual satisfaction through the sight and thought of safety pins. These experiences were related to complex partial seizures that were shown to arise from the left temporal lobe on EEG. The authors report that a temporal lobectomy relieved the seizures, the safety pin fetish, and returned the patient to normal sexual relations with his wife.

Davies and Morgenstern (1960) reported on a 36-year-old man who developed a complex partial seizure disorder followed by paroxysmal urges to put on women's clothes. Initially, this need was intermittent, but increased to become nearly constant. The etiology was thought to be cerebral cysticercosis because of the patient's travel history and the presence of cysts in his muscles. EEG was essentially normal. He was treated with anticonvulsants and psychotherapy. The authors present four other cases of seizure disorders associated with transvestism. Hunter et al. (1963) presented a similar case of a patient whose transvestism disappeared with anticonvulsants. His seizures recurred later without an associated desire to don women's clothing.

Trauma

Orbitofrontal lobe injury can result in disinhibited behavior, often manifesting as sexual disinhibition and consequent paraphilia. An illustrative case was reported by Miller and Cummings (1991), who described a 33-year-old man who suffered traumatic brain injury in an automobile accident and had burr holes placed in the post-traumatic period. Contusions of the frontal and temporal lobes were noted at operation. In the years after the surgery he became impulsive and had uncontrollable urges to expose himself in public and he joined a nudist colony.

Neurosurgery and brain tumors

Some of the most interesting and localizing information comes from the focal pathology seen in neurosurgical cases. In the review by Levine and Albert (1950) of sexual behavior in 40 patients with prefrontal lobotomy, the question of changes in sexual preference was directly addressed. Levine classified patients preoperatively as either heterosexual (14), autoerotic (6), autoerotic and heterosexual (6), or homosexual and heterosexual (2). There was inadequate information on the remaining patients (12). He noted that one of the heterosexual patients became autoerotic and three of the autoerotic patients remained so, with two becoming asexual and one with increased heterosexual activity. The two patients who engaged in some homosexual activity prior to the operation ceased to do so afterwards. The author also described three patients with exclusively heterosexual activity prior to the operation who also had homosexual fantasies which were associated with guilt. After the operation, two of these patients stopped having these fantasies and the third continued to have them but they were no longer associated with guilt. In this series there were no paraphilias, though one woman (described above) became 'crudely exhibitionistic,' probably related to disinhibition.

Brain tumors and the associated neurosurgery have also been noted to give rise to changes in sexual orientation. Regestein and Reich (1978) described a 56-year-old man who had a suprasellar meningioma removed via a right frontal craniotomy at the age of 49. He had an increased desire for sexual intercourse postoperatively, but was incapable of sustaining an erection. He was apathetic and without initiative; neuropsychological testing revealed attention deficits and poor performance on the Wisconsin Card Sorting Test. He sexually molested children of both genders on multiple occasions. In this case, the increased sexual urge combined with compromised erectile function may have contributed to the development of pedophilia.

A contribution of the hypothalamus in sexual orientation is indicated by the case of a 50-year-old man with a hypothalamic glioma described by Miller et al. (1986). At the age of 34, this man began displaying poor financial judgment and developed difficulty with erection and ejaculation. He also began collecting pornography and made sexual proposals toward his seven-year-old daughter and her friends. At the age of 44, he developed hydrocephalus, for which he received a ventriculoperitoneal shunt. His inappropriate sexual behavior worsened, and by the age of 48 he discussed sex continuously and was arrested for propositioning children in the neighborhood. He developed a left third nerve palsy, right hemiparesis, and hemiataxia, and eventually died at the age of 53. Autopsy revealed a brainstem glioma involving the thalamus, hypothalamus, ventral midbrain, and pons. The involvement of the hypothalamus in this patient is probably responsible for his erectile dysfunction and the markedly increased sexual urge with pedophilia.

Multiple sclerosis

There are two reported cases of altered sexual preference appearing in conjunction with multiple sclerosis. The first patient (Huws, Shubsachs and Taylor, 1991) had the sudden onset of excessive sexual demands and promiscuous behavior. Two years later, at the age of 25, he developed a transient quadraplegia, and one year later worsened hypersexuality and disinhibition appeared. He could attain erection but could not ejaculate. At the age of 28, he exhibited a foot fetish which, when acted on, caused him to be imprisoned. Despite treatment with counselling, behavior therapy, hormonal treatment, neuroleptics, and carbamazepine his problems persisted. Neuropsychological testing suggested frontal lobe dysfunction and magnetic resonance imaging (MRI) showed periventricular and frontal lobe white matter lesions.

Another multiple sclerosis patient with multiple paraphilias was described by Ortego et al. (1993). This woman had sustained a subdural hematoma after a head injury at the age of 5, but was normal until the age of 18, at which time she began experiencing numbness in her arms and legs. She was eventually diagnosed with multiple sclerosis and had progression of her symptoms despite intermittent treatment until the age of 22, at which time she was lost to follow-up. At the age of 31, she was arrested for multiple paraphilias including pedophilia, voyeurism, and zoophilia. Despite a clear diagnosis of multiple sclerosis with an MRI showing extensive white matter disease through the cerebrum, the patient was incarcerated for pedophilia. She died while in jail and pathology confirmed widespread demyelinating lesions.

Encephalitis

Many types of behavioral abnormality have been reported in association with postencephalitic parkinsonism (Cheyette and Cummings, 1995). In his paper of 1947, Fairweather described sexual deviations in a group of 275 institutionalized lowfunctioning postencephalitic parkinsonism patients. Of the 168 men, he noted that 22 engaged in mutual masturbation, five in masturbation of others, 51 in sodomy, 41 in fellatio, 24 in pedophilia with young girls, 15 in indecent exposures, 24 in sexual assaults with rape, and two in other forms of sexual misconduct. There were 11 cases of rectal masturbation, some with associated anal trauma. Thirty-five of the males had been convicted of sexual offences. Of the 107 women, four engaged in rectal masturbation, eight in sexual attacks on others, 12 in indecent exposure, and 13 had a history of illegitimate children. Though there was no comparison to a similarly handicapped institutionalized population, one can confidently say that deviant sex practices beyond simple disinhibition were common in postencephalitic parkinsonism patients.

The pathology in postencephalitic parkinsonism suggests that lesions of the basal ganglia, midbrain, and hypothalamus were responsible for the behavioral abnormalities. Inflammation, hemorrhage, cellular necrosis as well as chromatolysis, neuronophagia, and gliosis are seen in these areas in the acute infection. Chronically, cell loss is seen in these areas (see above) and there is depigmentation of the substantia nigra with neurofibrillary tangles, though without Lewy bodies. This supports the contribution of basal forebrain structures in the expression of paraphilias as well as in the tics, compulsions, chorea, tremor, and the myriad other behaviors exhibited by these patients.

Neuroanatomy of sexual behavior

We have discussed clinical cases which have provided clues as to the neuroanatomy of sexual behavior. These anecdotes are informative, but the conclusions to be drawn are limited because of the uncontrolled quality of these 'experiments of nature.' We now turn to a discussion of relevant animal studies that, despite the great differences between sexual behavior in people and other primates, confirm some observations made in humans.

Experimental observations

Klüver and Bucy (1939) defined Klüver–Bucy syndrome in monkeys in whom they had surgically ablated both temporal lobes. They described the hypersexuality in their male macaques as consisting of frequent penile erections, genital automanipulation, 'Presenting reactions' to human observers, and increased duration and frequency of heterosexual and homosexual activity. These generally occurred three to six weeks after bilateral surgery, in contrast to the 'psychic blindness,' oral tendencies, 'hypermetamorphosis,' and emotional placidity which can be observed almost immediately postoperatively. Klüver–Bucy syndrome only arose with extensive bilateral ablations involving the entire temporal lobe anterior to the vein of Labbe, including the amygdala and the hippocampus. An interpretation of the changes in sexual behavior occurring in Klüver–Bucy syndrome is a loss of the ability to recognize and remember usual sexual objects and therefore the loss of discriminatory control over sexual behavior.

Paul MacLean studied the neuroanatomy of sexual behavior over a number of years by stimulating various areas of mammalian brain. He found (MacLean, 1973) that electrical and chemical (with cholinergic agents) stimulation of the septum and caudal hippocampus resulted in enhanced grooming reactions and penile erection in cats. In male squirrel monkeys, he systematically stimulated various areas and studied the effects on penile erection. He found that erections could be readily elicited by stimulation in the septal area rostroventral to the anterior commissure as well as throughout the course of the medial forebrain bundle which connects the septum to various nuclei in the midbrain and pons. This area is of interest as it is implicated as a 'reward circuit' in that animals will self-stimulate this area electrically if given the opportunity (Olds and Milner, 1954). It is not surprising there should be this overlap of circuits involved in sexuality and motivational states, considering the strong drive and pleasure involved in sexual behavior and its necessity for the survival of a species. Other areas from which MacLean found penile erections could be elicited included the anterior and medial dorsal nuclei of the thalamus, the precallosal and subcallosal cingulate gyrus, and the caudal portion of the gyrus rectus.

Ejaculation did not occur with these stimulations, but instead occurred when the spinothalamic pathway and its ramifications within the caudal intralaminar region of the thalamus were stimulated. Ejaculation was associated with genital scratching, presumably because of the simultaneous elicitation of genital sensation by stimulation along this sensory pathway.

MacLean also studied the effects of manipulations of the basal ganglia on sexual behavior. He found that stimulation of the amygdala, a structure he included as part of the basal ganglia, induced salivation and chewing followed after a minute by erection. He performed various lesions in more than 70 monkeys and observed the effects on sexual display behavior. Lesions isolated to the amygdala, even when bilateral, had little, if any, effect on display behavior. MacLean described four monkeys in which extensive lesions of the globus pallidus eliminated sexual display behavior, perhaps in a manner analogous to the human surgical series of Meyers (1961) described above. MacLean's extensive work confirms a major role of the limbic system, a set of brain structures known to be involved in emotional and mnestic functions, in the orchestration of sexual behavior.

Lesions placed in the medial preoptic–anterior hypothalamic (MP-AH) area of male rhesus monkeys were associated with the reduction or complete elimination of mounting, intromission, and copulatory behavior without reducing masturbation, ejaculatory function, or nonsexual social behavior such as grooming (Slimp, Hart and Goy, 1978). Slimp et al. contrasted these effects and those of castration in which a gradual reduction of mounting behavior and ejaculatory function occurs. They concluded that the area lesioned (immediately posterior to the anterior commissure) was specifically involved in the expression of heterosexual behavior. In another study (Perachio, Marr and Alexander, 1979), electrical stimulation of the preoptic area (POA) and dorsomedial nucleus of the hypothalamus (DMH) of male rhesus monkeys led to increased mount duration and to an increased number of thrusts per mount. DMH stimulation caused increased frequency of ejaculation and thrusting rate, whereas POA stimulation caused a decrease of these measures.

In-vivo extracellular neurophysiological recordings from the medial preoptic area (MPOA) of the hypothalamus and the DMH in male rhesus monkeys help to elucidate the role of these areas in the sexual act (Oomura, Yoshimatsu and Aou, 1983). The activity of some MPOA neurons was maximal after visual contact with a sexual partner, but steadily declined with attainment of contact and the initiation of the sexual act. Their activity was minimal immediately after ejaculation and slowly increased in the next 25 minutes. This pattern could be interpreted as indicating a role for MPOA neurons in encoding sexual desire. The activity of DMH neurons, on the other hand, increased and ceased with the initiation and cessation of actual copulation.

Observations in humans

Neurophysiological recording and stimulation of deep brain structures relevant to sexual behavior have been performed on rare occasions in humans as well. Heath (1972) reported two patients with electrodes distributed in many parts of their cerebrum in which electrical activity was recorded during orgasm. In one male with temporal lobe epilepsy and depression, 2 Hz spike and slow-wave discharges with superimposed fast activity were recorded from the septal area during orgasm. Delta waves were concomitantly recorded from the amygdala and caudate leads. This investigator recorded similar epileptiform activity from the septal area of a nonepileptic woman on induction of orgasm by infusion of acetylcholine and levaterenol into this region. Extensive studies by Heath (1964) revealed a number of sites which, when stimulated, could produce pleasurable sensations. These included the centromedian nucleus of the thalamus, the caudate nucleus, the mesencephalic tegmentum, the amygdaloid nucleus, as well as the septal nucleus. Sexual feelings *per se* were most readily elicited by stimulation of the septal nuclei, defined by Heath as that region rostral to the anterior commissure extending to the anterior horn of the lateral ventricles and including the nucleus basalis, septal nuclei proper, the nucleus accumbens, the nucleus of the diagonal band of Broca, and the subcallosal gyrus.

Functional imaging techniques have been employed in the study of the physiology of human orgasm. One study (Tiihonen et al., 1994) looked at the HMPAO-SPECT during orgasm in eight right-handed male volunteers. A decrease in cerebral blood flow was found in all areas except in the right prefrontal cortex, where the flow was increased. Unfortunately, this technique is insensitive to the physiology of smaller anatomical structures such as subdivisions of the hypothalamus and the septal areas.

The aforementioned human cases and animal studies have produced converging information regarding the neural circuitry involved in sexual behavior. Though there are many differences in sexual behavior between species, between genders, and between individuals of the same gender, some general statements can be made. Portions of the frontal and temporal lobes as well as the cingulate gyrus serve a regulating role in sexual behavior, the ultimate expression of which is dependent on the hypothalamus and basal forebrain nuclei.

Treatment of altered sexual behavior in patients with neurological disease

Alterations in sexual behavior in neurological patients are not always troublesome and will not always require medical treatment. However if changes in sexuality lead to marital disharmony or illegal activities such as pedophilia, intervention is indicated. When therapies for the primary illness are available, as in the case of epilepsy and multiple sclerosis, these should be maximized before or in addition to specific management of the sexual disorder. Despite the fact that many medical and surgical treatments have been employed for many different sexual disorders, there are no large series of controlled trials to assess their efficacy, and data are particularly lacking in the context of focal brain lesions. The following is therefore necessarily based on anecdotal reports.

Medical treatment

Hormonal manipulations

Since testosterone is a prerequisite for sexual behavior in males and in females (Pardridge et al., 1982), treatments of hypersexuality are often aimed at reducing its level. Medroxyprogesterone acetate lowers serum testosterone levels by inducing its metabolism in the liver. Success has been noted in the treatment of general sexual offenders and dementia patients with sexual acting out (Bradford, 1988; Cooper, 1994), but its use in hypersexuality secondary of focal neurological disease has not been studied. A drawback to medroxyprogesterone acetate, especially in the context of neurological patients, is that it may increase the risk of cerebrovascular accidents (Biller and Saver, 1995).

Cyproterone acetate, an androgen receptor blocker, has been used to treat hypersexuality and paraphilias in both males and females (Mellor, Farid and Craig, 1988; Bradford, 1988).

Leuprolide and triptorelin, gonadotrophin-releasing hormone agonists, have been successfully employed in the treatment of exhibitionism in Huntington's disease and of other paraphilias (Cordier and Kuhn, 1993; Reich and Ovsiew, 1994).

Psychotropic medications

Hypersexuality and paraphilias may be manifestations of a separate underlying psychiatric disorder such as mania or obsessive–compulsive disorder. Many psychiatric medications have therefore been tried in different conditions expressed by pathological alteration of sexual behavior.

Serotonin reuptake inhibitors such as sertraline, fluvoxamine, and clomipramine have been used in the treatment of pedophilia, voyeurism, exhibitionism, as well as in depression associated with sexual masochism or transvestic fetishism, and in the demented elderly (Bianchi, 1990; Clayton, 1993; Massand, 1993; Zohar, Kaplan and Benjamin, 1994). Loss of sexual function, particularly erectile function in males (Piazza et al., 1997), is a common side-effect of serotonin reuptake inhibitors, suggesting that there is a direct effect of these medications on sexuality that is separate from their effects on the underlying psychopathology.

Buproprion, an atypical antidepressant, has been reported to have minimal sexual side-effects and may be useful in treating serotonin reuptake inhibitor-induced sexual dysfunction (Labbate and Pollack, 1994).

Surgical treatment

Castration

Castration, or surgical removal of the testes, causes a greater and more permanent decrease in testosterone than the above-mentioned drugs. It markedly reduced recidivism in male sexual offenders in Switzerland (Berlin, 1983).

Neurosurgery

Posterior hypothalamotomy has been promoted as a treatment of sexual offenders. The few centers that perform it have reported success (Dieckmann, Schneider-Jonietz and Schneider, 1988). Considering the data mentioned above, this target may minimize side-effects while achieving the desired loss of libido.

Conclusion

The literature regarding the treatment of sexual disorders resulting from focal brain lesions is limited to anecdotal reports, but one can conclude that behavioral alterations arising as a result of loss of brain tissue are generally treatment resistant. As no drug can hope to restore the function of lost brain, definitive treatment awaits progress in the fields of restorative neurological and neurosurgical science. In the meantime, the severity of the patient's problem will dictate the degree of intervention.

Acknowledgments

This project was supported by a National Institute on Aging Alzheimer's Disease Center grant (AG10123) and the Sidell–Kagan Foundation.

REFERENCES

Anson, J.A. and Kuhlman, D.T. (1993). Post-ictal Klüver–Bucy syndrome after temporal lobectomy. *J Neurol Neurosurg Psychiatry* 56: 311–13.

Bauer, H.G. (1958). Endocrine and metabolic conditions related to pathology in the hypothalamus: a review. *J Nerv Ment Dis* 128: 323–38.

Berlin, F.S. (1983). Sex offenders: a biomedical perspective and a status report on biomedical treatment. In *The Sexual Aggressor: Current Perspectives on Treatment*, ed. J.G. Greer and I.R. Stuart, pp. 83–123. New York: Van Nostrand Reinhold.

Bianchi, M.D. (1990). Fluoxetine treatment of exhibitionism. *Am J Psychiatry* 147: 1089–90.

Biller, J. and Saver, J.L. (1995). Ischemic cerebrovascular disease and hormone therapy for infertility and transsexualism. *Neurology* 45: 1611–13.

Blumer, D. (1970). Hypersexual episodes in temporal lobe epilepsy. *Am J Psychiatry* 126: 83–90.

Blumer, D. and Walker, A.E. (1967). Sexual behavior in temporal lobe epilepsy. *Arch Neurol* 16: 37–43.

Bradford, J.M.W. (1988). Organic treatment for the male sexual offender. *Ann N Y Acad Sci* 528: 193–202.

Bray, G.P., DeFrank, R.S. and Wolfe, T.L. (1981). Sexual functioning in stroke survivors. *Arch Phys Med Rehabil* 62: 286–8.

Calleja, J., Carpizo, R. and Berciano, J. (1988). Orgasmic epilepsy. *Epilepsia* 29: 635–9.

Cheyette, S.R. and Cummings, J.L. (1995). Encephalitis lethargica: lessons for contemporary neuropsychiatry. *J Neuropsychiatry Clin Neurosci* 7: 125–34.

Clayton, A.H. (1993). Fetishism and clomipramine. *Am J Psychiatry* 150: 673–4.

Cooper, A.J. (1994). Medroxyprogesterone acetate (MPA) treatment of sexual acting out in men suffering from dementia. *J Clin Psychiatry* 48: 368–70.

Cordier, T.F. and Kuhn, J.-M. (1993). Effect of a long-lasting gonadotrophin hormone-releasing hormone agonist in six cases of severe male paraphilia. *Acta Psychiatr Scand* 87: 445–50.

Coslett, H.B. and Heilman, K.M. (1986). Male sexual function: impairment after right hemisphere stroke. *Arch Neurol* 43: 1036–9.

Cummings, J.L. and Duchen, L.W. (1981). Klüver–Bucy syndrome in Pick disease: clinical and pathologic correlations. *Neurology* 31: 1415–22.

Cummings, J.L. and Mendez, M.F. (1984). Secondary mania with focal cerebrovascular lesions. *Am J Psychiatry* 141: 1084–7.

Davies, B.M. and Morgenstern, F.S. (1960). A case of cysticercosis, temporal lobe epilepsy, and transvestism. *J Neurol Neurosurg Psychiatry* 23: 247–9.

Dieckmann, G., Schneider-Jonietz, B. and Schneider, H. (1988). Psychiatric and neuropsychological findings after stereotactic hypothalamotomy, in cases of extreme sexual aggressivity. *Acta Neurochirgica* Suppl. 44: 163–6.

Epstein, A.W. (1961). Relationship of fetishism and transvestism to brain and particularly to temporal lobe dysfunction. *J Nerv Ment Dis* 133: 247–53.

Erickson, T.C. (1945). Erotomania (nymphomania) as an expression of cortical epileptiform discharge. *Arch Neurol* 53: 226–31.

Fairweather, D.S. (1947). Psychiatric aspects of the post-encephalitic syndrome. *J Ment Sci* 83: 201–54.

Federoff, J.P., Peyser, C., Franz, M.L. and Folstein, S. (1994). Sexual disorders in Huntington's disease. *J Neuropsychiatry Clin Neurosci* 6: 147–53.

Gorman, D.G. and Cummings, J.L. (1992). Hypersexuality following septal injury. *Arch Neurol* 49: 308–10.

Heath, R.G. (1964). Pleasure response of human subjects to direct stimulation of the brain: physiologic and psychodynamic considerations. In *The Role of Pleasure in Behavior*, ed. R.G. Heath, pp. 219–42. New York: Hoeber Medical Division, Harper & Row.

Heath, R.G. (1972). Pleasure and brain activity in man. *J Nerv Ment Dis* 154: 3–18.

Henn, F.A., Herjanic, M. and Vanderpearl, R.H. (1976). Forensic psychiatry: profiles of two types of sexual offenders. *Am J Psychiatry* 133: 694–6.

Hierons, R. and Saunders, M. (1966). Impotence in patients with temporal lobe lesions. *Lancet* 2: 761–3.

Hunter, R., Logue, V. and McMenemy, W.H. (1963). Temporal lobe epilepsy supervening on longstanding transvestism and fetishism. *Epilepsia* 4: 60–5.

Huws, R., Shubsachs, P.W. and Taylor, P.J. (1991). Hypersexuality, fetishism and multiple sclerosis. *Br J Psychiatry* 158: 280–1.

Isojarvi, J.I.T., Repo, M., Pakarinen, A.J., Lukkarinen, O. and Myllyla, V.V. (1995). Carbamazepine, phenytoin, sex hormones, and sexual function in men with epilepsy. *Epilepsia* 36: 366–70.

Kalliomaki, J.L., Markkanen, T.K. and Mustonen, V.A. (1961). Sexual behavior after cerebral vascular accident. *Fertil Steril* 12: 156–9.

Kaplan, D., Turner, G.S. and Warrell, D.A. (1986). *Rabies: the Facts.* Oxford: Oxford University Press.

Klein, R., Klein, B.E.K., Lee, K.R., Moss, S.E. and Cruickshanks, K.J. (1996). Prevalence of self-reported erectile dysfunction in people with long-term IDDM. *Diabetes Care* 19: 135–41.

Klüver, H. and Bucy, P.C. (1939). Preliminary analysis of functions of the temporal lobes in monkeys. *Arch Neurol Psychiatry* 42: 979–1000.

Kolarsky, A., Freund, M.D., Machek, J. and Polak, O. (1967). Male sexual deviation: association with early temporal lobe damage. *Arch Gen Psychiatry* 17: 735–43.

Labatte, L.A. and Pollack, M.H. (1994). Treatment of fluoxetine-induced sexual dysfunction with bupropion: a case report. *Ann Clin Psychiatry* 6: 13–15.

Levine, J. and Albert, H.S. (1950). Sexual behavior after lobotomy. In *Studies in Lobotomy*, ed. M. Greenblat, R. Arnot and H. Solomon, pp. 215–28. New York: Grune & Stratton.

Lilly, R., Cummings, J.L., Benson, D.F. and Frankel, M. (1983). The human Klüver–Bucy syndrome. *Neurology* 33: 1141–5.

MacLean, P.D. (1973). Special award lecture: new findings on brain function and sociosexual behavior. In *Contemporary Sexual Behavior: Critical Issues in the 1970s*, ed. J. Zubin & J. Money, pp. 53–74. Baltimore: Johns Hopkins University Press.

Massand, P.S. (1993). Successful treatment of sexual masochism and transvestic fetishism associated with depression with fluoxetine hydrochloride. *Depression* 1: 50–2.

Mattson, D., Petrie, M., Strivastava, D.K. and McDermott, M. (1995). Multiple sclerosis: sexual dysfunction and its response to medications. *Arch Neurol* 52: 862–8.

Mellor, C.S., Farid, N.R. and Craig, D.F. (1988). Female hypersexuality treated with cyproterone acetate. *Am J Psychiatry* 145: 1037.

Meyers, R. (1961). Evidence of a locus of the neural mechanisms for libido and penile potency in the septo-fornico-hypothalamic region of the human brain. *Trans Am Neurol Assoc* 80: 81–5.

Miller, B.L. and Cummings, J.L. (1991). How brain injury can change sexual behavior. *Med Aspects Hum Sex* 1: 54–62.

Miller, B.L., Cummings, J.L., McIntyre, H., Ebers, G. and Grode, M. (1986). Hypersexuality or altered sexual preference following brain injury. *J Neurol Neurosurg Psychiatry* 49: 867–73.

Mitchell, W., Falconer, M.A. and Hill, D. (1954). Epilepsy and fetishism relieved by temporal lobectomy. *Lancet* 2: 626–30.

Monga, T.N., Monga, M., Raina, M.S. and Hardjasudarma, M. (1986). Hypersexuality in stroke. *Arch Phys Med Rehabil* 67: 415–17.

Murialdo, G., Galimberti, C.A., Fonzi, S. et al. (1995). Sex hormones and pituitary function in male epileptic patients with altered or normal sexuality. *Epilepsia* 36: 360–5.

Olds, J. and Milner, P. (1954). Positive reinforcement produced by electrical stimulation of septal area and other regions of the rat brain. *J Comp Physiol Psychol* 47: 419–27.

Oomura, Y., Yoshimatsu, H. and Aou, S. (1983). Medial preoptic and hypothalamic neuronal activity during sexual behavior of the male monkey. *Brain Res* 266: 340–3.

Ortego, N., Miller, B.L., Itabashi, H. and Cummings, J.L. (1993). Altered sexual behavior with multiple sclerosis: a case report. *Neuropsychiatry, Neuropsychol Behav Neurol* 6: 260–4.

Pardridge, W.M., Gorski, R.A., Lippe, B.M. and Green, R. (1982). Androgens and sexual behavior. *Ann Int Med* 96: 488–501.

Penfield, W.G. and Rasmussen, T.B. (1950). *The Cerebral Cortex of Man.* New York: MacMillan.

Perachio, A.A., Marr, L.D. and Alexander, M. (1979). Sexual behavior in male rhesus monkeys elicited by electrical stimulation of preoptic and hypothalamic area. *Brain Res* 177: 127–44.

Piazza, L.A., Markowitz, J.C., Kocsis, J.H. et al. (1997). Sexual functioning in chronically depressed patients treated with SSRI antidepressants: a pilot study. *Am J Psychiatry* 154: 1757–9.

Pitt, D.C., Kriel, R.L., Wagner, N.C. and Krach, L.E. (1995). Klüver–Bucy syndrome following heat stroke in a 12-year-old girl. *Ped Neurol* 13: 73–6.

Poeck, K. and Pilleri, G. (1965). Release of hypersexual behavior due to lesion in the limbic system. *Acta Neurol Scand* 41: 233–44.

Regestein, Q.R. and Reich, P. (1978). Pedophilia occurring after onset of cognitive impairment. *J Nerv Ment Dis* 166: 794–8.

Reich, S.S. and Ovsiew, F. (1994). Leuprolide acetate for exhibitionism in Huntington's disease. *Mov Disord* 9: 353–7.

Remillard, G.M., Andermann, F., Testa, G.F. et al. (1983). Sexual ictal manifestations predominate in women with temporal lobe epilepsy: a finding suggesting sexual dimorphism in the human brain. *Neurology* 33: 323–30.

Richfield, E.K., Twyman, R. and Berent, S. (1987). Neurological syndrome following bilateral damage to the head of the caudate nuclei. *Ann Neurol* 22: 768–71.

Robinson, R.G., Kubos, K.L., Starr, L.B., Rao, D. and Price, T.R. (1984). Mood disorders in stroke patients. *Brain* 107: 81–93.

Sandel, M.E., Williams, K.S., Dellapietra, L. and Derogatis, L.R. (1996). Sexual functioning following traumatic brain injury. *Brain Inj* 10: 719–28.

Sawa, M., Ieki, Y., Arita, M. and Harada, T. (1954). Preliminary report on the amygdalectomy on the psychotic patients, with interpretation of oral–emotional manifestation in schizophrenics. *Folia Psychiatr Neurol Jpn* 7: 309–29.

Shukla, G.D., Srivastava, O.N. and Katiyar, B.C. (1979). Sexual disturbances in temporal lobe epilepsy: a controlled study. *Br J Psychiatry* 134: 288–92.

Slimp, J.C., Hart, B.L. and Goy, R.W. (1978). Heterosexual, autosexual and social behavior of adult male rhesus monkeys with medial preoptic–anterior hypothalamic lesions. *Brain Res* 142: 105–22.

Surridge, D. (1969). An investigation into some psychiatric aspects of multiple sclerosis. *Br J Psychiatry* 115: 749–64.

Terzian, H. and Dalle Ore, G. (1955). Syndrome of Kluver and Bucy reproduced in man by bilateral removal of the temporal lobes. *Neurology* 5: 373–80.

Tiihonen, J., Kuikka, J., Kupila, J. et al. (1994). Increase in cerebral blood flow of right prefrontal cortex in man during orgasm. *Neurosci Lett* 170: 241–3.

Uitti, R.J., Tanner, C.M., Rajput, A.H. et al. (1989). Hypersexuality with antiparkinsonian therapy. *Clin Neuropharmacol* 12: 375–82.

Van de Poll, N.E. and Van Goozen, S.H.M. (1992). Hypothalamic involvement in sexuality and hostility: comparative psychological aspects. *Prog Brain Res* 93: 343–61.

Walinder, J. (1965). Transvestism, definition and evidence in favor of occasional derivation from cerebral dysfunction. *Int J Neuropsychiatry* 1: 567–73.

Walker, A.E. (1972). The libidinous temporal lobe. *Archiv Suisse Neurol Neurochir Psychiatrie* 111: 473–84.

Walker, A.E. and Jablon, S. (1959). A follow-up of head-injured men of World War II. *J Neurosurg* 16: 600–10.

Zohar, J., Kaplan, Z. and Benjamin, J. (1994). Compulsive exhibitionism successfully treated with fluvoxamine: a controlled case study. *J Clin Psychiatry* 55: 86–8.

17

Anosognosia

Patrik Vuilleumier

Introduction

Anosognosia refers to the lack of awareness, misbelief, or explicit denial of their illness that patients may show following brain damage or dysfunction. Anosognosia may involve a variety of neurological impairment of sensorimotor, visual, cognitive or behavioral functions, as well as non-neurological diseases. The term was coined by Joseph Babinski in 1914 when he reported at the meeting of the Society of Neurology of Paris on two patients who had left hemiplegia after a right hemisphere stroke but 'were ignorant or seemed ignorant of the paralysis which affected them' (Babinski, 1914). Babinski emphasized the absence of confusion and major intellectual disturbance. During the discussion that followed his report, he and the neurologists who attended the meeting speculated on more than a half-dozen possible mechanisms to explain anosognosia. Babinski himself considered a deliberate protection of self-esteem and self-appearance as plausible but unlikely, and he pointed to the special role of right hemisphere lesions. He also stressed the possible role of a severe sensory loss. Déjerine and Souques agreed with the latter, while Ballet pondered on an underlying disorder of anterograde memory. Meige argued for a selective functional motor amnesia superimposed on hemiplegia. Claude raised the issue of a loss of representation of the affected limbs and, in addition, related anosognosia to cases with unilateral apraxia and topoanesthesia that would nowadays suggest some sort of interhemispheric disconnection syndrome. Finally, after a second report of Babinski in 1918, Pierre Marie put forward the role of spatial neglect. More than 80 years later, explanations for anosognosia appear not to have gone far beyond the above discussion; many of these speculations are still in place.

Anosognosia had actually been observed long before Babinski's report. While Seneca made mention of a woman who 'did not know that she was blind' (cited in Bisiach and Geminiani, 1991), and Montaigne (1588) discussed a similar disorder in a nobleman, unawareness of blindness was first described as a neurological condition in 1885 by Von Monakow in two patients with bilateral posterior brain damage. Others (e.g., Déjerine and Viallet, 1893; Rossolimo, 1896), described similar cases a few years later. However, Anton (1898) first theorized about the mechanisms of these disorders with respect to perceptual awareness. He described a patient who denied her cortical blindness, as well as two other patients who appeared unaware of their receptive aphasia and cortical deafness (Anton, 1898). He also first emphasized that the lack of awareness might result from focal brain lesions without a general decline in other cognitive functions. At the same time Pick (1898) described a patient with left hemiplegia, left hemianopia, and presumably left spatial neglect who denied any impairment. Another patient with left hemiplegia and delusional beliefs about his left hemibody was reported by Zingerle (1913), who termed this syndrome 'dyschiria', meaning 'impaired representation of one side' (see Bisiach and Geminiani, 1991). However, the term 'anosognosia', which was introduced one year later by Babinski (1914), has prevailed, literally meaning a 'lack of knowledge or lack of recognition about a disease.' Anosognosia is sometimes also refered to as the Anton–Babinski syndrome; Anton's syndrome specifically refers to unawareness of blindness. Babinski (1914) also introduced 'anosodiaphoria' as a related disorder in which patients appear aware of but indifferent to their impairment.

Anosognosia later took on a broader definition to include nonrecognition of a variety of other deficits, e.g., aphasia, apraxia, movement disorders, etc. (Fisher, 1989; McGlynn and Schacter, 1989), but it was recognized that the disorder could be limited to a specific defect; that is, some patients would admit to having blindness but not paralysis, or vice versa. Alajouanine and Lhermitte (1957) referred to such conditions as 'selective functional anosognosia' (anosognosies électives de fonctions). It was also emphasized that anosognosia entailed 'more than a mere ignorance of the paralysis . . . (but also) an obstinate determination not to accept it, a resistance to recognition that is striking and disconcerting' (Barré, Morin and Kaiser, 1923; see also Critchley, 1953). Yet, despite active negation, the behavior or discourse of some patients could betray some vague knowledge ('dunkle Kenntnis:' Anton, 1898) of their condition. This led Weinstein et al. (Weinstein and Kahn, 1950, 1955) to introduce the term 'denial of illness' and to suggest that anosognosia involved motivated psychodynamic defense mechanisms. These ideas were supported by the development of psychoanalytic theories and the finding that denial was reinstated during the injection of barbiturate (amytal test) in some patients who had recovered from transient anosognosia (Weinstein and Kahn, 1950; Guthrie and Grossman, 1952). Frederiks (1985) later distinguished anosognosia from denial and suggested that both could combine. However, neurological studies on anosognosia decreased following Weinstein and Kahn's (1955) review, until recent years (McGlynn and Schacter, 1989). The processes that subtend awareness and its disorders became a major issue in understanding brain–behavior relationships after observations in split-brain subjects, as well as evidence that certain brain lesions could make the processing of information occur without the patients' awareness, such as covert recognition of faces in prosopagnosics, or covert reading of words in alexics, unconscious perception in spatial neglect, and implicit learning in amnesics.

This chapter reviews the most common domains of anosognosia: hemiplegia, hemianopia, blindness, aphasia, and amnesia. Anosognosia for hemiplegia (AHP) is particularly emphasized because of its historical and clinical importance and because there is no systematic review available. However, unawareness of impairment has been observed for a variety of other disorders, e.g., alexia, prosopagnosia, apraxia, etc. (McGlynn and Schachter, 1989; Fisher, 1989; Berti, Ladavas and Della, 1996). Impaired awareness and lack of concern about deficits are important behavioral features of frontal dysfunction that are also dealt with elsewhere (e.g., Stuss and Benson, 1986). Finally, denial of illness occurs in patients without brain damage but with heart disease, cancer, AIDS, etc. While this shows that psychological and personality factors unrelated to cerebral damage do exist, it must be noted that such factors as cognitive fucntioning, belief-forming mechanisms, and elements of personality may certainly be altered after brain lesions.

Anosognosia for hemiplegia

Behavioral aspects

Given the dramatic nature of hemiplegia, it seems amazing that some patients fail to acknowledge and even deny it. This may actually take various forms, and the term 'anosognosic complex' has been used to describe a collection of symptoms composing the background out of which, it was proposed, anosognosia could develop (Gross and Kaltenbäck, 1955).

Typically, patients have no spontaneous complaints and further refuse to admit their weakness when asked. Some patients claim that nothing is wrong at all and argue that their stay in the hospital is due to some misunderstanding (Willanger, Danielsen and Ankergus, 1981). Others put forward irrelevant problems, for example rheumatism or phlebitis (like one of Babinski's patients). Still other patients admit a deficit but explain it away, saying that the limb is lazy or sleepy. Some volunteer the fact that they suffered a stroke, yet deny any impairment. When asked to make a movement with a paralyzed limb, the patient may move the contralateral healthy one or remain motionless but say 'Here it is . . . I am not paralyzed yet,' like one of Babinski's (1914) patients. This attitude can persist when the limb is passively moved and shown to the patient. 'Sometimes it's a bit stiff. It needs exercise,' one patient said (Cutting, 1978). Another one gave the excuse 'I have been sleeping on it' (Roth, 1949). Even when explicitly told and confronted with evidence, the patient remains reluctant: 'Doctors know more about it than I do' (Cutting, 1978). Patients may also deny ownership of the limb and claim that it belongs to another person, e.g., the doctor, another patient or a spouse (Gerstmann, 1942; Assal, 1983; Bisiach and Geminiani, 1991). Rarely, somesthetic hallucinations (Frederiks, 1985) or frank delusional beliefs (i.e., somatoparaphrenia: Gerstmann, 1942) regarding the affected limbs coexist with anosognosia for the paralysis. However, somatic illusions may exist without anosognosia (Lhermitte, 1939; Vuilleumier, Reverdin and Landis, 1997).

Remarkably, while some patients inappropriately attempt to get out of their bed to walk, many who verbally deny their hemiplegia accept staying in a bed or wheelchair (Bisiach and Geminiani, 1991). Conversely, other patients who verbally admit their hemiplegia attempt activities or express intentions (e.g., return to work) that are clearly inappropriate (Weinstein and Kahn, 1955). This suggests that anosognosia can be manifested independently at some verbal explicit level and at some other nonverbal behavioral level (Gainotti, 1972; Bisiach and Geminiani, 1991). One patient who experienced a supernumerary left arm after a right hemisphere stroke acknowledged his left paralysis but then used his right hand (but in an awkward way) when requested to write with his left one (Halligan, Marshall and Wade, 1993)! Another patient repeatedly rubbed her affected arm and rated her left limbs as weaker than the right on a ten-point scale although she denied any handicap (House and Hodges, 1988). Likewise, patients may deny their left paresis but complain of weakness or paresthesia on the right side (Roth, 1949; Gilliatt and Pratt, 1952; Starkstein et al., 1990; Bisiach and Geminiani, 1991), a phenomenon reminiscent of allesthesia and the 'dunkle Kenntnis' described by Anton (1898). This led several authors to identify different sorts of anosognosia. Gerstmann (1942) distinguished between 'complete' and 'incomplete' anosognosia, and Critchley (1953) between 'obstinate denial' and 'defect in appreciation'. Frederiks (1985) separated an explicit form of 'verbal anosognosia' and 'anosognosic behavioral disturbances' such as hemibody neglect, anosodiaphoria, and somatoparaphrenias. Other authors made related distinctions (Weinstein and Kahn, 1955; Cutting, 1978; Willanger et al., 1981; Bisiach and Geminiani, 1991), or argued that awareness of hemiplegia and awareness of handicap should be differentiated (House and Hodges, 1988). However, opinions as to the nature of such distinctions differ widely; they are considered as being a matter of degree (Willanger et al., 1981), dissociable cognitive disorders (House and Hodges, 1988; Bisiach and Geminiani, 1991), or distinct neurological and psychological levels of behavior (Critchley, 1953). The phenomenology of AHP should therefore be carefully assessed. Several studies used structured questionnaire or rating procedures, as shown in Table 17.1.

Interestingly, AHP can be dissociated from anosognosia for hemianopia (AHA)

(Willanger et al., 1981; Bisiach et al., 1986b; Celesia et al., 1997). In one study (Bisiach et al., 1986b) of 12 patients with both severe hemiparesis and hemianopia, four denied their visual defect but admitted motor impairment, while two showed the converse. AHP can similarly dissociate from anosognosia for cognitive deficits such as memory problems, dyslexia, or drawing apraxia (Berti et al., 1996). More surprisingly, some patients may show a different degree of awareness of the upper and lower limb deficit irrespective of its severity, e.g., acknowledging arm but not leg paralysis (Von Hagen and Ives, 1937; Bisiach et al., 1986b; Berti et al., 1996). One patient was very anxious about a left ptosis but denied his left hemiparesis (Roth, 1949).

Anosognosia is most common with acute cerebral disorders, e.g., strokes or head injuries, and is later often replaced by indifference or anosodiaphoria (Gilliatt and Pratt, 1952; Hier, Mondlock and Caplan, 1983b). However, in some cases, it persists for months or years (Babinski, 1914; Nathanson, Bergman and Gordon, 1952; House and Hodges, 1988). It also occurs with progressive impairment, e.g., brain tumors (Roth, 1949; Weinstein and Kahn, 1950), and with transient ischemic or epileptic attacks.

Incidence and hemispheric asymmetry

Babinski (1914) first pointed out that AHP most often follows a right hemisphere lesion. This asymmetry cannot be entirely explained by a bias due to language disturbances precluding assessment (Nathanson et al., 1952; Bisiach and Geminiani, 1991; Starkstein et al., 1992). AHP can occur after left hemisphere damage, although the strict unilateral focus of the lesion and the side of the dominant hemisphere remain questionable in many cases (Nathanson et al., 1952; Cutting, 1978) and it might be more often associated with acute and confusional disturbances.

Early studies of patients with mixed etiologies (Nathanson et al., 1952; Cutting, 1978), like more recent studies of stroke patients in whom lesions were confirmed by computed tomography (CT) or magnetic resonance imaging (MRI) (Starkstein et al., 1992; Stone, Halligan and Greenwood, 1993), found AHP in about 20–30% of consecutive hemiplegics, and 70–90% of them had a right-sided lesion (Table 17.2). Conversely, 32–58% of hemiplegics with a right hemisphere lesion have AHP, as opposed to 7–23% of those with a left hemisphere lesion. In several studies, a high number of patients with left hemisphere lesions were excluded because of severe aphasia or confusion. However, Cutting (1978) found no asymmetry for other abnormal attitudes, such as anosodiaphoria or nonbelonging, although others (Gainotti, 1972; Stone et al., 1993) found anosodiaphoria or minimization to be more frequent after right hemisphere damage. The frequency of anosognosia in other series of right-brain-damaged patients similarly ranges from 25% to 37% (Willanger et al., 1981; Hier, Mondlock and Caplan, 1983a; Bisiach et al., 1986b).

Table 17.1. Example of standardized procedures used in studies of anosognosia for hemiplegia

Structured interview of Nathanson et al. (1952)

Part I: awareness of illness

1. Why are you here? Why are you in the hospital?
2. What is the matter with you? Are you sick?
3. Is there anything wrong with it (the part involved)?
4. Is there anything wrong with it (the examiner points to or raises the part involved)?
5. Can you move it? Can you raise it?
6. Is it weak, paralyzed, numb? How does it feel?
7. What is this? (the examiner holds the part involved and shows it to the patient).

Part II: general mentation

Questions about orientation in time and place, ability to understand commands, general information, attempts to elicit confabulation (Have you seen me before? Where were you last night? etc.)

Structured questionnaire adapted from Cutting (1978)

If anosognosia elicited on previous questions:

1. You clearly have some problem with this? (arm picked up).
2. Can't you see that the two arms are not at the same level? (asked to lift arms).

Questions to elicit other anosognosic phenomena:

1. Anosodiaphoria: Is it a nuisance? How much trouble does it cause you? What caused it?
2. Nonbelonging: Do you ever feel that it doesn't belong? Do you feel that it belongs to someone else?
3. Strange feelings: Do you feel the arm is strange or odd?
4. Misoplegia: Do you dislike the arm? Do you hate it?
5. Personification: Do you ever call it names?
6. Somesthetic/kinesthetic hallucinations: Do you ever feel it moves without your moving it yourself? How big or strong is it? How is the other arm?
7. Phantom supernumerary illusion: Do you ever feel as if there was more than one arm/one hand? Do you ever feel a strange arm lying beside you? Do you ever feel your arm as separate from the real one/from you?

Rating procedure of Bisiach et al. (1986b) and Bisiach and Geminiani (1991)

Anosognosia is scored as:

0 = absent   The disorder is spontaneously reported or mentioned by the patient in reply to a general question about his complaints.

1 = mild   The disorder is reported only following a specific question about the affected function.

2 = moderate   The disorder is acknowledged only after its demonstration through routine techniques of neurological examination.

3 = severe   No acknowledgment of the disorder can be obtained.

Note: this can be used to assess awareness of any disorder.

Table 17.1. (*cont.*)

Assessment of direct/verbal and indirect/implicit knowledge after Berti et al. (1996)

I: direct report

Ask: 'Please touch my hand with your left hand' (examiner's hand in patient's right visual field). 'Now, have you done it?'

If answer is no: ask 'Why?' (verbal anosognosia rated 1, or mild).

If answer is yes: 'Are you sure? I have not seen it' (verbal anosognosia rated 2, or severe).

II: indirect report

Ask the patient to rate his/her ability to perform a number of different motor actions on a ten-point scale (0 = impossible; 10 = completely normal):

1. Unimanual actions (right and left hand): drinking from a glass; opening a door; eating with a fork; lifting a small object; hammering etc.
2. Bimanual actions: clapping hands; washing both hands; putting on gloves; opening a jam tin or a bottle; dealing the cards; making a knot etc.
3. Locomotor actions (i.e., lower limbs): walking; jumping; climbing the stairs; driving; riding a bicycle; shooting.

Note: Berti et al. (1996) considered self-rating scores between 5 and 10 as indicating the presence of anosognosia for paresis.

The association of unawareness of hemiplegia with right hemisphere dysfunction has been further confirmed during the Wada Test. Most observations show that the same subjects recall their left-side paralysis much less often than their right-side paralysis, even though they can recall other events equally (Adair et al., 1995a, 1995b; Breier et al., 1995; Carpenter et al., 1995; but see Dywan, McGlone and Fox, 1995, for opposite findings). Thus, 30/31 patients in one study (Adair et al., 1995a) and 27/31 patients in another one (Carpenter et al., 1995) denied left arm weakness after right hemisphere anesthesia, while 15/31 and 12/31 of them respectively, denied right arm weakness after left hemisphere anesthesia. This is not only a memory failure, because most subjects who cannot recall their paralysis are actually unaware of it when questioned during the Wada Test (Adair et al., 1995a, 1997; Carpenter et al., 1995). Further, unawareness of hemiplegia and aphasia can dissociate in left hemisphere anesthesia (Breier et al., 1995). AHP is not related to frontal inactivation, as inferred from the pattern of filling of the anterior cerebral arteries (Dywan et al., 1995).

In summary, much of the evidence supports a special link between AHP and right hemisphere dysfunction, although it is still to be determined how this relates to the brain asymmetry for spatial, attentional, and emotional processes, or to other

Table 17.2. Incidence of anosognosia for hemiplegia and hemispheric asymmetry

	Anosognosia (AHP)			No AHP		
	AHP cases	RHD	LHD	RHD	LHD	Not testable
Nonselected patients						
Nathanson et al. (1952)	28/100	19 (51%) =68% AHP	9 (23%) =32% AHP	18	30	24
Cutting (1978)	31/100	28 (58%) =90% AHP	3 (14%) =10% AHP	20	19	30
Starkstein et al. (1993)	27/86 (3 bilateral)	21 (46%) =77% AHP	3 (11%) =11% AHP	24	24	6
Stone et al. (1993)	24/131	19 (32%) =79%	4 (7%) =17%	41	51	55
RH-damaged patients						
Hier et al. (1983b)	15/41	=37%				
Bisiach et al. (1986b)	12/36	=33%	Moderate or severe AHP			
	6/36	=17%	Mild AHP			
Willanger et al. (1981)	14/55	=25%	'Systematic denial'			
	11/55	=20%	'Inconsistent denial'			
	8/55	=15%	'Inconsistent evaluation'			
Related disorders		RHD	LHD			
Cutting (1978)	Anosodiaphoria	9%	4%			
	Nonbelonging	14%	23%			
Stone et al. (1993)	Anosodiaphoria	30%	4%			
	Nonbelonging	45%	53%			

Notes:
RHD: right-hemisphere damage; LHD: left hemisphere damage. Percentages given in parentheses refer to the number of AHP cases/number of patients with RHD or LHD; percentages given below refer to the number of patients with RHD or LHD/number of AHP cases.

aspects of motor control such as handedness and functional asymmetries in motor pathways.

Anatomical aspects

While AHP tends to be more frequent in large cerebral lesions (Willanger et al., 1981; Hier et al., 1983a; Feinberg, Haber and Leeds, 1990; Levine, Calvanio and Rinn, 1991), this is not invariably the case (Starkstein et al., 1992; Feinberg et al., 1994; Small and Ellis, 1996), and it can occur with very restricted focal damage

(Bisiach et al., 1986b; House and Hodges, 1988). In a recent study of 80 stroke patients (Starkstein et al., 1992), a regression analysis showed that, among a variety of clinical and radiological features, lesion location (right temporoparietal or thalamic), and signs of subcortical atrophy (width of frontal ventricular horns) were the two most critical variables, accounting for 57% of the variance.

Indeed, early neurologists regarded 'the syncrome of unawareness of hemiplegia as one having highly accurate localizing value' (Nielsen, 1938). Many autopsy reports pointed to the association with lesions of the right hemisphere and the common involvement of either the posterior parietal lobe (Pick, 1898) or the thalamus (Barkman, 1925). Pötzl (1924) believed that AHP resulted from coincident damage to the parietal lobe and thalamus. Subsequent reports emphasized a disconnection of the thalamus from the overlying cortex, as it was found that some patients had cortical lesions extending into the white matter of the centrum ovale but sparing the thalamus, while other patients had destruction of the thalamus and posterior/retrolenticular internal capsule (Von Hagen and Ives, 1937; Sandifer, 1946). Based on ten autopsied cases, Nielsen (1938) distinguished 'anosognosia for hemiplegia' proper from 'amnesia' or 'illusion of absence' of the limbs. In his view, the critical lesion involved the thalamoparietal peduncle so as to prevent sensation from reaching the supramarginal gyrus, interfering with proprioceptive synthesis, and removing contralateral limbs from awareness; this produced amnesia or illusion of absence. If the patient could not recognize the illusion or if there was additional damage affecting the thalamus itself or separating the thalamus from other cortical areas in the parietal, frontal, and temporal lobes, then true anosognosia occurred. By contrast, later reports insisted more on the role of cortical parietal areas, in particular the supramarginal and angular gyri (Sandifer, 1946; Roth, 1949; Denny-Brown, Meyer and Horenstein, 1952; Critchley, 1953), and Gerstmann (1942) posited that the lesion had to be close to the intraparietal sulcus. These areas were implicated in a variety of disturbances of the 'body schema' (Head and Holmes, 1911).

Consistently, CT scan showed that the right temporoparietal junction was involved in 70% of right stroke patients with anosognosia (Hier et al., 1983a), though persistent anosognosia was associated with additional involvement of the right frontal lobe. In the Bisiach et al. (1986b) study, AHP was more frequent with cortical (6/13) than purely subcortical (3/15) lesions, and cortical lesions overlapped in the inferior posterior parietal lobe, both in patients with AHP and in those with anosognosia for hemianopia (Fig. 17.1). The three subcortical patients with AHP all had hematoma involving the thalamus, the posterior internal capsule, and the lenticular nucleus. Notably, while capsular-lenticular lesions were also common in patients without AHP, only 1/15 of the latter had thalamic damage. Starkstein et al. (1992) also found a higher frequency of lesions in both the inferior

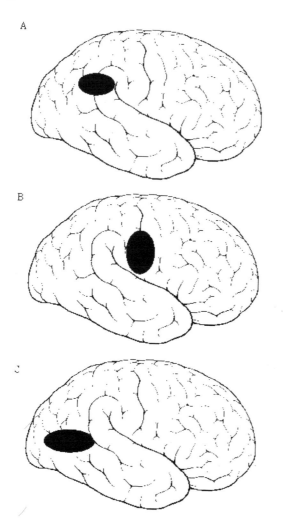

Fig. 17.1   Schematic representation of the cortical areas most commonly involved (A) in patients with anosognosia for either hemiplegia or hemianopia, and (B) in patients with hemiplegia but no anosognosia, or (C) hemianopia but no anosognosia. (Adapted from Bisiach et al., 1986b.)

parietal cortex (11/27 = 41% versus 8/41 = 20%) and the thalamus (5/27 = 19% versus 2/41 = 5%) in patients with AHP. Basal ganglia were often involved in moderate cases.

Like inferior posterior parietal lesions, focal lesions of the thalamus are frequently associated with unilateral spatial neglect (Watson, Valenstein and Heilman, 1982; Bogousslavsky, Regli and Assal, 1986; Vallar and Perani, 1986). Compared to patients with neglect but no AHP, those with AHP have greater involvement of the white matter, particularly the corona radiata (12/14 versus 3/7), as well as of the basal ganglia, particularly the caudate (11/14 versus 3/7) (Small and Ellis, 1996). A frequent involvement of the posterior corona radiata was noted in other CT studies as well (Levine et al., 1991; Feinberg et al., 1994). Also, patients who deny ownership of their paralyzed limb have more damage to the supramarginal gyrus and posterior corona radiata underneath it than other patients with right hemisphere damage and spatial neglect (Feinberg et al., 1990). Remarkably, two autopsy-confirmed cases showed that AHP can occur with lesions confined to the striatum (caudate and lenticular nucleus) and the deep white matter, particularly the corona radiata and posterior internal capsule (Healton et al., 1982; House and Hodges, 1988). Both cases also exhibited neglect. The role of the subcortical lesions themselves and remote diaschisis effects on cortical activity remain unclear. However, while severe neglect without AHP has been reported in patients with damage limited to the posterior internal capsule and widespread hypoactivity of the ipsilateral cortex (Bogousslavsky et al., 1988), both neglect and AHP occurred in a patient with similar diaschisis and a similar lesion except for additional involvement of the striatum and part of the amygdala (de la Sayette et al., 1995).

In summary, AHP is associated with damage to a variety of different brain areas, including the temporoparietal cortex, the thalamus, the striatum, as well as their interconnecting pathways in the posterior deep white matter. Each of these might make a different contribution to the disorder. Moderate signs of age-related subcortical atrophy might constitute a predisposing factor in some cases (Levine et al., 1991; Starkstein et al., 1992). Anosognosia for paralysis exceptionally occurred after nonhemispheric lesions associated with confusion or dementia, in particular brachial plexus damage (Laplane and Degos, 1984) or pedunculopontine stroke (Bakchine, Crassard and Seilhan, 1997), two conditions that cause sensorimotor deafferentation and may lead to phantom limb sensation (Melzack, 1990).

Symptomatic associations and dissociations

Some studies (Cutting, 1978; Starkstein et al., 1992; Small and Ellis, 1996) found no consistent correlation between the severity of weakness and the presence of AHP, but others did (Willanger et al., 1981; Hier et al., 1983a). Likewise, some investigators emphasized greater sensory loss, especially proprioceptive (Cutting, 1978; Levine et al., 1991), which was not confirmed by others (Willanger et al., 1981; Bisiach et al., 1986b; Starkstein et al., 1992; Small and Ellis, 1996). Some patients clearly had AHP despite preserved touch and position sensation (Pick, 1898; Nathanson et al, 1952; Bisiach et al., 1986b; House and Hodges, 1988; Small and Ellis, 1996). Primary sensory deafferentiation seems therefore neither sufficient nor necessary, but somatosensory processing might be altered at some higher level. In several cases (Gerstmann, 1942; Sandifer, 1946; Roth, 1949; Gilliatt and Pratt, 1952), pinching of the arm caused withdrawal, uneasiness, and vegetative reactions

Table 17.3. Frequency of unilateral spatial neglect in anosognosia for hemiplegia

	Patients with AHP	Patients without AHP
Extrapersonal neglect		
Cutting (1978)	16/31 (52%)	1/16 (6%)
Hier et al. (1983b)	13/15 (87%)	6/26 (23%)
Bisiach et al. (1986b) *moderate*	3/18 (17%)	1/18 (5%)
severe	11/18 (61%)	2/18 (11%)
Levine et al. (1991)	6/6 (100%)	4/7 (57%)
Starkstein et al. (1992)	15/27 (56%)	2/53 (4%)
Berti et al. (1996)	8/9 (89%)	19/25 (76%)
Personal neglect		
Cutting (1978)	10/31 (32%)	0/16 (0%)
Bisiach et al. (1986b) *mild*	8/18 (44%)	5/18 (28%)
moderate or severe	5/18 (28%)	1/18 (6%)
Maeshima et al. (1997)	12/12 (100%)	29/38 (76%)
Berti et al. (1996)	3/9 (33%)	0/9 (0%)
Tactile extinction		
Hier et al. (1983b)	15/15 (100%)	10/26 (38%)
Reading neglect		
Berti et al. (1996)	5/9 (56%)	5/25 (20%)

with no explicit acknowledgment of the stimulus. Allesthesia and extinction are also common (Roth, 1949; Gilliatt and Pratt, 1952; Hier et al., 1983a; Starkstein et al., 1992).

Anosognosia for hemiplegia is strongly associated with spatial neglect (Table 17.3). Neglect of extrapersonal space is present in 52% to 87% of patients with AHP, compared to 6% to 23% of those without AHP (Cutting, 1978; Hier et al., 1983a; Bisiach et al., 1986b; Starkstein et al., 1992). Conversely, 68–82% of patients with neglect have AHP, as opposed to 9–21% without neglect (Hier et al., 1983a; Bisiach et al., 1986b). Neglect for left personal space, demonstrated by the failure to direct the right hand across the midline to reach the left hand, is more frequent (Cutting, 1978; Bisiach et al., 1986a) or more severe (Starkstein et al., 1992) in patients with AHP. However, the two conditions are partially dissociable (Willanger et al., 1981; Small and Ellis, 1996; Feinberg, 1997). While many neglect patients have no AHP, a few patients with AHP have been observed who showed no signs of spatial neglect (Bisiach et al., 1986b; House and Hodges, 1988; Small and Ellis, 1996), and AHP during the Wada Test is rarely accompanied by personal neglect (Adair et al., 1995b). Further, vestibular stimulation can induce a transient remission of both neglect and AHP in some cases (Vallar et al., 1990), or improve only neglect without any effect on anosognosia (Cappa et al., 1987). This suggests that neglect is not sufficient to produce AHP, although the significance of these dissociations is still unclear, given the heterogeneity of spatial neglect, the limited tests used in most studies, and the small number of reported cases.

Babinski (1914, 1918) and other early neurologists (Barré et al., 1923; Barkman, 1925) emphasized that anosognosia was not related to confusion or other major intellectual disturbance. However, several investigators found evidence of significant impairment of higher cognitive functions (Weinstein and Kahn, 1950; Nathanson et al., 1952; Ullman et al., 1960; Cutting, 1978; Levine et al., 1991). Thus, in two large series, disorientation was present in 71–100% of the patients with AHP, but in only 6–37% of other patients (Nathanson et al., 1952; Cutting, 1978). As a group, anosognosics show greater deficits in some frontal lobe-related tasks (e.g., set shifting: Levine et al., 1991; Starkstein et al., 1992) but not in others (Small and Ellis, 1996). Motor impersistence (e.g., an inability to keep the eyes closed for more than a few seconds on command) is common (Hier et al., 1983a; Starkstein et al., 1993). However, there is no consistent impairment on the Mini Mental State Examination (Starkstein et al., 1992, 1993; Small and Ellis, 1996) or memory tests (Starkstein et al., 1992). Overall, a global cognitive impairment is clearly not an invariable prerequisite of anosognosia (McGlynn and Schacter, 1989; Bisiach and Geminiani, 1991).

Frederiks (1985) stated that emotional changes are more significant than cognitive deterioration. Cheerfulness and jocularity are noted (Goldstein, 1939; Gainotti, 1972), but apathy seems most common (Cutting, 1978; Levine et al., 1991). There is no significant relation to the occurrence of depression or anxiety (Cutting, 1978; Starkstein et al., 1990, 1992). Interestingly, anosognosic patients cope less well on tests involving the recognition of emotional expressions in faces and prosody in speech (Starkstein et al., 1993).

In summary, no consistent constellation of neurological and neuropsychological deficits has been elucidated. Sensory deafferentation and unilateral neglect are common, but not always present. While global confusion is far from being the rule, the existence of specific cognitive and affective disturbances remains to be confirmed.

Experimental studies of causative factors

One early direct inquiry into the mechanisms of AHP (Guthrie and Grossman, 1952) involved an 'arm-board test' that mechanically restrained the movements of the *intact* arm (eyes closed), and reported that two patients showed inappropriate appreciation of the induced dysfunction. Asked to use his intact but tied right hand, one patient said 'I can do it, just give me time.' Other investigators (Cole, Saexinger and Hard, 1968) used regional anesthesia to induce complete sensorimotor loss of the arm in patients with various brain diseases and elicited anosognosia for the paralysis in five of 22 subjects. Confabulations and ludic behavior were more common in these five cases than in others. Conversely, Ramachandran (1996) reported that a patient who denied his left hemiplegia would admit the paralysis after his left arm was injected with a placebo anesthetic, suggesting that denial might entail not only sensorimotor dysfunction but also belief construction. Another study (Feinberg et al., 1994) found an association with confabulations, that is, all patients with AHP who were briefly shown objects in their contralesional visual field produced more false responses and less admission of failure to perceive than patients with neglect but no AHP. Such a tendency was not found for tactile stimuli in patients with AHP during Wada Test, however (Lu et al., 1997).

Ramachandran (1995, 1996) described several observations, most of which, however, appear to have been poorly controlled. Thus, two patients with AHP were reported to deny the paralysis of another left hemiplegic patient facing them (so that their left limbs were in the intact visual field of the patients), suggesting impaired judgment for disability or a 'person-centered' disorder in body representation (Ramachandran and Rogers-Ramachandran, 1996). This was not the case in other anosognosics, however (Ramachandran, 1996). Further, the ability to appreciate different neurological disabilities (e.g., using pictures) was normal in a number of patients (House and Hodges, 1988; Small and Ellis, 1996). Of greater interest, two experiments (Ramachandran, 1995) assessed 'implicit' knowledge of the paralysis. First, when requested to lift an elongated object (i.e., a tray with glasses on it), patients with AHP inappropriately reached to the right side of the tray with their good hand (toppling the glasses), unlike other hemiplegics who reached for the center of the tray (Ramachandran, 1995). However, the role of spatial neglect was not specified. Second, when given a choice between a unimanual task (e.g., screwing in a light bulb) or a bimanual task (cutting paper with scissors), patients with AHP chose the latter in most (~90%) of the trials (Ramachandran, 1995); data from nonanosognosic hemiplegics were not provided. It is not clear why the patients should prefer the bimanual task rather than inappropriately selecting it as often as the unimanual one. These observations nonetheless imply that patients with AHP apparently intend to move and monitor their movements as if their limbs were good on both sides (see Halligan et al., 1993, for a different observation).

Some evidence suggests that AHP does not result only from a failure of visual appreciation, sensory loss, or spatial inattention. Having subjects move their (gloved) *right*, healthy hand in a box behind a mirror while the mirror reflected the (similarly gloved) hand of another hidden person who remained motionless, Ramachandran (1995, 1996) claimed that anosognosic patients nonetheless contended that they could see the hand moving. Others (Lapresle and Verret, 1978) and we (Vuilleumier and Landis, unpublished) have, however, observed patients in whom denial of ownership was reversed when the left limb was seen in a mirror placed in front of them or on their right side. For subjects who denied paralysis during the Wada Test, Adair et al. (1997) noted that passively moving the limb into the intact visual field did not allow for awareness of the deficit in most cases, whereas voluntary attempts to move sometimes did. This is consistent with the idea that awareness of the limb function might be related to 'feed-forward' mechanisms of motor intentions as much as to visual or proprioceptive feedback. In support of this hypothesis, Gold et al. (1994) recorded EMG activity in the pectoral muscles of patients while they were trying to squeeze either hand, taking advantage of the fact that axial muscles receive bilateral innervation; unlike normal controls and other hemiparetics with similar weakness, one of their patients with AHP produced no proximal contraction on either side during left hand attempts to squeeze. This suggests that AHP might involve a disturbance in motor intention, preventing the detection of a mismatch between intended and performed motor action (as no mismatch would be detected if a movement fails when there is no intention to move) (Heilman, 1991; Gold et al., 1994; Adair et al., 1997). However, other investigators (Hildebrandt and Zieger, 1995) found EMG responses in the affected limb of a left hemiplegic with AHP during tasks normally requiring both hands or during mental imagery of bimanual actions; yet the patient was unable to generate voluntary activation. All these findings suggest that AHP is associated with impaired access to action patterns and intentional motor control.

Possible mechanisms

Babinski (1914, 1918) and his students (Barré et al., 1923; Barkman, 1925) stressed sensory proprioceptive deafferentation depriving the patient of feedback about his weakness, although this explanation was subsequently felt to be insufficient. Other early investigators (Pick, 1898; Head and Holmes, 1911; Pötzl, 1924) considered AHP as a lack of conscious representation of the half-body subserved by special thalamo-parietal mechanisms, and Schilder (1935) ambiguously proposed this was caused by 'organic repression' in order to maintain the integrity of the self. Subsequent authors (Goldstein, 1939; Guthrie and Grossman, 1952; Ullman et al., 1960) viewed anosognosia as a biological adaptative mechanism to cope with a threatening condition, opposed to catastrophical reaction, and favored by a loss of abstract attitude after brain damage.

A motivated defense reaction was elaborated by Weinstein and Kahn (1950, 1955) on the basis that their patients often denied more than one defect, including vomiting or incontinence. In their view, brain damage gives way to stereotyped patterns of behavior, expressed in terms of needs and feelings, and anosognosia is the result of a basic drive to be well, the intensity of which is related to premorbid personality factors. Using interview ratings, Weinstein and Kahn found that anosognosia occurred in people with bland and affable attitudes who had compulsive and perfectionistic drives, a strong need for prestige, and a trend to regard illness as a failure. The predominance of right hemisphere lesions was explained by the fact that, unlike those with left hemisphere lesions and aphasia, patients with right hemisphere lesions were able to conceptualize their illness in metaphorical speech (Weinstein et al., 1964). In a recent study (Small and Ellis, 1996) in which a personality questionnaire was given to right brain-damaged patients with and without AHP and their relatives, no distinctive traits were found. But on a question of whether they could admit illness, more patients with AHP rated themselves as being unable to do so than in the control group. However, strict motivational accounts of anosognosia meet with a number of difficulties (McGlynn and Schacter, 1989; Bisiach and Geminiani, 1991; Berti et al., 1996). They cannot explain its usual occurrence with paralysis of central rather than peripheral origin; its association with specific anatomical sites; its frequent dissociation between certain defects and occasionally different limbs; its predominance in acute stage and its disappearance in chronic stage when motivated behavior would be more likely; or its transient remission during vestibular stimulation.

The same arguments mitigate explanations in terms of general cognitive impairment. Thus, although it is not constant, a memory disturbance was advocated on the basis that some patients may be led to admit their defect but deny it a few minutes later (Redlich and Dorsey, 1945). Others put forward a theory of general affective flattening (Gainotti, 1972) or hypoarousal (Heilman, Schwartz and Watson, 1978) in patients with right hemisphere lesions. Feinberg and colleagues (1994; Feinberg, 1997) related denial to confabulations in an attempt to fill in gaps in the patient's knowledge about his body parts or self. Geschwind (1965) also considered AHP as resulting from confabulations that might be produced by speech areas of the left hemisphere as they have become disconnected from sensorimotor information of the right hemisphere. The condition would be similar to the verbal responses offered by split-brain subjects for tactile or visual stimuli presented to their right hemisphere (Gazzaniga, 1992). However, AHP is not suppressed by passively showing the paralyzed limb to the left hemisphere's intact visual field (Adair et al., 1997). Cutting (1978) and Willanger et al. (1981) therefore regarded AHP as a true agnosia of the defect in the sense that its perception was not integrated with its meaning or other knowledge.

Following Lhermitte (1939) and Gerstmann (1942), several authors (Roth, 1949; Denny-Brown et al., 1952; Critchley, 1953) postulated a failure in a specific neural mechanism that integrates multiple sensory (tactile, kinesthetic, visual, vestibular) inputs into a conscious body image. According to this view, schemata stored in the posterior parietal cortex allow sensation to be referred to the body parts (Head and Holmes, 1911), so that their destruction or disconnection could result in the subjective disowning of the opposite hemibody. Denny-Brown et al. (1952) and Sandifer (1946) further expanded the view of Schilder (1935) that body awareness implies the representation of its position in space, and suggested that unilateral neglect of personal space might cause an agnosia of the body-half contained therein. Yet, anosognosia can dissociate from neglect and be domain specific (e.g., for hemiplegia versus hemianopia). Therefore, Bisiach and colleagues (1986b; Bisiach and Geminiani, 1991) proposed that anosognosia may result from the disruption of a modular representational network, holding both sensory-driven and internally generated signals, which subtends the conscious content of any specific function (Fig. 17.2). Such a disruption would cause a failure not only to perceive and attend to one half of the body but also to conceive and monitor its function (if the network is destroyed), or lead to abnormally constructed, or 'parasitic,' misrepresentations like somatoparaphrenia (if the network loses its normal inputs).

Other authors (Ullman et al., 1960; Frederiks, 1985; Levine, 1990; Levine et al., 1991) proposed that the absence of somatosensory and kinesthetic feedback from affected limbs might induce perceptual completion in the form of phantom limb sensations, misleading patients into the illusion that their limbs are intact. Indeed, phantom limbs in amputees or after cerebral damage attest to the existence of some network in the brain (a 'neuromatrix') whose patterns of neural activity may create the subjective experience of a body part, even in the absence of input from it (Melzack, 1990). Such a network undoubtedly involves a number of cortical and subcortical sites, including various areas in the parietal cortex that contribute to integrate somatosensory and spatial information and code for the position of body parts in space and in relation to each other (Berlucchi and Aglioti, 1997; Vuilleumier et al., 1997). While the superior parietal areas represent limbs and postures in terms of body-centered spatial coordinates, the inferior posterior parietal lobule brings together somatosensory and visual representations of the body and external space (Kalaska et al., 1997). Parietal or subcortical lesions impeding the correspondence between these representations might dissociate the subjective somatosensory experience of a deafferented limb from other sources of knowledge about its position (e.g., sight), eventually leading to denial of its ownership.

However, a patient may still recognize his or her arm but deny its weakness. A loss of motor intention might preclude the detection of a mismatch between motor expectancy and performed action (Heilman, 1991; Gold et al., 1994), and even prevent the patient gaining a conscious experience of the limb (Kinsbourne, 1995). Motor intention and commands have subjective correlates (Jeannerod, 1994) and these contribute to monitor action and perceive limb position (Kinsbourne, 1995). Thus, a patient with severe left motor neglect but no paralysis was reported to have

A. Normal state

Conscious representation

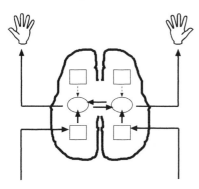

Sensory input

B. Awareness of a deficit

Conscious representation

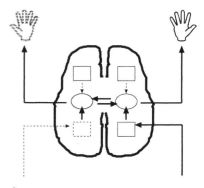

Sensory input

C. AHP and unilateral neglect

Conscious representation

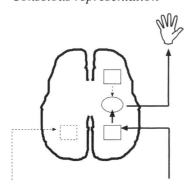

Sensory input

D. AHP and misrepresentation

Conscious representation

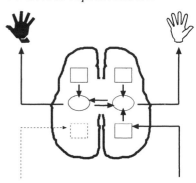

Sensory input

Fig. 17.2   A simplified version of the model proposed by Bisiach et al. (1986b, 1991) to account for (A) normal, (B) diseased, (C) lost, and (D) pathologic representations of one half-body and/or half-space. The lower and upper boxes in each hemisphere depict, respectively, a 'sensory transducer' that processes domain-specific inputs via bottom-up mechanisms, and a 'topologically corresponding cellular grouping' that provides internal reconstructive influences via top-down mechanisms. The ellipse in-between depicts a common network that is activated through both mechanisms and subserves a domain-specific representation, the latter being then available to conscious awareness. (C) and (D) correspond to different instances of anosognosia for hemiplegia (AHP). Bisiach et al. (1986b, 1991) suggested that the same modular organization might apply to different neurological domains (e.g., vision).

an inability to recognize his left hand which resolved when motor neglect disappeared, while his proprioceptive loss remained unchanged (Garcin, Varay and Dimo, 1938). This suggests that abnormal intentional premotor processes probably play a critical role in AHP, consistent with the feed-forward theory of Heilman et al. (Heilman, 1991; Gold et al., 1994). Impaired motor activation might be caused by damage to the basal ganglia or to their connections with cortical and thalamic structures within the white matter (Healton et al., 1982; Watson et al., 1982; Laplane and Degos, 1983).

Yet, while these mechanisms presumably deprive patients of a direct experience of their defect, explicit anosognosia also reflects an inability to become convinced of the fact. Nielsen (1938) posited that 'in all such cases there must, of course, be two lesions, one causing hemiplegia (of which, without a second lesion the patient would be aware), the other rendering the patient unaware of the fact,' and Nielsen added: 'What he believes . . . is another matter.' Ullman et al. (1960) made similar comments. Levine and colleagues (1991; Levine, 1990) proposed a 'discovery theory' of anosognosia according to which a defect may not cause any immediate experience but must be inferred, so that additional cognitive disorders will produce persistent denial. A lack of flexibility to adapt belief and resolve inconsistencies might be related to concomitant damage to striatal structures and subcortical–frontal circuits which participate in adaptive behavior and thought regulation (Cummings, 1993; Bhatia and Marsden, 1994). Further, while belief formation might depend on the left hemisphere capacity for making inference (Assal, 1983; Gazzaniga, 1992), belief change might require some affect-based drive and a capacity for detecting novelty that could be impaired after right hemisphere damage (Bear, 1982; Ramachandran, 1996; Berns, Cohen and Mintun, 1997).

In summary, AHP has been the subject of a myriad of explanations and speculations, suggesting that more than a single mechanism is probably involved. An impairment in parietal mechanisms that integrate somatosensory and spatial limb representations, as well as motor preparation, might create an abnormal experience of the paralyzed limbs, which could combine with an impaired ability to shift mental set and belief to result in denial of the defect (Bisiach and Geminiani, 1991).

Anosognosia for hemianopia and scotoma

Behavioral aspects and incidence

Although they may have similar visual field defects (i.e., homonymous hemianopia or quadranopia), some patients are aware of the fact and others are not. Because unaware patients do not complain, their visual loss sometimes goes unrecognized until it is specifically looked for. Also, it has long been known that patients who are aware of the defect may have different visual experiences (Critchley, 1949).

Rarely, they have a 'positive hemianopia' (or 'dark vision'), in which the objects or faces they fixate appear bisected in their midline, with one half of the visual field obscured. Most often, they have a 'negative hemianopia' (or 'null vision'), in which they realize that part of the visual field is missing without seeing bisected objects or a black scotoma.

Anosognosia for hemianopia also takes various forms. Some patients deny any visual problem even though they repeatedly bump into objects or people on the affected side (Gassel and Williams, 1963). Others complain of blurring or reading problems but deny any difference between the right and left sides (Koehler et al., 1986). Critchley (1949) scrupulously distinguished six possible levels of awareness of visual defect:

1 complete unawareness that remains unchanged even after repeated demonstration by the examiner;
2 unawareness of the defect itself while acknowledging its existence and its consequences;
3 awareness of a visual defect that is, however, rationalized and misattributed to another cause, e.g., insufficient lighting in the room;
4 relative awareness of the existence of a visual problem which cannot be adequately explained or described;
5 awareness of the defect, which can be described but in erroneous terms, e.g., a disturbance of vision affecting one eye only;
6 adequate awareness with correct description and attribution of the defect.

Most investigators have agreed that the first (or possibly first three) of these levels corresponds to obvious instances of anosognosia for hemianopia (Warrington, 1962; Gassel and Williams, 1963; Koehler et al., 1986; Celesia, Brigell and Vaphiades, 1997). The other levels entail more subtle disturbances that emphasize the multiple aspects of awareness of one's illness, and have been variably classified as complete (Warrington, 1962; Celesia et al., 1997) or partial (Gassel and Williams, 1963; Koehler et al., 1986) anosognosia. AHA is usually inferred from the patients' answer to questions such as 'Can you see well? Can you see equally to your left and right?' (Warrington, 1962; Koehler et al., 1986; Celesia et al., 1997). Few studies explicitly mention the impact of demonstrating the deficit during examination on the patients' appraisal of their visual function (Gassel and Williams, 1963). However, Bisiach and colleagues (1986a; Bisiach and Geminiani, 1991) assessed AHA using the same four-point rating scale as for AHP.

Anosognosia for hemianopia is even more common than AHP. Critchley (1949) estimated that it occurs in 25% of hemianopic patients. Gassel and Williams (1963) found that 10/35 patients (29%) had complete AHA, while only 4/35 (11%) showed full awareness. Other studies found comlete AHA in 55–63% of patients and partial awareness or misinterpretations in another 22–25% (Warrington, 1962; Koehler e al., 1986; Celesia et al., 1997). In right brain-damaged patients, AHA was noted in 71–87% of hemianopics (Willanger et al., 1981; Bisiach et al., 1986b). As mentioned earlier, anosognosia for hemianopia can be dissociated from anosognosia for hemiplegia. When both disorders were present, AHA existed without AHP in 5/9 cases in one study (Willanger et al., 1981) and 9/13 cases in another (Celesia et al., 1997); AHP less commonly occurs without AHA (Bisiach et al., 1986b).

Unawareness of acquired visual loss is also encountered with peripheral ophthalmological disorders, e.g., retinal scotoma or glaucoma (Critchley, 1949; Safran and Landis, 1996). Yet, visual defects caused by brain lesion appear more susceptible to denial than peripheral defects (Safran and Landis, 1996). A reported patient spontaneously complained about a right-eye visual loss due to retinal ischemia but denied a left homonymous hemianopia subsequent to a right parieto-occipital stroke (Bender, 1984). Contrary to Critchley's (1949) suggestions, AHA is not influenced by the rate of onset and macular sparing (Warrington, 1962; Gassel and Williams, 1963; Celesia et al., 1997).

Anatomical aspects

An early study of 122 brain-damaged patients (Battersby et al., 1956) reported that anosognosia could involve left and right visual field defects as well, although it appeared to be at least twice as frequent after lesions in the right hemisphere. Warrington (1962) noted a slight predominance of right hemisphere lesions with AHA found in 8/12 left hemianopics and 3/8 right hemianopics. In recent studies based on CT or MRI scans, one (Koehler et al., 1986) found that unawareness was more common with right than with left hemisphere damage (20/25 versus 3/10 cases), whereas another (Celesia et al., 1997) found no significant difference (16/26 versus 4/6 cases). However, both studies excluded left hemisphere patients with severe aphasia.

Early authors suggested that unawareness of hemianopia indicated a lesion that involved the visual cortex (Magitot and Hartmann, 1927) or its connection with the lateral geniculate body of the thalamus (Pötzl, 1924). These structures were held to be the critical substrate of conscious perception, so that their destruction would preclude awareness of missing sensory information. Critchley (1949) stated that AHA occurred with lesions in either cortical or subcortical visual areas. Two subsequent studies (Warrington, 1962; Koehler et al., 1986) found that, regardless of the side of damage, unawareness of hemianopia was more common in patients with parietal damage (11/13 and 14/15, respectively) than when lesions were restricted to the occipital lobe or spared the parietal areas (0/5 and 9/23, respectively) (Fig. 17.3). Sergent (1988) noted a similar trend. In right brain-damaged patients, Bisiach et al. (1986b) found a slightly higher proportion of AHA with lesions involving the cortex (6/13 patients) than purely subcortical lesions (4/15).

A

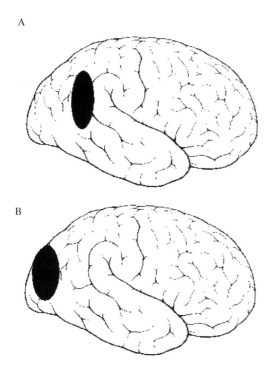

B

Fig. 17.3   Schematic representation of the cortical areas most commonly involved (A) in patients with anosognosia for hemianopia and (B) in patients with hemianopia but no anosognosia. Compare with Fig. 17.1. (Adapted from Koehler et al., 1986.)

Cortical lesions tended to overlap in the inferior parietal lobe in cases with AHA, as in those with AHP. Patients with subcortical lesions and AHA had thalamic or capsular-lenticular hematoma, one of whom was aware of his hemiplegia but denied his visual field defect. Another recent study (Celesia et al., 1997) failed to confirm an association between AHA and parietal lesions; however, patients with AHA had larger lesions and more involvement of anterior brain areas vascularized by the middle rather than the posterior cerebral artery. Moreover, involvement of the deep white matter was common, particularly in the paraventricular and retrolenticular regions, and sufficient to produce hemianopic anosognosia in some cases. Celesia et al. (1997) nonetheless pointed out that of eight patients with pure hemianopia and apparently similar occipital lesions, five fully acknowledged their deficit and the three others had anosognosia.

In summary, notwithstanding a number of inconsistencies and the fact that lesions causing hemianopia obviously involve different brain regions from those causing hemiplegia, there is a notable trend toward some overlap in parietal and subcortical areas of the right hemisphere in cases of AHA, as in cases of AHP.

Table 17.4. Frequency of unilateral spatial neglect in anosognosia for hemianopia (AHA)

	Patients with AHA	Patients without AHA
Extrapersonal neglect		
Warrington (1962)	8/11 (73%)	1/9 (11%)
Koehler et al. (1986)	11/25 (44%)	0/7 (0%)
Bisiach et al. (1986b)	20/28 (71%)	3/4 (75%)
Celesia et al. (1997)	17/20 (85%)	6/12 (50%)
Personal neglect		
Bisiach et al. (1986b)	4/28 (14%)	3/4 (75%)
Contralateral eye deviation		
Celesia et al. (1997)	12/20 (60%)	0/12 (0%)

Symptomatic associations and experimental studies

As Critchley (1949) emphasized, AHA is not related to general cognitive impairment or confusion (Warrington, 1962; Celesia et al., 1997). On the other hand, an association with unilateral spatial neglect has long been noted (Battersby et al., 1956). Across different studies (Warrington, 1962; Bisiach et al., 1986b; Koehler et al., 1986; Celesia et al., 1997), extrapersonal neglect was present in 44% to 85% of patients with AHA, as compared to 0% to 75% of hemianopics without anosognosia (Table 17.4). Personal neglect is uncommon (Bisiach et al., 1986a). However, again, clear dissociations are observed: several patients without spatial neglect are unaware of their hemianopia, whereas others who have neglect appear aware.

Perceptual completion has been noted with AHA since its first demonstration by Poppelreuter (1917). Completion refers to perceiving a figure as complete when it is presented in such a way that a part of it falls into the blind field (Fig. 17.4A). In some cases, this occurs only with physically complete forms, implicating some residual function in the blind field or an interaction between the normal and affected areas, but in many others it is obtained even with physically incomplete forms that project only onto the normal half-field. Either using geometric figures or asking patients whether they saw a whole or half face when fixating the examiner on a confrontation test, Warrington (1962) and Gassel and Williams (1963) demonstrated higher rates of completion in all of their patients with severe AHA and in none of the other hemianopics. Some of these patients also tended to give detailed reports at exposure time below the duration necessary for correct identification of the figures. Therefore, Warrington (1962), like Feinberg (1997), regarded completion as a form of visual confabulation.

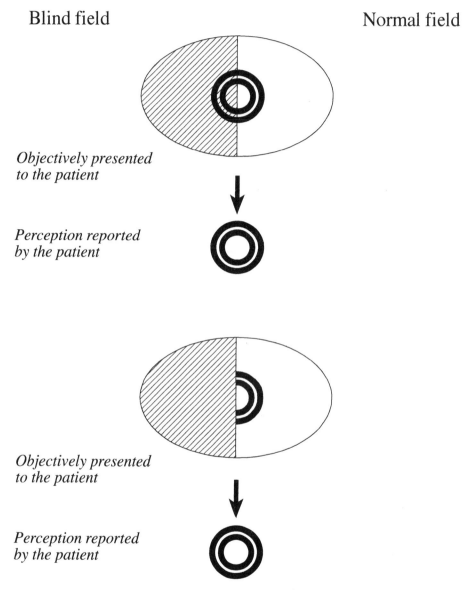

Fig. 17.4   Examples of perceptual completion in the blind field of hemianopic patients (A) and the divided fields of split-brain subjects (B).

(B) Completion in split-brain patients

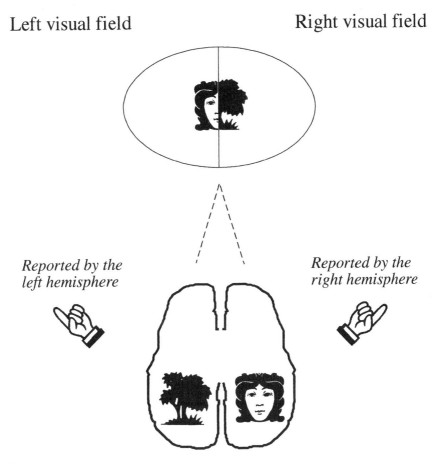

Left visual field   Right visual field

Reported by the
left hemisphere

Reported by the
right hemisphere

Fig. 17.4   (cont.).

Possible mechanisms

Critchley (1949) pointed out that the greater frequency of anosognosia for hemianopia than for hemiplegia, even though it is a far less incapacitating impairment,
reasonably rules out a simple account in terms of psychodynamic motivational
denial. On the other hand, as emphasized by Gassel and Williams (1963), 'the
hemianopic field is an area of absence which is discovered rather than sensed . . .
(its) presence is judged from some specific failure in function rather directly perceived.' Accordingly, Levine et al.'s (1991) 'discovery theory' posited that unawareness of hemianopia was common even in cognitively intact patients, because the
defect is not phenomenally immediate and difficult to discover. Anosognosia

ensues from superimposed disturbances which keep the patient unaware and unconvinced of his or her hemianopia. Concomitant involvement of parietal or subcortical structures might cause one or more additional disorders that combine with the primary visual loss so as to impede the ability to infer or monitor the impairment (Anton, 1898; Bisiach et al., 1986b; Levine et al., 1991). Thus, unilateral visual inattention or neglect might play a role although not constantly present. Residual visual functions within the hemianopic field ('blindsight') or through subcortical extrageniculate pathways could be implicated in yet undetermined ways, e.g., by influencing spatial coordinates of visual and orienting behavior (Rafal et al., 1990). Critchley (1949) also suggested that AHA was related to 'optic allesthesia,' whereby objects seen in the intact visual field are subjectively perceived in the contralateral blind field. Similarly, it is tempting to put forward perceptual completion as a major contributory factor (Poppelreuter, 1917; Gassel and Williams, 1963; Levine, 1990; Feinberg, 1997; Safran, 1997). Completion might involve filling-in processes, similar to those that make one unaware of the normal blind spot of each eye or retinal scotoma by perceptually filling them in with visual attributes (color, texture, etc.) of the surrounding field (Fig. 17.5; Safran and Landis, 1996). Filling-in processes have well-established neurophysiological correlates in the visual cortex; these include remapping of the receptive field of deafferented neurons, which then respond to new retinal areas, as well as long-range interactions through lateral cortical connections and perhaps subcortical connections (Spillmann and Werner, 1996). By creating patterns of neural activity that complete the missing information, the visual system might thus deprive patients of clues to their defect.

It must be noted, however, that perceptual completion is influenced by a variety of factors, suggesting that the blind field probably does not function as an extensive blind spot (Sergent, 1988). Completion can be suppressed when patients deliberately attend to the affected side or adopt a 'more critical attitude' (Gassel and Williams, 1963). It is facilitated by cognitive impairment and can be modulated by expectations, mental set, or the demonstration of errors (Gassel and Williams, 1963; Sergent, 1988). Gassel and Williams (1963) suggested that patients who explicitly deny their defect might be less susceptible to such effects. Remarkably, in those hemianopics who are only partially aware and misattribute their defect to the eye on the side of the hemifield loss, completion responses occurred more often or exclusively with the ipsilesional, subjectively 'better' eye when each eye was tested separately (Gassel and Williams, 1963). Belief formation and other cognitive factors, therefore, probably participate in the completion of hemianopia and presumably anosognosia as well. Finally, Sergent (1988) showed that completion occurred with verbal reports but not drawing responses, which might point to some underlying difference in terms of hemispheric processing. In split-brain

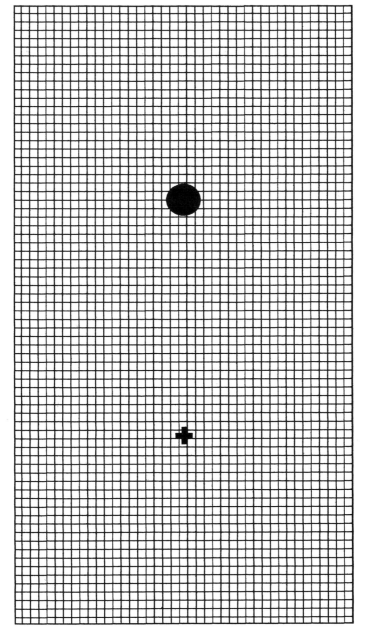

Fig. 17.5   Unawareness of the physiologic blind spot due to filling-in processes. When attentively fixating the left cross at a distance of about 20 cm and then closing the left eye, the right black dot will disappear without leaving any void in the reader's awareness.

subjects, each hemisphere is sufficient in itself to generate the missing half of chimeric stimuli simultaneously presented across the divided visual fields, and can produce independent completion responses (see Fig. 17.4B); both hemispheres remain unaware of the stimuli processed in the opposite hemisphere (Levy, Trevarthen and Sperry, 1972; Sergent, 1988). This suggests that completion is determined by the selection of a response, and probably occurs in the access to a conscious representation rather than at a lower level of primary visual processes.

Anosognosia for blindness (Anton's syndrome)

Behavioral aspects

Counter to commonsense expectations, some patients with cortical blindness are unaware that they cannot see anymore. Although totally unable to discriminate objects, shapes, colors, movement, and even light from dark, these patients maintain that they are not blind. Some patients will explicitly and actively deny any visual disturbance, contending that they see very clearly. Others will deny blindness but recognize some loss of visual function, which they attribute to another external cause (e.g., insufficient lighting). Like one patient of Von Monakow (1885), they often make excuses when confronted with their failures: 'The room is too dark' or 'I need my glasses' (Redlich and Dorsey, 1945); or, as the patient of Déjerine and Vialet (1893), 'I have a tear in my eyes.' Similarly, Anton's (1898) patient conceded that her vision was better in her younger days. Still other patients acknowledge their impaired vision but appear unconcerned about the fact and its consequences. Most patients report positive visual perceptions which they firmly refuse to dismiss as unreal (Anton, 1898; Redlich and Dorsey, 1945; Sandifer, 1946; Della Sala and Spinnler, 1988; Goldenberg, Mullbacher and Nowak, 1995). Clear descriptions are sometimes difficult to obtain. However, patients may unhesitatingly (yet incorrectly) describe their surroundings or misname objects shown to them (Anton, 1898; Guthrie and Grossman, 1952; Goldenberg et al., 1995); they may pretend to read the newspaper or watch television (Swartz and Brust, 1984), and try to grab things that they believe they see (Redlich and Dorsey, 1945; Goldenberg et al., 1995). While some patients attempt to walk and bump into objects, the behavior of others suggests some implicit knowledge of their condition, in that they make no objections to remaining in bed or request help from a companion to walk (Bergman, 1956; Feinberg, 1997).

Anton's syndrome is most common as a transient phenomenon in acute neurological injuries, often resolving into visual agnosia. Transient forms also occur during vertebrobasilar arteriography. In some cases, however, both blindness and anosognosia persisted for several years (Déjerine and Viallet, 1893; Celesia, Archer and Kuroiwa, 1980; Pérenin, Ruel and Hécaen, 1980). Many patients with both cortical blindness and hemiparesis present AHP together with Anton's syndrome (Redlich and Dorsey, 1945; Guthrie and Grossman, 1952), while others deny their blindness but complain of weakness (Symonds and MacKenzie, 1957), or complain of their associated speech disturbance (Anton, 1898). Exceptional cases may show dissociated awareness between the two visual hemifields, denying the loss of one side but acknowledging impaired vision in the other (Stengel and Steele, 1946).

Anatomical aspects

Anton's syndrome has diverse causes (Magitot and Hartmann, 1927; Redlich and Dorsey, 1945; Bergman, 1956; Angelergues, de Ajuriaguerra and Hécaen, 1960; Swartz and Brust, 1984). The first and most common is cortical blindness due to bilateral occipital damage, usually bilateral infarcts in the territory of the posterior cerebral artery (Aldrich et al., 1987). Because these cases are rare, so is Anton's syndrome, and no study allows a reliable comparison of lesions in those cortically blind patients who are aware of it and the others who are not. Bergman (1956) found denial in seven of 12 cases with blindness of cerebral origin; denial was associated with bilateral EEG abnormalities. Aldrich et al. (1987) noted that of 15 patients with cortical blindness, seven were not aware of their visual loss, yet only three of them exhibited explicit denial. Autopsy findings in early reports usually mentioned damage to both primary and associative visual areas (Von Monakow, 1885; Anton, 1898). Anton's (1898) patient had bilateral necrosis of the occipital cortex and angular gyri on both sides, extending into the white matter and the splenium of the corpus callosum. In addition to variable occipital damage, involvement of the cuneus and the lingual gyrus on one or both sides was common (Von Monakow, 1885; Déjerine and Viallet, 1893; Rossolimo, 1896). Thalamic, basal ganglia, or frontal lesions were all occasionally associated (Von Monakow, 1885; Rossolimo, 1896). Subsequent authors emphasized the destruction of white matter association tracts or thalamo-cortical pathways (Pötzl, 1924; Redlich and Dorsey, 1945), which were believed to be responsible for the integrated and conscious perception of self and environment. Others emphasized damage to medial temporal–limbic structures (Angelergues et al., 1960), responsible for a superimposed memory disorder. Only a few recent cases provided additional anatomical or neuroradiological data about lesions associated with anosognosia for cortical blindness (Celesia et al., 1980; Pérenin et al., 1980; Cusumano, Fletcher and Platel, 1981; Della Sala and Spinnler, 1988; Verslegers et al., 1991; Goldenberg et al., 1995). All had bilateral destruction of the calcarine cortex (area 17), with relative sparing of the lateral secondary visual cortex (areas 18 and 19) on one or both sides. Small isolated islands of intact visual cortex existed in some cases (Goldenberg et al., 1995). The medial temporo-occipital and parahippocampal gyri or the thalamic nuclei vascularized by the posterior cerebral arteries were often involved (Della Sala and Spinnler, 1988; Verslegers et al., 1991; Goldenberg et al., 1995).

The second most common cause of Anton's syndrome involves blindness of peripheral origin and raises interesting issues as to the mechanism of anosognosia. It typically occurs with traumatic lesions to the optic nerve and bilateral frontal contusions (Stuss and Benson, 1986; McDaniel and McDaniel, 1991), as well as with damage to the optic nerve by compression or intracranial hypertension in tumors of the frontal lobes, diencephalon, optic chiasm, skull base, or posterior fossa (Redlich and Dorsey, 1945; Sandifer, 1946; Stengel and Steele, 1946; Angelergues et al., 1960). The basal forebrain and orbito-medial frontal lobes appear to be most consistently involved in these cases. Neurosyphilis with optic neuropathy and general paresis has also been implicated (Pötzl, 1924; Angelergues et al., 1960).

Some authors (Redlich and Dorsey, 1945; Swartz and Brust, 1984) therefore claimed that Anton's syndrome may be associated with blindness due to lesions at any point along the visual pathways provided that it is accompanied by facilitating cognitive disorder.

Symptomatic associations

Severe cognitive dysfunction or confusion is common (Redlich and Dorsey, 1945; Oppenheimer and Weissman, 1951; Symonds and MacKenzie, 1957), and some patients who had peripheral or central blindness of which they were aware developed Anton's syndrome only as they became confused (Sandifer, 1946; Guthrie and Grossman, 1952; Bergman, 1956). However, denial can occur in the absence of confusion or significant dementia (Celesia et al., 1980; Stuss and Benson, 1986; McDaniel and McDaniel, 1991). One reported patient showed no significant change in her verbal IQ performance as denial abated (Goldenberg et al., 1995). Memory impairment is particularly frequent and severe, due to the involvement of medial temporal and/or thalamic structures in 'posterior' (occipital) cases and orbito-medial frontal lobe in 'anterior' (peripheral) cases, and prominent confabulations have been noted in virtually all cases of either type (Oppenheimer and Weissman, 1951; Castaigne et al., 1967; Aldrich et al., 1987; Della Sala and Spinnler, 1988; McDaniel and McDaniel, 1991). Redlich and Dorsey (1945) wrote: 'Anton's syndrome may be said to consist of a Korsakoff psychosis in a blind person.' Other authors emphasized personality changes and euphoria (Pötzl, 1924; Stengel and Steele, 1946; Angelergues et al., 1960).

Several patients with cortical blindness and Anton's syndrome had preserved mental imagery (e.g., to describe the visual appearance of objects or scenes from memory) in spite of occipital damage (Von Monakow, 1885; Anton, 1898; Magitot and Hartman, 1927; Redlich and Dorsey, 1945). Goldenberg et al. (1995) described a patient with intact imagery in whom pretended visual perceptions seemed to be provoked by meaningful information in other modalities, i.e., by auditory, verbal, or tactile stimulations. This suggests that synaesthetic phenomena might exist as in otherwise normal individuals and adventitiously blinded people (Levine et al., 1991). Frank visual hallucinations have also been reported (Redlich and Dorsey, 1945; Angelergues et al., 1960). Interestingly, in a man who had been blind since an old ocular trauma, transient episodes of Anton's syndrome were observed during hallucinosis periods due to alcohol withdrawal (Swartz and Brust, 1984). Curiously, while the patient believed that his vision had been restored and confabulated descriptions of the surroundings during the episodes, at the same time he recognized the unreality of other complex visual hallucinations (e.g., a dog in the room). He had no Korsakoff psychosis and had normal mentation outside the episodes. His belief of recovered vision might have arisen from the 'release' of visual mental images, somehow met with uncritical acceptance.

Possible mechanisms

Premorbid personality (Weinstein and Kahn, 1950, 1955; Guthrie and Grossman, 1952) or general cognitive factors (Oppenheimer and Weissman, 1951) do not adequately account for all cases of Anton's syndrome (McGlynn and Schacter, 1989; Redlich and Dorsey, 1945). Anton (1898) related anosognosia to the disruption of association fibers connecting the visual cortex to the rest of the brain in such a way that higher level areas could not detect the lack of sensory stimulation. Geschwind (1965) and Fisher (1989) similarly proposed that unawareness of the deficit and confabulatory responses resulted from the disconnection of all cortically mediated visual information from speech areas in the left hemisphere. This would be akin to the confabulations produced by the left hemisphere of split-brain subjects for visual stimuli that are projected to their right hemisphere (Levy et al., 1972; Gazzaniga, 1992). As suggested by Heilman (1991), impaired monitoring of visual function could, however, result not only from a disconnection between sensory and monitoring areas, but also from false feedback or disturbance in the monitor device itself.

According to Levine et al.'s (1991) theory, loss of vision may not cause any phenomenally immediate experience, but must be discovered by self-observation and inference. Like many blind subjects, patients with Anton's syndrome could have preserved visual imagery and subjective visual experiences triggered by other sensory modalities, memory, or various kinds of mental associations (Cohn, 1971). However, they might be unable to distinguish internally generated images from real percepts. A number of authors have made similar suggestions (Pötzl, 1924; Redlich and Dorsey, 1945; Heilman, 1991; Goldenberg et al., 1995). Whether mental imagery and visual awareness depend on the integrity of primary visual cortex in addition to secondary association areas has been controversial (Roland and Gulyás, 1994), but, importantly, not all patients with cortical blindness have preserved imagery. Some of these visual cortical areas could be spared, even in 'posterior' (occipital) cases of Anton's syndrome. Alternatively, other brain areas, e.g., the cuneus, might contribute to visual imagery. Preservation of imagery may also rely on asymmetric brain damage, because the generation of visual images involves the left more than the right hemisphere (Farah, 1989). Further, the lack of interference from actual afferent input might enhance spontaneous visual imagery, consistent with the fact that in several cases resolution of Anton's syndrome coincided with recovery of some functional sight (Redlich and Dorsey, 1945; Aldrich et al., 1987; McDaniel and McDaniel, 1991; Goldenberg et al., 1995), and not with the apparition of covert, nonconscious vision ('blindsight') (Pérenin et al., 1980). Unawareness would thus result because the patient has the subjective experience of not being blind.

Anosognosia and denial, however, imply the failure to discover and admit the defect. Levine et al. (1991) intimated that this can occur only in association with severe cognitive impairment, in particular of memory, attention, judgment, and flexibility abilities. Redlich and Dorsey (1945) insisted on the inability to learn and the existence of a fixed belief system which cannot be refuted in patients with Anton's syndrome. Angelergues et al. (1960) similarly emphasized that these patients uncritically accept their images. 'Anterior' (peripheral) cases of Anton's syndrome in patients who have peripheral blindness and no major cognitive loss other than confabulation (Stuss and Benson, 1986; McDaniel and McDaniel, 1991) point to the crucial role of frontal lobe systems. Medial and orbital prefrontal dysfunction might impair the ability to monitor the source of internally generated information, as well as the ability to adapt belief and mental set (Stuss and Benson, 1986; Frith, 1996; Johnson, 1997). Confabulations probably result from similar problems in monitoring memory. In 'posterior' (occipital) cases of Anton's syndrome, this could be secondary to concomitant involvement of the medial thalamic nuclei, which project to prefrontal regions, or of other areas in the limbic system, e.g., the medial temporal lobe or posterior cingulate. In particular, the posterior cingulate is involved in monitoring visual events and updating representations of the environment; it also has connections with anterior cingulate and prefrontal areas (Vogt, Finch and Olson, 1992). It might be implicated in monitoring signals that distinguish between externally and internally evoked visual representations.

Anosognosia for aphasia

Behavioral and anatomical aspects

As already noted by Wernicke (1874), some aphasics make no self-corrections of their deviant speech production and appear unaware of their errors. More rarely, they may be unaware that they have any speech problem at all and even explicitly deny it (Kinsbourne and Warrington, 1963; Weinstein and Lyerly, 1976). Others admit difficulties but remain unconcerned (Maher, Gonzalez Rothi and Heilman, 1994). Anosognosia typically occurs in patients with jargonaphasia. These patients, who have fluent aphasia of Wernicke's or transcortical sensory type, produce lengthy and digressive output replete with phonemic and semantic paraphasias, neologisms, and automatisms; yet they seemingly believe they communicate satisfactorily and may show anger when other people do not understand them. Jargonaphasia has been termed 'anosognosic aphasia' and compared to psychotic speech (Critchley, 1964). Some authors (Alajouanine, 1956; Weinstein et al., 1964; Weinstein and Lyerly, 1976) have suggested that jargon specifically results from the combination of aphasia and anosognosia. Thus, Weinstein and colleagues (1964; Weinstein and Lyerly, 1976) observed jargon only in patients who had both aphasia and manifestations of anosognosia but not in others who had aphasia without anosognosia. The same authors reported that 50% to 77% of patients with jargon denied any speech difficulty when directly questioned; the others were considered to show implicit denial in that they behaved or talked as if their speech was intact. However, anosognosia is not constant in jargonaphasia, and some of these patients do realize they have a language deficit (Rubens and Garrett, 1991). Gainotti (1972) noted that 25% of 16 Wernicke's aphasics were unaware of their language disturbances as compared to none of 19 patients with Broca's aphasia and 24 with anomia. Some patients with global aphasia also appear unaware of the lack of meaning of their repetitive stereotyped utterances, such as 'tan-tan-tan' (Alajouanine, 1956; Lebrun and Leleux, 1982; Cambier, Masson and Robine, 1993).

By contrast, other aphasics who appear aware of their failure show frequent self-corrections, halts, and occasional catastrophic reactions when they cannot be understood or understand others (Gainotti, 1972). They may use various deliberate strategies to facilitate or circumvent their difficulties, indicating that they are able to monitor their speech productions. However, it must be noted that the absence of self-correction does not necessarily imply unawareness or lack of detection of the errors: a patient may just give up struggling and be satisfied with approximations (Lebrun, 1987). On the other hand, a patient may be fully aware of having impaired linguistic abilities and behave appropriately while totally unable to perceive the nature of his or her errors (Shuren et al., 1995). Further, unawareness may be selective for one type of errors and not concern others. A patient could correct her phonemic errors but ignored her semantic errors (Marshall, Rappaport and Garcia-Bunuel, 1985). Others recognize their disturbance in writing better than in spoken language. Finally, contrary to the suggestions by Weinstein and colleagues (1964; Weinstein and Lyerly, 1976), anosognosia for speech errors and denial of aphasia often coexist with normal awareness of other deficits, such as hemiplegia or blindness, and vice versa (Kinsbourne and Warrington, 1963; McGlynn and Schacter, 1989; Maher et al., 1994). Anosognosia for linguistic and motor disturbances also dissociate during Wada procedure and left hemisphere anesthesia (Breier et al., 1995).

Jargonaphasia is associated with lesions of the posterior part of the left superior temporal gyrus that extend into the inferior parietal lobe, as well as the underlying white matter (Kertesz and Benson, 1970; Rubens and Garrett, 1991). It is particularly frequent in cases with bilateral lesions or associated diffuse brain dysfunction, such as head trauma (Weinstein and Lyerly, 1976; Rubens and Garrett, 1991). A double lesion involving both the superior temporal gyri and the third frontal gyrus of the left hemisphere was found in a patient who made stereotyped recurrent utterances of which she was unaware (Cambier et al., 1993). Marshall et al. (1985) suggested that anosognosia in Wernicke's aphasia might be related to the involvement of left parietal areas in addition to temporal lobe damage. Subcortical damage to the auditory radiations and basal ganglia is often associated (Marshall et al., 1985; Maher et al., 1994).

Experimental studies and possible mechanisms

Anosognosia for aphasic disorders may result from a number of different mechanisms which are not mutually exclusive (Lebrun, 1987; Rubens and Garrett, 1991; Maher et al., 1994). Weinstein and colleagues (1964; Weinstein and Lyerly, 1976) argued that jargon does not only reflect a language disorder but also an adaptation to the deficit which depends on premorbid personality factors. They stated that all patients had euphoric mood changes and that jargon occurred mostly in response to questions about their illness. This cannot account for the selectivity of anosognosia for some deficits or some speech errors, or for its greater occurrence in fluent rather than nonfluent aphasia. It is, however, plausible that some patients behave as if they ignored their errors to keep up social interaction and communication (Lebrun, 1987). Although many of Weinstein and colleagues' (1964; Weinsten and Lyerly, 1976) patients were confused, jargonaphasia and explicit denial may exist in the presence of preserved intellectual and reasoning abilities (Alajouanine, 1956; Kinsbourne and Warrington, 1963). Alajouanine noted that jargon, like Wernicke's aphasia, is associated with a severe comprehension deficit. Anosognosia for speech errors might therefore be a consequence of verbal deafness, as a loss of lexical phonological representations or impaired access to semantic representations would prevent comparing the output with correct templates of words (Heilman, 1991). However, several reported patients were unaware of their errors in spite of relatively intact comprehension and preserved lexical–semantic representations (Kinsbourne and Warrington, 1963; Maher et al., 1994; Shuren et al., 1995), whereas one patient with auditory agnosia and a severe comprehension deficit could recognize and correct her phonemic paraphasias (Marshall et al. 1985). Patients with jargon speech are also able to reject foreign language words (Rubens and Garrett, 1991). In addition, although patients appear unaware of their jargon and judge most of their paraphasic responses as correct when questioned immediately after their production, they will detect most of the same errors when these are reproduced by the examiner (Alajouanine, 1956; Kinsbourne and Warrington, 1963; Maher et al., 1994; Shuren et al., 1995). Kinsbourne and Warrington (1963) observed that the patients nonetheless judged their verbal or written productions as satisfactory when played back in their own voices or presented in their own handwriting. This was also found in the patient of Maher et al. (1994), who rejected more errors in someone else's voice than in his own voice, but not in the patient of Shuren et al. (1995).

Since comprehension and error detection are preserved under some conditions, unawareness of speech errors might result from a failure of 'on-line' monitoring processes. Impaired auditory feedback in jargonaphasics is suggested by the fact that, unlike normal subjects and most other aphasics, their performance is little affected by having their speech played back to them after a short delay (e.g., 100–400 ms) during a concurrent language task (e.g., naming) (Boller et al., 1978; Shuren et al., 1995). However, conduction aphasics are less affected by delayed feedback than Wernicke's aphasia patients and yet much more proficient in self-monitoring and self-correcting (Boller et al., 1978). Lebrun (1987) and Rubens and Garrett (1991) suggested that unawareness might rather stem from the patient's inability to listen and speak at the same time because of a reduced attentional capacity. Consistently, Shuren et al. (1995) reported a jargonaphasic patient who was worse at detecting spoken nonwords during a simultaneous naming task but still able to detect anomalous rhythms during a tapping task. Impaired verbal working memory might contribute to a reduced processing capacity (Cambier et al., 1993). Finally, on the basis that both jargonaphasics and normal subjects have greater difficulty in monitoring semantic than phonemic errors, Rubens and Garrett (1991) also related unawareness of speech errors to mechanisms of 'perceptual reconstruction' during semantic decoding, somewhat akin to perceptual completion at the sensory level. However, studies on self-correction behavior in aphasic patients suggest that speech monitoring does not only operate on comprehension-based input processes. Despite worse comprehension abilities. Wernicke's aphasia patients do not differ from other aphasic groups in the amount or type of self-corrections they make (Farmer, 1977; Marshall and Tompkins, 1982; Schlenck, Huber and Willmes, 1987). In particular, they do not generate fewer 'repairs' of incorrect preceding utterances. On the other hand, their self-corrections are clearly less successful (Marshall and Tompkins, 1982) and they are less likely to use delays or pauses (Farmer, 1977; Schlenck et al., 1987). Patients with poorer comprehension also make fewer anticipatory searching corrections, or 'prepairs' (Schlenck et al., 1987). Monitoring processes can occur at pre-articulatory stages of speech production, involving complex interactions between cortical language areas and several thalamo-based ganglia loops that control the release of planned speech segments (Crosson, 1985). An impairment in these monitoring stages caused by additional damage to these loops might foster the release of copious unedited utterances. This might contribute to jargonaphasia and unawareness of speech errors, particularly so in the presence of impaired comprehension and reduced attentional abilities, resulting in the 'self-imposed receptive loss' in monitoring suggested by Kinsbourne and Warrington (1963). Further dysfunction in the basal ganglia–frontal systems might also hinder adapting behavior and beliefs, so as to result in anosognosia with explicit denial.

Anosognosia for amnesia and confabulations

Behavioral aspects

Korsakoff (1889) remarked that many of his patients were ignorant not only of having lost memory but also of producing false memories instead. Yet, neither un-awareness of impaired memory nor confabulation is an obligatory feature of amnesia; they cannot be regarded as merely resulting from the patient's 'inability to remember that he cannot remember' (Whitlock, 1981). The purest cases of amnesia, like patient HM of Milner, Corkin and Teuber (1968) who had bilateral temporal lobectomy, or patients with transient global amnesia who have a selective memory dysfunction, are aware of their defect and do not confabulate. 'My memory is a blank,' said an amnesic patient (Volpe and Hirst, 1983); 'I try to remember and I can't,' said another, though he was unable to recall any specific instance of his failure (Schacter, 1991).

By contrast, anosognosia is manifest in amnesic patients who claim that nothing is wrong with their memory. Other patients may admit some difficulties but remain little concerned and assert that their memory had always been poor (Talland, 1961). In addition, many (but not all) patients with anosognosia produce confabulations, i.e., they claim to remember fictitious episodes, sometimes in minute details. Confabulations are classified into a provoked/momentary type (plausible fabrications in response to questions, sometimes with real but distorted features) and a spontaneous/fantastic type (grandiose fabrications without relation to the patient's past or reality), but it is unclear whether this corresponds to a difference in degree or distinct disorders (Kapur and Coughlan, 1980; Dalla Barba, 1993). Anosognosia for amnesia seems to be a prerequisite for the occurrence of confabulations, rather than the converse (Fisher, 1989). Confabulations may abate even though patients remain unaware of their memory loss or little concerned (Talland, 1961; Alexander and Freedman, 1984), but most often resolve as the patient regains some awareness of the impairment (Mercer et al., 1977; Victor, Adams and Collins, 1989).

Deficient awareness can be more precisely assessed using a variety of questionnaires specifically developed for that purpose (Parkin, Bell and Leng, 1988; Schacter, 1991; Van der Linden and Bruyer, 1992). By comparing patients' subjective rating for their own memory or their self-prediction of performance on a given test with their actual performance or the rating and predictions made by a relative (e.g., a spouse), one can derive both qualitative and quantitative indices of self-awareness. Further indices of bias or general judgment capabilities can be derived by other comparisons, including patients' rating and prediction for their relative's performance, the relative's self-rating and prediction for his or her own performance, or the patients' prediction for different test conditions such as easy/difficult items or long/short delay (Schacter, 1991). Denial of memory impairment may coexist with intact awareness of other cognitive or physical disabilities (McGlynn and Schacter, 1989).

Although anosognosia and confabulations usually occur in the context of acute neurological impairment of memory and then tend to clear, the lack of insight may at times persist indefinitely (Schacter, 1991). On the other hand, there is always a full awareness of acute impairment in transient global amnesia. Thus, impaired awareness cannot be ascribed solely to abruptness of memory loss.

Anatomic and etiologic aspects

Anosognosia and confabulations are typically associated with amnesic disorders that result from damage to the diencephalon, e.g., alcoholic Korsakoff's syndrome and focal thalamic lesions, or damage to the basal forebrain and frontal lobes, e.g., following ruptured anterior communicating artery aneurysms or severe traumatic head injuries. In contrast, they are usually not seen when amnesia results from damage restricted to the temporal lobes, e.g., selective hippocampal ischemia or herpetic encephalitis (Parkin and Leng, 1993). Exceptions to the latter case may occur when damage extends to other limbic structures in the basal forebrain and the orbital and medial frontal lobes (Damasio et al., 1985b). In infarction of the medial temporal lobe, amnesia is not associated with anosognosia and confabulation except when there is concomitant involvement of thalamic nuclei supplied by paramedian or tuberothalamic branches from the posterior cerebral artery (Servan et al., 1994).

Most patients with Korsakoff's syndrome lack awareness of their problem and exhibit confabulations in the earliest stage (Talland, 1961). The disorder is caused by bilateral lesions in the mamillary bodies and midline nuclei of the thalamus, in particular the dorsomedial nucleus, yet the most critical site remains disputed (Brion, Mikol and Plas, 1985; Victor et al., 1989). Whereas lesions to the mamillary bodies or to the mamillothalamic tract might be sufficient to impair memory, varying involvement of the dorsomedial (Victor et al., 1989), laterodorsal (Brion et al., 1985), or intralaminar nuclei (Mennemeier et al., 1992) has been put forward to explain additional disorders such as confabulations, temporal order confusions, or susceptibility to interference. The dorsomedial nucleus receives connections from limbic structures, e.g., the amygdala, and projects to orbital and medial frontal lobe in a circuit which runs in parallel to the hippocampal–mamillothalamic memory pathways. Accordingly, patients with Korsakoff's syndrome have significant orbitofrontal atrophy, as shown by MRI, compared to nonamnesic alcoholics (Jernigan et al., 1991), and superimposed frontal cognitive dysfunction compared to other amnesics (Parkin and Leng, 1993). Decreased blood flow in both the medial thalamus and orbitomedial frontal regions was shown by single photon emission computerized tomography (SPECT) in one patient during the acute stage of amnesia with severe anosognosia and confabulation, whereas only the medial thalamus was implicated in a later stage when amnesia persisted but insight had improved and confabulation stopped (Benson, 1996).

Similarly, focal lesions (e.g., stroke) in either the paramedian or anterior part of the thalamus can disrupt mamillothalamic tract and cause amnesia, but lack of insight and confabulations both appear more common in the former case (Gentilini, de Renzi and Crisi, 1987; Stuss et al., 1988). Further, one patient suffered a profound amnesia with severe anosognosia and confabulations after a unilateral right inferior capsular genu, which presumably disconnected the orbitofrontal cortex from the dorsomedial nucleus of the thalamus and the amygdala, as it involved the anterior and inferior thalamic peduncles (Schnider et al., 1996a). These findings also point to the role of dorsomedial nucleus and orbitomedial frontal systems in awareness and monitoring of memory functions.

In series of anterior communicating artery aneurysm patients, denial of amnesia and confabulations are mentioned in 30% to 50% of the cases (Logue et al., 1968; Alexander and Freedman, 1984; Vilkki, 1985; Van der Linden and Bruyer, 1992). Whereas damage to the basal forebrain is sufficient to cause amnesia, this does not preclude intact awareness in some patients (Volpe and Hirst, 1983), and anosognosia probably ensues from additional involvement of adjacent frontal areas. Patients with combined lesions of the basal forebrain and the orbital cortex produce more intrusion errors in memory tests than those with lesions restricted to the basal forebrain (Irle et al., 1992). Virtually all patients with confabulations have concomitant infarction in the territory of the anterior cerebral artery on either side, namely the orbital and medial frontal lobe and the anterior cingulate, as well as in the ventral caudate and the genu of the corpus callosum (Alexander and Freedman, 1984; Damasio et al., 1985a; Vilkki, 1985; Deluca and Diamond, 1995). Other anterior communicating artery aneurysm patients who have damage limited to frontal structures and no amnesia do not confabulate however (Van der Linden and Bruyer, 1992; Deluca and Diamond, 1995). In a study of nine amnesic anterior communicating artery aneurysm patients (Fischer et al., 1995), all of five patients with spontaneous/grandiose confabulations had striatal damage on one side, and four of them also had medial frontal damage on both sides; the other four, with only provoked/momentary confabulations, had lesions restricted to the basal forebrain, except for one who had bilateral orbital and polar frontal damage. Involvement of the frontal lobes is also common in patients with amnesia of mixed etiologies who lack awareness of their impairment (Jahro, 1973; Luria, 1980; McGlynn and Schacter, 1989) or demonstrate confabulations (Shapiro et al., 1981; Schnider, von Däniken and Gutbrod, 1996b), in particular, patients with head trauma who often have orbital frontal damage. In many reported cases of confabulations, lesions appear predominantly bilateral or right sided (Shapiro et al., 1981; Alexander and Freedman, 1984; DeLuca and Cicerone, 1991), whereas unilateral left lesions are much less common (Kapur and Coughlan, 1980). Also, confabulations and false recognitions have been observed in the absence of a major amnesic disorder in a few patients with bilateral but right-predominant medial frontal lesions (Delbecq-Derouesné, Beauvois and Shallice, 1990; De Villiers et al., 1996; Papagno and Baddeley, 1997), and false recognitions without confabulation were observed in a patient with right dorsolateral frontal infarct (Schacter et al., 1996). This is consistent with several recent positron emission tomography (PET) studies in normal subjects which revealed activation in various ventral and dorsolateral areas of the right prefrontal cortex (e.g., Brodmann's areas 10/46) during the retrieval of episodic memories (Shallice et al., 1994). It has been suggested that these areas might be critical in the evaluation and verification processes that determine whether the retrieved information is accepted as memories.

Experimental studies and possible mechanisms

Unawareness of memory loss has long been related to frontal lobe dysfunction and imputed to deficient critical attitude and affective indifference (Sachs, 1927; Jahro, 1973; Luria, 1980). More recent theories put forward a failure of 'metacognitive' processes which entail the knowledge and supervision of one's own cognitive abilities, presumably related to other frontal executive functions such as integration, organizational strategies, and response monitoring (Stuss and Benson, 1986; Schacter, 1991). Indeed, patients with Korsakoff's and anterior communicating artery aneurysms often show frontal executive disorders (Parkin and Leng, 1993). Hippocampal amnesics are accurate in their self-rating judgments and prediction of memory performance, but not Korsakoff's syndrome and anterior communicating artery aneurysm amnesics, or nonamnesic patients with focal frontal lesions

(Parkin et al., 1988; Van der Linden and Bruyer, 1992). Likewise, the 'feeling-of-knowing' (i.e., the prediction of being able subsequently to recognize given information when spontaneous recall fails) is inaccurate in Korsakoff's syndrome patients and those with frontal lesions, but not in hippocampal amnesics (Shimamura and Squire, 1986; Janowsky, Shimamura and Squire, 1989). This suggests that amnesics who lack insight cannot use searching cues and make appropriate inferences to monitor accessible information in memory. Schacter (1991) speculated that this could result from a disruption within the frontal executive system or its disconnection from the (hippocampal) memory system. Alternatively, frontal dysfunction might result in a failure to initiate and engage searching procedures in memory (Damasio et al., 1985a). This might prevent patients from realizing their memory failure, especially in the presence of concomitant cognitive and belief inflexibility, to which disturbed frontal systems also contribute.

Another possibility is that patients might lack awareness of memory loss and exhibit inappropriate feeling-of-knowing because they can still access *some* stored information. Unlike in the case of patients who have damage to hippocampal and temporal lobe structures (Damasio et al., 1985a; Moscovitch, 1992), the preservation of associative memory links or binding codes coupled with abnormal retrieval processes might enable patients with anterior communicating artery aneurysms or diencephalic amnesia to evoke information yielding a subjectively compelling yet incorrect experience that they can remember. Whitlock (1981) and Schacter (1991) also suggested that anosognosic patients might base their responses on knowledge and memories dating from before their illness, perhaps owing to impaired temporal tagging secondary to frontal dysfunction. However, even new or irrelevant associations could be incorrectly attributed to memory retrieval, as automaticity in evoking processes might be sufficient to generate subjective familiarity signals (Jacoby, Kelley and Dywan, 1989). Episodic memory traces might become less distinct from other representations after damage to orbitofrontal and dorsomedial thalamic structures which probably provide temporal contextual and personal relevance tagging (Schnider et al., 1996a). Postretrieval verification processes would then be required to dismiss incorrectly retrieved information.

Confabulations might therefore ensue from additional failure in the verification processes (Delbecq-Derouesné et al., 1990; Moscovitch, 1992). Although these processes have still to be specified, they are presumably subserved by distinct right-sided prefrontal areas (Shallice et al., 1994; Schacter et al., 1996). Overall, confabulations are clearly not related to the severity of amnesia (Talland, 1961; Logue et al., 1968; Victor et al., 1989; De Villiers et al., 1996; Papagno and Baddeley, 1997) and do not necessarily correlate with the severity of frontal lobe dysfunction (Dalla Barba, 1993; Schnider et al., 1996b), even though decreased response latencies, lack of inhibition of inappropriate responses, inability to use external cues, and perseverations have been noted (Mercer et al., 1977; Kapur and Coughlan, 1980; Shapiro et al., 1981). A study in one Korsakoff's syndrome patient showed confabulatory responses to brief visual presentation of incomplete pictures (Wyke and Warrington, 1960). However, confabulations do not result from suggestibility or a tendency to fill gaps because patients tend to answer 'I don't know,' as do normal subjects, to questions for which the response is unknown (Mercer et al., 1977; Dalla Barba, 1993; Schnider et al., 1996b). On the other hand, confabulations have been related to impaired recognition of the temporal context or source of registered information (Talland, 1961; Whitlock, 1981; Schnider et al., 1996b). Such impairment could also indicate an inability to discriminate between different sources of familiarity during recognition and retrieval processes. Confabulations and false recognitions might thus reflect abnormal acceptance of subjective familiarity signals, in particular as contextual recall fails and memory attributions must rely on familiarity (Delbecq-Derouesné et al., 1990). Medial and/or dorsolateral prefrontal areas might be critically involved in monitoring the source of familiarity and internally generated information for memory attributions (Shallice et al., 1994; Johnson, 1997). Hence, confabulations could partly arise from imagination and thought associations uncritically mistaken for memories.

Therapeutic aspects

Anosognosia has obvious but still little-investigated implications in the prognosis and rehabilitation of patients with cerebral lesions. A patient who lacks awareness and denies a defect is not likely to accept therapy or benefit from it. AHP is clearly associated with poorer motor recovery and less benefit from rehabilitation, independently of other factors such as the presence of unilateral spatial neglect (Hier et al., 1983a, 1983b; Gialanella and Mattioli, 1992). Rehabilitation of speech disorders (Farmer, 1977; Lebrun, 1987) or visual defects (Krantz, 1992) is also greatly influenced by impaired awareness. Although few investigators have specifically addressed therapeutic issues and proposed structured approaches for rehabilitation in these patients (Prigatano, 1986; Calvanio et al., 1993), managing problems of unawareness is part of most neurological therapy programs, both in the sensorimotor and cognitive domains (Diller, 1987; Robertson, 1994; Brockmann-Rubio, 1998), and only a brief overview is provided here. Moreover, therapeutic approaches to unawareness in neuropsychology have usually been more concerned with the dysexecutive and behavioral sequels after frontal or diffuse traumatic head injury than with modality-specific deficits due to focal lesions.

Given that anosognosia can encompass a variety of underlying mechanisms and clinical manifestations, therapeutic approaches must often be tailored to the particular conditions and patients. Awareness of deficits often increases in the postacute stage of brain damage, and specific remedial procedures usually take place in chronic rehabilitation programs. However, it is important to initiate appropriate therapeutic management as soon as possible in order to enhance recovery and benefits from other physical treatments. There are no standardized guidelines (AHCPR Manual/Gresham et al., 1995), but a few general principles are useful to consider.

A first step is to characterize the dimensions of anosognosia, e.g., whether it is domain specific or more generalized; whether it is relatively encapsulated or accompanied by other cognitive, behavioral or emotional disturbances; whether it affects one or more distinct levels, including intellectual knowledge and appraisal, subjective experience and monitoring, or integration and adaptation responses (Allen and Ruff, 1990; Barco et al., 1991; Giacino and Cicerone, 1998). Clinical observation and neuropsychological examination must evaluate not only overt behavior and reports of the patient, but also the patient's ability to use compensatory strategies, anticipation of failure, and response to feedback signals. This can be complemented by semistructured interviews (e.g., Fleming, Strong and Ashton, 1996; Giacino and Cicerone, 1998) and rating questionnaires (e.g., Allen and Ruff, 1990; Sherer et al., 1998) given to the patient, relatives, or caregivers. General cognitive abilities and possible contributing factors such as mood disorders and sedative drug effects must be carefully evaluated.

A second step is to determine the functional implications of anosognosia for the patient's activities and the therapeutic interventions most appropriate to overcome its effects. Management strategies can be restorative or compensatory (Diller, 1987; Calvanio et al., 1993). Restorative treatments are aimed at directly training the impairment and enhancing awareness, including educational and experiential procedures. Experiential therapies typically involve retraining or substituting a function through repetitive exercises, with appropriate supervision and feedback about performance, which allow patients to experience changes in their abilities and provide a basis for increasing insight and developing an adapted behavior. The most useful techniques are probably those integrating multiple modalities and in which patients are given a sense of correct acts and error signals that they otherwise lack, so that they can eventually form new internal cues to guide and monitor self-initiated behavior. Psychotherapeutic intervention directed toward affective symptoms and appreciation of self may be also necessary. Educational therapy provides patients with information to modify their knowledge, interpretation, and beliefs about deficits using a systematic, structured approach; this may involve repetitive but empathic confrontation with failures as well as residual capabilities, review of medical documents, comparison of ratings by the patient or others, use of video, or other formal teaching methods. Counselling of relatives and caregivers is also important. On the other hand, compensatory treatments aim at maximizing functioning in daily activities while bypassing the lack of awareness, and are typically oriented to a specific task or behavior, usually in patients with severe anosognosia and indifference about their deficits. This may include training functional routines and exploiting residual abilities in order to increase the use of compensation strategies, modifying the linkage between a behavior and its outcome, prosthetic devices (motor or cognitive), and modification in the environment (Calvanio et al., 1993).

Motor rehabilitation in patients with AHP emphasizes tasks using both sides of the body, e.g., bimanual action, and sensorimotor activation of the affected limbs to increase awareness and integration of their function. Passive guided movements or voluntary supervised movements are useful to provide proprioceptive inputs and innervatory patterns, and may help to overcome hemispatial neglect. Sensory stimulation (e.g., applying lotions, bathing, massage, tactile vibration, or even acupuncture) is often used to redirect attention to the affected limb and increase arousal (Robertson, 1994; Brockmann-Rubio, 1998). Caloric vestibular stimulation can induce a transient improvement in sensorimotor function, with remission of spatial neglect, anosognosia, and even delusional somatoparaphrenia (e.g., Cappa et al., 1987; Vallar et al., 1990). Optokinetic stimulation, limb or neck vibration, and visual prisms can all also produce transient improvements of neglect behavior (from a few minutes to hours). However, there is no evidence that even repeated use of these techniques yields long-lasting benefits. Training of arousal and sustained attention using a self-alerting procedure may also produce lasting improvements in visuomotor neglect (Robertson, 1994). Drugs such as dopamine agonists have been used in an attempt to enhance motor preparation and exploration, with variable success.

Rehabilitation of AHA, like AHP, is closely linked to that of hemispatial neglect (Diller, 1987; Robertson, 1994). Patients with hemianopia and visual neglect may benefit from visual training procedures which include a variety of tasks, such as visual scanning, searching, reading, anchoring techniques, or complex visual perceptual organization. Occupations using multiple modalities and allowing the integration of vision with movement and other senses appear particularly useful (Gordon et al., 1985).

Awareness-enhancing rehabilitation in apahasia is particularly difficult because awareness of the deficit is not easy to determine (Brockmann-Rubio, 1998). In Wernicke's aphasia patients, specific drills can be given such as detecting syntactic and semantic incongruities in the patient's own speech or in the therapist's speech. Using other modalities (e.g., gestures, drawing, or even writing) may help to direct and organize the discourse. Improving semantic comprehension, as well as working memory, attention, and concentration is also useful to increase integration and monitoring competences in linguistic functions.

Rehabilitation attempts for unawareness of amnesia have probably been more systematic than in other domains (Schacter, 1991; Wilson, 1992). A variety of cognitive strategies and external aids (notebooks, tape-recorders, alarm beepers, computers) can be used to supplement and supervise memory failures. Better subjective appraisal can be obtained by repetitive confrontation of self-rating of performance by the patient with ratings made by others, as well as by specific feedback training to predict recall performance in comparison to actual task performance, and by learning to anticipate situations likely to result in memory failures. However, enhanced knowledge and improved realistic appraisal may not generalize flexibly in other real-life situations (Schacter, 1991). Procedural or implicit learning can be successfully exploited to teach new skills and strategies. Finally, drug therapy (donezepil, physostigmine, norepinephrine, or clonidine) has been reported to facilitate both memory function and insight in a few anecdotal cases, but side-effects may occur.

Conclusion

Anosognosia is one of the most intriguing consequences of focal brain lesions because it affects the unity of one individual in such a way that 'the I or me part, the sentient part has no way of detecting and recognizing the deficit' (Fisher, 1989). Thus, a hemiplegic patient may claim that he can move his four limbs and walk, and a blind patient may contend that he can see; an aphasic may believe that his speech is correct, and an amnesic may think that his memory is normal. A number of questions about the anatomical and cognitive bases of these conditions are unresolved. Also, a number of questions about definitions and methods of assessment should be clarified (Galin, 1992). Over the past century, the terms anosognosia, denial, and unawareness of deficit have been used and have become interchangeable (not to mention insight, imperception, and unconcern) (McGlynn and Schacter, 1989). Yet, the different words might well pinpoint the different facets of the complex interplay of brain processes that allow normal and impaired awareness. Anosognosia might be something of both unawareness and denial rather than one or other of them. The diversity and variability of anosognosic phenomenon probably reflect the implication of multiple levels or steps in the organization of cerebral functions which clearly have to be teased out.

As a first rule, anosognosia entails a disorder in the subjective experience that a patient has of one specific function (e.g., moving, seeing, remembering) which makes him or her unaware that the function is impaired; the modular sequential (McGlynn and Schacter, 1989) or parallel distributed (Levine, 1990) organization of brain functions might account for it. As a second rule, anosognosia entails a disorder in monitoring operations that allow interpretation, belief, and doubt about subjective experiences (Bisiach and Geminiani, 1991; Halligan and Marshall,

1996); a higher level of processing subserved by frontal–striatal and limbic systems might be implicated in this adaptive behavior (Bear, 1982; Cummings, 1993). A better understanding of the neurological and cognitive factors that bring about unawareness and denial of deficits is not only of great theoretical interest for the neurology of behavior and consciousness, but is also clearly warranted to improve therapeutic interventions in patients with brain lesions.

Acknowledgment

This work was supported by a grant from the Swiss National Science Foundation (grant no. 81-GE-50080).

REFERENCES

Adair, J.C., Gilmore, R.L., Fennell, E.B., Gold, M. and Heilman, K.M. (1995a). Anosognosia during intracarotid barbiturate anesthesia: unawareness or amnesia for weakness. *Neurology* 45: 241–3.

Adair, J.C., Na, D.L., Schwartz, R.L. et al. (1995b). Anosognosia for hemiplegia: test of the personal neglect hypothesis. *Neurology* 45: 2195–9.

Adair, J.C., Schwartz, R.L., Na, D.L. et al. (1997). Anosognosia: examining the disconnection hypothesis. *J Neurol Neurosurg Psychiatry* 63: 798–800.

AHCPR Manual/Gresham, G.E. et al. (1995). Post-stroke rehabilitation, Vol. 16. Rockville, MA: Agency for Health Care Policy and Research.

Alajouanine, T. (1956). Verbal realization in aphasia. *Brain* 79: 1–28.

Alajouanine, T. and Lhermitte, F. (1957). Des anosognosies électives. *Encéphale* 46: 505–19.

Aldrich, M.S., Alessi, A.G., Beck, R.W. and Gilman, S. (1987). Cortical blindness: etiology, diagnosis, and prognosis. *Ann Neurol* 21: 149–58.

Alexander, M.P. and Freedman, M. (1984). Amnesia after anterior communicating artery aneurysm rupture. *Neurology* 34: 752–7.

Allen, C. and Ruff, R.M. (1990). Self-rating versus neuropsychological performance of moderate versus severe head-injured patients. *Brain Inj* 4: 7–17.

Angelergues, R., de Ajuriaguerra, J. and Hécaen, H. (1960). La négation de la cécité au cours des lésions cérébrales. *J Psychol Normale Pathol* 57: 381–404.

Anton, G. (1898). Ueber Herderkrankungen des Gehirns, welche vom Patienten selbst nicht wahrgenommen werden. *Wien Klin Wochenschr* 11: 227–9.

Assal, G. (1983). Non, je ne suis pas paralysée, c'est la main de mon mari. *Schweizer Archiv Neurol Neurochir Psychiatrie* 133: 151–7.

Babinski, J. (1914). Contribution a l'étude des troubles mentaux dans l'hémiplégie organique (anosognosie). *Rev Neurol* 27: 845–8.

Babinski, J. (1918). Anosognosie. *Rev Neurol* 31: 365–7.

Bakchine, S., Crassard, I. and Seilhan, D. (1997). Anosognosia for hemiplegia after a brainstem haematoma: a pathological case. *J Neurol Neurosurg Psychiatry* 63: 686–7.

Barco, P.P., Crosson, B., Bolesta, M.M., Werts, D. and Stout, R. (1991). Training awareness and compensation in post-acute head injury rehabilitation. In *Cognitive Rehabilitation for Persons with Traumatic Brain Injury: a Functional Approach*, ed. J.S. Kreutzer and P.H. Wehman. Baltimore: Paul Brookes.

Barkman, A. (1925), De l'anosognosie dans l'hémiplégie cérébrale: contribution clinique à l'étude de ce symptome. *Acta Med Scand* 62: 235–54.

Barré, J.A., Morin, L. and Kaiser, J. (1923). Etude clinique d'un nouveau cas d'anosognosie de Babinski. *Rev Neurol* 39: 500–3.

Battersby, W.S., Bender, M.B., Pollack, M. and Kahn, R.L. (1956). Unilateral spatial agnosia ('inattention') in patients with cerebral lesions. *Brain* 79: 68–93.

Bear, D.M. (1982). Hemisphere specialization and the neurology of emotion. *Arch Neurol* 40: 195–202.

Bender, M.B. (1984). Dissociated perception of a visual defect. *J Ment Nerv Dis* 172: 364–8.

Benson, D.F. (1996). Neural basis of confabulation. *Neurology* 46: 1239–43.

Bergman, P.S. (1956). Cerebral blindness. *Arch Neurol Psychiatry* 78: 568–84.

Berlucchi, G. and Agliotti, S. (1997). The body in the brain: neural bases of corporeal awareness. *Trends Neurosci* 20: 560–4.

Berns, G.S., Cohen, J.D. and Mintun, M.A. (1997). Brain regions responsive to novelty in the absence of awareness. *Science* 276: 1272–5.

Berti, A., Ladavas, E. and Della, C.M. (1996). Anosognosia for hemiplegia, neglect dyslexia, and drawing neglect: clinical findings and theoretical considerations. *J Int Neuropsychol Soc* 2: 426–40.

Bhatia, K.P. and Marsden, C.D. (1994). The behavioral and motor consequences of focal lesions of the basal ganglia in man. *Brain* 117: 859–76.

Bisiach, E. and Geminiani, G. (1991). Anosognosia related to hemiplegia and hemianopia. In *Awareness of Deficit after Brain Injury: Clinical and Theoretical Issues*, ed. G.P. Prigatano and D.L. Schacter, pp. 17–39. New York: Oxford University Press.

Bisiach, E., Perani, D., Vallar, G. and Berti, A. (1986a). Unilateral neglect: personal and extra-personal. *Neuropsychologia* 24: 759–67.

Bisiach, E., Vallar, G., Perani, D., Papagno, C. and Berti, A. (1986b). Unawareness of disease following lesions of the right hemisphere: anosognosia for hemiplegia and anosognosia for hemianopia. *Neuropsychologia* 24: 471–82.

Bogousslavsky, J., Miklossy, J., Regli, F. et al. (1988). Subcortical neglect: neuropsychological, SPECT, and neuropathological correlations with anterior choroidal artery territory infarction. *Ann Neurol* 23: 448–52.

Bogousslavsky, J., Regli, F. and Assal, G. (1986). The syndrome of unilateral tuberothalamic artery territory infarction. *Stroke* 17: 434–41.

Boller, F., Vrtrunski, P.B., Kim, Y. and Mack, J.L. (1978). Delayed auditory feedback and aphasia. *Cortex* 14: 212–26.

Breier, J.I., Adair, J.C., Gold, M. et al. (1995). Dissociation of anosognosia for hemiplegia and aphasia during left-hemisphere anesthesia. *Neurology* 45: 65–7.

Brion, S., Mikol, J. and Plas, J. (1985). Neuropathologie des syndromes amnésiques chez l'homme. *Rev Neurol* 141: 627–43.

Brockmann-Rubio, K. (1998). Treatment of neurobehavioral deficits: a function-based approach. In *Stroke Rehabilitation: a Function-based Approach*, ed. G. Gillen and A. Burkhard, pp. 334–52. St Louis: Mosby.

Calvanio, R., Levine, D. and Petrone, P. (1993). Elements of cognitive rehabilitation after right hemisphere stroke. *Neurol Clin* 11: 25–57.

Cambier, J., Masson, C. and Robine, B. (1993). Préservation dissociée de l'expression écrite dans une aphasie à stéréotypes. *Rev Neurol* 149: 455–61.

Cappa, S., Sterzi, R., Vallar, G. and Bisiach, E. (1987). Remission of hemineglect and anosognosia during vestibular stimulation. *Neuropsychologia* 25: 775–82.

Carpenter, K., Berti, A., Oxbury, S. et al. (1995). Awareness of and memory for arm weakness during intracarotid sodium amytal testing. *Brain* 118: 243–51.

Castaigne, P., Cambier, J., Escourolle, R., Masson, M. and Lechevalier, B. (1967). Anosognosie d'une cécité par atrophie optique au cours d'un syndrome de Korsakoff consécutif à une nécrose bilatérale de l'hippocampe. *Rev Neurol (Paris)* 117: 576–85.

Celesia, G.G., Archer, C.R. and Kuroiwa, Y. (1980). Visual function of the extrageniculo-calcarine system in man. *Arch Neurol* 37: 704–6.

Celesia, G.G., Brigell, M.G. and Vaphiades, M.S. (1997). Hemianopic anosognosia. *Neurology* 49: 88–97.

Cohn, R. (1971). Phantom vision. *Arch Neurol* 25: 468–71.

Cole, M., Saexinger, H.G. and Hard, A. (1968). Anosognosia: studies using regional intravenous anesthesia. *Neuropsychologia* 6: 365–71.

Critchley, M. (1949). The problem of awareness or non-awareness of hemianopic field defects. *Trans Ophthalmol Soc UK* 69: 95–109.

Critchley, M. (1953). *The Parietal Lobes.* New York: Hafner.

Critchley, M. (1964). The neurology of psychotic speech. *Br J Psychiatry* 110: 353–64.

Crosson, B. (1985). Subcortical functions in language: a working model. *Brain Lang* 25: 257–92.

Cummings, J.L. (1993). Frontal–subcortical circuits and human behavior. *Arch Neurol* 50: 873–80.

Cusumano, J.V., Fletcher, J.W. and Platel, B.K. (1981). Scintigraphic appearance of Anton's syndrome. *J Am Med Assoc* 245: 1248–9.

Cutting, J. (1978). Study of anosognosia. *J Neurol Neurosurg Psychiatry* 41: 548–55.

Dalla Barba, G. (1993). Different patterns of confabulation. *Cortex* 29: 567–81.

Damasio, A., Graff-Radford, N.R., Eslinger, P.J., Damasio, H. and Kassel, N. (1985a). Amnesia following basal forebrain lesions. *Arch Neurol* 42: 263–71.

Damasio, A.R., Eslinger, P.J., Damasio, H., Van Hoesen, G.W. and Cornell, S. (1985b). Multimodal amnesic syndrome following bilateral temporal and basal forebrain damage. *Arch Neurol* 42: 252–9.

Déjerine, J. and Vialet, N. (1893). Sur un cas de cécité corticale. *Comptes Rendus Soc Biol* 11: 983–97.

de la Sayette, V., Petit Taboue, M.C., Bouvier, F. et al. (1995). Infarctus dans le territoire de l'artère choroïdienne antérieure droite et syndrome de l'hémisphère mineur: étude clinique et métabolique par tomographie à émission de positons. (Infarction in the territory of the right choroidal artery and minor hemisphere syndrome: case report and brain glucose utilisation study.) *Rev Neurol* 151: 24–35.

Delbecq-Derouesné, J., Beauvois, M.F. and Shallice, T. (1990). Preserved recall versus impaired recognition. *Brain* 113: 1045–74.

Della Sala, S. and Spinnler, H. (1988). Anton's (–Redlich–Babinski's) syndrome associated with Dide–Botacazo's syndrome: a case report of denial or cortical blindness and amnesia. *Schweizer Arch Neurol Neurochir Psychiatrie* 139: 5–15.

DeLuca, J. and Cicerone, K.D. (1991). Confabulation following aneurysms of the anterior communicating artery. *Cortex* 29: 639–47.

DeLuca, J. and Diamond, B.J. (1995). Aneurysm of the anterior communicating artery: a review of neuroanatomical and neuropsychologic sequelae. *J Clin Exp Neuropsychol* 17: 20–8.

Denny-Brown, D., Meyer, J.S. and Horenstein, S. (1952). The significance of perceptual rivalry resulting from parietal lesion. *Brain* 75: 433–71.

De Villiers, C., Zent, R., Eastman, R.W. and Swingler, D. (1996). A flight of fantasy: false memories in frontal lobe disease. *J Neurol Neurosurg Psychiatry* 61: 652–7.

Diller, L. (1987). Neuropsychological rehabilitation. In *Neuropsychological rehabilitation*, ed. M.J. Meier, A.L. Benton and L. Diller, pp. 3–17. New York: Guilford Press.

Dywan, C.A., McGlone, J. and Fox, A. (1995). Do intracarotid barbiturate injections offer a way to investigate hemispheric models of anosognosia? *J Clin Exp Neuropsychol* 17: 431–8.

Farah, M.J. (1989). The neural basis of mental imagery. *Trends Neurosci* 12: 395–9.

Farmer, A. (1977). Self-correctional strategies in the conversational speech of aphasic and non-aphasic brain damaged subjects. *Cortex* 13: 327–34.

Feinberg, T.E. (1997). Anosognosia and confabulation. In *Behavioral Neurology and Neuropsychology*, ed. T.E. Feinberg and M.J. Farah, pp. 369–90. New York: McGraw-Hill.

Feinberg, T.E., Haber, L.D. and Leeds, N.E. (1990). Verbal asomatognosia. *Neurology* 40: 1391–4.

Feinberg, T.E., Roane, D.M., Kwan, P.C., Schindler, R.J. and Haber, L.D. (1994). Anosognosia and visuoverbal confabulation. *Arch Neurol* 51: 468–73.

Fischer, R.S., Alexander, M.P., D'Esposito, M. and Otto, R. (1995). Neuropsychological and neuroanatomical correlates of confabulation. *J Clin Exp Neuropsychol* 17: 20–8.

Fisher, C.M. (1989). Neurologic fragments. II. Remarks on anosognosia, confabulation, memory, and other topics; and an appendix on self-obseration. *Neurology* 39: 127–32.

Fleming, J.M., Strong, J. and Ashton, R. (1996). Self-awareness of deficits in adults with traumatic brain injury: how best to measure? *Brain Inj* 10: 1–15.

Frederiks, J.A.M. (1985). Disorders of the body schema. In *Handbook of Clinical Neurology*, Vol. 45, ed. J.A.M. Frederiks, pp. 373–404. Amsterdam: Elsevier.

Frith, C. (1996). The role of the prefrontal cortex in self-consciousness: the case of auditory hallucinations. *Philosoph Trans R Soc Lond* B 351: 1505–12.

Gainotti, G. (1972). Emotional behavior and hemispheric side of the lesion. *Cortex* 8: 41–55.

Galin, D. (1992). Theoretical reflections on awareness, monitoring, and self in relation to anosognosia. *Consciousness & Cognition* 1: 152–62.

Garcin, R., Varay, A. and Dimo, H. (1938). Document pour servir à l'étude des troubles du schéma corporel. *Rev Neurol* 69: 498–510.

Gassel, M.M. and Williams, D. (1963). Visual function in patients with homonymous hemianopia. Part III: The completion phenomenon; insight and attitude to the defect; and visual functional efficiency. *Brain* 86: 229–60.

Gazzaniga, M.S. (1992). Brain modules and belief formation. In *Self and Consciousness: Multiple Perspectives* ed. F.S. Kessel, P.M. Cole and D.L. Johnson, pp. 88–102. Hillsdale, NJ: Lawrence Erlbaum Associates.

Gentilini, M., de Renzi, E. and Crisi, G. (1987). Bilateral paramedian thalamic artery infarcts: report of eight cases. *J Neurol Neurosurg Psychiatry* 50: 900–9.

Gerstmann, J. (1942). Problems of imperception of disease and of impaired body territories with organic lesions: relation to body scheme and its disorders. *Arch Neurol Psychiatry* 48: 890–913.

Geschwind, N. (1965). Disconnexion syndromes in animals and man. Parts I and II. *Brain* 88: 237–94; 634–54.

Giacino, J.T. and Cicerone, K.D. (1998). Varieties of deficit unawareness after brain injury. *J Head Trauma Rehabil* 13: 1–15.

Gialanella, B. and Mattioli, F. (1992). Anosognosia and extrapersonal neglect as predictors of functional recovery following right hemisphere stroke. *Neuropsychol Rehabil* 2: 169–78.

Gilliatt, R.W. and Pratt, R.T.C. (1952). Disorders of perception and performance in a case of right-sided cerebral thrombosis. *J Neurol Neurosurg Psychiatry* 15: 264–71.

Gold, M., Adair, J.C., Jacobs, D.H. and Heilman, K.M. (1994). Anosognosia for hemiplegia: an electrophysiologic investigation of the feed-forward hypothesis. *Neurology* 44: 1804–8.

Goldenberg, G., Mullbacher, W. and Nowak, A. (1995). Imagery without perception – a case study of anosognosia for cortical blindness. *Neuropsychologia* 33: 1373–82.

Goldstein, K. (1939). *The Organism: a Holistic Approach to Biology Derived from Pathological Data in Man.* New York: American Book Co.

Gordon, W., Hibbard, M., Egelko, S. et al. (1985). Perceptual remediation in patients with right brain damage: a comprehensive program. *Arch Phys Med Rehabil* 66(6): 353–9.

Gross, H. and Kaltenbäck, E. (1955). Die Anosognosie. *Wien Zeitschr Nervenheilkunde* 11: 374–418.

Guthrie, T.C. and Grossman, E.M. (1952). A study of the syndromes of denial. *Arch Neurol Psychiatry* 68: 362–71.

Halligan, P.W., and Marshall, J.C. (1996). The wise prophet makes sure of the event first: hallucinations, amnesia, and delusions. In *Method in Madness: Case Studies in Cognitive Neuropsychiatry*, ed. P.W. Halligan and J.C. Marshall, pp. 237–66. Hove, UK: Psychology Press.

Halligan, P.W., Marshall, J.C. and Wade, D.T. (1993). Three arms: a case study of supernumerary phantom limb after right hemisphere stroke. *J Neurol Neurosurg Psychiatry* 56: 159–66.

Head, H. and Holmes, G. (1911). Sensory disturbance from cerebral lesions. *Brain* 34: 102–254.

Healton, E.B., Navarro, C., Bressman, S. and Brust, J.C. (1982). Subcortical neglect. *Neurology* 32: 776–8.

Heilman, K.M. (1991). Anosognosia: possible neuropsychological mechanisms. In *Awareness of Deficit after Brain Injury: Clinical and Theoretical Issues*, ed. G.P. Prigatano and D.L. Schacter, pp. 53–62. New York: Oxford University Press.

Heilman, K.M., Schwartz, H.D. and Watson, R.T. (1978). Hypoarousal in patients with the neglect syndrome and emotional indifference. *Neurology* 28: 229–32.

Hier, D.B., Mondlock, J. and Caplan, L.R. (1983a). I. Behavioral abnormalities after right hemisphere stroke. *Neurology* 33: 337–44.

Hier, D.B., Mondlock, J. and Caplan, L.R. (1983b). II. Recovery of behavioral abnormalities after right hemisphere stroke. *Neurology* 33: 345–50.

Hildebrandt, H. and Zieger, A. (1995). Unconscious activation of motor responses in a hemiplegic patient with anosognosia and neglect. *Eur Arch Psychiatry Clin Neurosci* 246: 53–9.

House, A. and Hodges, J. (1988). Persistent denial of handicap after infarction of the right basal ganglia: a case study. *J Neurol Neurosurg Psychiatry* 51: 112–15.

Irle, E., Wowra, B., Kunert, H.J., Hampl, J. and Kunze, S. (1992). Memory disturbance following anterior communicating artery rupture. *Ann Neurol* 31: 473–80.

Jacoby, L.L., Kelley, C.M. and Dywan, J. (1989). Memory attributions. In *Varieties of Memory and Consciousness: Essays in Honour of Endel Tulving*, ed. H.L.I. Roediger and F.I.M. Craik, pp. 391–442. NJ: Lawrence Erlbaum Associates.

Jahro, L. (1973). Korsakoff-like amnesic syndrome in penetrating brain injury. *Acts Neurol Scand* 49: 44–67.

Janowsky, J.S., Shimamura, A.P. and Squire, L.R. (1989). Memory and metamemory: comparisons between patients with frontal lobe lesions and amnesic patients. *Psychobiology* 17: 3–11.

Jeannerod, M. (1994). The representing brain: neural correlates of motor intention and imagery. *Behav Brain Sci* 17: 187–245.

Jernigan, T.L., Schafer, K., Butters, N. and Cermak, L.S. (1991). Magnetic resonance imaging of alcoholic Korsakoff patients. *Neuropsychopharmacology* 4: 175–86.

Johnson, M.K. (1997). Source monitoring and memory distorsion. *Philosoph Trans R Soc Lond* B 352: 1733–45.

Kalaska, J.F., Scott, S.H., Cisek, P. and Sergio, L.E. (1997). Cortical control of reaching movements. *Curr Opin Neurobiol* 7: 849–59.

Kapur, N. and Coughlan, A.K. (1980). Confabulation and frontal lobe dysfunction. *J Neurol Neurosurg Psychiatry* 43: 461–3.

Kertesz, A. and Benson, D. (1970). Neologistic jargon: a clinicopathologic study. *Cortex* 6: 362–86.

Kinsbourne, M. (1995). Awareness of one's body: an attentional theory of its nature, development, and brain basis. In *The Body and the Self*, ed. J.L. Bermúdez, A. Marcel and N. Eilan, pp. 205–23. Cambridge, MA: MIT Press.

Kinsbourne, M. and Warrington, E.K. (1963). Jargon aphasia. *Neuropsychologia* 1: 27–37.

Koehler, P.J., Endtz, L.J., Te Velde, J. and Hekster, R.E. (1986). Aware or non-aware: on the significance of awareness for the localization of the lesion responsible for homonymous hemianopia. *J Neurol Sci* 75: 255–62.

Korsakoff, S.S. (1889). Étude medico-psychologique sur une forme des maladies de la mémoire. *Rev Philosoph* 28: 501–30.

Krantz, J.L. (1992). Psychosocial aspects of vision loss associated with head trauma. *J Am Optometric Assoc* 63: 589–91.

Laplane, D. and Degos, J.D. (1983). Motor neglect. *J Neurol Neurosurg Psychiatry* 46: 152–8.

Laplne, D. and Degos, J.D. (1984). Troubles inhabituels du schéma corporel par désafférentation périphérique. *Rev Neurol* 140: 45–8.

Lapresle, J. and Verret, J.M. (1978). Syndrome d'Anton–Babinski avec reconnaissance du membre supérieur gauche dans le miroir. *Rev Neurol* 134: 709–13.

Lebrun, Y. (1987). Anosognosia in aphasics. *Cortex* 23: 251–63.

Lebrun, Y. and Leleux, C. (1982). Anosognosie et aphasie. *Schweizer Archiv Neurol Neurochirurgie und Psychiatrie*, 130: 25–38.

Levine, D.N. (1990). Unawareness of visual and sensorimotor defects: a hypothesis. *Brain Cogn* 13: 233–81.

Levine, D.N., Calvanio, R. and Rinn, W.E. (1991). The pathogenesis of anosognosia for hemiplegia. *Neurology* 41: 1770–81.

Levy, J., Trevarthen, C. and Sperry, R.W. (1972). Perception of bilateral chimeric figures following hemispheric deconnexion. *Brain* 95: 61–78.

Lhermitte, J. (1939). *L'image de Notre Corps*. Paris: Nouvelle Revue Critique.

Logue, V., Durward, M., Pratt, R.T., Piercy, M. and Nixon, W.L.B. (1968). The quality of survival after rupture of anterior cerebral artery aneurysm. *Br J Psychiatry* 114: 137–60.

Lu, L.H., Barrett, A.M., Schwartz, R.L. et al. (1997). Anosognosia and confabulation during the Wada test. *Neurology* 49: 1316–22.

Luria, A.R. (1980). *Higher Cortical Functions in Man*. New York: Basic Books.

Maeshima, S., Dohi, N., Funahashi, K. et al. (1997). Rehabilitation of patients with anosognosia for hemiplegia due to intracerebral haemorrhage. *Brain Inj* 11(9): 691–7.

Magitot, A. and Hartmann, E. (1927). La cécité corticale. *Bull Soc d'Ophthalmol* 8: 427–546.

Maher, L.N., Gonzalez Rothi, L.J. and Heilman, K.M. (1994). Lack of awareness in an aphasic patient with relatively preserved auditory comprehension. *Brain Lang* 46: 402–18.

Marshall, R.C., Rappaport, B.Z. and Garcia-Bunuel, L. (1985). Self-monitoring behavior in a case of severe auditory agnosia with aphasia. *Brain Lang* 24: 297–313.

Marshall, R.C. and Tompkins, C.A. (1982). Verbal self-correction behaviors of fluent and nonfluent aphasic subjects. *Brain Lang* 15: 292–306.

McDaniel, K.D. and McDaniel, L.D. (1991). Anton's syndrome in a patient with posttraumatic optic neuropathy and bifrontal contusions. *Arch Neurol* 48: 101–5.

McGlynn, S.M. and Schacter, D.L. (1989). Unawareness of deficits in neuropsychological syndromes. *J Clin Exp Neuropsychol* 11: 143–205.

Melzack, R. (1990). Phantom limbs and the concept of a neuromatrix. *Trends Neurosci* 13: 88–92.

Mennemeier, M., Fennel, E., Valenstein, E. and Heilman, K.M. (1992). Contributions of the left intralaminar and medial thalamic nuclei to memory: comparisons and report of a case. *Arch Neurol* 49: 1050–8.

Mercer, B., Wapner, W., Gardner, H. and Benson, D.F. (1977). A study of confabulation. *Arch Neurol* 34: 429–33.

Milner, B., Corkin, S. and Teuber, H.L. (1968). Further analysis of the hippocampal amnesic syndrome: 14-year follow-up study of H.M. *Neuropsychologia* 6: 215–34.

Montaigne, M. de (1588). *Les Essais*. Livre II, Chapter 12. (Édition 1965). Paris: Presses Universitaires de France.

Moscovitch, M. (1992). Memory and working-with-memory: a component process model based on modules and central systems. *J Cogn Neurosci* 4: 257–67.

Nathanson, M., Bergman, P.S. and Gordon, C.G. (1952). Denial of illness: its occurrence in one hundred consecutive cases of hemiplegia. *Arch Neurol Psychiatry* 68: 380–7.

Nielsen, J.M. (1938). Disturbances of the body scheme: their physiologic mechanism. *Bull Los Angeles Neurol Soc* 3: 127–35.

Oppenheimer, H. and Weissman, M. (1951). On anosognosia: report of a case of anosognosia for blindness. *Am J Psychiatry* 108: 337–42.

Papagno, C. and Baddeley, A. (1997). Confabulation in a dysexecutive patient: implication for models of retrieval. *Cortex* 33: 743–52.

Parkin, A.J., Bell, W.P. and Leng, N.R.C. (1988). Metamemory in amnesic and normal subjects. *Cortex* 24: 141–7.

Parkin, A.J. and Leng, N.R.C. (1993). *Neuropsychology of the Amnesic Syndrome*. Hove, UK: Lawrence Erlbaum Associates.

Pérenin, M.T., Ruel, J. and Hécaen, H. (1980). Residual visual capacity in a case of cortical blindness. *Cortex* 16: 605–12.

Pick, A. (1898). *Beiträge zur Pathologie und pathologische Anatomie des Zentralnervensystems mit Bemerkungen zur normalen Anatomie desselben*. Berlin: Karger.

Poppelreuter, W. (1917). *Die psychische Schädigungen durch Kopfschuss im Krieg 1914/16*. Leipzig: Leopold Voss.

Pötzl, O. (1924). Über Störungen der Selbstwahrnehmung bei linksseitiger Hemiplegie. *Zeitschr Neurol Psychiatrie* 93: 117–68.

Prigatano, G.P. (1986). *Neuropsychological Rehabilitation after Brain Injury*. Baltimore: Johns Hopkins University Press.

Rafal, R., Smith, J., Krantz, J., Cohen, A. and Brennan, C. (1990). Extrageniculate vision in hemianopic humans: saccade inhibition by signals in the blind field. *Science* 29: 118–20.

Ramachandran, V.S. (1995). Anosognosia in parietal lobe syndrome. *Conscious Cogn* 4: 22–51.

Ramachandran, V.S. (1996). What neurological syndromes can tell us about human nature: some lesions from phantom limbs. Capgras syndrome, and anosognosia. *Cold Spring Harbor Symp Quant Biol* 61: 115–34.

Ramachandran, V.S. and Rogers-Ramachandran, D. (1996). Denial of disabilities in anosognosia. *Nature* 382: 501.

Redlich, F.C. and Dorsey, J.F. (1945). Denial of blindness by patients with cerebral disease. *Arch Neurol Psychiatry* 53: 407–17.

Robertson, I.H. (1994). Persisting unilateral neglect: compensatory processes within multiply-interacting circuits. *Neuropsychol Rehabil* 4(2): 193–7.

Roland, P.E., and Gulyás, B. (1994). Visual imagery and visual representation. *Trends Neurosci* 17: 281–7.

Rossolimo, G. (1896). Ueber Hemianopsie und enseitige Ophtalmoplegie vasculären Ursprungs. *Neurol Centralb* 15: 626–37.

Roth, M. (1949). Disorders of the body image caused by lesions of the right parietal lobe. *Brain* 72: 89–111.

Rubens, A.B. and Garrett, M.F. (1991). Anosognosia of linguistic deficits in patients with neurological deficits. In *Awareness of Deficit after Brain Injury: Clinical and Theoretical Issues*, ed. G.P. Prigatano and D.L. Schacter, pp. 40–52. New York: Oxford University Press.

Sachs, E. (1927). Symptomatology of a group of frontal lobe lesions. *Brain* 50: 474–9.

Safran, A.B. (1997). Unperceived visual field defects. *Arch Ophthalmol* 115: 686–7.

Safran, A.B. and Landis, T. (1996). Plasticity in the adult visual cortex: implications for the diagnosis of visual field defects and visual rehabilitation. *Curr Opin Ophthalmol* 7: 53–64.

Sandifer, P.H. (1946). Anosognosia and disorders of the body scheme. *Brain* 69: 122–37.

Schacter, D.L. (1991). Unawareness of deficit and unawareness of knowledge in patients with memory disorders. In *Awareness of Deficit after Brain Injury: Clinical and Theoretical Issues*, ed. G.P. Prigatano and D.L. Schacter, pp. 126–51. New York: Oxford University Press.

Schacter, D.L., Curran, T., Galluccio, L., Milberg, W. and Bates, J. (1996). False recognition and the right frontal lobe: a case study. *Neuropsychologia* 34: 793–808.

Schilder, P. (1935). *The Image and Appearance of the Human Body*, Vol. 4. London: Kegan, Paul, Trench, Trubner, and Company.

Schlench, K.J., Huber, W. and Willmes, K. (1987). 'Prepairs' and repairs: different monitoring functions in aphasic language production. *Brain Lang* 30: 226–44.

Schnider, A., Gutbroad, K., Hess, C.W. and Schroth, G. (1996a). Memory without context: amnesia with confabulations following infarction of the right capsular genu. *J Neurol Neurosurg Psychiatry* 61: 186–93.

Schnider, A., von Däniken, C. and Gutbrod, K. (1996b). The mechanisms of spontaneous and provoked confabulations. *Brain* 119: 1365–75.

Sergent, J. (1988). An investigation into perceptual completion in blind areas of the visual field. *Brain* 111: 347–73.

Servan, J., Verstichel, P., Catala, M. and Rancurel, G. (1994). Syndromes amnésiques et fabulations au cours d'infarctus du territoire de l'artère cérébrale postérieure. *Rev Neurol* 150: 201–8.

Shallice, T., Fletcher, P., Frith, C.D. et al. (1994). Brain regions associated with acquisition and retrieval of verbal episodic memory. *Nature* 368: 1587–96.

Shapiro, B.E., Alexander, M.P., Gardner, H. and Mercer, B. (1981). Mechanisms of confabulation. *Neurology* 31: 1070–6.

Sherer, M., Bergloff, P., Boake, C., High, W.J.R. and Levin, E. (1998). The Awareness Questionnaire: factor structure and internal consistency. *Brain Inj* 12: 63–8.

Shimamura, A.P. and Squire, L.R. (1986). Memory and metamemory: a study of the feeling-of-knowing phenomenon in amnesic patients. *J Exp Psychol Learn Mem Cogn* 12: 452–60.

Shuren, J.E., Hammond, C.S., Maher, L.M., Rothi, L.J. and Heilman, K.M. (1995). Attention and anosognosia: the case of a jargonaphasic patient with unawareness of language deficit. *Neurology* 45: 376–8.

Small, M. and Ellis, S. (1996). Denial of hemiplegia: an investigation onto the theories of causation. *Eur Neurol* 36: 353–63.

Spillmann, L. and Werner, J.S. (1996). Long-range interactions in visual perception. *Trends Neurosci* 19: 428–34.

Starkstein, S.E., Berthier, M.L., Fedoroff, P., Price, T.R. and Robinson, R.G. (1990). Anosognosia and major depression in 2 patients with cerebrovascular lesions [see comments]. *Neurology* 40: 1380–2.

Starkstein, S.E., Fedoroff, J.P., Price, T.R., Leiguarda, R. and Robinson, R.G. (1992). Anosognosia in patients with cerebrovascular lesions: a study of causative factors. *Stroke* 23: 1446–53.

Starkstein, S.E., Fedoroff, J.P., Price, T.R. et al. (1993). Neuropsychological deficits in patients with anosognosia. *Neuropsychiatry Neuropsychol Behav Neurol* 6: 43–8.

Stengel, E. and Steele, G.D.F. (1946). Unawareness of physical disability (anosognosia). *Br J Psychiatry* 92: 379–88.

Stone, S.P., Halligan, P.W. and Greenwood, R.J. (1993). The incidence of neglect phenomena and related disorders in patients with an acute right or left hemisphere stroke. *Age Ageing* 22: 46–52.

Stuss, D.T. and Benson, F.D. (1986). *The Frontal Lobes*. New York: Raven Press.

Stuss, D.T., Guberman, A., Nelson, R. and La Rochelle, S. (1988). The neuropsychology of thalamic infarction. *Brain Cogn* 7: 1–31.

Swartz, B.E. and Brust, J.C. (1984). Anton's syndrome accompanying withdrawal hallucinosis in a blind alcholic. *Neurology* 34: 969–73.

Symonds, C. and MacKenzie, I. (1957). Bilateral loss of vision from cerebral infarction. *Brain* 80: 415–55.

Talland, G.A. (1961). Confabulation in the Wernicke–Korsakoff syndrome. *J Nerv Ment Disord* 132: 361–81.

Ullman, M., Ashenhurst, E.M., Hurwitz, L.J. and Gruen, A. (1960). Motivational and structural factors in the denial of hemiplegia. *Arch Neurol* 3: 306–18.

Vallar, G. and Perani, D. (1986). The anatomy of unilateral neglect after right-hemisphere stroke lesions: a clinical/CT-scan correlation study in man. *Neuropsychologia* 24: 609–22.

Vallar, G., Sterzi, R., Bottini, G. et al. (1990). Temporary remission of left hemianesthesia after vestibular stimulation: a sensory neglect phenomenon. *Cortex* 26: 123–31.

Van der Linden, M. and Bruyer, R. (1992). Troubles de la mémoire et signes de dysfonctionnement frontal chez vingt-neuf patients opérés d'un anévrysme de l'artère communicante antérieure. *Acta Neurol Belg* 92: 255–77.

Verslegers, W., De Deyn, P., Saerens, J. et al. (1991). Slow progressive bilateral posterior artery infarction presenting as agitated delirium, complicated with Anton's syndrome. *Eur Neurol* 31: 216–19.

Victor, M., Adams, R.D. and Collins, G.H. (1989). *The Wernicke–Korsakoff Syndrome and Related Neurological Disorders due to Chronic Alcoholism and Malnutrition*. Philadelphia: Davis.

Vilkki, J. (1985). Amnesic syndromes after surgery of anterior communicating artery aneurysms. *Cortex* 21: 421–44.

Vogt, B.A., Finch, D.M. and Olson, C.R. (1992). Functional heterogeneity in the cingulate cortex: the anterior executive and the posterior evaluative regions. *Cereb Cortex* 2: 435–43.

Volpe, B.T. and Hirst, W. (1983). Amnesia following rupture and repair of an anterior communicating artery aneurysm. *J Neurol Neurosurg Pyychiatry* 46: 704–9.

Von Hagen, K.O. and Ives, E.R. (1937). Anosognosia (Babinski) imperception of hemiplegia: report of six cases, one with autopsy. *Bull Los Angeles Neurol Soc* 2: 95–103.

Von Monakow, C. (1885). Experimentelle und pathologisch-anatomische Untersuchungen über die Beziehungen der sogenannten Sehphäre zu den infrakortikalen Opticuscentren und zum N. opticus. *Archiv Psychiatie Nervenkr* 16: 151–99.

Vuilleumier, P., Reverdin, A. and Landis, T. (1997). Four legs: illusory reduplication of the lower limbs after bilateral parietal lobe damage. *Arch Neurol* 54: 1543–7.

Warrington, E.K. (1962). The completion of visual forms across hemianopic field defects. *J Neurol Neurosurg Psychiatry* 25: 208–17.

Watson, R.T., Valenstein, E. and Heilman, K.M. (1982). Thalamic neglect: possible role of the medial thalamus and nucleus reticularis in behavior. *Arch Neurol* 38: 501–6.

Weinstein, E.A., Cole, M., Mitchell, M.S. and Lyerly, O.G. (1964). Anosognosia and aphasia. *Arch Neurol* 10: 376–86.

Weinstein, E.A. and Kahn, R.L. (1950). The syndrome of anosognosia. *Arch Neurol Psychiatry* 64: 772–91.

Weinstein, E.A. and Kahn, R.L. (1955). *Denial of Illness: Symbolic and Physiological Aspects.* Springfield, IL: Charles C. Thomas.

Weinstein, E.A. and Lyerly, O.G. (1976). Personality factors in jargon aphasia. *Cortex* 12: 122–33.

Wernicke, C. (1874). *Der Aphasische Symptomen Komplex.* Breslau: Cohn & Weigert.

Whitlock, F.A. (1981). Some observations on the meaning of confabulation. *Br J Med Psychol* 54: 213–18.

Willanger, R., Danielsen, U.T. and Ankergus, J. (1981). I. Denial and neglect of hemiparesis in right-sided apoplectic lesions. II. Visual neglect in right-sided apoplectic lesions. *Acta Neurol Scand* 64: 310–26; 327–36.

Wilson, B. (1992). Clinical management of memory problems, 2nd edn. San Diego: Singular Publishing Group, Inc.

Wyke, M. and Warrington, E. (1960). An experimental analysis of confabulation in a case of Korsakoff's syndrome using a tachystoscopic method. *J Neurol Neurosurg Psychiatry* 23: 327–33.

Zingerle, H. (1913). Ueber Störungen der Wahrnehmung des eigenen Körpers bei organischen Gehirnerkrankungen. *Monatschr Psychiatrie Neurol* 34: 13–36.

18

Acute confusional states and delirium

Louis R. Caplan

Introduction: terminology and definitions

The terms *delirium, confused,* and *confusional state* have been used differently by neurologists and psychiatrists and authors in the past. The criteria for delirium in DSM-IV include (Folstein and Caplan, 1996):

1 a disturbance in consciousness with reduced ability to focus and sustain shifts of attention;

2 a change in cognition or the development of a perceptual disturbance that is not better accounted for by a preexisting, established, or evolving dementia;

3 the disturbance develops over a short period of time (usually hours to days) and tends to fluctuate during the course of the day;

4 there is evidence from the history, physical examination, or laboratory findings that the disturbance is caused by direct physiological consequences of a general medical condition.

These criteria incorporate several very different elements, including acuteness, altered thinking and concentrating, level of consciousness, and cause. Confusion is defined by Adams, Victor and Ropper (1997) as:

denoting the patient's incapacity to think with customary speed, clarity, and coherence. Its most conspicuous attributes are an inner sense of bewilderment, impaired attention and concentration, an inability to properly register immediate events and to recall them later, and a diminution of all mental activity including the normally constant inner ideation . . . Reduced perceptiveness with visual and auditory illusions and even hallucinations and paranoid delusions are variable features.

Confusion, in their terminology, is an essential component of delirium. Adams et al. use the term delirium to denote a special type of confusional state: 'Delirium is marked by a prominent disorder of perception, terrifying hallucinations and vivid dreams, a kaleidoscopic array of strange and absurd fantasies and delusions, inability to sleep, a tendency to convulse, and intense emotional reactions.' Lipowski defined the acute confusional state as 'an organic mental syndrome featuring global cognitive impairment, attentional abnormalities, a reduced level of consciousness, increased or decreased psychomotor activity, and a disordered wake–sleep cycle' (Lipowski, 1990; Young, 1998).

Some authors, including Adams et al. (1997), reserve the term delirium to describe an overactive state of heightened alertness that includes agitation, frenzied excitement, and trembling, while others, including many psychiatrists, include both hypoactive and hyperactive behavior with confusion within the spectrum of delirium. Many simply reserve the term delirium for behavioral and cognitive states that closely resemble the most familiar form of delirium – delirium tremens that develops in alcoholics after they withdraw from alcohol.

These terms are very difficult to apply practically. The word confused is used in common parlance to mean *mixed up*. Confusion refers to altered thinking ability. It is not a technical term. Because the terms delirium and confusional state are used so differently and include so many disparate features, their use only serves to confuse physicians. Instead, simple, direct English descriptions of (1) the acuteness or chronicity of the disorder, (2) the level and amount of activity, (3) the nature of the altered thinking, and (4) the cause, are greatly preferred.

It is well known and appreciated that individuals who are sleepy or stuporous cannot pay attention or concentrate normally and cannot think as clearly as those who are wide awake and alert. For that reason, I believe it serves little purpose to apply the term delirium to individuals who have decreased alertness. The discussion in this chapter is limited to hyperactive behavioral states in which thinking and concentration are abnormal. In my opinion it is best to consider etiology as a separate issue and not to incorporate it into the definition of the clinical state. Diffuse brain dysfunction characterized by altered level of consciousness, poor ability to concentrate, and altered cognitive functions when caused by potentially reversible biochemical and physiological changes is usually referred to as *encephalopathy*. When the dysfunction relates to endogenous, usually biochemical, abnormalities in various internal organs, the term *metabolic encephalopathy* is used, while dysfunction due to exogenous factors such as drugs and toxic substance exposure is usually called *toxic encephalopathy*. As this book is concerned mostly with the neuroanatomy and neurophysiology of various behavioral and mood disorders, discussion here is limited to hyperactive states with accompanying confusion associated with focal central nervous system pathology, and the encephalopathies are not discussed.

Neuroanatomical substrate of hyperactivity

Miller Fisher (1983) reviewed his extensive personal experience with two behavioral states that appeared to be polar opposites – abulia and agitated behavior. Abulic patients were hypoactive. They were apathetic and lacked initiative and exploratory behavior. They were slow to respond and their responses were brief. In contrast, were patients who were hyperactive and agitated. These individuals were often restless, excited, and hyperalert, and had an increased amount of speech (logorrhea) and behavior (Fisher, 1983). The brain lesions in patients with abulia were located in the upper mesencephalic tegmentum, substantia nigra, medial thalami, striatum, and frontal lobes. Many of the lesions involved or interrupted the ascending reticular activating system in the rostral brainstem or target destinations in the frontal lobes. Fisher postulated that lesions of a mesencephalo-frontal activating system which was mostly dopaminergic was the basic pathological anatomy of hypoactive, abulic states. In contrast, when hyperactive agitated patients had focal brain lesions, the location was most often in the posterior portions of the cerebral hemispheres in the temporal, occipital, and inferior parietal lobes (Fisher, 1983). Many of the agitated patients had infarcts or inflammatory lesions that involved limbic cortex in these regions.

Localization of lesions in reported series of patients with focal brain lesions

Top of the basilar artery embolism

Horenstein, Chamberlain, and Conomy, at the 1962 Annual Meeting of the American Neurological Association, reported nine patients who presented with hyperactive agitated behavior and sudden-onset visual loss. The authors described the behavior of their patients as 'restlessness, agitation, forced crying out, and extreme distractability.' These patients were very talkative and their conversations tended to flow from one topic to another. All had infarctions in the unilateral or bilateral territory supplied by the posterior cerebral arteries. The infarcts most often involved the fusiform and lingual gyri (Horenstein et al., 1962). Later Medina, Rubino, and Ross (1974) described the clinical and pathological findings in a 78-year-old man who had sudden onset of an agitated, excited state. The man was described as being previously quiet, stable, and kind, despite a prior stroke that caused a transient left hemiparesis and left hemisensory loss, and a persistent left hemianopia. His niece found him in an agitated state, and he cursed and struck her. On admission to hospital, he was described as extremely agitated, perspiring profusely, and screaming, biting, and spitting. He was also blind and had defective memory. The man remained agitated and shouted most responses to queries until his death about five months after his stroke. Necropsy showed an old infarct in the territory of the inferior division of the right middle cerebral artery involving the superior temporal gyrus and the inferior parietal lobe. The left posterior cerebral artery territory was also infarcted, including the entire lingual gyrus and portions of the adjacent fusiform, parahippocampal, and calcarine gyri (Medina et al., 1974). The left hippocampus and portions of the left thalamus were also involved, including the mamillary bodies and the pulvinar. The anatomy of the thalamic infarct was not described or illustrated in any further detail (Medina et al., 1974).

I later reviewed other reports of patients who developed an agitated delirious state caused by embolism to the rostral basilar artery and its posterior cerebral artery branches (Caplan, 1980, 1996). Necropsy and neuroimaging in these patients showed bilateral infarcts, invariably involving occipital and temporal lobe cortex below the calcarine sulcus, including the lingual and fusiform gyri. Bilateral visual field defects and memory loss usually accompanied the agitated, hyperactive state. Some patients also had infarcts in the rostral brainstem and superior cerebellar artery territory of the cerebellum; however, no patient with an isolated rostral brainstem infarct had an agitated hyperactive state. The patients with bilateral rostral brainstem tegmental infarcts were, in contrast, first sleepy and had reduced behavior and activity. Infarction of the posterior cerebral artery territory on the lower bank of the calcarine sulcus was a necessary component in these patients with posterior circulation brain embolism (Caplan, 1980, 1996).

A hyperactive agitated state also occasionally develops after vertebral artery angiography (Caplan, 1996). These patients become hyperactive and restless, have markedly reduced vision, and poor memory. The confusional disturbance and other neurological signs usually remit within several hours. In most patients the angiography is normal and the patients have received a relatively large amount of iodinated contrast. This syndrome is probably caused by a dye reaction in the bilateral territories of the posterior cerebral arteries.

Unilateral temporo-occipital infarcts in the territory of one posterior cerebral artery

Devinsky, Bear and Volpe (1988) reported the clinical and imaging abnormalities in four patients with left posterior cerebral artery territory infarcts and an agitated confusional state, and reviewed prior reports of confusional states in patients with unilateral posterior cerebral artery territory infarcts. All four patients had lesions of the left occipital and posteromedial temporal lobes. Three had infarcts in the distribution of the left posterior cerebral artery that were probably due to cardiogenic embolism. One patient probably had dural sinus and cortical venous thrombosis with left posteromedial temporal lobe and occipital lobe infarction. Three of the patients had agitated states, sometimes alternating with lethargy. One patient had the sudden onset of 'confusion, agitated disorientation, and aggressive behavior' (Devinsky et al., 1988). This patient shouted curses and threats and threw objects at the wall. He was 'distractable and shifted the focus of his attention to virtually any novel stimulus.' Another agitated patient had speech that was described as 'fluent but tangential with difficulty finding words.' In some patients, the agitated confusional state was temporary. Devinsky and colleagues reviewed prior reports of patients with unilateral posterior cerebral artery territory infarcts who had acute confusional states. Eighteen of the 19 patients (95%) described in ten different reports had left posterior cerebral artery territory infarcts, whereas only one had a right posterior cerebral artery territory infarct. Fisher (1983) also commented that when an agitated delirium developed in patients with unilateral posterior cerebral artery territory infarcts, the lesion was predominantly in the dominant left cerebral hemisphere.

Infarcts in the territory of the inferior division of the middle cerebral arteries

Boudin et al., in 1963, described ten patients who had sudden onset of confusion with agitated behavior. Two of the patients died and were found to have right temporal lobe infarcts. In the other patients, the clinical findings and EEG abnormalities suggested to the authors that the vascular lesions involved the right temporal lobe (Boudin et al., 1963). This report antedated modern neuroimaging.

A year later, Juillet and colleagues (1964) described four patients who had visual and mental confusion, often with agitation. In two of these patients, the clinical and EEG abnormalities suggested right temporal lobe infarction. Mesulam et al., in 1976, reported on three patients who had acute confusion with agitation related to infarction in the territory of the right middle cerebral artery. The abnormal behavior in these patients began abruptly and the patients showed extreme distractibility, incoherent streams of thought, restlessness, agitation, and hyperactive behavior (Mesulam et al., 1976). In one patient, an early-generation computed tomography (CT) scan showed a lesion in the inferior right frontal lobe, although this patient had no motor or sensory signs. In the other two patients, a radionuclide scan showed lesions in the right temporal and inferior parietal lobes. Angiography in one patient showed an occlusion of the right angular artery branch of the middle cerebral artery, but was normal in the patient with the CT-documented frontal lobe infarct. These patients all had emboli to the right middle cerebral artery. Although the authors posited that right parietal lobe infarction was the likely explanation for the agitated state, the localization of the ischemic lesions in their patients was quite vague and all probably also had temporal lobe infarcts.

Schmidley and Messing (1984) reviewed the clinical and imaging findings in 46 patients who had infarction in the territory of the right middle cerebral artery. Two patients presented with agitation and confusion. Each had a left hemianopia and minor left limb motor signs. CT scans in one of these patients were normal, and showed an enhancing right temporal–parietal infarct in the other. Angiography in the agitated patient who had a normal CT scan showed delayed filling of the temporal and inferior parietal branches of the inferior trunk of the right middle cerebral artery. The other 44 patients had more severe motor and sensory signs, indicating that they had more anterior and/or deep infarcts.

A clinicopathological conference in Paris ('Confrontation de la Salpetriere') concerned a 68-year-old man who had sudden onset of abnormal behavior (Awada, Poncet and Signoret, 1984). This man was agitated and could not attend to tasks. He spoke incessantly and incoherently. He had a left hemianopia but no motor, sensory, or reflex abnormalities. CT showed an infarct that involved the right inferior parietal and temporal lobes in the territory of the inferior division of the right middle cerebral artery.

In 1986, my colleagues in the Stroke Data Bank project and I searched the Stroke Data Bank registry and their own patient files for patients with acute strokes that involved the inferior division of the right middle cerebral artery (Caplan et al., 1986). The purpose was to characterize the findings in this syndrome. All ten patients reported had left visual field abnormalities. Motor abnormalities were slight and transient. Three of the patients had a severe agitated delirium at onset. One patient moaned continuously, and repeatedly removed all treatment lines, tubes, and catheters despite four-limb restraints. He became less restless after 12 hours, but continued to call out apparently random names, spoke incoherently and his conversation incessantly flitted from one topic to another. The wife of this patient said that her husband had reported that people were coming into his room through the windows and so he often hid under the covers to avoid them. Four other patients were restless and had difficulty concentrating for neurologic testing (Caplan et al., 1986). The restless, agitated patients had abnormal drawing and copying skills. The anatomical localization of infarcts was plotted in the five agitated, restless patients and compared with those of the five other patients who were not agitated. Figures 18.1 and 18.2 show this reconstruction. The agitated patients all had right temporal lobe infarcts. The authors concluded that infarction of the right temporal lobe was the likely explanation for the agitation that may accompany right middle cerebral artery territory infarcts.

Mori and Yamadori (1987) reviewed their experience with patients who had right middle cerebral artery territory infarcts associated with acute confusional states and agitated delirium. They characterized the acute confusional state as a failure to maintain a coherent stream of thought or action, with inattention and easy distractability. Among the 41 patients with right middle cerebral artery territory infarcts, 25 had an acute confusional state and six had an acute agitated state that the authors called an acute agitated delirium. This hyperactive state was characterized by extreme agitation, irritability, vivid hallucinations, delusions, insomnia, and signs of autonomic nervous system overactivity. The six patients with agitation had infarcts in the distribution of the inferior division of the right middle cerebral artery, involving the territories of the middle and posterior temporal artery branches in five of the six patients. Mori and Yamadori (1987) attributed confusion to right frontal and basal ganglionic dysfunction and agitated delirium

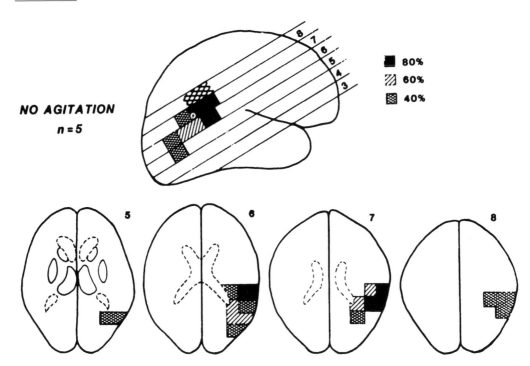

NO AGITATION
n = 5

■ 80%
▨ 60%
▧ 40%

Fig. 18.1   Five CT scans from patients without agitation were analyzed. The lesions tended to extend mostly into the inferior parietal lobe, sparing the temporal lobe. Solid black shading indicates involvement of the area in 80% of patients; diagonal striped shading indicates involvement in 60% of patients; and cross-hatched shading indicates involvement in 40% of patients. (Reproduced from Caplan et al., 1986, with permission.)

to temporal lobe infarction. They posited a limbic–sensory disconnection as the mechanism of the agitated state.

Agitation, anger, and paranoia are sometimes observed in patients with Wernicke's aphasia. These patients usually have embolic infarctions involving the inferior branch of the left middle cerebral artery and temporal lobe infarcts. Patients with aphasia who are irascible and show anger usually have Wernicke-type aphasia (Fisher, 1970). These behavioral changes are probably related to dysfunction of limbic cortex and its connections that lie medial to the convexal temporal lobe infarcts that cause the aphasia. Logorrhea has long been recognized as a common feature of the speech output in patients with Wernicke's aphasia.

The studies cited provide conclusive data that infarcts involving the right temporal lobe in the territories of the temporal artery branches of the right middle cerebral artery are an important cause of an agitated, hyperactive, restless state associated with logorrhea. Recall that logorrhea and excessive speech production are also features in patients with Wernicke's aphasia. Excessive loquaciousness may

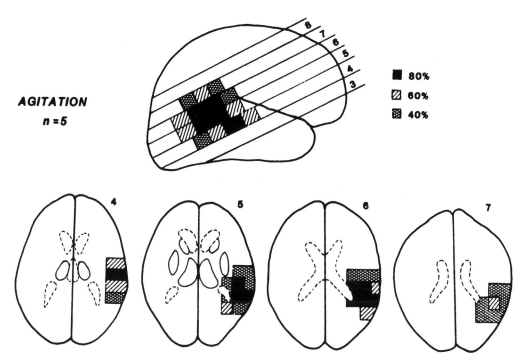

Fig. 18.2   Five CT scans from patients with agitation were analyzed. The lesions tended to extend into the temporal lobe. Shading as in Fig. 18.1. (Reproduced from Caplan et al., 1986, with permission.)

be a characteristic of temporal lobe dysfunction involving either hemisphere and may be present without aphasia.

Caudate nucleus infarcts and hemorrhages

Stein and colleagues, in 1984, first reported the findings in patients with hemorrhages that involved the caudate nucleus. Several of their patients were restless and agitated and had memory dysfunction and confusion. These hemorrhages often dissected into the anterior horn of the lateral ventricle, and the restlessness and agitation could have been related to the subarachnoid blood. Restlessness, irritability, and agitation had long been a known feature in patients who had subarachnoid hemorrhages.

Mendez, Adams, and Lewandowski, in 1989, reported the neurobehavioral abnormalities found among 12 patients with caudate infarcts, 11 unilateral and one bilateral. Five of the 12 patients had 'affective symptoms with psychotic features.' One of these patients was extremely anxious and had difficulty sleeping and had feelings of panic. She was suspicious and paranoid and heard voices that commented on 'activities in the atmosphere.' During examination she was very restless and 'fidgety' (Mendez et al., 1989). Patients with agitation and psychotic features had lesions that involved mostly the ventromedial portion of the caudate nucleus. Three other patients were disinhibited, inappropriate, and impulsive; one of these patients was unkempt, distractable, loquacious, unconcerned, and sexually disinhibited. These three patients had larger lesions that included most of the caudate nucleus and spread to adjacent structures. Mendez et al. pointed to the similarities of the behavioral and cognitive abnormalities found in their patients with those associated with Huntington's chorea, another disorder known to involve the caudate nucleus. They pointed out that the ventromedial caudate – the 'limbic striatum' (Nauta and Domesick, 1984; Nauta, 1986) – was topographically connected to orbito-frontal cortex.

In 1990, my colleagues and I reported the neurological findings in 18 patients with caudate infarcts (Caplan et al., 1990). The infarcts often extended into the adjacent anterior limb of the internal capsule and the anterior portion of the putamen. The cause was probably occlusion of the medial lenticulostriate arterial branches of the proximal middle cerebral artery or the recurrent artery of Heubner branches of the anterior cerebral arteries. Seven of these patients had transient or persistent restlessness and hyperactivity; three of these seven patients had left caudate infarcts, and the other four had right-sided lesions. In these patients, apathy and abulia often alternated with hyperactivity. Two patients with right caudate infarcts had severe hyperactivity. They were restless, talked and moved incessantly, and often called out loudly. The authors reviewed the anatomical connections of the caudate nucleus in an attempt to explain the behavioral abnormalities. The anatomical studies were the work of Alexander, DeLong, and Strick (1986), and Walle Nauta (Nauta and Domesick, 1984; Nauta, 1986). A lateral orbitofrontal circuit exists which projects from the orbitofrontal cortex (Brodman area 10) to the ventromedial portion of the caudate nucleus. This portion of the caudate nucleus also receives input from temporal lobe visual and auditory association cortex. An anterior cingulate circuit originates in the anterior cingulum (Brodman area 24) and in limbic temporal lobe structures, including the hippocampi, amygdala, and enterorhinal and perirhinal cortex structures, and projects to the ventral striatum (nucleus accumbens septi, olfactory tubercle, and ventromedial caudate nucleus). The caudate nuclei have reciprocal connections with the internal segment of the globus pallidus, the rostromedial substantia nigra, and the ventral anterior and dorsomedial thalamic nuclei (Alexander et al., 1986; Caplan et al., 1990). To my knowledge, however, an agitated state has not yet been described in patients with lesions limited to the globus pallidus or putamen. Although sleep abnormalities and apathetic abulic states do occur in patients with thalamic hemorrhages and infarcts, I am not aware of the presence of an agitated delirious state in patients with lesions limited to the thalamus.

Frontal lobe and other location vascular and other lesions

Occasional reports describe patients with frontal lobe lesions that contain some features of the behavioral abnormalities described in patients with agitated hyperactive delirious states. In 1988, Starkstein, Boston, and Robinson reported 12 patients with manic-like behavior after brain lesions. The lesions in these patients clustered in limbic and limbic-related areas with strong frontal lobe projections. The authors also reviewed reports of similar patients. They posited that dysfunction of the orbitofrontal region might underlie the production of the somatic and mood abnormalities found in patients with mania due to organic brain lesions (Starkstein et al., 1988, 1990).

Two years later, Starkstein and colleagues (1990) described a second group of patients with mania after brain injuries, a consecutive series of eight patients. All eight patients were elated and had pressured speech and grandiose delusions. Seven were hyperactive and had insomnia and flights of ideas, five were irritable, and six were hypersexual. All of the lesions involved the right cerebral hemisphere. One patient had an infarct involving the head of the caudate, medial temporal gyrus, and basotemporal and dorsolateral frontal regions. Another had an infarct involving the head of the caudate, amygdala, hippocampus, and basotemporal cortex. Another patient developed an infarct after embolization of a right basotemporal vascular malformation. One had a right temporal lobe hemorrhage. One patient had bilateral orbitofrontal contusions. Three patients had subcortical lesions including: contusion that on CT and MRI was shown to involve the white matter of the anterior frontal lobe, an infarct of the ventromedial caudate head and adjacent anterior limb of the capsule white matter, and a larger infarct of the caudate nucleus and anterior limb. PET scans in the three patients with subcortical lesions showed abnormal metabolism in the right lateral basotemporal regions in all.

Bakchine and colleagues (1989) reported a manic-like state in a patient with bilateral orbitofrontal and right temporoparietal lobe contusions. This patient had a reduced amount of spontaneous behavior when left alone but became manic when stimulated. She had reduced sleep time, and frequent outbursts of anger. When spoken to, she became logorrheic and constantly switched conversation from one topic to another. She was easily distracted and often told jokes with a sexual content. Fisher (1983) included a brief citation of two early reports (Hyland, 1933; Amyes and Nielsen, 1955) of hyperactivity in relation to frontal lobe lesions in his discussion of abulia versus agitation behavior. Amyes and Nielsen (1955) reported two patients who had hyperactivity in relation to infarcts that involved the left cingulate gyrus and the bilateral medial orbitofrontal cortex in the distribution of the anterior cerebral arteries. Hyland (1933) reported a patient who had thrombosis of an azygous-type anterior cerebral artery and developed a left hemiparesis accompanied by hypersexuality and incessant talking. Lesions of the orbitofrontal cortex have been shown to cause distractability, overactivity, and motor disinhibition. A so-called 'inhibitory control of interference' is lost in patients with orbitofrontal lesions (Stuss et al., 1982). The patients seem unable to ignore even trivial stimuli and cannot maintain attention to tasks and ideas if there are any alternative external stimuli.

I have also seen agitation with hypersexuality, aggressiveness, and anger in patients with brain injuries that had involvement of the orbitofrontal regions. Accompanying basotemporal contusions could not be excluded from the neuroimaging tests performed.

Finally, Arseni and Danaila (1977) described hyperative behavior in relation to pontine brainstem disease. Their patients showed logorrhea with a flow of ideas and content and hyperactivity (Arseni and Danaila, 1977; Fisher, 1983). One of Arseni and Danaila's patients with a basilar artery aneurysm and a clinical deficit localizable to the pons and upper brainstem showed logorrhea with a flow of ideas and content and hyperactivity (Arseni and Danaila, 1977). They posited that a lesion that stimulated the ascending reticular activating system could cause increased speech and behavior. They also emphasized that logorrhea and hyperkinesis did not always to go together. Among their 13 patients, six had both logorrhea and hyperactivity, whereas one had logorrhea without hyperactivity, and six were hyperkinetic but mute (Arseni and Danaila, 1977). I have seen one patient with a dolichoectatic basilar artery and an infarct in the territory of a penetrating pontine artery branch who suddenly became loquacious and had persistent logorrhea after she developed a hemiparesis caused by her pontine infarct (Pessin et al., 1989).

Conclusion

Hyperactive agitated states can develop after focal brain lesions. Accompanying the overactive behavior are other features that are found in some but not all patients. These include: logorrhea, press of ideas with flitting quickly from one idea and one topic to another, distractability, insomnia, shouting, aggressive sometimes violent behavior, disinhibition, hypersexuality, hallucinations, delusions, and paranoia. The full syndrome is most apparent in patients with right temporal lobe infarcts that include the basotemporal structures including the hippocampus, amygdala, enterorhinal and perirhinal cortex and their underlying white matter. Patients with bilateral lesions involving the fusiform and lingual gyri within the medial basal temporal lobes have a similar agitated delirium. This syndrome is also found in some patients with predominantly left fusiform and lingual gyri infarcts. Lesions of the ventromedial caudate nucleus and its underlying white matter can also produce a similar syndrome, perhaps more often when the lesions are on the right side of the brain. Although orbitofrontal lesions might also produce similar findings, this occurrence is unusual.

The unifying theme of these lesions is involvement of structures that relate closely to the limbic cortex of the temporal lobes and the orbitofrontal regions. The right basotemporal lobe and its connections with the right ventral limbic striatum and the left lingual and fusiform gyri are preferred sites for lesions that cause an overactive, restless, talkative state. Occasional brainstem lesions might also produce logorrhea and hyperactivity, but usually without an accompanying confusional state.

REFERENCES

Adams, R.D., Victor, M. and Ropper, A.H. (eds.) (1997). Delirium and other acute confusional states. In *Principles of Neurology*, 6th edn, pp. 405–16. New York: McGraw-Hill.

Alexander, G.E., DeLong, M.R. and Strick, P.L. (1986). Parallel organization of functionally segregated circuits linking basal ganglia and cortex. *Ann Rev Neurosci* 9: 357–81.

Amyes, E.W. and Nielsen, J.M. (1955). Clinicopathological study of the vascular lesions of the anterior cingulate region. *Bull Los Angeles Neurol Soc* 20: 112–30.

Arseni, C. and Danaila, L. (1977). Logorrhea syndrome with hyperkinesia. *Eur Neurol* 15: 183–7.

Awada, A., Poncet, M. and Signoret, J. (1984). Troubles de comportement soudains avec agitation chez un homme de 68 ans. *Rev Neurol* 140: 446–51.

Bakchine, S., Lacomblez, L., Benoit, N. et al. (1989). Manic-like state after bilateral orbitofrontal and right temporoparietal injury: efficacy of clonidine. *Neurology* 39: 777–81.

Boudin, G., Barbizet, J., Lauras, A. and Lortat-Jacob, O. (1963). Ramollissements temporaux droit: manifestations psychiques rélévatrices. *Rev Neurol* 108: 470–4.

Caplan, L.R. (1980). Top of the basilar syndrome: selected clinical aspects. *Neurology* 30: 72–9.

Caplan, L.R. (1996). Posterior circulation disease; clinical findings, diagnosis, and management. Boston: Butterworth–Heinemann.

Caplan, L.R., Kelly, M., Kase, C.S. et al. (1986). Infarcts of the inferior division of the right middle cerebral artery: mirror image of Wernicke's aphasia. *Neurology* 36: 1015–20.

Caplan, L.R., Schmahmann, J.D., Kase, C.S. et al. (1990). Caudate infarcts. *Arch Neurol* 47: 133–43.

Devinsky, O., Bear, D. and Volpe, B.T. (1988). Confusional states following posterior cerebral artery territory infarction. *Arch Neurol* 45: 160–3.

Fisher, C.M. (1970). Anger associated with dysphasia. *Trans Am Neurol Assoc* 95: 240–2.

Fisher, C.M. (1983). Honored guest presentation: abulia minor vs. agitated behavior. *Clin Neurosurg* 31: 9–31.

Folstein, M. and Caplan, L.R. (1996). Delirium. In *Neurological Disorders, Course and Treatment*, ed. T. Brandt, L.R. Caplan, J. Dichgans, H.C. Diener and C. Kennard, pp. 237–44. San Diego: Academic Press.

Horenstein, S., Chamberlain, W. and Conomy, J. (1962). Infarctions of the fusiform and calcarine regions with agitated delirium and hemianopsia. *Trans Am Neurol Assoc* 92: 85–9.

Hyland, H.H. (1933). Thrombosis of intracranial arteries. Report of three cases involving respectively the anterior cerebral, basilar, and internal carotid arteries. *Arch Neurol Psychiatry* 30: 342–56.

Juillet, P., Savelli, A., Rigal, J., Sabourin, M. and Jenny, B. (1964). Confusion mentale et lobe temporale droit: a propos de quatre observations. *Rev Neurol* 111: 430–4.

Lipowski, Z.J. (1990). *Delirium. Acute Confusional States.* New York: Oxford University Press.

Medina, J.L., Rubino, F.A. and Ross, E. (1974). Agitated delirium caused by infarctions of the hippocampal formation and fusiform and lingual gyri: a case report. *Neurology* 24: 1181–3.

Mendez, M.F., Adams, N.L. and Lewandowski, K.S. (1989). Neurobehavioral changes associated with caudate lesions. *Neurology* 39: 349–54.

Mesulam, M., Waxman, S., Geschwind, N. and Sabin, T. (1976). Acute confusional states with right middle cerebral artery infarctions. *J Neurol Neurosurg Psychiatry* 39: 84–9.

Mori, E. and Yamadori, A. (1987). Acute confusional state and agitated delirium. Occurrence after infarction in the right middle cerebral artery territory. *Arch Neurol* 44: 1139–43.

Nauta, H.J.W. (1986). The relationship of the basal ganglia to the limbic system. In *Handbook of Clinical Neurology*, Vol. 49, *Extrapyramidal Disorders*, ed. P.J. Vinken, G.W. Bruyn and H.L. Klawans, pp. 19–31. Amsterdam: Elsevier Science.

Nauta, W.J.H. and Domesick, V.B. (1984). Afferent and efferent relationships of the basal ganglia. In *Functions of the Basal Ganglia*, ed. D. Evered and M. O'Connor, pp. 3–29. *Ciba Foundation Symposium* Vol. 107. London: Pitman.

Pessin, M.S., Chiumowitz, M.I., Levine, S.R. et al. (1989). Stroke in patients with fusiform vertebrobasilar aneurysms. *Neurology* 39: 16–21.

Schmidley, J. and Messing, R. (1984). Agitated confusional states in patients with right hemispheral infarctions. *Stroke* 15: 883–5.

Starkstein, S.E., Boston, J.D. and Robinson, R.G. (1988). Mechanisms of mania after brain injury: 12 case reports and review of the literature. *J Nerv Ment Dis* 176: 87–100.

Starkstein, S.E., Mayberg, H.S., Berthier, M.L. et al. (1990). Mania after brain injury: neuroradiological and metabolic findings. *Ann Neurol* 27: 652–9.

Stein, R.W., Kase, C.S., Hier, D.B. et al. (1984). Caudate hemorrhage. *Neurology* 34: 1549–54.

Stuss, D.T., Kaplan, E.F., Benson, D.F. et al. (1982). Evidence for the involvement of the orbitofrontal cortex in memory function – an interference effect. *J Comp Physiol* 96: 913–25.

Young, G.B. (1998). Major syndromes of impaired consciousness. In *Coma and Impaired Consciousness*, ed. G.B. Young, A.H. Ropper, and C.F. Bolton, pp. 38–50. New York: McGraw-Hill.

Index

Note: page numbers in *italics* refer to figures and tables.